Clinical Urology

Clinical Urology

Editor: Ezra Martin

FOSTER ACADEMICS
www.fosteracademics.com

www.fosteracademics.com

FOSTER ACADEMICS

Cataloging-in-Publication Data

Clinical urology / edited by Ezra Martin.
p. cm.
Includes bibliographical references and index.
ISBN 978-1-63242-823-3
1. Urology. 2. Genitourinary organs--Diseases. 3. Clinical medicine. I. Martin, Ezra.
RC871 .C55 2019
616.6--dc23

Foster Academics,
118-35 Queens Blvd., Suite 400,
Forest Hills, NY 11375, USA

ISBN 978-1-63242-823-3 (Hardback)

Printed and bound in China.

Contents

Preface

The world is advancing at a fast pace like never before. Therefore, the need is to keep up with the latest developments. This book was an idea that came to fruition when the specialists in the area realized the need to coordinate together and document essential themes in the subject. That's when I was requested to be the editor. Editing this book has been an honour as it brings together diverse authors researching on different streams of the field. The book collates essential materials contributed by veterans in the area which can be utilized by students and researchers alike.

Urology, also known as genitourinary surgery, is a study of the diseases related to the urinary-tract system. It also involves the study of the disorders associated with the male reproductive organs. Organs which come under the scope of urology include the bladder, kidneys, urethra, ureters, prostate, seminal vesicles, vas deferens, epididymis, adrenal glands, testes and penis. Some of the sub-disciplines of urology include endourology, neurourology, reconstructive urology, urologic oncology, female urology, among others. Some of the fields that are closely linked with urology are andrology, gynaecology, nephrology, gastroenterology and endocrinology. Surgeons and medical practitioners, whose area of specialization is urology, are called urologists. This book is a valuable compilation of topics, ranging from the basic to the most complex advancements in the field of clinical urology. It brings forth some of the most innovative concepts and elucidates the unexplored aspects of urology. This book with its detailed analyses of data, will prove immensely beneficial to professionals and students involved in this area at various levels.

Each chapter is a sole-standing publication that reflects each author´s interpretation. Thus, the book displays a multi-facetted picture of our current understanding of application, resources and aspects of the field. I would like to thank the contributors of this book and my family for their endless support.

Editor

Predictors of survival outcomes in native sub Saharan black men newly diagnosed with metastatic prostate cancer

Jibril Oyekunle Bello

Abstract

Background: Though it is well established that black men are at higher risk of prostate cancer (PCa) very little is known about the disease in native sub Saharan black men. Newly diagnosed metastatic PCa patients treated with primary androgen deprivation therapy were identified and predictors of progression-free survival (PFS) assessed.

Methods: Patients diagnosed with metastatic PCa between 2010 and 2015 in a sub Saharan black population were included in the study. Primary outcome measure was PFS defined as time from primary androgen deprivation therapy to clinical progression or death. Demographic, clinical and PSA kinetic variables were evaluated for their prognostic power using Cox proportional hazard regression models.

Results: Seventy-nine patients met the eligibility criteria and were analyzed. Median age, median overall survival and PFS was 69 years, 40 months and 27 months respectively. A PSA nadir >4 ng/mL was found to predict an earlier clinical progression. Median PFS was shorter in those with PSA nadir >4 ng/mL (15 months) compared to those with PSA nadir ≤4 ng/mL (29 months); log rank p value = 0.003.

Conclusions: The PSA nadir achieved following primary androgen deprivation therapy predicts progression-free survival in sub Saharan black men newly diagnosed with metastatic PCa. PSA nadir >4 ng/mL was found to be associated with a more rapid clinical progression.

Keywords: Prostate cancer, Androgen deprivation therapy, PSA kinetics, PSA nadir, Black men, Sub Saharan Africa

Background

Although the exact burden of Prostate cancer (PCa) in sub Saharan Africa remains largely unknown [1]; the region is home to the largest populations of black men, a well-established high risk group for PCa. Unfortunately, despite this, very little is known about the basic and clinical aspects of the disease in these native black men. This is probably due to weak health systems, poor cancer registries and a hostile research environment with poor funding [2]. In the few studies that are available, findings have supported the widely-held view that significantly higher proportion of men in the region present late with advanced disease compared to most other regions of the world [3]. This may be attributable to a near lack of any established systematic screening practices in the region during the early PSA era when PCa screening was encouraged up to current times when population screening has become controversial. In our practice, well over half of newly diagnosed patients have locally advanced or metastatic disease.

Primary androgen deprivation therapy (PADT) is the most widely used and most potent systemic treatment for newly diagnosed hormone sensitive metastatic PCa. It is probably the most common form of treatment for PCa received by black men of sub Saharan Africa largely due to the much higher proportion of men with advanced disease. PADT is often in the form of bilateral orchiectomy with or without antiandrogens for the majority of these men mainly due to cost considerations as health insurance coverage are generally low. Despite PADT, most men progress biochemically and clinically eventually to castrate resistant disease and or death. Wide variability in clinical progression of metastatic PCa has been observed and though certain demographic,

Correspondence: jabarng@yahoo.com
Department of Surgery, University of Ilorin Teaching Hospital, Ilorin, Nigeria

PSA kinetic and histopathological markers have been reported to be associated with higher mortality risk, most of the studies were done with moderate to fair representation of black men generally but scarcely inclusive of any native sub Saharan black men [4–7]. There is thus a need to determine surrogate markers of aggressive progressive disease and impaired survival in our very peculiar and under studied high risk population. This retrospective study queried the clinical records of post-PADT native black men newly diagnosed with metastatic disease to assess progression-free survival (PFS) and overall survival (OS) and determine possible early surrogate markers of rapidly progressive disease. Although OS is the standard endpoint in survival analysis, PFS is also a relevant endpoint in the setting of metastatic PCa as patients often eventually die of disease progression.

Methods

This cohort was generated from clinical records of newly diagnosed black men with metastatic PCa who presented for care at a tertiary care hospital in North Central Nigeria, West Africa between June 2010 and July 2015. To be eligible for inclusion in the study, patients must have had metastatic bone disease confirmed with radiological investigations and subsequently agreed to androgen deprivation therapy (orchiectomy or luteinizing hormone-releasing hormone with or without anti androgens). Patients would also have had a pretreatment PSA and at least 2 post treatment PSA readings done less than 12 months' post androgen deprivation therapy with at least one assay between the third and eighth month. Patients who had prior primary surgery (prostatectomy) or radiotherapy were excluded from the study. Demographic and clinical information retrieved include age, use of Non-steroidal anti-inflammatory drugs (NSAID), pretreatment PSA, PSA decline, Post treatment PSA nadir and Gleason score. Post treatment PSA nadir was defined as the lowest PSA reported during the first 12 months following androgen deprivation therapy. PSA decline was defined as the relative change of PSA nadir from baseline (pretreatment PSA). This study's primary outcome measure was progression-free survival (PFS). PFS was defined as time from commencement of androgen deprivation therapy to clinical progression or censure. Clinical progression was defined as a composite outcome of the occurrence of new metastases or skeletal related events or death from PCa. Categorical and continuous variables were summarized using percentages and medians (interquartile range) respectively. Univariate logistic and multivariate Cox proportional hazard models with backward elimination were used to explore the impact of potential predictors. PFS was estimated using the Kaplan-Meier method with significance determined by log rank test. All analyses were performed with SPSS software, version 22.0 (SPSS Inc), p value <0.05 was considered to be statistically significant. Institutional ethics board approval was obtained for the study.

Results

Seventy-nine patients met the eligibility criteria and were analyzed. The baseline characteristics of the patients are shown in Table 1. The median age and pretreatment PSA at diagnosis were 69 years (IQR: 65 – 73 years) and 94 ng/mL (IQR: 50 – 124 ng/mL) respectively. Majority of the men 65(82.3%) had orchiectomy with or without anti androgens. The median PSA nadir was 4 ng/mL (IQR: 1.0 – 9.0 ng/mL) and 60 (75.9%) patients achieved a PSA decline of ≥ 90%. The median time from PADT to PSA nadir was 7 months (IQR: 5-8). The median OS and PFS was 40.3 months (95%CI 24.3-49.7 months) and 26.8 months (95% 19.1 – 28.9 months) respectively. After a median follow-up of 15 months (IQR: 12 – 24 months) clinical progression was documented in 35 (44.3%) patients and of these 19 (23.8%) died. Prognosticators of clinical progression found on univariate analysis (Table 2) were analgesic consumption (NSAID use) and PSA nadir. Pretreatment PSA and PSA decline were not significant prognosticators; waterfall plots (Fig. 1) of

Table 1 Baseline characteristics of study cohort (n = 79)

Variables	n (%)	median[a](IQR)
Age		69.0 (65.0 – 73.0)
Place of residence		
Urban	56 (70.9)	
Rural	23 (29.1)	
Initial Clinical presentation		
LUTS	69 (87.3)	
[b]NSAID use	51 (64.6)	
Anaemia (<10 g/dL)	25 (31.6)	
PADT received		
Orchiectomy	65(82.3)	
LH-RH analogues	14 (17.7)	
PSA kinetics		
Pre-treatment PSA(ng/mL)		94.0 (50.0 – 124.0)
PSA nadir (ng/mL)		4.0 (1.0 – 9.0)
PSA decline		
≥ 90%	60 (75.9)	
< 90%	19 (24.1)	
Biopsy Gleason score		
3 + 3	24 (30.4)	
3 + 4	10 (12.7)	
4 + 3	20 (25.3)	
≥ 8	25 (31.7)	

[a]Interquartile range, [b]Non-steroidal anti-inflammatory drugs

Table 2 Cox proportional hazards models for progression-free survival following primary androgen deprivation therapy

Variables	Univariate			Multivariate		
	HR	95% CI	p	HR	95% CI	p
Age	1.01	0.96-1.06	0.706			
Urban residence	1.44	0.59-3.48	0.421			
LUTS	2.15	0.70-6.57	0.181			
[a]NSAID use	3.80	1.43-10.10	0.007	3.40	0.74-15.66	0.117
Anaemia	1.89	0.77-4.64	0.162			
Pretreatment PSA	1.00	0.99-1.01	0.913			
PSA decline						
< 90%	1.00 (Reference)					
≥ 90%	0.36	0.13-1.10	0.063			
[a]PSA nadir						
≤ 4 ng/mL	1.00 (Reference)					
> 4 ng/mL	3.86	1.49-10.04	0.006	2.85	1.06-7.67	0.038
Biopsy Gleason score						
6	1.00 (Reference)					
7	0.82	0.35-1.91	0.648			
8-10	1.26	0.56-2.80	0.579			

[a]significant at univariate analysis and carried onward to multivariate analysis

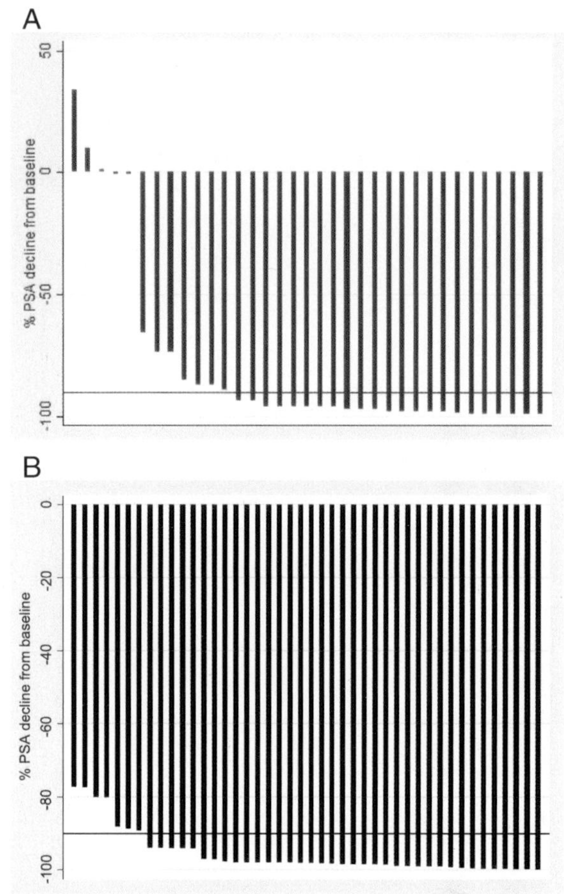

Fig. 1 Waterfall plots of relative PSA decline from baseline for patients with (**a**) and without (**b**) clinical progression during study follow-up (median 15 months). A decline of ≥90% was seen in 23 (65.7%) and 37 (84.1%) patients in (**a**) and (**b**) respectively. This was not statistically significant (p = 0.06). The bold reference line represents PSA decline of 90%

PSA decline for patients with (A) and without (B) clinical progression during study follow-up show that a decline of ≥ 90% was not significantly different in both groups (p = 0.06). PSA nadir was dichotomized at median (4 ng/mL) and this was also found to be predictive. On multivariate analysis (Table 2), only PSA nadir remained as statistically significant predictor with reduced PFS apparent in patients with PSA nadir >4 ng/mL (HR = 2.85, 95% CI: 1.06-7.67). Kaplan Meier plot of PFS by PSA nadir (Fig. 2) illustrated the differences between the two survival distributions (PSA nadir ≤4 ng/mL versus PSA nadir >4 ng/mL) with the median PFS for patients with PSA nadir ≤4 ng/mL of 29 months (95%CI 19.3 – 38.7) significantly longer than that of those with PSA nadir >4 ng/mL which was found to be 15 months (95%CI 8.3 – 21.7), log-rank p-value = 0.003.

Discussion

In sub Saharan Africa, urologists are often faced with the dilemma of how to interpret prostate cancer guidelines mostly derived with suboptimal representation of black men (and scarcely any native sub-Saharan African men). This problem is compounded by the dearth of research on the basic and clinical aspects of PCa from sub Saharan Africa and the weak healthcare system of the region which offers fewer options in the treatment of PCa. The resulting knowledge gap is particularly remarkable taking to consideration the high-risk status of the population and the fact that a large majority of native African black men currently present with aggressive disease and at a late stage with metastases [3, 8, 9]. As observed in other populations, wide variability exists in the clinical course of metastatic PCa in sub Saharan African men. This study of a cohort of sub Saharan African men thus examined the role of some demographic and clinical (including PSA kinetics) variables in predicting clinical progression following PADT.

Median age of our study cohort was 69 years which is similar to that found in similarly studied sub Saharan African populations [3, 8, 9]. There are no available studies of sub Saharan black men that evaluated the relationship between age and survival for comparison with this study. However, a study carried out in the United States, in which African Americans formed 10% of the study population found that the prognostic power of age though significant at univariate analysis was lost at multivariate analysis that controlled for treatment modality [4]. This suggests that where treatments are

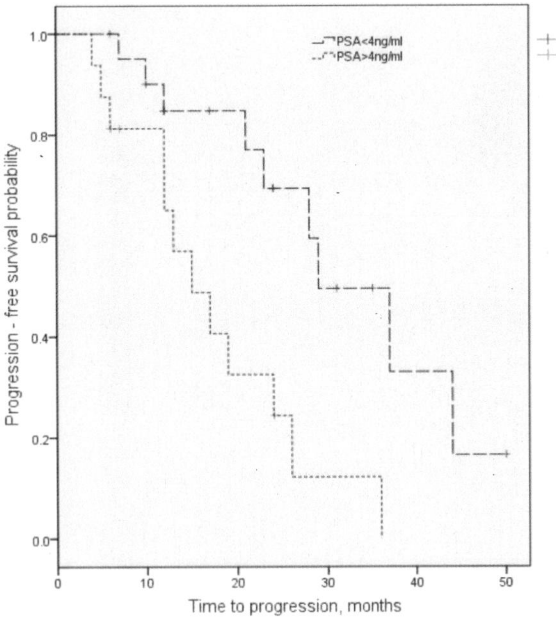

At risk:

≤ 4 ng/mL	38	22	10	4
> 4 ng/mL	20	8	2	0

Fig. 2 Progression-free survival probability of patients with metastatic prostate cancer following primary androgen deprivation therapy. Kaplan-Meier analysis showed significant differences between patients with PSA nadir ≤4 ng/mL Vs > 4 ng/mL, log-rank *p*-value = 0.003

similar survival outcomes would probably not be different across age groups. Another study from the same region in which blacks were about one-sixth of the study population found that younger men, who were more likely to be black, were at higher risk of all cause and cancer specific death [5]. This could be interpreted to mean that young black men were more likely to die than other groups. This current study done exclusively in native black men of sub Saharan Africa found no such relationship though it investigated the broader outcome of PFS; and it corroborates Koff et al. findings of no relationships between age, race and PFS [10]. NSAID use was found to be associated with decreased PFS at univariate analysis in this study but this association was lost when PSA nadir was included in multivariate analysis. About two-thirds of the patients studied required analgesia for pains related to metastasis. No association was found between Gleason score and PFS in this study.

While pretreatment PSA, PSA velocity and Gleason score have been found to be important predictors of response to therapy and survival in the setting of localized disease [11, 12]; alkaline phosphatase, PSA nadir and time to PSA nadir, PSA half-life have been reported to predict survival following PADT for advanced or metastatic disease [6, 7, 10, 13–17]. The importance of these variables has never been investigated in a native African black population. While many studies have reported that lower PSA nadir reflects a good prognosis with slower clinical progression, there are no agreed values of optimum PSA nadir above which prognosis worsens. Reported values include 0.1 ng/mL, 0.2 ng/mL, 2 ng/mL and 4 ng/mL [7, 10, 13, 15]; these different values may be attributable to the dissimilar cohorts studied. Some cohorts included patients who had prior treatment with curative intent (prostatectomy or radiotherapy), some included only newly diagnosed metastatic PCa patients while others included a mix of patients with localized, locally advanced or metastatic disease. This current study includes only newly diagnosed metastatic PCa patients and found that a PSA nadir >4 ng/mL was associated with earlier clinical progression; this is similar to findings of Hussain et al. in their study cohort of metastatic PCa patients who were treated with 7-month "induction" course of Goserelin and bicalutamide [7]. Hussain et al. assessed for OS and found a median OS of 13 months for patients with PSA nadir of more than 4 ng/mL which was significantly differently from those in their cohort with PSA less than 4 ng/mL or less than 0.2 ng/mL [7]. In contrast, the current study assessed PFS (clinical progression and or death as endpoints) and found a PFS of 15 months in cohort members with PSA nadir >4 ng/mL which was significantly less than the PFS of 29 months found in those with PSA nadir ≤4 ng/mL. Unlike PSA nadir, evaluations of the prognostic value of time to PSA nadir (TTN) have produced inconsistent results [6, 14, 16–18]. Both shorter and longer TTN have been found to be associated with worse outcomes. These varied results may be due to dissimilar cohorts or inappropriate statistical analysis; more frequent PSA measurements done at similar intervals would be required for appropriate analysis of TTN. This was unavailable in the current study and TTN was not analyzed.

There are some important limitations to this study. Admittedly it is a retrospective study and cohort size is not large. Additionally, predictors of PFS and not OS were assessed because of the relatively few events (deaths) that occurred during the study period. Despite these limitations, this is the first study to report on the predictors of clinical progression in native sub Saharan African black men with metastatic PCa. Findings from this study may help identify patients likely to develop early clinical progression and these patients may benefit from early commencement of other therapies aimed at delaying clinical progression and prolonging survival. In our resource-limited setting, patients commonly receive chemohormonal therapy with docetaxel added to PADT following clinical progression to castrate-resistant PCa. The high costs associated with newer drugs, abiraterone and enzalutamide, make them out-of-reach for patients in our low- and middle- income region where payments for health care are mainly out-of-pocket and health insurance coverage is low.

Conclusions

The PSA nadir achieved following primary androgen deprivation therapy predicts progression-free survival in sub Saharan black men newly diagnosed with metastatic PCa. PSA nadir >4 ng/mL was found to be associated with a more rapid clinical progression.

Abbreviations

NSAID: Non-Steroidal anti-inflammatory drugs; OS: Overall survival; PADT: Primary androgen deprivation therapy; PCa: Prostate cancer; PFS: Progression-free survival; PSA: Prostate-specific antigen; TTN: Time to PSA nadir

Acknowledgements

Mr. Joshua helped in retrieving the records of patients.

Funding

None.

Authors' contributions

JOB collated the Data used, performed the Data analysis, wrote and approved the manuscript.

Competing interests

The author declares that there are no competing interests.

References

1. Adeloye D, David RA, Aderemi AV, Iseolorunkanmi A, Oyedokun A, Iweala EE, et al. An Estimate of the Incidence of Prostate Cancer in Africa: A Systematic Review and Meta-Analysis. PLoS One. 2016;11(4):e0153496.
2. Bello JO. Urological research in sub-Saharan Africa: a retrospective cohort study of abstracts presented at the Nigerian Association of Urological Surgeons conferences. BMC Urol. 2013;13:59.
3. Zeigler-Johnson CM, Rennert H, Mittal RD, Jalloh M, Sachdeva R, Malkowicz SB, et al. Evaluation of prostate cancer characteristics in four populations worldwide. Can J Urol. 2008;15(3):4056–64.
4. Bechis SK, Carroll PR, Cooperberg MR. Impact of age at diagnosis on prostate cancer treatment and survival. J Clin Oncol. 2011;29(2):235–41.
5. Lin DW, Porter M, Montgomery B. Treatment and survival outcomes in young men diagnosed with prostate cancer: a Population-based Cohort Study. Cancer. 2009;115(13):2863–71.
6. Choueiri TK, Xie W, D'Amico AV, Ross RW, Hu JC, Pomerantz M, et al. Time to PSA nadir independently predicts overall survival in metastatic hormone sensitive prostate cancer patients treated with androgen deprivation therapy. Cancer. 2009;115(5):981–7.
7. Hussain M, Tangen CM, Higano C, Schelhammer PF, Faulkner J, Crawford ED, et al. Absolute prostate-specific antigen value after androgen deprivation is a strong independent predictor of survival in new metastatic prostate cancer: data from Southwest Oncology Group Trial 9346 (INT-0162). J Clin Oncol. 2006;24(24):3984–90.
8. Tindall EA, Monare LR, Petersen DC, van Zyl S, Hardie RA, Segone AM, et al. Clinical presentation of prostate cancer in black South Africans. Prostate. 2014;74(8):880–91.
9. Kirakoya B, Hounnasso PP, Pare AK, Mustapha AB, Zango B. Clinico-pathological features of prostate cancer at the University hospital Yalgado Ouedraogo, Ouagadougou, Burkina Faso. J West Afr Coll Surg. 2014;4(4):70–81.
10. Koff SG, Connelly RR, Bauer JJ, McLeod DG, Moul JW. Primary hormonal therapy for prostate cancer: experience with 135 consecutive PSA-ERA patients from a tertiary care military medical center. Prostate Cancer Prostatic Dis. 2002;5(2):152–8.
11. Cooperberg MR, Pasta DJ, Elkin EP, Litwin MS, Latini DM, Du Chane J, et al. The University of California, San Francisco Cancer of the Prostate Risk Assessment score: a straightforward and reliable preoperative predictor of disease recurrence after radical prostatectomy. J Urol. 2005;173(6):1938–42.
12. D'Amico AV, Renshaw AA, Sussman B, Chen MH. Pretreatment PSA Velocity and Risk of Death from Prostate Cancer Following External Beam Radiation Therapy. JAMA. 2005;294(4):440–7.
13. Tomioka A, Tanaka N, Yoshikawa M, Miyake M, Anai S, Chihara Y, et al. Nadir PSA level and time to nadir PSA are prognostic factors in patients with metastatic prostate cancer. BMC Urol. 2014;14:33.
14. Sasaki T, Onishi T, Hoshina A. Nadir PSA level and time to PSA nadir following primary androgen deprivation therapy are the early survival predictors for prostate cancer patients with bone metastasis. Prostate Cancer Prostatic Dis. 2011;14(3):248–52.
15. Stewart AJ, Scher HI, Chen MH, McLeod DG, Carroll PR, Moul JW, et al. Prostate-specific antigen nadir and cancer-specific mortality following hormonal therapy for prostate-specific antigen failure. J Clin Oncol. 2005;23(27):6556–60.
16. Kim KH, Han KS, Kim KH, Kim DK, Koo KC, Rha KH, et al. The prognostic effect of prostate-specific antigen half-life at the first follow-up visit in newly diagnosed metastatic prostate cancer. Urol Oncol. 2015;33(9):383.e17–22.
17. Hong SY, Cho DS, Kim SI, Ahn HS, Kim SJ. Prostate-specific antigen nadir and time to prostate-specific antigen nadir following maximal androgen blockade independently predict prognosis in patients with metastatic prostate cancer. Kor J Urol. 2012;53(9):607–13.
18. Chung CS, Chen MH, Cullen J, McLeod D, Carroll P, D'Amico AV. Time to prostate-specific antigen nadir after androgen suppression therapy for postoperative or postradiation PSA failure and risk of prostate cancer-specific mortality. Urology. 2008;71(1):136–40.

2

Psychometric properties of the expanded prostate cancer index composite - 26 instrument in a cohort of radical prostatectomy patients: theoretical and practical examinations

Karol Axcrona[1], Rasmus Nilsson[2], Bjørn Brennhovd[3], Øystein Sørebø[4], Sophie D. Fosså[5,6] and Alv A. Dahl[5,6*]

Abstract

Background: Recently, the Expanded Prostate Cancer Index Composite 26-item version (EPIC-26) was recommended for the assessment of adverse effects after the treatment of prostate cancer without clear reasons. This decision encouraged us to review the questionnaire development from the UCLA Prostate Cancer Index (UCLA-PCI) to the EPIC-16 CP with a focus on psychometric properties. We also reviewed PubMed for papers concerning such properties of the EPIC-26 since 2012 (latest review in 2011). Finally, we examined the psychometric properties of the EPIC-26 in a sample of Norwegian males treated with robot-assisted laparoscopic prostatectomy (RALP).

Methods: This study used three methods: (1) Comparison of the content of the UCLA-PCI, EPIC-50, EPIC-26, and EPIC-16 CP; (2) Review of EPIC-26 and EPIC-16 CP papers in PubMed from 2012 to 2016, identifying papers reporting on the psychometric properties of these questionnaires; and (3) Psychometric examination of the EPIC-26 rating in 651 Norwegian men treated with RALP at a mean of 3.2 years post-surgery.

Results: The questionnaire development showed a significant increase in bother versus function items, and the EPIC-26 contains eight function and 18 bother items. Twelve papers concerning the EPIC-26 available on PubMed since 2012 support the psychometric properties of the EPIC-26. The Norwegian EPIC-26 findings supported the psychometric properties of the EPIC-26, but suggested six subdomains both by exploratory and confirmatory factor analyses.

Conclusions: In general our examinations supported the adequate psychometric properties of the EPIC-26, although the factor structure, construct and predictive validity of the instrument should be examined further.

Keywords: Prostate cancer, Adverse effects, Patient-reported outcome measures, The expanded prostate cancer index composite 26 item version, The UCLA prostate cancer index

Background

There is an increasing understanding within the uro-oncological community that the endpoints of prostate cancer (PCa) treatment should not only reflect disease recurrence and survival but also include patient-reported outcome measures (PROMs). In particular, PCa is a disease wherein the health-related quality of life (HRQoL)-related issues are crucial, since most patients live with the malignancy for many years. A major point of discussion regarding the introduction of PCa screening has been the diminished HRQoL affecting patients because of the diagnosis itself or of radical treatment for the disease [1, 2].

The development and increased use of PROMs for PCa have proliferated for many years, and this has continued in recent years. In addition, most physician-reported outcome measures show discrepancies with the

* Correspondence: a.a.dahl@ibv.uio.no
[5]National Resource Center for Late Effects after Cancer Treatment, Oslo University Hospital, The Norwegian Radium Hospital, P.O. Box 4453, Nydalen, 0424 Oslo, Norway
[6]Faculty of Medicine, University of Oslo, Oslo, Norway
Full list of author information is available at the end of the article

patients' experience of adverse effects after treatment [3]. PROMs are covered by questionnaires, which should document sufficient psychometric properties in their development process, including reliability and validity. In addition, PROMs should be founded on pre-diagnostic levels in a relevant population for such adverse effects, and should cover adverse effects that significantly affect the patients' HRQoL. The validity of PROMs is based on continuous development over time reflecting improvements in treatment techniques, health-care delivery, and the changing priorities of society [4]. Importantly, PROMs also seem to be dependent on language and the cultural background of the samples studied [5]. Hamoen et al. [6] give a concentrated overview of psychometric key concepts for urologists and uro-oncologists, and the concepts relevant for this paper are given in Table 1.

Recently, two international working groups recommended the Expanded Prostate Cancer Index Composite 26-question short form (EPIC-26) [7] as a Standard Set of Patient-centered Outcome for men with both localized [8] and advanced PCa [9]. Interestingly, the groups hardly provided any reasons for their choice, except indirectly stating that the EPIC-26 covered post-radiation rectal bleeding and therefore was preferred over the 16 items Expanded Prostate Cancer Index Composite for Clinical Practice (EPIC-16 CP) [10]. In a review by Rnic et al. [11] analyzing the psychometric properties of 29 PROMs for localized PCa, the EPIC-26 was rated among the top three instruments together with the UCLA Prostate Cancer Index (UCLA-PCI) [12], while the EPIC-50 [13] got lower ratings. Hamoen et al. [6] published a more extensive psychometric evaluation of 20 PROMs for HRQoL in PCa patients including the UCLA-PCI and the EPIC-50, and they recommended the UCLA-PCI, which according to them had been used in 268 studies of 135,366 patients. They also pointed out the problem of making recommendations when one instrument was an extended version of another, such as the EPIC-50 in relation to the UCLA-PCI. Comparisons were also considered more difficult since not all psychometric properties were tested in the validation studies of these two instruments. The same problem of comparison also concerned the reduced versions of the EPIC-26 and the EPIC-16 CP based on the EPIC-50. Using the Evaluating Measures of Patient-Reported Outcomes examining eight instruments, Schmidt et al. [14] recommended the EPIC-50 versus the UCLA-PCI due to a better overall methodology score. Considering these three psychometric reviews, the abovementioned international recommendation [8, 9] of the EPIC-26 appeared problematic, particularly in the absence of a detailed rationale supporting the recommendation.

Methods

The current paper examines three issues relevant for the validity of the EPIC-26 recommendation: (1) The developmental history of the UCLA-PCI and EPIC instruments; (2) Review of psychometric studies of the EPIC-26 published since 2012; and (3) Psychometric testing of the EPIC-26 in a Norwegian sample of PCa patients treated by robot-assisted prostatectomy (RALP) at a median of 3 years post-surgery.

Results

Development of the UCLA-PCI and the EPIC PROMs (Table 2)

The UCLA-PCI

The American urologist Mark S. Litwin and the CaPSURE-group have led the development and psychometric testing of PCa-relevant PROMs. They first developed the UCLA Prostate Cancer Index (UCLA-PCI) [12]

Table 1 Explanations of key psychometric concepts described in this paper

Explanatory factor analysis	Statistical exploration of the underlying number of factors included in a questionnaire. The factor structure is the described by the number of factors, the items' loading and the overall explained variance
Confirmatory factor analysis	Statistical analysis testing whether the data fit a hypothesized measurement model of the questionnaire. Indicators of adequate model fit are given in the text.
Feasibility	Indicates whether test persons find the questionnaire easy or complicated to complete.
Internal consistency	Describes how well subscale items of the questionnaire go together, and eventually subscales in relation to the total questionnaire.
Criterion validity	The questionnaire's correlation with 'gold standard' questionnaires for the same concepts.
Convergent validity	High correlations with other questionnaires covering the same concepts.
Divergent validity	Low correlations with questionnaires covering other concepts.
Construct validity	How well the questionnaire corresponds to other ways of measuring the construct i.e. various adverse effects.
Predictive validity	The ability of the questionnaire score to predict important future outcome.
Responsiveness to change	The ability of the questionnaire to identify clinical changes in the domains covered by the questionnaire.

Table 2 Item distribution of the UCLA-PCI and EPIC PROMs

Items	UCLA-PCI	EPIC 50	EPIC-26	EPIC-16 CP
Urinary domain				
Function				
Leakage	1	1	1	0
Control	1	1	1	1
Pad use	1	1	1	1
Hematuria	0	1	0	0
Pain or burning	0	1	0	0
Bother				
Urinary symptom bother	2	6	5	4
Overall urinary bother	1	1	1	1
Bowel domain				
Function				
Rectal urgency	1	1	0	0
Loose or liquid stools	1	0	0	0
Uncontrolled leakage	0	1	0	0
Bloody stools	0	1	0	0
Painful movements	0	1	0	0
Frequency of movements	0	1	0	0
Cramping pain	1	1	0	0
Bother				
Bowel symptom bother	1	6	5	2
Overall bowel bother	1	1	1	1
Sexual domain				
Function				
Sexual desire	1	1	0	0
Ability to have erections	1	1	1	0
Ability to reach orgasm	1	1	1	1
Quality of erections	1	1	1	1
Frequency of erection	1	1	1	0
Awakening with erection	1	1	0	0
Overall sexual function	0	1	1	0
Any sexual activity	0	1	0	0
Had intercourse	1	1	0	0
Bother				
Sexual symptom bother	0	3	0	0
Overall sexual bother	1	1	1	1
Hormonal domain				
Function				
Hot flashes	0	1	0	0
Breast tenderness	0	1	0	0
Depression	0	1	0	0
Lack of energy	0	1	0	0
Weight change	0	1	0	0
Bother				
Hormonal side effects bother	0	6	5	3
Overall hormonal bother	0	0	0	0

that included 20 items covering both function and bother items (experienced problems) within the urinary, bowel, and sexual domains, with 17 items covering function (85% of all items) and 3 items covering bother, one for each of the domains (15% of all items). The item distribution is shown in Table 2.

As demonstrated by the reviews [6, 11, 14], the psychometric documentation of the UCLA-PCI is extensive. All the three reviews recommend the UCLA-PCI as compared to other PROMs for PCa. The main criticism has been poor coverage of irritative voiding symptoms and lacking coverage of adverse effects related to neo-adjuvant or adjuvant androgen deprivation therapy (ADT) [11].

The EPIC-50

The Expanded Prostate Cancer Index Composite (EPIC-50) was developed since the UCLA-PCI addressed neither irritative and obstructive voiding symptoms nor specific symptoms related to ADT. However, the main expansion concerned additional bother items corresponding to each of the symptom items, without any reasons given for their introduction [13]. The three overall bother items of the UCLA-PCI were kept, while no corresponding item for the hormonal domain was included. The item distribution of the EPIC-50 is displayed in Table 2.

Compared to the 20 items of the UCLA-PCI, the EPIC-50 represented a considerable expansion of items and, accordingly, longer completion time for the patients. The balance between function and bother items was changed since 48% of the items now concerned bother. Most items' responses offered rating alternatives from worst (bad) to best (good). The item on the frequency of bowel movements (item #18), however, had no best or worst alternatives, and concerning the sexual symptom items, the best and worst alternatives were not stated explicitly. The relations between the overall and function bother scores were nowhere specified. For the urinary incontinence and irritation/obstruction subscales, the function and bother items were combined without any explanation. Since ≥40% of the sample scored maximum on the urinary function and irritation/obstruction subscales, a problem with ceiling effects could be relevant [13]. In spite of these weaknesses, all the three reviews [6, 11, 14] recommended the EPIC-50 in comparison with other relevant PCa PROMs.

The EPIC-26

The development of the EPIC-26 was motivated by a presumed better clinical utility of a shortened version of the EPIC-50 [7]. The main procedure for item reduction was item-scale correlations geared by reliability rather than validity considerations. The items distribution is shown in Table 2. With 8 function items and 18 symptom bother and overall bother items, the proportion of bother items increased to 69% in the EPIC-26. The EPIC-26 included 12 (60%) of the original 20 UCLA-PCI items [7]. The EPIC-26 was the top recommendation of the review by Rnic et al. [11], while the two other reviews did not include the EPIC-26.

The EPIC-16 CP

Inspired by successful PROMs measuring lower urinary tract symptoms and erectile dysfunction as well as given the need for improving weaknesses of the EPIC-26, the EPIC-16 CP was developed [10]. With 4 function items and 12 symptom bother and overall bother items, the proportion of bother items increased to 75% in the EPIC-16 CP. The item distribution is shown in Table 2.

Review of recent psychometric studies of the EPIC-26 (Table 3)

The psychometric properties of the EPIC-50 and the UCLA-PCI have been reviewed recently [6, 14]. Concerning the psychometric review of the EPIC-26, Rnic et al. [11] included papers published before the end of 2011. Therefore, in March 2016, we performed a PubMed search with the term "Expanded Prostate Cancer Index Composite" retrieving 266 papers; of these, 161 of them were published in 2012 or later and therefore were not included in the review by Rnic et al. Two of the authors (RN and AAD) read the 161 abstracts, of which 22 full papers were examined. Among them, 13 papers included psychometric data on the EPIC-26 (Table 3). Only the paper by Chipman et al. [15] contained psychometric data on the EPIC-16 CP.

Our review confirmed the good feasibility, internal consistencies, and test-retest reliability previously demonstrated for the EPIC-26 [16–26]. In addition, responsiveness to change over time was amply demonstrated [20, 23, 27, 28]. The convergent, divergent, and criterion validity of the EPIC-26 were also supported [22–24]. However, the stronger types of construct and predictive validity were hardly covered. Predictive validity with future HRQoL (the Short Form 12) was documented by Evans et al. [23]. Interestingly, the hormonal subscale of the EPIC-26 predicted future suicidal ideation [26].

Psychometric examination of the EPIC-26 in a Norwegian sample

The database for our psychometric testing comprised the complete EPIC-26 ratings from 651 men operated with robot-assisted laparoscopic prostatectomy for PCa at the Oslo University Hospital, The Norwegian Radium Hospital, between January 1, 2005 and July 31, 2010 [29, 30]. Initially, 982 primary operated men were invited to a cross-sectional, mailed questionnaire study in March 2011, and 777 of them responded (79% response rate) at a median of 2.9 (range, 0.5–6.1) years postoperatively. However, only 651 (83%) had completed all items of the EPIC-26, and this sample was used for our psychometric analyses. Among them, 142 patients (22%) self-reported relapse, and 104 patients described that they had been treated with radiotherapy and 53 with ADT. The questionnaire also included the Hospital Anxiety and Depression Scale (HADS) [31], the Short Form-12 (SF-12) Measuring HRQoL [32], and a 6-item scale examining the personality trait of neuroticism [33].

The following statistical analyses were performed on our EPIC-26 sample: internal consistencies with Cronbach's coefficient alpha and correlation coefficients with Spearman's coefficient rho. Explained variance was the second power of the correlation coefficient. Exploratory factor analysis (EFA) was performed as principal component analysis with Oblimin rotation with Kaiser normalization including EPIC-26 items with a factor loading of ≥0.30. Confirmatory factor analysis (CFA) was done with LISREL analyses (i.e., Maximum Likelihood estimation). The fit of the CFA model was evaluated through examination of the sizes of the factor loadings and values for the fit indices. Acceptable fit was shown by Root Mean Square Error of Approximation <0.07; Standardized Root Mean Square Residual <0.08; The Comparative Fit Index ≥0.95 and a Parsimonious Normed Fit Index > .50 [34, 35]. There is, however, no exact threshold for PNFI in the literature but a value above .50 indicates a parsimonious model. In addition to these fit indices, we also included the Akaike Information Criterion with the purpose to compare alternative measurement models.

Satisfactory Cronbach's coefficients alphas were observed for all EPIC-26 domain scales (Table 4). The proportion of scores with floor effects was satisfactory; however, 62.5% of the men showed ceiling effects on the bowel subscale (Table 4).

All EPIC-26 domain scales, except for the hormonal one, showed satisfactory discriminant validity in relation to the HADS anxiety and depression, the SF-12 PCS and MCS, and neuroticism scores (Table 4B). In contrast,

Table 3 Studies examining the psychometric properties of the EPIC-26 since 2012

Study (reference)	Psychometric findings
Korzeniowski et al. 2016 [16]	Informative and useful for patient communication as judged by clinicians
Sharma et al. 2016 [17]	Good feasibility both on paper and electronically
Skolarus et al. 2012 [18]	Good feasibility both on paper and automatic telephone response
Sampurno et al. 2015 [19]	Good feasibility both on paper and interactive voice method
Fosså et al. 2016 [20]	Internal consistencies alpha 0.64–0.91 of the 5 domains
Skolarus et al. 2012 [18]	Good test-retest reliability
Sampurno et al. 2015 [19]	Good test-retest reliability
Ellison et al. 2013 [21]	Criterion validity with the Incontinence Severity Index
Fosså et al. 2016 [20]	Criterion validity with the International Prostate Symptom Score
Punnen et al. 2013 [22]	Convergent validity of urinary and sexual bother scores and Generalized Anxiety Disorders Screener (GAD-7) and Distress Thermometer, and sexual bother with Patient Health Questionnaire-9 (depression)
Evans et al. 2015 [23]	Convergent validity with the SF-12 (quality of life)
Watson et al. 2015 [24]	Convergent validity of urine and bowel domains with health (EQ-5D-5 L), unmet needs (SCNS-SF34), anxiety/depression (HADS), and self-efficacy (Cancer Survivors Self Efficacy Scale)
Schofield et al. 2012 [25]	Divergent validity with unmet needs (SCNF-SF 34)
Evans et al. 2015 [23]	Predictive validity with the SF-12 (quality of life)
Recklitis et al. 2014 [26]	Predictive validity of hormonal subscale score and more suicidal ideation
Evans et al. 2015 [23]	Responsiveness to change (minimally important differences)
Skolarus et al. 2015 [27]	Responsiveness to change (minimally important differences)
Tavlarides et al. 2015 [28]	Responsiveness to change documented
Fosså et al. 2016 [20]	Responsiveness to change documented

testing the EPIC-26 domain scales in relation to major PCa outcome characteristics that were registered at baseline, demonstrated small correlation coefficients (Table 4C).

The EFA showed an explained variance of 67% for a six factor solution (Table 5). The bowel and sexual domain scales of the EPIC-26 were supported (factors 1 and 3), while the urinary and hormonal domain scales showed two factors each (1 and 6 versus 4 and 5), respectively. The urinary factors corresponded to the incontinence and irritation/obstruction subscales described for the EPIC-26 [7], while no such correspondence was shown for the two factors of the hormonal domain.

Item 12 showed a factor loading (factor 3) and a cross-loading (factor 5) that were approximately equal, while item 13E showed up with a substantial cross loading (factor 4 and 5). The two identified cross loadings indicate that there may be discriminant validity problem on the item level regarding items 12 and 13E. We, however, decided to test the EFA generated six-factor solution with CFA before we conclude on the issue of discriminant validity.

As demonstrated in Fig. 1, item 12 showed a relatively low factor loading (0.39) in the CFA while item 13E showed an acceptable loading (0.72). Item 12 seems not to fit well with the EPIC-26 measurement model. The wording on item 12 deals with an "overall problem with sexual function" which indicates a global wording that is less specific than the other items of the EPIC-26. Hence, this may explain the low factor loading and the identified problem with discriminant validity.

The CFA showed adequate fit values for the six-factor solution (Fig. 1 and Table 6). The four-factor solution, however, showed some fit values that were outside the threshold values (Fig. 2 and Table 6).

Discussion

Development of the UCLA-PCI and the EPIC PROMs

In 1994, Litwin was inspired by the urinary questionnaire from the Olmsted County studies, in which 12 items concerning functions and symptoms had 12 corresponding bother items [36]. Accordingly, Litwin stated that PCa-related PROMs must cover both function and bother: "Function and bother must be measured, and the distinction between these two dimensions is important to recognize. Some men with significant sexual dysfunction were minimally bothered, while others with only mild dysfunction may be miserable... Therefore, while sexual function and bother are undeniably linked, they are independent domains and must be measured separately ([37], page 1884)." In the light of this statement, 15% bother

Table 4 A-C Norwegian sample findings on EPIC-26 ($N = 651$)

A. Characteristics of EPIC-26 domain-specific scores

Domain	Mean (SD)	% Minimum	% Maximum	Median (range)	Cronbach's α
Urinary					
Incontinence	71.8 (27.8)	1.5	27.9	79.3 (0.0–100.0)	0.89
Irritation	86.7 (15.1)	0.0	29.8	90.0 (10.0–100.0)	0.72
Bowel	93.7 (12.5)	0.0	62.5	100.0 (12.5–100.0)	0.82
Sexual	32.9 (27.7)	11.8	1.1	23.7 (0.0–100.0)	0.78
Hormonal	86.9 (17.5)	0.3	41.8	95.0 (0.3–100.0)	0.78

B. Correlation matrix of EPIC-26 domains and psychosocial scales (*$p < 0.001$)

EPIC domains	HADS-A	HADS-D	SF-12 PCS	SF-12 MCS	Neuroticism
Urinary					
Incontinence	−0.16*	−0.17*	0.27*	0.13*	−0.22*
Irritation	−0.24*	−0.26*	0.34*	0.21*	−0.30*
Bowel	−0.27*	−0.26*	0.28*	0.20*	−0.26*
Sexual	−0.06	−0.16*	0.15*	0.11*	−0.16*
Hormonal	−0.48*	−0.53*	0.47*	0.58*	−0.66*
Urinary bother	−0.17*	−0.19*	0.29*	0.20*	−0.26*
Bowel bother	−0.23*	−0.21*	0.24*	0.15*	−0.21*
Sexual bother	−0.14*	−0.13*	0.15*	0.15*	−0.18*

C. Correlation matrix of EPIC-26 domains and prostate cancer variables (*$p < 0.02$)

EPIC-26 domains	D'Amico risk score	Positive margins	Prostate volume	Nerve-sparing	Relapse
Urinary					
Incontinence	−0.14*	−0.03	−0.12*	0.16*	−0.08
Irritation	−0.13*	−0.07	−0.02	0.15*	−0.13*
Bowel	−0.11*	−0.07	−0.02	0.09*	−0.06
Sexual	−0.19*	−0.08	−0.19*	0.28*	−0.10*
Hormonal	−0.10*	−0.08	0.04	0.16*	−0.20*
Urinary bother	−0.11*	−0.05	−0.06	0.11*	−0.13*
Bowel bother	−0.11*	−0.10*	−0.03	0.09*	−0.05
Sexual bother	−0.10*	−0.13*	−0.16*	0.16*	−0.02

items in the UCLA-PCI seem a small proportion which is compensated by 48% bother items in the EPIC-50. This equality was then changed over again with 69% bother items in the EPIC-26 and 75% of such items in the EPIC-16 CP. During the development of these PROMs, the proportion of bother items increased at the cost of functional items (Table 2). However, the instrument developers did not explain this conceptual change towards reduced interest in the functional results of the patients. From a clinical point of view, Litwin's original statement of equal relevance of function and bother seems to be reasonable, and it is difficult to gauge the reasons for the increased focus on bother problems in the later instruments. In addition, the measurement of functional outcomes enables a more objective assessment of the effectiveness of treatment modifications.

Review of recent psychometric studies of the EPIC-26

The PubMed update from 2012 on the EPIC-26 showed considerable popularity of this PROM, but only 8% (13/161 publications) contained psychometric data (Table 3). The update confirmed the good feasibility, internal consistencies, and test-retest reliability and responsiveness to change of the EPIC-26. The reliability of the EPIC-26 has been further supported, although factor analytic studies remain infrequent.

The demonstration of various types of validity is a continually ongoing process [4]. *Content validity* concerns the extent to which the EPIC-26 adequately covers the expectable adverse effects related to the treatment of PCa. For example, the UCLA-PCI lacked some content validity since that PROM omitted the hormonal domain included in the EPIC-26. On the other hand, the focus on bother rather than function could represent a

Table 5 Explorative principal component analysis with direct oblimin rotation of the EPIC-26 scores of the Norwegian sample ($N = 651$)

EPIC-26 items	Factors					
	1	2	3	4	5	6
1. Leaked urine	**0.90**					
2. Urinary control	**0.86**					
3. Number of pads	**0.89**					
4 A. Dripping or leaking of urine	**0.92**					
B. Pain or burning on urination						**0.89**
C. Bleeding with urination						**0.88**
D. Weak urine stream or incomplete emptying						**0.44**
E. Need to urinate frequently	**0.42**					
5. Overall problem with urinary function	**0.81**					
6 A. Bowel urgency		**0.82**				
B. More frequent bowel movements		**0.84**				
C. Loosing control over stools		**0.77**				
D. Bloody stools		**0.48**				
E. Abdominal/pelvic/rectal pain		**0.50**				
7. Overall problem with bowel habits		**0.87**				
8 A. Ability to have an erection			**0.93**			
B. Ability to reach orgasm			**0.76**			
9. Quality of erections			**0.91**			
10. Frequency of erections			**0.91**			
11. Ability to function sexually			**0.91**			
12. Overall problem with sexual function			0.39		0.40	
13 A. Hot flashes				**0.67**		
B. Breast tenderness/enlargement				**0.78**		
C. Feeling depressed					**0.82**	
D. Lack of energy					**0.81**	
E. Change in body weight				**0.56**	0.41	
Per cent explained variance	26.7	10.2	13.5	7.1	5.3	4.2

Coefficients below .30 were supressed
Bold texts represent factor loading > 0.40

weakened content validity of the EPIC-26 as compared to the EPIC-50.

Convergent validity confirms that the domains of the EPIC correlate highly with other established PROMs covering the same domains. Correspondingly, *divergent validity* relates to low correlation with established PROMs measuring unrelated concepts. In our update, we found support for both these types of validity in relation to the EPIC-26 [20–23]. *Criterion validity* (which includes convergent and divergent validity) involves the assessment of the EPIC-26 against more well-established questionnaires covering all or some of the same treatment-related domains. Both the previous review of Rnic et al. [11] and our update (references #18 and 19) supported such validity of the EPIC-26.

Construct validity concerns the relationship of the EPIC-26 to theoretical constructs about adverse effects related to the treatment modalities of PCa. A problem in this regard is the construction of the EPIC-26 as a multidimensional PROM covering adverse effects related to surgery, radiotherapy, and hormonal treatment. One construct is erectile dysfunction related to nerve damage during prostatectomy or radiotherapy, while another is proctitis after radiotherapy. We must therefore question whether construct validity is a meaningful concept for the total EPIC-26, or that such validity only can be studied for each of its domains (subscales). For example, many studies have examined the relationship between nerve sparing and post-surgical erectile dysfunction and found a considerable correlation [38], which supported the construct validity of the sexual domain of the EPIC-26. We conclude that future studies of the construct validity of the EPIC-26 on the domain level should be performed.

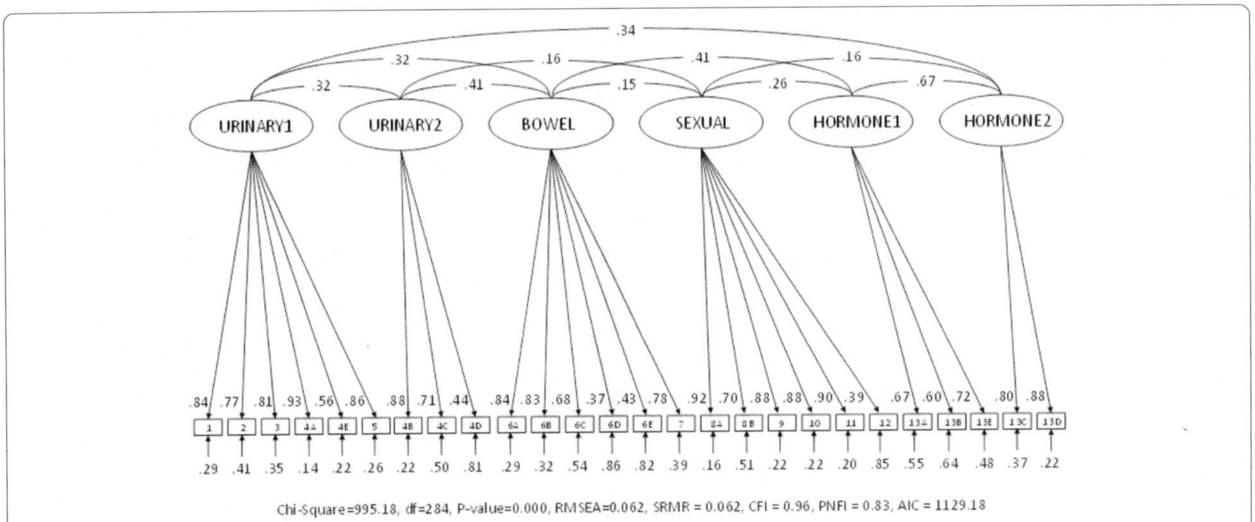

Fig. 1 Confirmatory factor analysis of the 6-factor EPIC-26 in the Norwegian sample ($N = 651$)

Predictive validity concerns the ability of the EPIC-26 to predict future health status, test results, or events in PCa patients. Urologists and uro-oncologists are familiar with this concept from the D'Amico risk index based on the pre-treatment prostate-specific antigen (PSA) level, Gleason score, and tumor stage [39] concerning biochemical outcomes for localized PCa. Additional prognostic factors include PSA velocity and doubling time (biochemical failure), BMI, primary Gleason score/grading system, the number of positive biopsy cores, and, in the case of radical prostatectomy, the presence of a positive surgical margin and the presence of perineural invasion [40, 41]. Baseline HRQoL scores also predicted PCa outcome in one study [42]. Thus far, the relationship between the EPIC-26 and these prognostic factors hardly has been studied.

Among the update studies, Evans et al. [23] observed that better baseline HRQoL scores predicted better EPIC-26 domain scores at 2 years post-treatment in a considerable sample treated with stereotactic body radiotherapy. Another update study found that suicidal ideation at a mean of 5 years after treatment was significantly predicted by the EPIC-26 hormonal domain score [26]. A reasonable explanation is that the hormonal items of depression, lack of energy, and changes in body weight are typical symptoms of a depressive disorder, which is a strong risk factor for suicidal ideation [43].

Table 6 Measurement model fit for EPIC-26 scores of the Norwegian sample ($N = 651$)

Fit-indexes	Six-factor solution	Four-factor solution	Threshold values
Chi-Square	995.18	1637.19	–
df	284	293	–
P-value	0.000	0.000	–
RMSEA (95% CI)	0.062 (0.058;0.066)	0.084 (0.080;0.088)	0.07
SRMR	0.062	0.077	0.08
CFI	0.96	0.93	0.95
PNFI	0.83	0.83	0.50
AIC	1129.18	1753.19	Lowest value are optimal

Psychometric findings of the EPIC-26 in the Norwegian sample

Similar to the results of Szymanski et al. [7] and another recent study from Norway [20], we observed adequate internal consistencies (Cronbach's coefficients alpha, 0.65–0.90) for the EPIC-26 domains (Table 4). Our mean domain scores and floor/ceiling proportions (Table 4) were both close to those observed in these previous studies [7, 20].

The present study confirmed the previous finding [24] that the EPIC-26 hormonal domain scores have a considerably strong correlation with anxiety/depression, HRQoL, and neuroticism, with explained variances ranging from 22% to 44% (Table 4B). With a maximum of 12% explained variance for the other EPIC-26 domain scores, discriminant validity in relation to such variables was confirmed.

The maximum explained variance of 8% for relevant predictors of PCa outcome variables at surgery and those concerning relapse indicated a lack of predictive validity for the EPIC-26 domain scores in this regard.

To the best of our knowledge, we have presented here the first factor analyses of the EPIC-26. In our sample, the optimal EFA solution identified six rather than the expected four factors showing the highest explained variance of 67%. This new solution was due to two factors (1and 6) within the urinary domain of the EPIC-26, defining items #4B (pain), 4C (bleeding with urination),

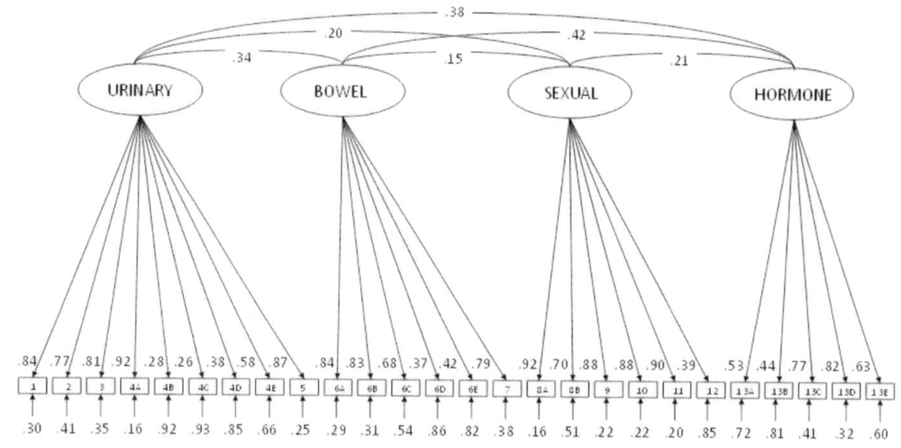

Chi-Square=1637.19, df=293, P-value=0.000, RMSEA=0.084, SRMR = 0.077, CFI = 0.93, PNFI = 0.83, AIC = 1753.19

Fig. 2 Confirmatory factor analysis of the 4-factor EPIC-26 in the Norwegian sample ($N = 651$)

and 4D (weak stream and incomplete emptying) as a second irritative urinary factor (Table 5). Correspondingly, two factors were identified within the hormonal domain (factors 4 and 5). Our EFA identified 2 EPIC-26 items with factor loading on two factors items #12 and 13E, that are in need of further investigation as relevant EPIC-26 items.

An EFA model of the EPIC-26 with 67% explained variance should be considered as reasonably good. Comparing fit values favors our six-factor solution (Table 6). There are, however, some issues that need to be considered before such a conclusion is drawn. The four-factor solution has some support in previous studies, and it appears as theoretically valid and parsimonious. The six-factor solution is based on an exploratory empirical approach (EFA) that may have generated a setting specific solution due to the composition of our sample. The EPIC instruments were meant to assess HRQOL after treatment for PCa by all modalities not just RP. A major limitation of our psychometric analyses is the absence of in our sample of patients who received radiation either alone or with ADT as their primary treatment.

Conclusions

In this paper we have presented the development and psychometrics of the EPIC-26 and the problems associated with the recent recommendations of that questionnaire. The literature unanimously supports the reliability of the EPIC-26, although two items are of doubtful value in our study. Further studies of the EFA and CFA in other samples are needed. The content, discriminant and convergent validities of the EPIC-26 appear good, while the construct and predictive validities remain in need of further examination and development with different treatments.

Abbreviations

CFA: Confirmatory factor analysis; EFA: Exploratory factor analysis; EPIC-16CP: Expanded Prostate Cancer Index Composite for Clinical Practice 16 items; EPIC-26: Expanded Prostate Cancer Index Composite 26 items; EPIC-50: Expanded Prostate Cancer Index Composite 50 items; HRQoL: Health-related quality of life; PCa: prostate cancer; PROMs: Patient-rated outcome measures; SF-12 MCS: Short Form 12: Mental composite scale; SF-12 PCS: Short Form 12: Physical composite scale; UCLA-PCI: University of California at Los Angeles Prostate Cancer Index

Acknowledgements

We have no acknowledgements for this study.

Funding

The authors had no funding for this study.

Authors' contributions

KA has made substantial contributions to the design, acquisition of data and manuscript revising. He approved the submitted version. RN has made substantial contributions to assessment of new papers on the EPIC-26 and manuscript revision. He has been involved in drafting and revising the manuscript and approved the submitted version. BB has made substantial contributions to the design, acquisition of data and manuscript revising. He approved the submitted version. ØS made substantial contributions to the statistical analyses, made Fig. 1 and manuscript revising. He approved the submitted version. SDF has made substantial contributions to conception and design and manuscript revising. She approved the submitted version. AAD has made substantial contributions to conception and design, and data analysis. He has drafted the manuscript and approved the submitted version. All authors read and approved the final manuscript.

Competing interest

The authors declare that they have no competing interests.

Author details

[1]Department of Urology, Akershus University Hospital, Lørenskog, Norway. [2]Department of Urology, Telemark Hospital, Skien, Norway. [3]Department of Urology, Oslo University Hospital, The Norwegian Radium Hospital, Oslo, Norway. [4]School of Business and Social Sciences, University College of Southeast Norway, Hønefoss, Norway. [5]National Resource Center for Late Effects after Cancer Treatment, Oslo University Hospital, The Norwegian Radium Hospital, P.O. Box 4453, Nydalen, 0424 Oslo, Norway. [6]Faculty of Medicine, University of Oslo, Oslo, Norway.

References

1. Schröder FH, Hugosson J, Roobol MJ, Tammela TL, Ciotto S, Nelen V, et al. Screening and prostate cancer mortality in a randomized European study. N Engl J Med. 2009;360(13):1320–8.
2. Schröder FH, Hugosson J, Roobol MJ, Tammela TL, Ciotto S, Nelen V, et al. Prostate cancer mortality at 11 years of follow-up. N Engl J Med. 2012;366(11):981–90.
3. Steinsvik EA, Fosså SD, Axcrona K, Fransson P, Widmark A, Dahl AA. Do perceptions of adverse events differ between patients and physicians? Findings from a randomized controlled trial of radical treatment of prostate cancer. J Urol. 2010;184(2):525–31.
4. Fayers PM, Machin P. Quality of life. The assessment, analysis and interpretation of patient-reported outcomes. 2nd ed. Chichester, UK: Wiley; 2007.
5. Storås AH, Sanda MG, Boronat OG, Chang P, Patil D, Crociani C, et al. Erectile dysfunction and sexual problems two to three years after prostatectomy among American, Norwegian, and Spanish patients. Clin Genitourin Cancer. 2016;14(3):e265–73.
6. Hamoen EH, De Rooij M, Witjes JA, Barentsz JO, Rovers MM. Measuring health-related quality of life in men with prostate cancer: A systematic review of the most used questionnaires and their validity. Urol Oncol. 2015;33(2) 69.e19–28
7. Szymanski KM, Wei JT, Dunn L, Sanda MG. Development and validation of an abbreviated version of the expanded prostate index composite instrument for measuring health-related quality of life among prostate cancer survivors. Urology. 2010;76(5):1245–50.
8. Martin NE, Masey L, Stowell C, Bangma C, Briganti A, Bill-Axelson A, et al. Defining a standard set of patient-centered outcomes for men with localized prostate cancer. Eur Urol. 2015;67(3):460–7.
9. Morgans AK, van Bommel AC, Stowell C, Abrahm JL, Basch E, Bekelmann JE, et al. Development of a standardized set of patient-centered outcomes for advanced prostate cancer: an international effort for a unified approach. Eur Urol. 2015;68(5):891–8.
10. Chang P, Szymanski KM, Dunn RL, Chipman JJ, Litwin MS, Nguyen PL, et al. Expanded prostate cancer index composite for clinical practice: development and validation of a practical health related quality of life instrument for use in the routine clinical care of patients with prostate cancer. J Urol. 2011;186(3):865–72.
11. Rnic K, Linden W, Tudor I, Pullmer R, Vodermaier A. Measuring symptoms in localized prostate cancer: a systematic review of assessment instruments. Prost Cancer Prost Dis. 2013;16(2):111–22.
12. Litwin MS, Hays RD, Fink A, Ganz PA, Leake B, Brook RH. The UCLA prostate index: development, reliability, and validity of a health-related quality of life measure. Med Care. 1998;36(7):1002–12.
13. Wei JT, Dunn RL, Litwin MS, Sandler HM, Sanda MG. Development and validation of the expanded prostate cancer index composite (EPIC) for comprehensive assessment of health-related quality of life in men with prostate cancer. Urology. 2000;56(6):899–905.
14. Schmidt S, Garin O, Pardo Y, Valderas JM, Alonso J, Rebollo P, et al. Assessing quality of life in patients with prostate cancer: a systematic and standardized comparison of available instruments. Qual Life Res. 2014;23(8):2169–81.
15. Chipman JJ, Sanda MG, Dunn RL, Wei JT, Litwin MS, Crociani CM, et al. Measuring and predicting prostate cancer related quality of life changes using EPIC for clinical practice. J Urol. 2014;191(3):638–45.
16. Korzeniowski M, Kalyvas M, Mahmud A, Shenfield C, Tong C, Zaza K, et al. Piloting prostate cancer patient-reported outcomes in clinical practice. Support Care Cancer. 2016;24(5):1983–90.
17. Sharma P, Dunn RL, Wei JT, Monite JE, Gilbert SM. Evaluation of point-of-care PRO assessment in clinical settings: integration, parallel-forms reliability, and patient acceptability of electronic QOL measures during clinical visits. Qual Life Res. 2016;25(3):575 83.
18. Skolarus TA, Holmes-Rovner M, Hawley ST, Dunn RL, Barr KL, Willard NR, et al. Monitoring quality of life among prostate cancer survivors: the feasibility of automated telephone assessment. Urology. 2012;80(5):1021–6.
19. Sampurno F, Ruseckaite R, Millar JL, Evans SM. Comparison of patient-reported quality-of-life and complications in men with prostate cancer, between two modes of administration. Clin Genitourin Cancer. 2016;14(4):284–9.
20. Fosså SD, Holck Storås A, Steinsvik EA, Myklebust TA, Eri LM, Loge JH, et al. Psychometric testing of the Norwegian version of the expanded prostate cancer index composite 26-item version (EPIC-26). Scand J Urol. 2016;50(4):280–5.
21. Ellison JS, He C, Wood DP. Stratification of postprostatectomy urinary function using expanded prostate cancer index composite. Urology. 2013;81(1):56–60.
22. Punnen S, Cowan JE, Dunn LB, Shumay DM, Carroll PR, Cooperberg MRA. Longitudinal study of anxiety, depression and distress as predictors of sexual and urinary quality of life in men with prostate cancer. BJU Int. 2013;112(2):E67–75.
23. Evans JR, Zhao S, Daignault S, Sanda MG, Michalski J, Sandler HM, et al. Patient-reported quality of life after stereotactic body radiotherapy (SBRT), intensity modulated radiotherapy (IMRT), and brachytherapy. Radiother Oncol. 2015;116(2):179–84.
24. Watson E, Shinkins B, Frith E, Neal D, Hamdy F, Walter F, et al. Symptoms, unmet needs, psychosocial well-being and health status in survivors of prostate cancer: implications for redesigning follow-up. BJU Int. 2016;117(6B):E10–9.
25. Schofield P, Gough K, Lotfi-Jam K, Aranda S. Validation of the supportive care needs survey-short form 34 with a simplified response format in men with prostate cancer. Psycho-Oncologia. 2012;21(10):1107–12.
26. Recklitis CJ, Zhou ES, Zwerner EK, JC H, Kantoff PW. Suicidal ideation in prostate cancer survivors: understanding the role of physical and psychological health outcomes. Cancer. 2014;120(21):3393–400.
27. Skolarus TA, Dunn RL, Sanda MG, Chang P, Greenfield TK, Litwin MS, et al. Minimally important difference for the expanded prostate cancer index composite short form. Urology. 2015;85(1):101–6.
28. Tavlarides AM, Ames SC, Thiel DD, Diehl NN, Parker AS. Baseline and follow-up association of the MAX-PC in men with newly diagnosed prostate cancer. Psycho-Oncologia. 2015;24(4):451–7.
29. Brennhovd B, Axcrona K, Fosså SD, Giercksky KE, Vlatkovic L, Dahl AA. Robot- assisted radical prostatectomy of clinical high-risk patients with prostate cancer: a controlled study of operative and short-term post-operative events. Scand J Urol. 2013;47(6):449–55.
30. Østby-Deglum M, Brennhovd B, Axcrona K, Fosså SD, Dahl AAA. Comparative study of erectile function and use of erectile aids in high-risk prostate cancer patients after robot-assisted laparoscopic prostatectomy. Scand J Urol. 2015;49(6):433–9.
31. Bjelland I, Dahl AA, Haug TT, Neckelmann D. The validity of the hospital anxiety depression scale. An updated literature review. J Psychosom Res. 2002;52(2):69–77.
32. Gandek B, Ware JE, Aaronson NK, Apolone B, Bjorner JB, Bullinger M, et al. Cross-validation of item selection and scoring for the SF-12 Health Survey in nine countries: results from the IQOLA Project. International Quality of Life Assessment. J Clin Epidemiol. 1998;51(11):1171–8.
33. Grov EK, Fosså SD, Bremnes RM, Dahl O, Klepp O, Wist E, et al. The personality trait of neuroticism is strongly associated with long-term morbidity in testicular cancer survivors. Acta Oncol. 2009;48(6):842–9.
34. Hooper D. Exploratory factor analysis. In: Chen H, editor. Approaches to quantitative research – theory and its practical application: a guide to dissertation students. Cork, Ireland: Oak Tree Press; 2012.
35. Hu L, Bentler PM. Cutoff criteria for fit indexes in covariance structure analysis: conventional criteria versus new alternatives. Struct Equat Model. 1999;6:1–55.
36. Jacobsen SJ, Girman CJ, Guess HA, Panser LA, Chute CB, Oesterling JE, et al. Natural history of prostatism: factors associated discordance between frequency and bother of urinary symptoms. Urology. 1993;42(6):663–71.
37. Litwin MS. Measuring health related quality of life in men with prostate cancer. J Urol. 1994;152(5 Pt 2):1882–7.
38. Briganti A, Gallina A, Suardi N, Capitanio U, Tutolo M, Bianci M, et al. Predicting erectile function recovery after bilateral nerve sparing radical prostatectomy: a proposal of a novel preoperative risk stratification. J Sex Med. 2010;7(7):2521–31.

39. D'Amico AV, Whittington R, Malkowicz SB, Schultz D, Blank K, Broderick GA, et al. Biochemical outcome after radical prostatectomy, external beam therapy, or interstitial radiation therapy for clinically localized prostate cancer. JAMA. 1998;280(11):969–74.
40. Crook J, Ots AF. Prognostic factors for newly diagnosed prostate cancer and their role in treatment selection. Sem. Radiat Oncol. 2013;23(3):165–72.
41. Martin NE, Mucci LA, Loda M, Depinho RA. Prognostic determinants in prostate cancer. Cancer J. 2011;17(6):429–37.
42. Braun DP, Gupta D, Staren ED. Predicting survival in prostate cancer: the role of quality of life assessment. Support Care Cancer. 2012;20(6):1267–74.
43. American Psychiatric Association. Practice guideline for the treatment of patients with major depressive disorder. 3rd ed. Washington, DC: American Psychiatric Press; 2010.

3

A retrospective feasibility study of biweekly, reduced-dose docetaxel in Asian patients with castrate-resistant, metastatic prostate cancer

Hae Su Kim[1,2], Ji Yun Lee[1], Su Jin Lee[1], Ho Yeong Lim[1], Hyun Hwan Sung[3], Hwang Gyun Jeon[3], Byong Chang Jeong[3], Seong Il Seo[3], Seong Soo Jeon[3], Hyun Moo Lee[3], Han-Yong Choi[3] and Se Hoon Park[1*]

Abstract

Background: The aim of this retrospective study was to evaluate the clinical outcomes of reduced dose, biweekly docetaxel chemotherapy for Korean patients with castrate-resistant prostate cancer (CRPC).

Methods: We retrospectively reviewed the medical records of 48 patients with metastatic CRPC who were treated with a biweekly regimen (intravenous docetaxel 40 mg/m^2 on day 1 plus prednisolone 5 mg twice daily) between 2012 and 2015 at Samsung Medical Center (Seoul, Korea). Prior to the adoption of a biweekly regimen in Oct 2013, our institutional standard chemotherapy was docetaxel 75 mg/m^2 every 3 weeks for patients with CRPC (n = 24). After Oct 2013, all chemotherapy-naïve patients with CRPC received a 40 mg/m^2 biweekly regimen (n = 24). The primary end point was a PSA response, defined as a greater than 50% decline in PSA level from baseline.

Results: The baseline characteristics of the patients in the two treatment groups were similar. The most common cause of treatment discontinuation was disease progression, which was exhibited by 17 patients (71%) in the 3-weekly group and 20 (75%) in the biweekly group. PSA responses were observed in 12 (50%) and 11 (46%) patients in the 3-weekly and biweekly groups, respectively (p = 0.683). Time to treatment failure (TTTF, 4.5 vs 3.9 months) and time-to-progression (TTP, 5.0 vs 4.2 months) were not significantly different between the 3-weekly and biweekly groups.

Conclusions: Within the limitations of a retrospective study, the biweekly reduced dose docetaxel regimen was active and well-tolerated in Korean patients with metastatic CRPC.

Keywords: Castrate-resistant prostate cancer, Docetaxel, Biweekly

Background

Prostate cancer is one of the most rapidly rising malignancies in Korea [1]. In patients with advanced or metastatic disease, androgen-deprivation therapy (ADT) or surgical castration is regarded as the standard treatment. After years of treatment, however, medically or surgically castrated prostate cancer eventually transforms into castration-resistant prostate cancer (CRPC) [2]. Although the prognosis of patients with CRPC has typically been very poor [3], two randomized clinical trials demonstrated a survival benefit with docetaxel chemotherapy in patients with metastatic CRPC [4, 5]. Docetaxel is usually administered at a dose of 75 mg/m^2 every 3 weeks based on the results from the TAX-327 study [5, 6], in which 3-weekly docetaxel conferred a clear survival benefit over mitoxantrone (median, 19.2 vs 17.8 months; P = 0.004), but was also associated with significant hematologic toxicity.

As a result of these two landmark trials, docetaxel was approved in Korea for the treatment of CPRC. Moreover, a retrospective study [7] demonstrated that the standard regimen (docetaxel 75 mg/m^2 every 3 weeks plus prednisolone

* Correspondence: hematoma@skku.edu
[1]Division of Hematology-Oncology, Department of Medicine, Samsung Medical Center, Sungkyunkwan University School of Medicine, 81 Irwon-Ro Gangnam-gu, Seoul 135-710, South Korea
Full list of author information is available at the end of the article

5 mg twice daily) was feasible in Asian patients with CRPC and yielded a manageable toxicity profile. However, based on a pharmacokinetics study conducted in Japan [8] and the belief that treatment safety and tolerability are indispensable in the treatment of solid tumors in a palliative setting [7], docetaxel is most commonly administered in Asian countries at a lower dose (60 mg/m^2 every 3 weeks).

Another way to circumvent docetaxel-induced hematologic toxicity is to use different administration schedules, such as weekly or biweekly regimens. In support of this strategy, weekly administration of docetaxel has been shown to yield lower hematologic toxicity than the standard 3-weekly regimen [9]. Moreover, grade 3 or 4 neutropenia occurred in 75% of all Asian patients with CRPC who were treated with 3-weekly docetaxel [10]. Furthermore, the median survival duration in the weekly docetaxel arm of the TAX-327 study [6] was shorter than in the mitoxantrone arm (median, 17.8 vs 16.3 months; $p = 0.09$), although this difference was not significant. In contrast, biweekly administration of docetaxel 50 mg/m^2 resulted in a longer time-to-treatment failure (TTTF; median, 5.6 vs 4.9 months; $p = 0.014$) than 3-weekly docetaxel [11]. As expected, the biweekly regimen was better tolerated than the 3-weekly docetaxel regimen; importantly, efficacy was not compromised.

Based on these considerations, in Oct 2013 we adopted a biweekly low dose docetaxel regimen (40 mg/m^2 every 2 weeks) as an institutional standard chemotherapy regimen for patients with chemotherapy-naïve CPRC. Here we retrospectively investigated and compared the clinical outcomes of biweekly 40 mg/m^2 docetaxel plus prednisolone with those of 75 mg/m^2 docetaxel every 3 weeks in korean patients with CRPC.

Methods

Patients

We retrospectively collected and reviewed the medical records of 48 patients with metastatic CRPC who were consecutively treated with docetaxel plus prednisolone as the first-line chemotherapy regimen between March 2012 and February 2015. Patients with histologically-proven adenocarcinoma of the prostate whose disease had progressed after maximal ADT were eligible for the study. Disease progression was defined as 1) radiologic evidence of a new metastatic lesion or aggravated measurable disease, or 2) serial increases in the prostate-specific antigen (PSA) level on 2 or more occasions at least 2 weeks apart. Patients were required to have a castrate level of serum testosterone while receiving ADT, an Eastern Cooperative Oncology Group (ECOG) performance status of 0 to 2, and adequate major organ functions. We excluded all patients who were enrolled in clinical trials to ensure that the study population reflected our daily clinical practice. The choice of biweekly docetaxel was solely at the discretion of the treating oncologists. Other exclusion criteria were as follows: (1) prior chemotherapy for advanced or metastatic disease, (2) histologic evidence of neuroendocrine carcinoma, (3) another malignancy within 5 years, and (4) inappropriate laboratory findings or any severe comorbidity.

Procedures

Prior to the adoption of a biweekly regimen in Oct 2013, our institutional standard chemotherapy was docetaxel 75 mg/m^2 every 3 weeks for patients with CRPC. After Oct 2013, all chemotherapy-naïve patients with CRPC at our institution received a biweekly regimen. Docetaxel was administered intravenously over 1 h on day 1 with dexamethasone and anti-emetics. Oral prednisolone 5 mg was administered twice daily from day 1 and continued throughout treatment. Supportive care, including the administration of blood products, bisphosphonates, and the use of analgesics was given if judged appropriate by the treating physicians. Before initiating the first dose of docetaxel, a complete history was taken from each patient. In addition, complete blood counts, serum chemistry analyses, chest x-rays, bone scans, and computed tomography (CT) scans of all involved sites were performed. Patients were seen every 2 or 3 weeks; during these visits, a brief history was taken, a physical examination was performed, and adverse events, blood counts, and PSA levels were assessed. In both groups, treatment was repeated on an outpatient basis and continued until objective disease progression, unacceptable toxicity, deterioration of clinical conditions, or patient refusal. Radiologic responses were evaluated every 6 weeks (3-weekly group) or 8 weeks (biweekly group) by bone scan, chest and abdominopelvic CT, or the same tests that were used for initial tumor staging. Adverse events were collected and graded according to the National Cancer Institute criteria (CTCAE) version 4.0.

Statistical analysis

The primary end point was a PSA response, defined as a ≥ 50% decline in the PSA level from baseline with no clinical or radiologic evidence of disease progression. PSA progression was defined as an increase of ≥25% and ≥2 ng/ml above the nadir that was confirmed by a second value 3 or more weeks later. If no decline from baseline was observed, PSA progression was defined as an increase of ≥25% and ≥2 ng/ml after 12 weeks according to the Prostate Cancer Working Group 2 (PCWG2) criteria [12]. Secondary end points included TTTF, time to progression (TTP), duration of PSA response, and toxicity profile. TTTF was defined as the time from the first administration date to the date of disease progression (PSA or radiologic progression), unacceptable toxic effects, death, or discontinuation of chemotherapy for any reason. TTP was defined as the time from the first administration date to the date of disease progression or death. TTTF and TTP were calculated using the Kaplan-Meier method. Categorical variables were compared using Pearson's chi-square test or Fisher's exact test. Continuous variables were compared with the Mann-Whitney U test. TTTF and TTP were calculated using the Kaplan-Meier method and compared using the log-rank test. An unstratified Cox regression model was used to estimate hazard ratios (HRs) with 95% confidence intervals (CIs). All p values were two-sided, with $p < 0.05$ taken to indicate statistical significance. All analyses were performed using R for Windows, v2.11.1 (R Core Team, Vienna, Austria; http://www.Rproject.org).

Results

Patient characteristics

From March 2012 to Feb 2015, 58 patients with CRPC underwent screening, 48 (83%) of whom were eligible for the current study. Each group contained 24 patients. The patient baseline characteristics were not significantly different between the two treatment groups (Table 1). The median patient age was 68 years (range, 52–84 years) and the most common site of metastasis was bone (100%), followed by lymph node (58%) and bladder (8%). A total of 42 (88%) patients had received prior hormonal therapy, and 8 (17%) patients had undergone prostatectomy. The median follow-up duration after the first chemotherapy treatment was 11 months (range, 2.5–36.3 months).

Table 1 Baseline characteristics according to docetaxel regimens

Characteristic	3-weekly docetaxel (n = 24)	2-weekly docetaxel (n = 24)	P value
Median age (years) (range)	69.5 (52.3–83.9)	64.6 (56.6–80.0)	0.110
Site of metastasis			
Bone	24 (100%)	24 (100%)	1.000
Liver	2 (8.3%)	1 (4.2%)	0.500
Lung	1 (4.2%)	2 (8.3%)	0.500
Lymph node	10 (41.7%)	18 (75%)	0.019
Bladder	1 (4.2%)	3 (12.5%)	0.609
Gleason score			0.190
≤ 7	5 (20.8%)	3 (12.5%)	
8	6 (25.0%)	5 (20.8%)	
≥ 9	7 (29.2%)	16 (66.7%)	
Unknown	6 (25.0%)	0 (0%)	
Median PSA (ng/mL)			
Baseline	34.7	31.2	0.279
Nadir	15.1	11.6	0.279
Previous therapy			
Prostatectomy	4 (16.7%)	4 (16.7%)	0.500
Prostate radiotherapy	2 (8.3%)	1 (4.2%)	0.500
Total dose (mg/m^2), median	395	320	0.011
Total # cycles, median (range)	6 (1–11)	8 (2–23)	0.023
Mean dose (mg/m^2) at each cycle, median	68 (58–75)	40 (35–40)	<0.001
Initial dose (mg/m^2), median	75 (60–75)	40 (35–40)	<0.001

Abbreviations: PSA prostate-specific antigen

PSA response

A PSA response was observed in 12 (50%) patients in the 3-weekly group and 11 (45.8%) patients in the biweekly group (p = 0.683) (Table 2). Among the patients with a PSA response, the median time to PSA response was 1.4 months in both groups (p = 0.839). The median response durations were 4.0 and 3.7 months in the 3-weekly and biweekly groups, respectively (p = 0.342).

TTTF and TTP

The median TTTF was longer in the 3-weekly group than in the 2-weekly group; however, this difference was not significant (4.5 months, 95% CI 3.1–5.9 in the 3-weekly group vs 3.9 months, 95% CI 3.2–4.6 in the 2-weekly group, p = 0.542; Fig. 1). Similarly, the TTP were not significantly different between the two groups (5.0 months, 95% CI 3.9–6.1in the 3-weekly group vs 4.2 months, 95% 3.5–4.9 in the 2-weekly group, p = 0.530; Fig. 2). At the time of data cut-off (July 2015), six (25%) patients in the 3-weekly group and four (17%) patients in the 2-weekly group had died. The median OS had not been reached in either group.

Toxicities

The median numbers of cycles per patient were six (range, 1–11) in the 3-weekly group and 8 (range, 2–23) in the 2-weekly group (Table 1). The most common cause of treatment discontinuation was disease progression (17 [71%] in the 3-weekly group; 18 (75%) in the 2-weekly group), followed by adverse events (4 [17%] and 1 [4%]), patient refusal of treatment (2 [8%] and 0), and unknown reasons (1 [4%] and 3 [13%]). The median cumulative doses of docetaxel were 395 mg/m^2 in the 3-weekly group and 320 mg/m^2 in the 2-weekly group. Fourteen (58%) patients in the 3-weekly group and 4 (17%) in the 2-weekly group required dose reduction. Toxic effects requiring dose reduction included fatigue (61%), neutropenia (22%), thrombocytopenia (11%), and nausea (6%). The hematological and non-hematological toxic effects for each group are listed in Table 3. No patient died from any therapy-related toxic effect. The most common hematologic toxicity was anemia. Four patients (17%) who received 3-weekly docetaxel had grade 3–4 neutropenia; among them, 3 (13%) experienced neutropenic infections. In contrast, no patient who received 2-weekly docetaxel exhibited

Table 2 Summary of primary and secondary outcomes

Outcome	3-weekly docetaxel (95% CI)	2-weekly docetaxel (95% CI)	*P*-value	Hazard ratio (95% CI)	*P*-value
Overall PSA response			0.683		
Objective response[a]	12 (50.0%)	11 (45.8%)	..	..	..
Stable disease	10 (41.7%)	9 (37.5%)	..	..	..
Disease progression	2 (8.3%)	4 (16.7%)	..	..	..
Median response duration months, (95% CI)	4.0 (3.2–8.1)	3.7 (2.7–6.0)	0.342		
Median TTTF, months, (95% CI)	4.5 (3.1–5.9)	3.9 (3.2–4.6)	0.542	1.2 (0.7–2.2)	0.551
Median TTP, months, (95% CI)	5.0 (3.9–6.1)	4.2 (3.5–4.9)	0.530	1.2 (0.6–2.3)	0.536

Abbreviation: *CI* confidence interval; *PSA* prostate-specific antigen; *TTTF* time to treatment failure; *TTP* time to progression; *PSA* prostate-specific antigen
Medians and 95% CIs were estimated from Kaplan-Meier analyses
[a]Objective responses include only partial responses; no complete responses were observed

febrile neutropenia. Eight (33%) patients in the 3-weekly group and 3 (13%) in the 2-weekly group had grade 3–4 fatigue.

Discussion

The purpose of the present retrospective study was to evaluate the feasibility of biweekly docetaxel 40 mg/m^2 in patients with metastatic CRPC. Patients who received docetaxel every 2 weeks showed similar PSA responses, TTTFs, TTPs, and fewer occurrences of grade 3–4 adverse events compared with patients who received docetaxel 75 mg/m^2 every 3 weeks.

Several treatment options are available for men with progressing metastatic CRPC, including docetaxel plus estramustine [4], cabazitaxel plus prednisone [13], abiraterone plus prednisone [14], enzalutamide [15], radium-223 [16], and sipuleucel-T [17]. However, docetaxel with prednisone has been the standard first-line drug for men with metastatic CRPC for more than 10 years, based on two landmark studies showing a 20–30% improvement in OS compared with mitoxantrone chemotherapy [4, 5]. The GETUG-AFU-15 and CHAARTED studies, both of which assessed the efficacy and tolerability of ADT (with or without docetaxel), also suggested that ADT plus docetaxel should be considered as a standard treatment in men with metastatic hormone-sensitive prostate cancer [18, 19].

Now that docetaxel has been approved as a first-line treatment for metastatic CRPC, it is particularly relevant to determine whether administering a lower dose of docetaxel over a shorter interval yields improved efficacy and tolerability compared with the standard regimen of 75 mg/m^2 docetaxel every 3 weeks. The TAX 327 trial showed significantly longer survival for patients treated with 75 mg/m^2 docetaxel every 3 weeks compared with 12 mg/m^2 mitoxantrone every 3 weeks (OS 19.2 months vs 17.8 months, respectively); however, patients treated with 30 mg/m^2 docetaxel once weekly (OS 17.8 months) did not exhibit any significant difference in survival compared with patients treated with the mitoxantrone regimen [6]. Although the 3-weekly docetaxel regimen yielded a slightly longer OS than the weekly docetaxel regimen, 32% of the 332 patients who received 3-weekly

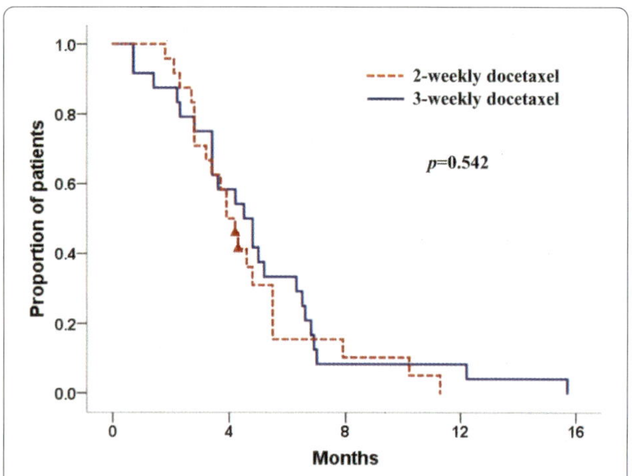

Fig. 1 Kaplan-Meier survival analysis according to time to treatment failure (log-rank $p = 0.542$)

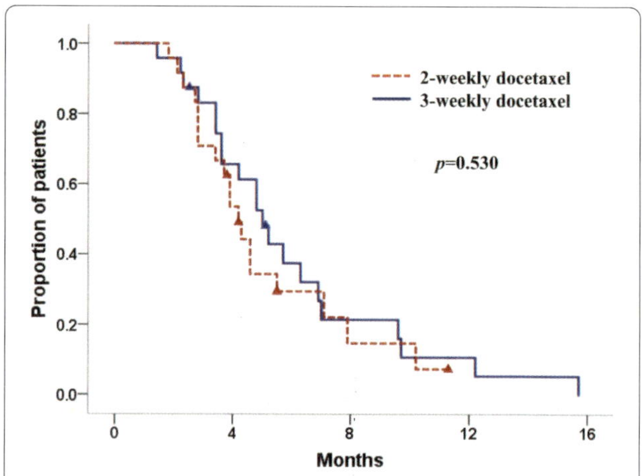

Fig. 2 Kaplan-Meier survival analysis according to time to progression (log-rank $p = 0.530$)

Table 3 Treatment-related adverse events

	3-weekly docetaxel (n = 24)		2-weekly docetaxel (n = 24)	
	Grade 1–2	Grade 3–4	Grade 1–2	Grade 3–4
Neutropenia	7 (30%)	4 (17%)	5 (21%)	0
Febrile neutropenia	..	3 (13%)	..	0
Anemia	23 (96%)	1 (4%)	15 (63%)	1 (4%)
Thrombocytopenia	4 (17%)	2 (8%)	2 (8%)	0
Fatigue	8 (33%)	8 (33%)	5 (21%)	3 (13%)
Peripheral neuropathy	0	0	1 (4%)	0
Allergic reaction	0	0	1 (4%)	0
Arthralgia	8 (33%)	0	6 (25%)	0
Diarrhea	6 (25%)	0	7 (29%)	0
Nausea	4 (17%)	1 (4%)	5 (21%)	0
AST elevation	1 (4%)	0	0	0
ALT elevation	1 (4%)	0	0	0

docetaxel experienced grade 3–4 neutropenia, whereas only 2% of the 330 patients who received weekly docetaxel had grade 3–4 neutropenia [5].

Few studies have determined the optimal schedule for docetaxel-based chemotherapy so that it is both efficacious and safe. In one phase III study, 170 patients were treated with docetaxel 50 mg/m^2 administrated every 2 weeks, whereas another 176 patients were treated with docetaxel 75 mg/m^2 every 3 weeks [11]. Although the total doses in both groups were identical over the 12 weeks, 2-weekly administration was found to be associated with significantly longer TTTF than 3-weekly administration (5.6 vs 4.9 months; HR 1.3, p = 0.014). Moreover, 2-weekly administration of docetaxel was also associated with improved OS and fewer occurrences of neutropenia, leucopenia, and febrile neutropenia. In another study, 94 patients with metastatic CRPC were treated with docetaxel 45 mg/m^2 every 2 weeks with estramustine [20]. A PSA response was observed in 45 (53%) of the 84 patients, and the median time to PSA progression was 5.0 months. In another study by Karavasillis et al., 16 patients with metastatic CRPC were treated with a regimen of biweekly docetaxel 30 mg/m^2, and 6 patients (38%) showed a PSA response over a median duration of 4.5 months [21]. The patient characteristics, TTTF, and PSA responses in both groups in the present study were highly similar to those in a previous phase III study [11]. In the previous study, 2-weekly 50 mg/m^2 docetaxel resulted in a significantly longer TTTF than 3-weekly docetaxel; however, no significant differences were observed between patients treated with 2-weekly 40 mg/m^2 docetaxel versus 3-weekly 75 mg/m^2 docetaxel in present study. We observed similar PSA responses and TTTFs in the 2-weekly and 3-weekly docetaxel groups; this result may be due to the relatively small dose of docetaxel in the 2-weekly group and the small number of patients. Therapy-related adverse effects and comorbidities are common in elderly patients and play important roles in determining the optimal approach to palliative chemotherapy for individuals with CRPC [22]. Our results show that a 2-weekly docetaxel chemotherapy regimen is well tolerated, safe, and yields results comparable to those achieved with a 3-weekly docetaxel regimen.

The current study has several limitations. First, 17% of the patients treated with docetaxel were not included in the present study, leading to potential selection bias. Second, given the retrospective nature of the study, some of the data may be missing, especially data regarding adverse events. Finally, patient-reported outcomes, such as quality-of-life factors, could not be determined.

Conclusions

In conclusion, a biweekly reduced dose docetaxel regimen is active and well-tolerated in Korean patients with metastatic CRPC. Thus, a biweekly docetaxel regimen should be considered as an additional option for Asian patients and men with comorbidities. Our results warrant further large prospective studies of biweekly reduced dose docetaxel.

Abbreviations

ADT: androgen-deprivation therapy; CRPC: castration-resistant prostate cancer; PSA: prostate-specific antigen; TTP: time to progression; TTTF: time-to-treatment failure

Acknowledgements

None.

Funding

No funding was obtained for this study.

Authors' contributions

HSK, JYL, SJL conceived and designated the study; SHP, HYL and HHS helped to conceive the study and revised manuscript critically for important intellectually content; HGJ, BCJ, SIS and SSJ critically revised the manuscript; HML, and HC helped acquisition and interpretation of data; HSK and JYL participated in statistical analysis and interpretation of data; HSK, SHP conceived the study, participated in the design of it and coordination. All authors read and approved the final manuscript.

Competing interests

The authors declare that they have no competing interests.

Author details

[1]Division of Hematology-Oncology, Department of Medicine, Samsung Medical Center, Sungkyunkwan University School of Medicine, 81 Irwon-Ro Gangnam-gu, Seoul 135-710, South Korea. [2]Department of Hematology-Oncology, Department of Medicine, Veterans Health Service Medical Center, Seoul, South Korea. [3]Department of Urology, Samsung Medical Center, Sungkyunkwan University School of Medicine, Seoul, South Korea.

References

1. Jung KW, Won YJ, Kong HJ, Oh CM, Cho H, Lee DH, et al. Cancer statistics in Korea: incidence, mortality, survival, and prevalence in 2012. Cancer Res Treat. 2015;47:127–41.
2. Damber JE, Aus G. Prostate cancer. Lancet. 2008;371:1710–21.
3. Eisenberger MA, Simon R, O'Dwyer PJ, Wittes RE, Friedman MA. A reevaluation of nonhormonal cytotoxic chemotherapy in the treatment of prostatic carcinoma. J Clin Oncol. 1985;3:827–41.
4. Petrylak DP, Tangen CM, Hussain MH, Lara PN Jr, Jones JA, Taplin ME, et al. Docetaxel and estramustine compared with mitoxantrone and prednisone for advanced refractory prostate cancer. N Engl J Med. 2004;351:1513–20.
5. Tannock IF, de Wit R, Berry WR, Horti J, Pluzanska A, Chi KN, et al. Docetaxel plus prednisone or mitoxantrone plus prednisone for advanced prostate cancer. N Engl J Med. 2004;351:1502–12.
6. Berthold DR, Pond GR, Soban F, de Wit R, Eisenberger M, Tannock IF. Docetaxel plus prednisone or mitoxantrone plus prednisone for advanced prostate cancer: updated survival in the TAX 327 study. J Clin Oncol. 2008;26:242–5.
7. Lee JL, Kim JE, Ahn JH, Lee DH, Lee J, Kim CS, et al. Efficacy and safety of docetaxel plus prednisolone chemotherapy for metastatic hormone-refractory prostate adenocarcinoma: single institutional study in Korea. Cancer Res Treat. 2010;42:12–7.
8. Taguchi T, Furue H, Niitani H, Ishitani K, Kanamaru R, Hasegawa K, et al. Phase I clinical trial of RP 56976 (docetaxel) a new anticancer drug. Gan To Kagaku Ryoho. 1994;21:1997–2005.
9. Park SH, Choi SJ, Kyung SY, An CH, Lee SP, Park JW, et al. Randomized phase II trial of two different schedules of docetaxel plus cisplatin as first-line therapy in advanced nonsmall cell lung cancer. Cancer. 2007;109:732–40.
10. Shimazui T, Kawai K, Miyanaga N, Kojima T, Sekido N, Hinotsu S, et al. Three-weekly docetaxel with prednisone is feasible for Japanese patients with hormone-refractory prostate cancer: a retrospective comparative study with weekly docetaxel alone. Jpn J Clin Oncol. 2007;37:603–8.
11. Kellokumpu-Lehtinen PL, Harmenberg U, Joensuu T, McDermott R, Hervonen P, Ginman C, et al. 2-weekly versus 3-weekly docetaxel to treat castration-resistant advanced prostate cancer: a randomised, phase 3 trial. Lancet Oncol. 2013;14:117–24.
12. Scher HI, Halabi S, Tannock I, Morris M, Sternberg CN, Carducci MA, et al. Design and end points of clinical trials for patients with progressive prostate cancer and castrate levels of testosterone: recommendations of the prostate cancer clinical trials working group. J Clin Oncol. 2008;26:1148–59.
13. de Bono JS, Oudard S, Ozguroglu M, Hansen S, Machiels JP, Kocak I, et al. Prednisone plus cabazitaxel or mitoxantrone for metastatic castration-resistant prostate cancer progressing after docetaxel treatment: a randomised open-label trial. Lancet. 2010;376:1147–54.
14. Ryan CJ, Smith MR, de Bono JS, Molina A, Logothetis CJ, de Souza P, et al. Abiraterone in metastatic prostate cancer without previous chemotherapy. N Engl J Med. 2013;368:138–48.
15. Tran C, Ouk S, Clegg NJ, Chen Y, Watson PA, Arora V, et al. Development of a second-generation antiandrogen for treatment of advanced prostate cancer. Science. 2009;324:787–90.
16. Parker C, Nilsson S, Heinrich D, Helle SI, O'Sullivan JM, Fossa SD, et al. Alpha emitter radium-223 and survival in metastatic prostate cancer. N Engl J Med. 2013;369:213–23.
17. Kantoff PW, Higano CS, Shore ND, Berger ER, Small EJ, Penson DF, et al. Sipuleucel-T immunotherapy for castration-resistant prostate cancer. N Engl J Med. 2010;363:411–22.
18. Gravis G, Fizazi K, Joly F, Oudard S, Priou F, Esterni B, et al. Androgen-deprivation therapy alone or with docetaxel in non-castrate metastatic prostate cancer (GETUG-AFU 15): a randomised, open-label, phase 3 trial. Lancet Oncol. 2013;14:149–58.
19. Sweeney CJ, Chen YH, Carducci M, Liu G, Jarrad DH, Eisenberger M, et al. Chemohormonal Therapy in Metastatic Hormone-Sensitive Prostate Cancer. N Engl J Med. 2015;373:737–46.
20. Bamias A, Bozas G, Antoniou N, Poulias I, Katsifotis H, Skolarikos A, et al. Prognostic and predictive factors in patients with androgen-independent prostate cancer treated with docetaxel and estramustine: a single institution experience. Eur Urol. 2008;53:323–31.
21. Karavasilis V, Briasoulis E, Siarabi O, Pavlidis N. Biweekly administration of low-dose docetaxel in hormone-resistant prostate cancer: pilot study of an effective subtoxic therapy. Clin Prostate Cancer. 2003;2:46–9.
22. Droz JP, Aapro M, Balducci L, Boyle H, Van den Broeck T, Cathcart P, et al. Management of prostate cancer in older patients: updated recommendations of a working group of the International Society of Geriatric Oncology. Lancet Oncol. 2014;15:e404–14.

Transperineal cryotherapy for unresectable muscle invasive bladder cancer: preliminary experience with 7 male patients

Qing Zhang†, Shiwei Zhang†, Shun Zhang, Wei Wang, Xiaozhi Zhao, Yongming Deng, Huibo Lian and Hongqian Guo*

Abstract

Background: Radical cystectomy (RC) with pelvic lymph node dissection (PLND) and urinary diversion (UD) is considered the standard treatment for muscle invasive bladder cancer (MIBC). In a part of patients, RC procedure is aborted due to unresectable disease, other followed treatment like systemic chemotherapy, radiotherapy or cryotherapy may be a better option. The aim of present study was to report the preliminary results of transperineal cryotherapy for unresectable muscle invasive bladder cancer.

Methods: From January 2011 to August 2013, 7 male patients with pT4b unresectable bladder cancer underwent bilateral ureterocutaneostomy. Two performed a pelvic lymph node dissection (PLND). Then primary transperineal cryosurgery for preserved bladder at the guidance of transrectal ultrasound (TRUS) was performed. All patients underwent a dual freeze-thaw cycle using third-generation cryotechnology with ultrathin 17-gauge cryoneedles. Computer tomography (CT) and/or magnetic resonance image (MRI)were performed at 3 month intervals after cryosurgery to determine whether progression or recurrence occurred.

Results: All cryosurgery was performed successfully, mean operation time was 76.43 ± 25.12 min (range 50-120 min), mean blood loss was 19.29 ± 15.92 ml (range 5-50 ml). Mean hospital stay was 3.86 ± 1.68 day (range 2-7 days). No operative related deaths occurred. Four patients dead due to the metastasis disease at the follow up time of 8, 15, 18 and 37 months, respectively. Six patients received postoperative therapy, of whom 5 patients were treated with combined chemoradiation, and the other one received chemotherapy alone. The progression free survival (PFS) of the 7 patients was 22.00 ± 14.61 months (range 3-40 months). The one, two and three year overall survival (OS) was 85.7%, 57.1% and 42.9%, respectively.

Conclusion: Our results suggest that cryosurgery combination with chemoradiotherapy provide a safe and effective alternative method for unresectable pT4b bladder cancer. Longer follow-up is necessary to determine the sustained efficacy.

Keywords: Cryotherapy, Invasive bladder cancer, Progression free survival, Transperineal cryoablation, Unresectable

Background

Bladder cancer (BC) is a common human malignancy and is the second most common genitourinary malignancy [1]. About 20-40% of patients with BC present or develop a muscle invasive bladder cancer (MIBC). Currently, radical cystectomy (RC) with pelvic lymph node dissection (PLND) and urinary diversion (UD), although associated with significant morbidity, is considered the standard treatment for MIBC [2]. In a part of patients, RC procedure is aborted due to unresectable disease, either the presence of gross palpable nodes (pN2-3) or tumor fixation to the pelvis or rectum (pT4b). In these patients, RC will be aborted intraoperatively, other followed treatment like systemic chemotherapy, radiotherapy or cryotherapy may be a better option.

Cryosurgery, which can induce tissue necrosis by ice ball formation, has been used as an alternative therapeutic

* Correspondence: dr.ghq@nju.edu.cn
†Equal contributors
Department of Urology, Drum Tower Hospital, Medical School of Nanjing University, Institute of Urology, Nanjing University, 321 Zhongshan Road, Nanjing 210008, Jiangsu, People's Republic of China

approach in bladder cancer for half a century. The effects of cryoablation on the bladder were investigated in dogs by McDonald et al. in 1950 and typical necrotic lesions were produced [3]. Several reports recently described the utility of cryosurgery in the treatment of bladder cancer through percutaneous or transurethral route and concluded that this precudure could be used as a novel therapeutic approach to the treatment of benign and malignant bladder tumors, especially unresectable tumors and metastatic bladder cancer [4, 5].

Since 2011, we have performed transperineal cryotherapy in patients who had aborted RC with unresectable disease secondary to fixation to the pelvis and/or rectum and followed ureterocutaneostomy. The aim of the current study was to analyze the preliminary results and to investigate the safety and efficacy of transperineal cryotherapy in our 7 male patients.

Methods

Patients

Between January 2011 to August 2013, 7 male patients with unresectable bladder cancer underwent transperineal cryotherapy in our institution were enrolled in the study. All patients had an aborted RC due to unresectable disease secondary to fixation to the pelvis and/or rectum (pT4b) then the followed ureterocutaneostomy was performed. Preoperative work-ups were performed, including serum blood tests, chest X-ray, abdomen/pelvis computed tomography scans (CT) (Fig. 1a and b), and bone scans if clinically indicated. Moreover, each patient underwent a staging cystoscopy with transurethral resection of bladder tumor (TURBT). Preoperative CT and/or MRI scans were negative for pelvic adenopathy, metastasis, or evidence of clinically unresectable disease (Fig. 1a and b). The pre-anesthetic risk was quantified using the American Society of Anesthesiologist's physical status classification score. No neoadjuvant chemotherapy was applied. Then cryoablation was performed on the preserved bladder at the second time and the followed adjuvant chemoradiotherapy or chemotherapy alone was performed (Gemcitabine and cisplatin regimens chemotherapy were added to patients 3 months later after cryoablation, followed local radiotherapy for bladder cancer). Each patient provided written informed consent, and the study was approved by Ethics Committee of Nanjing Drum Tower Hospital. Patient demographics were summarized in Table 1.

Ureterocutaneostomy and PLND

RC with appropriate LND and UD was the preferred treatment for patients with MIBC. However, RC could not be achieved due to the diseases of the fixation to the pelvis and/or rectum (pT4b) or the presence of gross palpable nodes (pN2-3) according intraoperative findings. All the patients were pT4b stage and urinary diversion was performed with bilateral ureterocutaneostomy. Two of the 7 patients had a PLND, and 5 did not at the discretion of the treating surgeon in our study. Ureterocutaneous anastomosis was performed according to the technique originally described by Glenn [6].

Cryosurgery procedure

All cryosurgery procedures were performed using the Cryo-Hit System (Galil Medical Ltd., Israel) by a single urologist. All patients were placed in a modified lithotomy position under spinal anesthesia. The scrotum was elevated off the perineum after a 18F Foley catheter was inserted into bladder. The template was placed in stepper, approximate to perineum, and the grid was overlaid on ultrasound screen (Fig. 2a). The template and ultrasound grid were verified alignment with first needle. All needles were tested before insertion. Under transrectal ultrasound (TRUS) guidance, 1.47-mm 17G IceSeed cryoneedles were placed transperineally into the bladder tumor (Fig. 2b and c). Two single-point temperature monitoring probes were placed at tumor around and rectum, respectively. The number and position of cryoneedles varied with bladder cancer size and location. Freezing with argon gas to < − 40 °C was initiated and monitored using the temperature-monitoring probes, and TRUS guidance, which revealed an acoustic shadow as the ice-ball formed (Fig. 2d). The tumor around and rectum was maintained at temperatures greater than 0 °C, and freezing was stopped when the iceball reached the anterior rectal wall was at least 20 °C. After maintaining −40 °C or the lowest temperature below −25° Cfor 10 min, a passive thaw was initiated until the temperature reached a plateau. At this point, active thawing with helium was started. Two cycles of rapid freeze-thaw were carried out, ensuring the temperature in the bladder cancer and just outside it was below a therapeutic value of −40 °C. At the end of the procedure, the needles and probes were removed and pressure applied to the perineal area for 10 min to reduce bruising.

Follow up evaluation and statistical analysis

Radiographic local tumor control was assessed using image-guided tumor ablation criteria [7]. Follow-up CT and MRI were performed at 3-month intervals after cryotherapy procedure. Two diagnostic radiologists reviewed CT and MRI scans for every case to determine whether progression or recurrence had occurred. Progression free survival (PFS) and overall survival (OS) were calculated from the date of cryosurgery. Data are presented as the mean ± standard deviation (SD). Analyses were performed with Statistical Package for Social Sciences, version 17 (SPSS, Chicago, IL).

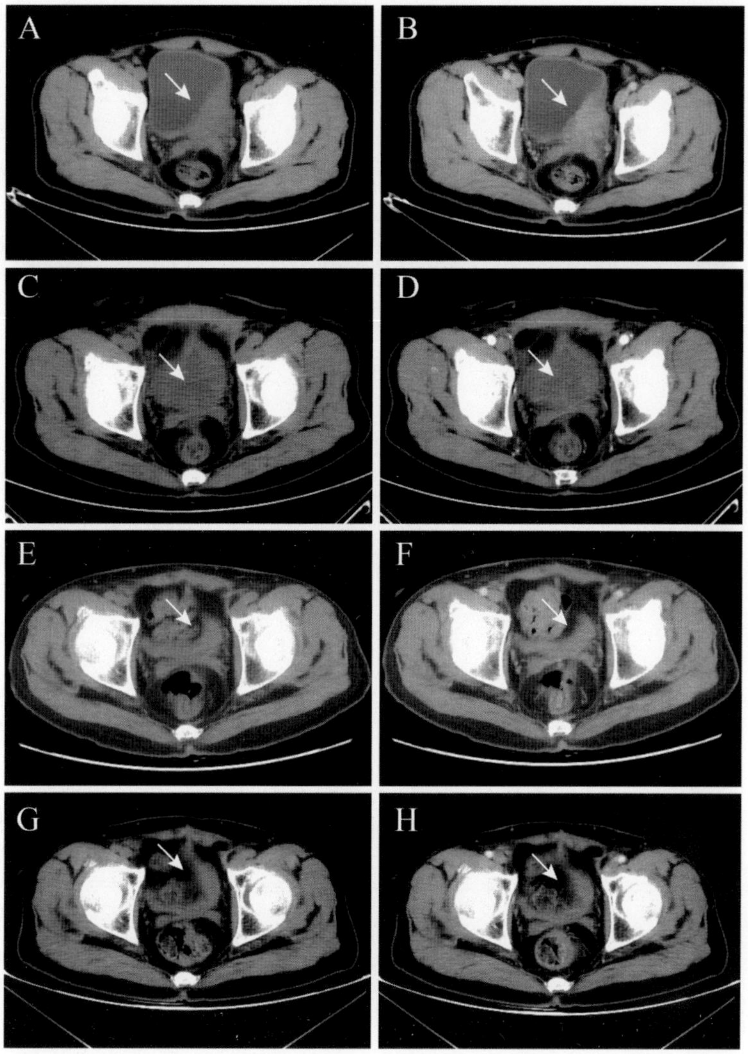

Fig. 1 CT images of a patient with cancer in the left wall of the bladder (patient number 5)Non-contrast (**a**) and contrast-enhanced arterial phase images (**b**) of CT scans indicated that the tumor (white arrow) located on left wall of bladder, the longest diameter of tumor was 8.1 cm before cryosurgery. One months after cryosurgery, non-contrast (**c**) and contrast-enhanced arterial phase images (**d**) of CT show the structure of the bladder wall remained intact and tumor (white arrow) inside and outside the bladder had no obviously enchancement. One year after cryosurgery, non-contrast (**e**) and contrast-enhanced arterial phase CT images (**f**) show the bladder (white arrow) contraction and no urinary filling. There was no obviously enchancement in the preserved bladder. Three year after cryosurgery, non-contrast (**g**) and contrast-enhanced arterial phase images (**h**) of CT show the bladder (white arrow) shrink further and no obviously enchancement in the shrinked bladder. No progression and local recurrence happened in this patient at the follow up time of 40 months

Results

Totally 7 male patients were included in this study. The clinical characteristics of the 7 patients are summarized in Table 1. The mean age of patients was 60.14 ± 9.04 years (range from 47 to 73 years) with a mean follow-up of patients alive of 28.43 ± 14.25 months (range from 8 to 43 months). Five patients were found to have hydronephrosis, either unilateral or bilateral. Histology showed all these patients were high grade urothelial carcinoma according to TURBT and the followed biopsy. Tumors were located in the right, left or back wall of the bladder in two, four, and one cases, respectively. The mean tumor longest diameter was 7.87 ± 1.79 cm (range from 5.8 to 11.4 cm). All 7 patients planned to cystectomy, but underwent aborted cystectomy due to unresectable disease secondary to fixation to the pelvis and/or rectum (pT4b stage) according to the intraoperative findings and the followed ureterocutaneostomy was performed. Mean time from ureterocutaneostomy to cryosurgery was 6.00 ± 1.63 months (ranging from 4 to 9 months). Two of the 7 patients had a PLND, and the other 5 had no PLND at the discretion of the treating surgeon. No positive pelvic lymph nodes were found in followed histopathological examination of the two patients.

Table 1 Data for 7 male patients (age range from 47 to 73 years) who underwent transperineal cryotherapy for high grade MIBC

Patients	TLD(cm)	OP(min)	PFS(month)	Location	Initial symptom	Complications Post-cryosurgery	Additional Treatment
1	7.5	55	11	Left wall	Hematuria	None	Chemoradiotherapy
2	8.3	70	25	Left wall	Urinary irritation	Urinary irritation	Chemoradiotherapy
3	6.5	50	35	Left wall	Hematuria, Urinary irritation, Abdominal pain	Abdominal pain	Chemotherapy
4	11.4	120	3	Right wall	Hematuria	None	None
5	8.1	100	40	Left wall	Hematuria, Abdominal pain	None	Chemoradiotherapy
6	5.8	75	8	Back wall	Hematuria	None	Chemoradiotherapy
7	7.5	65	32	Right wall	Hematuria, Urinary irritation	None	Chemoradiotherapy

Note: *TLD* tumor longest diameter, *PFS* progression free survival, *OP* operation time

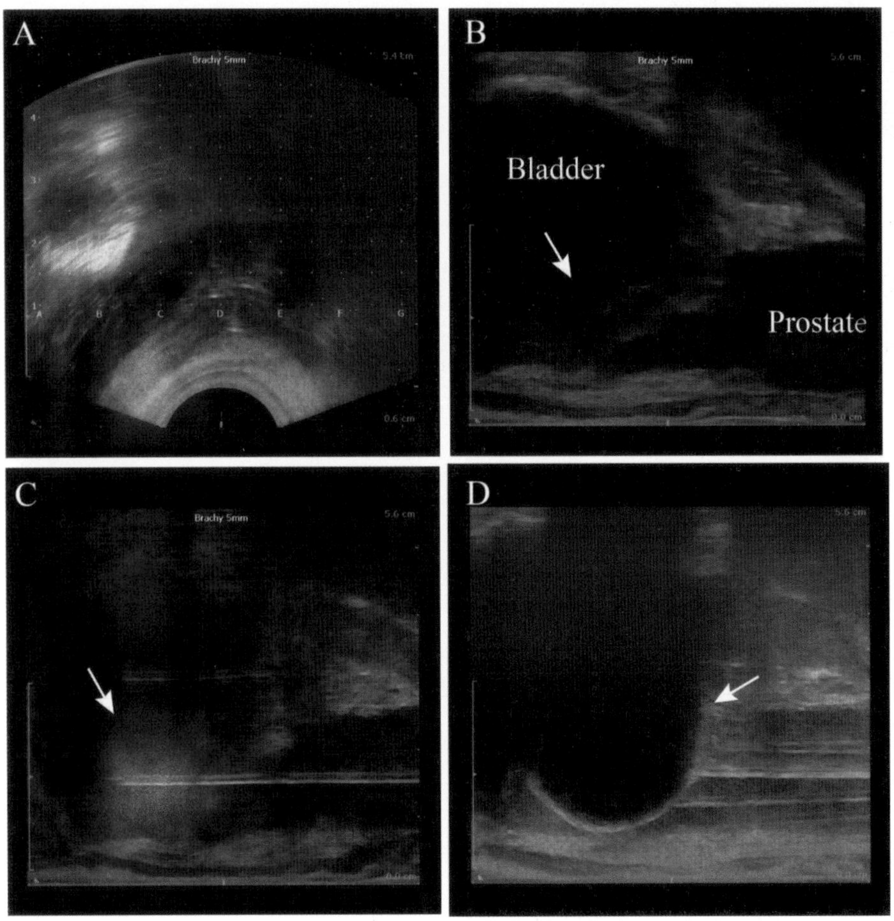

Fig. 2 Images of transperineal cryotherapy procedure for unresectable muscle invasive bladder cancer under the real-time guidance of TRUS (patient number 5). The template was placed in stepper, approximate to perineum, and the grid was overlaid on ultrasound screen (**a**). Bladder tumor (white arrow) and other nearby tissues and organs including prostate and rectum were identified by TRUS (**b**). Under TRUS guidance, two 1.47-mm 17G IceSeed cryoneedles were placed transperineally into the bladder tumor (white arrow) (**c**). Two single-point temperature monitoring probes were placed at tumor around and rectum, respectively. Freezing with argon gas to < − 40 °C was initiated and monitored using the temperature-monitoring probes, and TRUS guidance, which revealed an acoustic shadow as the ice-ball formed (white arrow) (**d**)

All the cryosurgery procedures were performed successfully and all patients well tolerated with the transperineal cryosurgery, and with minimal requirements for pain medication and without the need for blood transfusions. No operative-related deaths occurred in these patients. The mean operative time of transperineal cryosurgery was 76.43 ± 25.12 min (range from 50 to 120 min). The mean bleed loss was 19.29 ± 15.92 ml (range from 5 to 50 ml). The mean length of hospital stay for the patients after cryosurgery was 3.86 ± 1.68 days (range from 2 to 7 days). In the process of follow-up, all patients have abandoned freezing treatment again, and two patients' dead due to pulmonary metastasis disease at the follow up time of 8 and 37 months, the other two patients' dead due to extensive abdominal and pelvic metastasis at 15 and 18 months after cryosurgery respectively. The other three patients were alive at 43, 40 and 38 months after cryosurgery and no progression of disease at the follow up examination of CT (Fig. 1c–h). There were minor complications but no major complications of the treatment. These new treatment-related symptoms are not considered as complications and no other minor or severe complications were noticed. All complications had disappeared completely after 2 weeks. Six of 7 patients received postoperative therapy, of whom 5 patients were treated with combined identical chemoradiation, while the other one received chemotherapy alone. The PFS of the 7 patients was 22.00 ± 14.61 months (range 3-40 months). The one, two and three-year OS was 85.7%, 57.1% and 42.9%, respectively.

Discussion

BC is currently one of the tumors with the most rapid increase in incidence. At the time of diagnosis, approximately 15% of patients who present with bladder cancer will be found to have regional or distant metastasis [8–10]. Radical cystectomy with PLND and UD continues to be the gold standard for MIBC [11]. It is a clinical and therapeutic dilemma when these tumors are found to be unresectable (pN2-3 or pT4b) on surgical exploration. In this situation, chemotherapy and/or radiotherapy are the only treatment that has been shown to improve survival as described previously [12, 13]. However, systemic chemotherapy and radiotherapy may have severe side effects, such as significant hematologic, mucosal toxicity or gastrointestinal bleeding or perforation [14], or lead to treatment-related death [15].

Faysal A. Yafi et al. addressed the outcomes of thirty-one patients who underwent aborted RC due to unresectable disease. The outcome of patients with unresectable disease is dismal. The 2- and 5-year OS was 41% and 0%, respectively. They get the conclusion that patients who had an aborted cystectomy due to unresectable disease may benefit from PLND and upfront chemotherapy [11]. Recently, a study included 35 patients who had an aborted radical cystectomy for intraoperative findings of metastatic bladder cancer [16]. It showed a poor prognosis for these patients with a median time to cancer-specific survival of 26.5 months, and OS at one, two, and three years of 67%, 43%, and 18% respectively. Other several literatures reported that adjuvant radiotherapy also has the ability to improve the OS and PFS in patients with MIBC [14, 17]. From these results of previous studies, the survival enhancement was not very satisfying in combined chemoradiation or chemotherapy/radiotherapy alone.

Cryosurgery, also known as cryoablation, is widely used as primary or salvage treatment for various urological malignances like renal cell carcinoma (RCC) and prostate cancer (PC) in recent years [18–21]. It is reported that cryosurgery offers benefits with fewer complications, shorter hospitalization times, and allows for quicker convalescence in the treatment of RCC and PC [22–25]. Transperineal cryosurgery for prostate cancer has been carried out since 2006 in our hospital. Lian et al. addressed the preliminary results of 102 patients underwent primary cryoablation for clinically localized PCa from January 2006 to December 2009 in Nanjing Drum Tower Hospital. The early results of their study suggest that cryoablation offers a safe and effective alternative for the primary treatment of localized prostate cancer [24]. Recently, Zhou et al. analysed the results of a study of 23 patients with metastatic BC under percutaneous cryosurgery. No severe complications occurred in the study. The PFS of these patients was 14 ± 8 months, and indicated that percutaneous cryosurgery may be a safe and efficacious therapeutic option in the treatment of metastatic BC [5].

In the present study, we attempted to manage the aborted RC due to unresectable disease secondary to fixation to the pelvis and/or rectum (pT4b stage) and cryosurgery for these unresectable bladder cancer throuth transperineal approach. In this retrospective study, the longest 43 months of follow-up data from 7 patients obtained from our hospital's database were analyzed to determine the safety and efficacy of this procedure in bladder cancer (Fig. 1). In the study, all cryosurgical procedures for bladder cancer were performed successfully, with no treatment-related deaths. No severe preoperative, intraoperative or postoperative complications were happened. The therapeutic effect of transperineal cryoablation was evaluated by means of PFS. The PFS of the 7 patients who underwent comprehensive cryosurgery for unresectable bladder cancer was 22.00 ± 14.61 months, which was better than that reported for cisplatin monotherapy and M-VAC combination chemotherapy [26]. The 1-, 2- and 3-year OS was 85.7%, 57.1% and 42.9% in the study, respectively. This study indicated that transperineal cryoablation may be an attractive alternative treatment for unresectable pT4b stage bladder cancer. This technique also could applicable to patients who could not tolerate cystectomy due to the minimal invasion.

According to our preliminary experience of transperineal cryosurgery for unresectable MIBC of 7 male patients, we believe that the following is the key to ensure cryotherapy successful. Firstly, the use of TRUS to monitor the appearance of the ice ball as well as to guide cryoprobe placement to avoid any injury to other tissues, especially rectum. Secondly, the placement of temperature monitoring probes around tumor and rectum to enhance the temperature information provided by TRUS. Moreover, the success of this procedure benefits from the previous experience of transperineal cryosurgery for prostate cancer in our hospital. Furthermore, patient selection is also very important.

In this study, we describe a cryosurgery alone, cryo-chemoradiation or cryo-chemotherapy combination as an alternative treatment in unresectable pT4b stage bladder cancer. We believe that reduction local tumor burden through cryosurgery and followed with chemoradiation or chemotherapy will benefit more than chemoradiation or chemotherapy alone for locally advanced BC. Moreover, we believe that patients with the pT4b stage unresectable disease will benefited more from this procedure than pN2-3 patients. However, the retrospective design raises the issue of potential selection bias which are likely to have influenced the results of the present study. Moreover, it is limited by its small series and single-institution study design. Future prospective, large-scale and long-term studies are needed in multiply centers.

Conclusions

Transperineal cryoablation combination with chemoradiotherapy may be an option in the treatment of unresectable invasive bladder cancer due to unresectable disease secondary to fixation to the pelvis and/or rectum (pT4b) and these patients who could not tolerate cystectomy. The side effects were relatively mild and a PFS of 22.00 ± 14.61 months can be achieved. A larger number of cases is required, however, and long-term survival following this therapy and its role in combination with other therapies awaits further research.

Abbreviations

BC: bladder cancer; CT: computed tomography; MIBC: muscle invasive bladder cancer; OS: overall survival; PFS: Progression free survival; PLND: pelvic lymph node dissection; RC: radical cystectomy; TRUS: transrectal ultrasound; TURBT: transurethral resection of bladder tumor; UD: urinary diversion

Acknowledgements

The authors would like to thank all our participants for their gracious participation in this study.

Funding

No funding was obtained for this study.

Authors' contributions

QZ conception and design, acquisition of data, analysis and interpretation of data; drafting of manuscript. SWZ conception and design, acquisition of data, analysis and interpretation of data; drafting of manuscript. SZ conception and design, acquisition of data, or analysis and interpretation of data; drafting of manuscript. WW acquisition of data, analysis and interpretation of data. XZ acquisition of data, analysis and interpretation of data. YD analysis and interpretation of data. HL analysis and interpretation of data. HG conception and design, analysis and interpretation of data; drafting of manuscript, supervision. All authors have read and approved the final version of this manuscript.

Authors' Information

Department of Urology, Drum Tower Hospital, Medical School of Nanjing University, Institute of Urology, Nanjing University, 321 Zhongshan Road, Nanjing 210,008, Jiangsu, PR China.

Competing interests

The authors declare that they have no competing interests.

References

1. Siegel R, Ma J, Zou Z, Jemal A. Cancer statistics, 2014. CA Cancer J Clin. 2014;64(2014):9–29.
2. Kaufman DS, Shipley WU, Feldman AS. Bladder cancer. Lancet. 2009; 374(2009):239–49.
3. McDONALD JH, TAYLOR CB, HECKEL NJ. Rapid freezing of the bladder: an experimental and clinical study. J Urol. 1950;64(1950):326–37.
4. Logan C, Brown M, Hayne D. Intravesical therapies for bladder cancer - indications and limitations. BJU Int. 2012;110(Suppl 4):12–21.
5. Liang Z, Fei Y, Lizhi N, Jianying Z, Zhikai Z, Jibing C, Jialiang L, Kecheng X. Percutaneous cryotherapy for metastatic bladder cancer: experience with 23 patients. Cryobiology. 2014;68(2014):79–83.
6. Glenn JF, Alyea EP. Ureterocutaneous anastomosis. I. Experimental use of a surgical splint to prevent stricture. J Urol. 1960;83(1960):602–5.
7. Goldberg SN, Grassi CJ, Cardella JF, Charboneau JW, Dodd GD 3rd, Dupuy DE, Gervais DA, Gillams AR, Kane RA, Lee FT Jr, Livraghi T, McGahan J, Phillips DA, Rhim H, Silverman SG, Solbiati L, Vogl TJ, Wood BJ, Vedantham S, Sacks D. Image-guided tumor ablation: standardization of terminology and reporting criteria. J Vasc Interv Radiol. 2009;20(2009):S377–90.
8. Bellmunt J, Albiol S. Chemotherapy for metastatic or unresectable bladder cancer. Semin Oncol. 2007;34(2007):135–44.
9. Stein JP, Lieskovsky G, Cote R, Groshen S, Feng AC, Boyd S, Skinner E, Bochner B, Thangathurai D, Mikhail M, Raghavan D, Skinner DG. Radical cystectomy in the treatment of invasive bladder cancer: long-term results in 1,054 patients. J Clin Oncol. 2001;19(2001):666–75.
10. Herr HW, Donat SM. Outcome of patients with grossly node positive bladder cancer after pelvic lymph node dissection and radical cystectomy. J Urol. 2001;165(2001):62–4. discussion 64
11. Yafi FA, Duclos M, Correa JA, Tanguay S, Aprikian AG, Cury F, Souhami L, Rajan R, Kassouf W. Contemporary outcome and management of patients who had an aborted cystectomy due to unresectable bladder cancer. Urol Oncol. 2011;29(2011):309–13.
12. Dunst J, Rodel C, Zietman A, Schrott KM, Sauer R, Shipley WU. Bladder preservation in muscle-invasive bladder cancer by conservative surgery and radiochemotherapy. Semin Surg Oncol. 2001;20(2001):24–32.
13. Custodio S, Joaquim A, Peixoto V, Macedo JE, Faria AL, Macias E, Rego S, Araujo A. Metastatic renal cell carcinoma: the importance of immunohistochemistry in differential diagnosis. Case Rep Oncol. 2012; 5(2012):30–4.
14. Chen B, Zeng ZC, Wang GM, Zhang L, Lin ZM, Sun LA, Zhu TY, Wu LL, Zhang JY, Ji Y. Radiotherapy may improve overall survival of patients with T3/T4 transitional cell carcinoma of the renal pelvis or ureter and delay bladder tumour relapse. BMC Cancer. 2011;11(2011):297.
15. von der Maase H, Hansen SW, Roberts JT, Dogliotti L, Oliver T, Moore MJ, Bodrogi I, Albers P, Knuth A, Lippert CM, Kerbrat P, Sanchez RP, Wersall P, Cleall SP, Roychowdhury DF, Tomlin I, Visseren-Grul CM, Conte PF. Gemcitabine and cisplatin versus methotrexate, vinblastine, doxorubicin,

and cisplatin in advanced or metastatic bladder cancer: results of a large, randomized, multinational, multicenter, phase III study. J Clin Oncol. 2000; 18(2000):3068–77.
16. Guzzo TJ, Rogers CG, Deng CY, Bivalacqua TJ, Palapattu GS, Bastian PJ, Eisenberger MA, Schoenberg MP, Gonzalgo ML. Outcomes of patients after aborted radical cystectomy for intraoperative findings of metastatic disease. BJU Int. 2008,102(2008):1539–43.
17. Nagele U, Anastasiadis AG, Merseburger AS, Corvin S, Hennenlotter J, Adam M, Sievert KD, Stenzl A, Kuczyk MA. The rationale for radical cystectomy as primary therapy for T4 bladder cancer. World J Urol. 2007;25(2007):401–5.
18. Rodriguez SA, Arias FF, Bueno BC, Rodriguez-Patron RR, Sanz ME, Palacios VH, Burgos RFJ. Cryotherapy for primary treatment of prostate cancer: intermediate term results of a prospective study from a single institution. Prostate Cancer. 2014;2014(2014):571576.
19. Autran-Gomez AM, Scarpa RM, Chin J. High-intensity focused ultrasound and cryotherapy as salvage treatment in local radio-recurrent prostate cancer. Urol Int. 2012;89(2012):373–9.
20. Marcus DM, Canter DJ, Jani AB, Dobbs RW, Schuster DM, Carthon BC, Rossi PJ. Salvage therapy for locally recurrent prostate cancer after radiation. Can J Urol. 2012;19(2012):6534–41.
21. Sverrisson EF, Nguyen H, Kim T, Pow-Sang JM. Primary cryosurgery for clinically localized prostate cancer–do perioperative tumor characteristics correlate with post-treatment biopsy results. Urology. 2014;83(2014):376–8.
22. Schiffman M, Moshfegh A, Talenfeld A, Del PJJ. Laparoscopic Renal Cryoablation. Semin Intervent Radiol. 2014;31(2014):64–9.
23. Sverrisson E, Jones JS, Pow-Sang JM. Cryosurgery for prostate cancer: a comprehensive review. Arch Esp Urol. 2013;66(2013):546–56.
24. Lian H, Guo H, Gan W, Li X, Yan X, Wang W, Yang R, Qu F, Ji C. Cryosurgery as primary treatment for localized prostate cancer. Int Urol Nephrol. 2011; 43(2011):1089–94.
25. Hartman JB, Bhojwani N, Corn DJ, Cooney MM, Haaga J, Ponsky L, Abouassaly R, Paspulati A, Prologo JD. Incidence of hypercoagulable events after image-guided percutaneous cryoablation of renal tumors: a single-center experience. J Vasc Interv Radiol. 2014;25(2014):776–9.
26. Sr LPJ, Einhorn LH, Elson PJ, Crawford ED, Kuebler P, Tannock I, Raghavan D, Stuart-Harris R, Sarosdy MF, Lowe BA, et al. A randomized comparison of cisplatin alone or in combination with methotrexate, vinblastine, and doxorubicin in patients with metastatic urothelial carcinoma: a cooperative group study. J Clin Oncol. 1992;10(1992):1066–73.

Increasing bladder capacity by foot stimulation in rats with spinal cord injuries

Guoqing Chen[1,2], Limin Liao[1,2*], Zhaoxia Wang[1,2], Xing Li[1,2] and Wenjuan Du[1,2]

Abstract

Background: This study was to explore the possibility that foot stimulation increased bladder capacity(BC) in rats with neurogenic bladder secondary to T10 spinal cord injuries.

Methods: In 20 awake rats (stimulation group) with T10 spinal cord injuries, 5 repeat cystometrograms (CMGs) were recorded. The 1st and 2nd CMGs were performed without stimulation. The 3rd, 4th, and 5th CMGs were done separately with 1 T, 2 T, and 4 T stimulation, respectively, through a pair of pad electrodes on the skin of the hind foot. In the control group of 20 rats, 5 repeat CMGs were recorded without foot stimulation. The threshold (T) was the minimal stimulation intensity to induce an observable toe twitch.

Results: In the stimulation group, foot stimulation with 2 T significantly increased the BC an additional 68.9% ± 20.82% ($p < 0.05$). Foot stimulation with 4 T increased the BC an additional 120.9% ± 24.82% ($p < 0.05$). Compared with the control group, BC in the 1st, 2nd, and 3rd (1 T) CMG had no significant difference in the stimulation group, but the 4th (2 T) and 5th (4 T) CMGs were significantly increased ($p < 0.05$).

Conclusions: Electrical stimulation of the foot was effective in inhibiting reflex bladder activity and increasing bladder capacity in spinal cord injury rats.

Keywords: Foot stimulation, Spinal cord injury, Rat, Cystometrogram, Bladder capacity

Background

In the supra-sacral spinal cord injury (SCI) patients, the loss of supraspinal control leads to neurogenic detrusor overactivity (NDO) and detrusor sphincter dyssynergia (DSD), which can result in small bladder capacity、- high bladder pressure during micturition, vesicoureteral reflux and renal impairment. The target of treatment must meet the following three points: urine storage with low pressure, voiding with low pressure and adequate bladder emptying [1]. Clean intermittent catheterization (CIC) with muscarinic receptor antagonists is the gold standard treatment for neurogenic lower urinary tract dysfunction (NLUTD), but the drug has a few side effects which prompt urologists to select new therapeutic method [2].

Recently, sacral neuromodulation (SNM) [3], pudendal nerve stimulation (PNS) [4]and tibial nerve stimulation (TNS) [5] are considered very valuable for the treatment of NDO secondary to SCI; but, SNM and PNS need to implant an electrode and an stimulator, and TNS need to insert a needle electrode near to the nerve.

Stimulation of the foot using skin surface electrodes is a new, non-invasive, easily accessible, convenient way to inhibit bladder activity and increase bladder capacity, which has been verified in cats with overactive bladders [6] and healthy humans [7]. In our previous study, we reported that electrical stimulation of somatic afferent nerves in the feet can increase bladder capacity in patients with neurogenic bladders after sigmoid cystoplasty [8]. Although a positive effect was shown in those patients, we need to do further research in patients with other types of neurogenic bladder.

In this study we explored the possibility that foot stimulation with surface electrodes increased bladder capacity in rats with neurogenic bladder secondary to T10 SCI.

* Correspondence: lmliao@263.net
[1]Department of Urology, China Rehabilitation Research Center, Beijing 100068, China
[2]Department of Urology, Capital Medical University, Beijing, China

Methods

Ethics statement

All protocols involving the use of animals in this study were approved by the Ethics Committee of Capital Medical University, China.

Animal model

A total of 40 adult female Sprague-Dawley rats weighing 236–270 g were used. To produce a SCI, the rats were anesthetized with pentobarbital (30 mg/kg i.p.). We performed T10 laminectomy and open the dura of the rats, transected the T10 spinal cord with scissors and placed an absorbable gelatin sponge between the cut ends, then sutured the muscle and skin. Rats were then put on an electric warmer to maintain body temperature until recovering from anesthesia. SCI animals were treated postoperatively with ampicillin (100 mg/kg i.m.) for 5 days. As we known, detrusor areflexia persist during spinal shock period after suprasacral spinal cord injury, so the bladder need to be emptied by abdominal compression twice a day until reflex detrusor contraction recovered, often 10–14 days after surgery. Then SCI rats were divided into two groups: 1) control group, SCI rats without foot stimulation (n = 20); and 2) stimulation group, SCI rats with foot stimulation (n = 20).

Surgical procedure for experiments

Three weeks after SCI when reflex detrusor contraction recovered, the animals in both groups were anesthetized with 2% isoflurane, and the abdomen was opened via a midline laparotomy. The ureters were cut and drained externally and the urethra was secured by a ligature. A PE-90 catheter was inserted into the bladder for recording the intravesical pressure through the bladder dome. The catheter was connected to a pressure transducer (MP150; Biopac, Goleta, CA, USA) and micro-infusion pump (Stoelting, Wood Dale, IL, USA) through a three-way stopcock. After the abdomen was closed, the rats were placed in a restrainer and were allowed to recover from anesthesia for 1–2 h. After removing the fur, a pair of surface self-adhesive pad electrodes (Grass F- E10ND, diameter = 1 cm; Astro-Medical Inc., Mentor, OH, USA) were attached to the skin area on both hind feet. A Grass S88 stimulator (Grass Medical Instruments, West Warwick, RI, USA) with stimulus isolator (SIU5; Grass Medical Instruments) was used to generate stimulus pulses.

Experiment: Cystometry in an awake condition (n = 20 each of two groups).

After the rats recovered from anesthesia, the bladder was infused with physiologic saline at a rate of 0.08 ml/min until repetitive detrusor contractions were elicited. After at least two stable micturition cycles were observed, cystometric parameters can be recorded.

In the control group, five cystometrograms (CMGs) were performed without stimulation. In the stimulation group, five CMGs were performed as follows: 1 and 2, control CMG without stimulation; 3, CMG during 1 T stimulation; 4, CMG during 2 T stimulation; and 5, CMG during 4 T stimulation. A 3–5 min rest period was performed after each CMG to allow the detrusor to recover from dilatation. Foot stimulation was done with uniphasic rectangular pulses (5 Hz frequency, 0.2 ms pulse width) according the previous research [6]. The threshold (T) stimulation intensity (3–16 V), which was defined as the minimal intensity to induce an observable toe twitch, was determined by slowly increasing the stimulation intensity at the beginning of the experiment.

The bladder capacity (BC) was defined as the bladder volume threshold to induce a bladder reflex contraction of large amplitude (>30 cmH_2O) and long duration (>20 s) [9, 10].

Statistical analysis

Statistical analysis was performed using graph pad prism 6.0. For the repeated CMG recordings, BC was normalized to the initial saline control capacity in the same animal to allow comparisons between animals. Capacity measurements under the same conditions were averaged and reported as the mean ± standard error of the mean. Statistical significance ($P < 0.05$) was detected by ANOVA, followed by Dunnett or Bonferroni post-tests.

Results

In the control group, BC did not differ significantly in five repeat continuous CMGs ($p > 0.05$) (Fig. 1a). In the stimulation group (Fig. 1b), the 1st and 2nd CMGs without stimulation were not significantly different with respect to BC ($p > 0.05$). Although foot stimulation with 1 T increased BC an additional 36.2% ± 11.75%, this difference was not significantly different compared with the 1st and 2nd CMG (p > 0.05). Foot stimulation with 2 T significantly increased BC an additional 68.9% ± 20.82% ($p < 0.05$). Foot stimulation with 4 T significantly increased BC an additional 120.9% ± 24.82% ($p < 0.05$). Compared with the control group (Fig. 2), BC in the 1st, 2nd, and 3rd (1 T) CMG did not differ significantly in the stimulation group, but the 4th (2 T) and 5th (4 T) CMG increased significantly ($p < 0.05$).

Discussion

Neurogenic bladder (NB) dysfunction after SCI is a major medical and social problem. The ultimate goal of any urologic treatment is to prevent upper urinary tract damage and renal failure [1]. Currently, the gold standard treatment for NDO is clean intermittent catheterization (CIC) combined with muscarinic receptor antagonists; however, many patients are often refractory to the medication

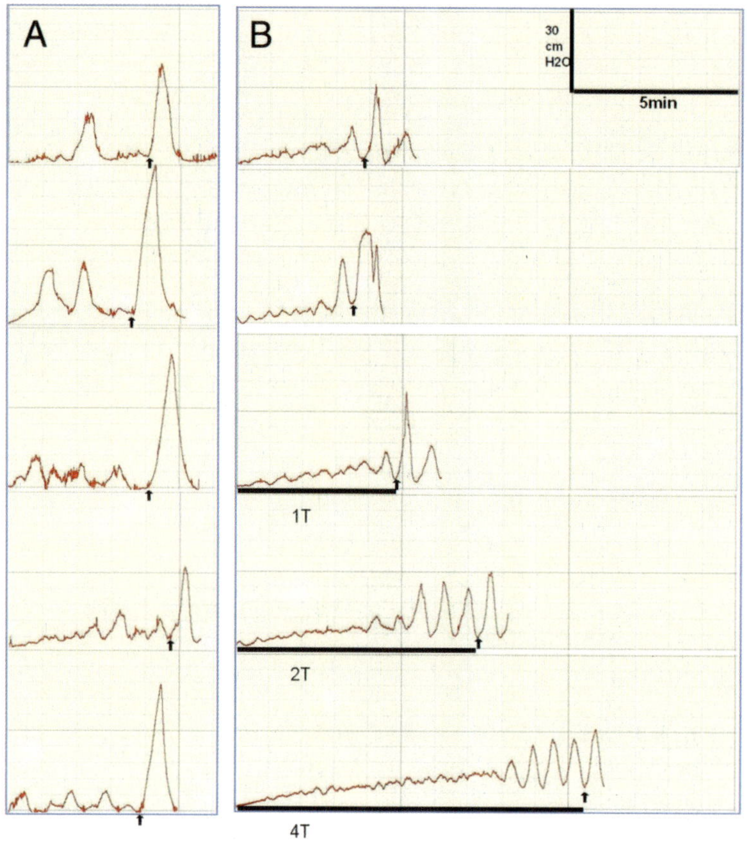

Fig. 1 **a**: In control group, bladder capacity was not significantly changed during repeated CMGs in the absence of foot stimulation. **b**: In treatment group, the 1st and 2nd was the BC without stimulation. The 3rd, 4th and 5th were the BC with 1 T, 2 T and 4 T stimulation. The arrows indicatethe stop of bladderinfusion. The black bars under the pressure traces indicate the stimulation duration

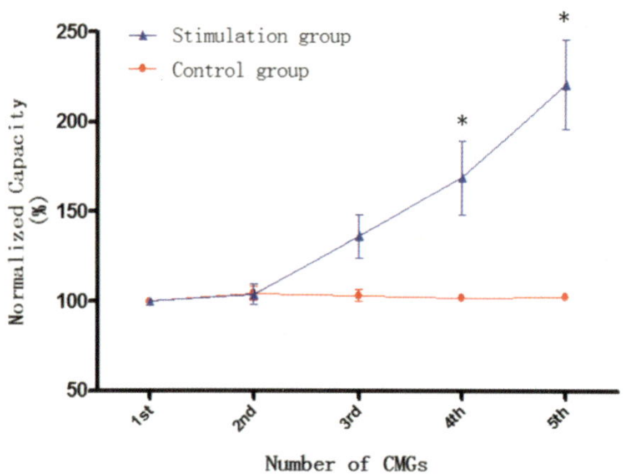

Fig. 2 BC in control and stimulation group. Asterisk indicates control vs treatment statistically significantly different ($p < 0.05$). In treatment group, the 1st and 2nd was the BC without stimulation. The 3rd、4th and 5th were the BC with 1 T、2 T and 4 T stimulation. In control group, all the five BC were not with stimulation. T was stimulation intensity (3–16 V)

because of side effects [2]. So somatic nerve stimulation was proposed to treat bladder dysfunction for complement medication in recently [11].

Previous studies have shown that foot stimulation with surface electrode can inhibit reflex micturition, significantly increase BC, and induce post-stimulation inhibition of reflex bladder activity that persists for 1–2 h in cats [6]. Actually, the same effect can be found in healthy volunteers [7]. It showed that foot stimulation with surface electrode can delay bladder filling sensation and significantly increase BC > 50% in healthy humans.

In our previous study [8], we found that foot stimulation delayed the bladder filling sensation and significantly increased BC in the patients after bladder augmentation. Comparing with baseline, the volume per CIC was significantly increased, and this long-lasting effect persisted nearly 1 day. This is the first clinical trial in which electrical stimulation of the foot was used to treat patients. Although a positive effect was shown in the current study, the patients did not represent all types of lower urinary tract disorders.

Thus, in this study we used BC to evaluate the effect of foot stimulation on bladder function by CMG in rats secondary to T10 spinal cord injury. In the control group, BC did not differ significantly in the five continuous CMGs which means repeated CMG did not increase BC. In the stimulation group, the 1st and 2nd CMGs without stimulation did not differ significantly. Although foot stimulation with 1 T increased the BC an additional 36.2% ± 11.75%, this difference was not significant ($p > 0.05$). Foot stimulation with 2 T significantly increased the BC an additional 68.9% ± 20.82% ($p < 0.05$). Foot stimulation with 4 T significantly increased the BC an additional 120.9% ± 24.82% ($p < 0.05$). Compared with the control group, this enlargement was the effect of foot stimulation, but not repeated bladder infusion.

The mechanism underlying foot stimulation is unknown, but may be mediated by the nerves in the foot [6–8]. The stimulation electrodes were placed on the skin surface rather than directly on the nerves. Which nerves were activated? The tibial nerve courses from the inner ankle inferiorly to the plantar surface of the foot and branches into the lateral and medial plantar nerves at the location of the electrodes. These nerves further branch into multiple small nerves that course toward the toes. Thus, it is highly likely that foot stimulation activates afferent branches of the tibial nerve in the lateral and medial plantar aspects of the foot.

A previous study in cats showed that the inhibitory effect on BC elicited by electrical stimulation of the nerves from the hind limb muscles was lost after chronic spinal cord transection at the thoracic level, indicating a possible role of the supra-spinal mechanisms in somatovesical inhibition [12]. In the current study, the complete T10 SCI model was used. The previous research showed sacral neuromodulation (SNM) [3], pudendal nerve stimulation (PNS) [4], and tibial nerve stimulation [5] all inhibit bladder overactivity in complete SCI patients. Thus, we suggest that foot stimulation should inhibit detrusor overactivity and increase BC in complete SCI patients as in animal models. It is highly likely that foot stimulation activates afferent branches of the tibial nerve in the lateral and medial plantar aspects of the foot.

In this study, 4 T stimulation achieved a good result in BC, but the foot twitched strongly under this intensity. If we use this intensity in patients in the future, it may induce discomfort in patients. Thus, we will investigate whether or not low-intensity stimulation combined with low-dose drug can increase BC as high-intensity stimulation, but no adverse event occurred which induced by high-intensity stimulation and high-dose drug.

Conclusions

Foot stimulation with surface electrode was effective to inhibit reflex bladder activity and increase BC in SCI rats. These results showed that electrical stimulation of the foot might be an effective treatment for neurogenic bladder secondary to SCI.

Abbreviations

BC: Bladder capacity; CIC: Clean intermittent catheterization; CMGs: Cystometrograms; DSD: Detrusor sphincter dyssynergia; NDO: Neurogenic detrusor overactivity; NLUTD: Neurogenic lower urinary tract dysfunction; PNS: Pudendal nerve stimulation; SCI: Spinal cord injury; SNM: Sacral neuromodulation; T: Threshold; TNS: Tibial nerve stimulation

Acknowledgements

Not applicable.

Funding

This study was funded by Chinese national natural science foundation (Grant Number 81270847).

Authors' contributions

GC, ZW, XL and WD participated in all procedure. They were responsible for data gathering and writing papers. LL was responsible for guiding work, as well as modifications to the thesis. All authors read and approved the final manuscript.

Competing interests

The authors declare that they have no competing interests.

References

1. Liao L. Evaluation and Management of Neurogenic Bladder: what is new in China? Int J Mol Sci. 2015;16:18580–600.
2. Cameron AP. Medical management of neurogenic bladder with oral therapy. Transl Androl Urol. 2016;5:51–62.
3. Sievert KD1, Amend B, Gakis G, Toomey P, Badke A, Kaps HP, et al. Early sacral neuromodulation prevents urinary incontinence after complete spinal cord injury. Ann Neurol. 2010;67:74–84.
4. Chen G, Liao L, Dong Q, Ju Y. The inhibitory effects of Pudendal nerve stimulation on bladder Overactivity in spinal cord injury dogs: is early stimulation necessary? Neuromodulation. 2012;15:232–7. discussion 237
5. Schneider MP, Gross T, Bachmann LM, Blok BF, Castro-Diaz D, Del Popolo G, et al. Tibial nerve stimulation for treating neurogenic lower urinary tract dysfunction: a systematic review. Eur Urol. 2015;68:859–67.
6. Chen G, Larson JA, Ogagan PD, Shen B, Wang J, Roppolo JR, et al. Post stimulation inhibitory effect on reflex bladder activity induced by activation of somatic afferent nerves in the foot. J Urol. 2012;187:338–43.
7. Chen ML, Chermansky CJ, Shen B, Roppolo JR, de Groat WC, Tai C. Electrical stimulation of somatic afferent nerves in the foot increases bladder capacity in healthy human subjects. J Urol. 2014;191:1009–13.
8. Chen G, Liao L, Miao D. Electrical stimulation of somatic afferent nerves in the foot increases bladder capacity in neurogenic bladder patients after sigmoid cystoplasty. BMC Urol. 2015;15:26.
9. Jia C, Yoshimura N, Liao L. Herpes simplex virus vector-mediated gene transfer of kynurenine aminotransferase improves detrusor overactivity in spinal cord-injured rats. Gene Ther. 2014;21:484–9.
10. Schwen Z, Matsuta Y, Shen B, Wang J, Roppolo JR, de Groat WC, Tai C. Inhibition of bladder overactivity by duloxetine in combination with foot stimulation or WAY-100635 treatment in cats. Am J Physiol Renal Physiol. 2013;305:F1663–8.
11. Sanford MT, Suskind AM. Neuromodulation in neurogenic bladder. Transl Androl Urol. 2016;5:117–26.
12. McPherson A. The effects of somatic stimuli on the bladder in the cat. J Physiol. 1966;185:185–96.

The influence of prior laparoscopic experience on learning laparoendoscopic single site surgery: a prospective comparative preliminary study using cystorraphy in a live porcine model

U-Syn Ha[1], Kyu Won Lee[1], Sun Wook Kim[1], Seung Hyun Jeon[2], Tae Gyun Kwon[3], Hyung Keun Park[4] and Sung-Hoo Hong[1*]

Abstract

Background: The purpose of this study is to assess the impact of prior laparoscopic experience on the ability to learn laparoendoscopic single site surgery (LESS) skills.

Methods: A total of 33 urologists who completed a training program in LESS surgery were recruited for this study. After completing the educational course and training, the study participants demonstrated LESS suturing and knot-tying via a 2-cm cystotomy in a live porcine model for 15 min. An objective structured assessment of technical skills (OSATS) was used to evaluate videos of each participant's procedure. The participants were divided according to laparoscopic experience; advanced experienced group (AS), intermediate experienced group (IS), novice group (NS).

Results: Three participants in the NS group completed the porcine cystorrhaphy in 15 min (30.0%), 3 (25.0%) completed the task in the IS group, and 3 (27.2%) completed it in the AS group. There were no statistically significant differences in the mean total OSATS quality score (NS; 16.7, IS; 18.5, AS; 16.8) among the 3 groups. Concerning all each assessment, there were also no statistically significant difference. Additionaly, the mean total OSATS quantity score (NS; 4.1, IS; 3.5, AS; 4.3) did not differ significantly among groups. The NS group succeeded a mean of 1.4 knots, the IS group succeeded 0.9, and the AS group 1.3 ($p = 0.727$).

Conclusions: There was no significant difference among the groups in LESS proficiency after training. Surgeons who were novices in conventional laparoscopic surgery reached comparable scores to those of experienced laparoscopic surgeons after training.

Keywords: Laparoscopic surgery, Learning curve, Minimally invasive surgery

Background

Minimally invasive surgeries are becoming more widely accepted and popular procedures. Advanced surgical techniques and new instruments allow surgeons to minimize surgery's invasiveness. Most recently, laparoendoscopic single-site surgery (LESS) has become an effective surgical alternative to conventional laparoscopic surgery [1, 2].

The surgical techniques required to perform LESS are different from those required during conventional laparoscopic surgery [3]. LESS is technically challenging because the surgeon must pass all of his instruments through a single port to provide limited triangulation [4]. To overcome this challenge, surgeons can operate either using one instrument, or using articulating instruments that cross over each other [5]. These limitations increase the challenge of learning LESS, which requires considerable practice.

The LESS learning curve can be influenced by several factors, including technical advances, education and prior surgical experience. Simulation is a common learning tool used to teach surgeons the basic technical skills of conventional laparoscopy [6]. It allows surgeons to acquire skills for laparoscopic surgery without the risk of harming patients. It is expected that simulation could also be a valuable learning tool for LESS. We investigated how a surgeon's prior experience influences the LESS learning curve.

* Correspondence: toomey@catholic.ac.kr
[1]Department of Urology, Seoul St. Mary's Hospital, College of Medicine, The Catholic University of Korea, 222, Banpo-daero, Seocho-gu, Seoul 06591, Republic of Korea
Full list of author information is available at the end of the article

Proficiency in LESS likely requires experience with minimally invasive surgery, including laparoscopic surgery. Therefore, experience in laparoscopic surgery could shorten the LESS learning curve. However, several prior studies have found conflicting results. Lewis et al. [7] demonstrated that previous laparoscopic experience improved the ability to perform LESS. In contrast, a comparative study evaluating the LESS learning curves of novices by Sodergren et al. [8] found that prior training in conventional laparoscopy does not influence LESS learning or proficiency.

However, the Sodergren et al. study has limitations. For example, the tasks used as assessments are basic laparoscopic skills that may not have provided a sufficient challenge to experienced laparoscopic surgeons. Therefore, more complex tasks may have exposed differences. In addition, this study did not provide proper time for learning, because the tasks were tested on a single attempt, without prior training or education (3). The group also used a box trainer, with which they could not assess performance under biological conditions. In addition, the study is so insufficient not to draw conclusion in view of the results so far achieved. Given the limitations of the prior research in this area, our aim was to conduct an optimized study, and to provide more satisfactory results.

Surgeons who participated in this study had completed a training program and were assessed using difficult tasks, such as cystorrhaphy. The purpose of this study was to assess whether prior laparoscopic surgical experience affects the ability to learn LESS skills.

Methods

Subjects

The study was approved by the Institutional Animal Care and Use Committee of Samsung Biomedical Research Institute (H-B2–001). The animals for this study were used for LESS training courses, in which the bladder had been preserved intact.

Of 36 urology specialists who received surgical training program in the LESS workshop, 33 were suitable for this study, and were recruited. The suitable participants included novices with LESS experience and surgeons with varying laparoscopic experience. Before survey, written informed consent had been taken from all participants. We surveyed participants for prior laparoscopic surgical experience during registration for the workshop (Figure 3 in Appendix). In order to be included, participants must have completed the training program and taken the test.

Training

The workshop was composed of 3 parts under the supervision of tutors. The first part involved theoretical instruction, while the second part included training in basic surgical skills including instrument handling, cutting, grasping, clipping and suturing in the live porcine model and box trainer. During the third part of the workshop, the participants practiced their surgical skills by performing nephrectomy, partial nephrectomy, pyeloplasty, and ureter anastomosis in live porcine models. Each participant had the opportunity to practice his/her respective training format for at least 90 min using the porcine model. All procedures were performed through a single port device that was made from a size 7 surgical glove and an Alexis wound retractor (Applied Medical, Rancho Santa Margarita, CA). Three trocars were inserted through the glove finger site (Fig. 1). The participants were supplied with standard and roticulating dissectors, scissors, and needle holders.

Performance assessment

After finishing the educational course and training, the study participants performed LESS suturing and knot tying via a 2-cm cystotomy in a live porcine model (Fig. 2). Cystorrhaphy was performed for 15 min using closed 2–0 polyglactin sutures. Each participant was recorded while performing cystorrhaphy. Participant videos were blinded with an identifying code. Recorded videos were conveyed to the assessor to be selected for objective structured assessment of technical skills (OSATS).

Two assessors with experience in laparoscopic surgery and LESS scored the cystorrhaphy performances. The OSATS evaluation was used to assess the videos for quantity (time to close the cystostomy, number of knots required, and each step of procedure) and quality (see Appendix). These methods were adopted and edited from Martin et al. [9]. We used the same OSATS that McDougall et al. [10] used to score porcine laparoscopic cystorrhaphy. The participants were assessed on task success, and on whether the closure was watertight or not. The closure's watertight seal was assessed at the end of the procedure by instilling 150 cm^3 of saline into the bladder under laparoscopic visualization. A successful

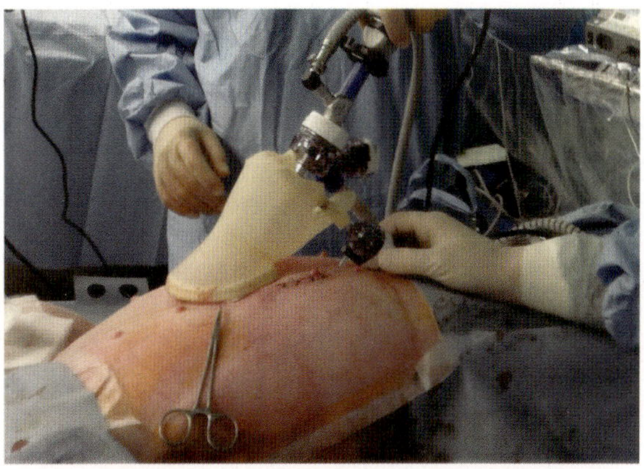

Fig. 1 External view of Laparoendoscopic single site surgery homemade single-port device using a surgical glove, wound retractor (Alexis, Applied Medical), and trocars

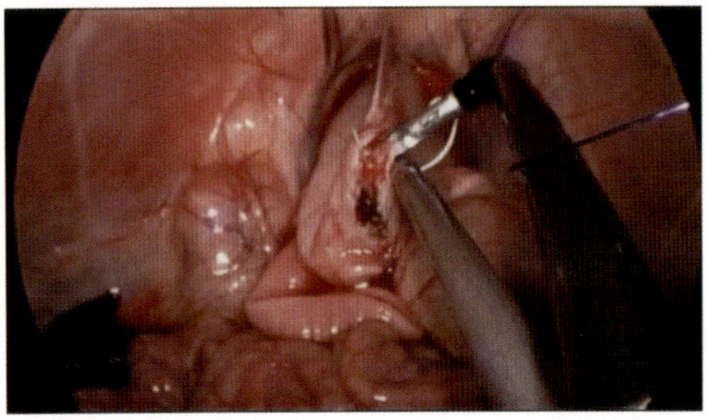

Fig. 2 The view of of Laparoendoscopic single site cystorraphy in a live porcine model

cystorrhaphy was one that was completed in 15 min and produced bladder closure with no saline leakage.

Statistical analysis

The participants were divided into 3 groups according to their prior laparoscopic experience: the novice surgeon group (NS), the intermediate experienced surgeon group (IS), and the advanced experienced surgeon group (AS). Participants with no prior experience as primary operators were placed in the NS group. Primary surgeon with experience in laparoscopic surgery including nephrectomy and cyst marsupialization, but not in reconstructive surgery were placed in the IS group. Finally, primary surgeons with experience in 30 or more cases of laparoscopic reconstructive surgery, including partial nephrectomy, pyeloplasty, and prostatectomy, were placed in the AS group. Data were analyzed statistically and expressed as means ± standard deviations. The scores of each group were compared using ANOVA. Tukey's test was used for multiple comparisons. Pearson's chi-square test was used to compare the 3 groups with regard to their success. *P*-values <0.05 were considered statistically significant. Since this was a pilot study, power analysis was not performed.

Results

Thirty-six urologists participated in workshop. Of these, 33 participants who completed the suture task survey were enrolled. Ten participants were placed in the NS group, 12 in the IS group, and 11 in the AS group. Some participants in group AS had performed over 100 laparoscopic partial nephrectomies. Three participants in the NS group completed the porcine cystorrhaphy in 15 min (30.0%), 3 (25.0%) completed the task in the IS group, and 3 (27.2%) completed it in the AS group with no significant difference. Table 1 shows the mean and total OSATS quality scores from each assessment. There were no statistically significant differences in the mean total OSATS quality score among the 3 groups. Concerning all each assessment, there were also no

Table 1 Results of OSATS quality on each variable and total score

	Novice (n = 10)	Intermediate (n = 12)	Advanced (n = 11)	p-value
Respect	2.8 ± 1.3	3.4 ± 1.2	2.8 ± 1.5	0.577
Time and motion	2.0 ± 1.0	2.3 ± 0.5	2.3 ± 1.3	0.779
Instrument	2.6 ± 1.1	2.4 ± 0.8	2.5 ± 1.2	0.945
Use of assistant	2.3 ± 1.1	2.7 ± 0.8	2.4 ± 1.3	0.709
Non-dominant hand	2.5 ± 0.8	3.0 ± 0.8	2.9 ± 1.4	0.656
Flow of operation	2.3 ± 1.1	2.7 ± 0.5	2.7 ± 1.3	0.642
Total	16.7 ± 6.0	18.5 ± 4.0	16.8 ± 7.6	0.774

statistically significant difference. The results of quantity assessment from each group are summarized in Table 2. There was also no statistically significant difference in the mean total OSATS quantity score among the groups. The NS group succeeded a mean of 1.4 knots, the IS group succeeded 0.9, and the AS group 1.3 (p = 0.727).

Discussion

There were several main findings from this study. First, there was no significant difference among the groups in LESS proficiency after training. Experienced surgeons did not perform significantly better than less experienced surgeons with regard to their OSATS scores. Previous laparoscopic experiences did not change the outcomes. After a brief training course, surgeons who were novices in conventional laparoscopic surgery reached comparable scores to those of experienced laparoscopic surgeons. The educational program used in this study effectively trains surgeons of varying experience in LESS skills.

One might expect LESS proficiency to require experience in minimal invasive surgery, including laparoscopic surgery. Therefore, it is reasonable to hypothesize that experience in laparoscopy surgery would shorten the LESS learning curve. However, our results are to the contrary. These results may be explained by the fact that suturing was selected as the main task. Distinctions in the suturing method between conventional laparoscopy and LESS may have reduced the score gap. The standard suturing and tying methods in conventional laparoscopy are triangular instrumental composition and the "smiley-face" knot technique [11]. However, during LESS, a single incision limits the range of motion and angle of the laparoscopic instruments and causes instrument crowding. These limitations during LESS suturing make triangular instrumental composition difficult. Therefore, experienced laparoscopic surgeons who are familiar with wide triangular compositions during conventional laparoscopy had trouble adjusting to the more limited triangulation in LESS suturing. The instruments were extremely limited during intracorporeal needling and knotting. Crossing manipulation of articulating instruments requires another learning curve that needs to be overcome [5]. These factors had a big impact on all the course of procedure, and which could make no

Table 2 Results of OSATS quantity, total number of knots and success rate on the each variable and total score

	Novice ($n = 10$)	Intermediate ($n = 12$)	Advanced ($n = 11$)	p-value
Needle directed at a 90-degree angle to tissues	0.14 ± 0.38	0.20 ± 0.42	0.40 ± 0.52	0.305
Needle passed through tissue using a rotation of the wrist/hand motion	0.14 ± 0.38	0.20 0.42	0.30 ± 0.48	0.605
Suture pulled through to leave a ¼"–½" tail	0.14 ± 0.38	0.00 0.00	0.20 ± 0.42	0.329
A single knot throw performed	0.43 ± 0.53	0.20 ± 0.42	0.20 ± 0.42	0.695
Knot tied down squarely	0.43 ± 0.53	0.20 ± 0.42	0.20 ± 0.42	0.695
A second knot throw performed	0.43 ± 0.53	0.20 ± 0.42	0.30 ± 0.48	0.716
A third knot throw performed	0.71 ± 0.49	0.40 ± 0.52	0.70 ± 0.48	0.263
Knots tied snuggly (no air knots)	0.57 ± 0.53	0.40 ± 0.52	0.40 ± 0.52	0.923
suturing with evenly spaced throws	0.57 ± 0.53	0.90 ± 0.32	0.80 ± 0.42	0.408
closure smooth – no bunching of tissues	0.57 ± 0.53	0.80 ± 0.42	0.80 ± 0.42	0.695
Total score	4.14 ± 3.62	3.50 ± 3.14	4.30 ± 2.41	0.475
Total No. of knots	1.4 ± 1.6	0.9 ± 0.6	1.3 ± 1.5	0.727

difference among groups. There was no significant difference in total number of knots between the groups. The lower the OSATS quantity score, the better the procedure. Paradoxically, the total OSATS quantity score was highest in the AS group (2). The intrinsic LESS attributes, such as narrow range of motion and crossing manipulation, are very different from those of conventional laparoscopy. Therefore, these skills were novel for all LESS novices, and made the learning curve steep. Although experienced laparoscopic surgeons may be proficient in skills such as depth perception in the operating field, they still had to learn new skills for LESS. Learning the intrinsic technical difficulties of LESS seems to transcend the benefits of having experience in minimally invasive surgery.

LESS surgery may at first seem to be more technically challenging than conventional laparoscopic surgery. However, there are effective educational tools to train surgeons in LESS. Fransen et al. [12] found that short-term box training significantly improved novice trainees' basic skills in LESS. Sodergren et al. [8] showed that prior training in conventional laparoscopy did not influence learning or proficiency in LESS for novice surgeons. These previous reports agree with our findings that prior surgical experience in laparoscopic surgery does not make it easier to obtain LESS proficiency.

A distinctive feature of this study is that participants were evaluated under biological conditions using a porcine model, which is most similar to the intracorporeal procedure. In contrast, other studies used the dry box trainer to evaluate participants. Under the dry box condition, it is almost impossible to evaluate tissue handling and task performance with regard to space and depth.

Another distinctive feature of this study is that both quantitative and qualitative analyses were performed. Qualitative analyses allowed us to assess parameters like careful tissue/instrument handling, efficient time/motion, and operative flow. These parameters cannot be evaluated through quantitative analysis alone.

A potential limitation of this study was the level of difficulty of the task itself. Cystorrhaphy demands both basic and relatively advanced surgical skills with high dexterity. The LESS cystorrhaphy may have been so difficult that participants in the AS group could not even complete the task. The reason why we selected cystorrhaphy is that it was necessary to increase the task's difficulty based upon prior findings in the literature. Researchers who conducted previous studies [7] indicated that the basic tasks that were used may not have provided a sufficient challenge to experienced laparoscopic surgeons [7, 13]. If this is true, it limits a study's assessment function. Two different studies [7, 13] that were conducted using similar tasks produced contrary results. Increasing the complexity of the task should have led to variation between performances. Therefore, we selected cystorrhaphy as the main task. Analyses included those of suturing, needle handling, knotting and the total number of knots. Quantitative analysis was used to assess the whole step, and basic skills including tissue and instrument handling, motion, and operative flow.

Similar results have been observed between LESS and robotic surgery with regard to prior experience in conventional laparoscopic surgery. Regardless of the differences between these types of surgery, experience in conventional laparoscopic surgery does not appear to affect the learning curve in robotic surgery [14, 15]. These results suggest that conventional laparoscopy does not have to be a transitional step to learning another type of minimally invasive surgery.

Conclusions

Our results suggest that surgical skills acquired in conventional laparoscopy could not appear to transfer directly to LESS. In addition, a surgeon who is a novice in conventional laparoscopic surgery can acquire comparable proficiency in LESS via training compared to more experienced laparoscopic surgeons.

Appendix
Quality assessment

Objective	Point	1	2	3	4	5
Respect for tissue		Frequently used unnecessary force or caused damage with inappropriate instruments	Occasional unnecessary force or inappropriate instrument used	Careful handling of tissues but occasionally caused inadvertent tissue damage	Careful handling of tissues but on 1 occasion caused inadvertent tissue damage	Consistently handled tissues appropriately with minimal tissue damage
Time and Motion		Many unnecessary moves	Occasional unnecessary moves	Efficient time/motion but some unnecessary moves	Efficient time/motion but 1 unnecessary move	Clear economy of movement and maximum efficiency
Instrument Handling		Repeated tentative or awkward moves or inappropriate use of instruments	Occasional tentative or awkward moves or inappropriate use of instruments	Competent use of instruments but occasional stiff or awkward moves	Used appropriate instruments but made 1 awkward move	Fluid moves with instruments and no awkwardness
Use of Assistant		Failed to use retraction or assistant at all for exposure during the case	Failed to use retraction or assistant effectively for exposure during the case	Used retraction and assistant occasionally-could have been better	Used retraction and assistant quite well when necessary	Used retraction and assistant to best advantage all the time
Use of Non-dominant hand		Failed to non-dominant hand at all for exposure during the case	Failed to use non-dominant hand effectively for exposure during the case	Used non-dominant hand occasionally-could have been better	Used non-dominant hand quite well when necessary	Used non-dominant hand to best advantage all the time
Flow of Operation		Frequently stopped operating and seemed unsure	Occasionally stopped operating or seemed unsure	Had forward planning with reasonable progression	Had forward planning with only 1 unsure episode	Well planned operation with effortless flow of moves

Abbreviations
LESS: Laparoendoscopic single-site surgery; SATS: Objective structured assessment of technical skills

Acknowledgments
The authors acknowledges the members of the Korean Endourological Society who have participated as tutor and assessors.

Funding
This work was supported by the Catholic Medical Center Research Foundation.

Authors' contributions
Each author had participated in the work as follows: study conception and design (USH, SWK), acquisition of data (USH, KWL, SWK, SHJ, TGK, HKP), analysis and interpretation of data (USH, SWK), drafting of manuscript (USH, KWL, SWK), and critical revision (SHJ, TGK, HKP, SHH). All authors read and give approval of the final manuscript.

Competing interests
The authors declare that they have no competing interests.

Author details
[1]Department of Urology, Seoul St. Mary's Hospital, College of Medicine, The Catholic University of Korea, 222, Banpo-daero, Seocho-gu, Seoul 06591, Republic of Korea. [2]Department of Urology, School of Medicine, Kyung Hee University, Seoul, Republic of Korea. [3]Department of Urology, College of Medicine, Kyungpook National University, Daegu, Republic of Korea. [4]Department of Urology, Asan Medical Center, University of Ulsan College of Medicine, Seoul, Republic of Korea.

References
1. Desai MM, Berger AK, Brandina R, Aron M, Irwin BH, Canes D, et al. Laparoendoscopic single-site surgery: initial hundred patients. Urology. 2009;74:805–12.
2. White WM, Haber GP, Goel RK, Crouzet S, Stein RJ, Kaouk JH. Single-port urological surgery: single-center experience with the first 100 cases. Urology. 2009;74:801–4.
3. Cox DR, Zeng W, Frisella MM, Brunt LM. Analysis of standard multiport versus single-site access for laparoscopic skills training. Surg Endosc. 2011; 25:1238–44.
4. Chow A, Purkayastha S, Aziz O, Paraskeva P. Single-incision laparoscopic surgery for cholecystectomy: an evolving technique. Surg Endosc. 2010;24: 709–14.
5. Khanna R, Stein RJ, White MA, Isac W, Laydner H, Autorino R, et al. Single institution experience with robot-assisted laparoendoscopic single-site renal procedures. J Endourol. 2012;26:230–4.
6. Kneebone R. Simulation in surgical training: educational issues and practical implications. Med Educ. 2003;37:267–77.
7. Lewis T, Aggarwal R, Kwasnicki R, Darzi A, Paraskeva P. Does previous laparoscopic experience improve ability to perform single-incision laparoscopic surgery? Surg Endosc. 2012;26:1214–9.
8. Sodergren M, McGregor C, Farne HA, Cao J, Lv Z, Purkayastha S, et al. A randomised comparative study evaluating learning curves of novices in a basic single-incision laparoscopic surgery task. J Gastrointest Surg. 2013;17: 569–75.
9. Martin JA, Regehr G, Reznick R, MacRae H, Murnaghan J, Hutchison C, et al. Objective structured assessment of technical skill (OSATS) for surgical residents. Br J Surg. 1997;84:273–8.
10. McDougall EM, Kolla SB, Santos RT, Gan JM, Box GN, Louie MK, et al. Preliminary study of virtual reality and model simulation for learning laparoscopic suturing skills. J Urol. 2009;182:1018–25.
11. Gill IS. Textbook of Laparoscopic Urology. New York: Informa Healthcare; 2006.
12. Fransen SA, Mertens LS, Botden SM, Stassen LP, Bouvy ND. Performance curve of basic skills in single-incision laparoscopy versus conventional laparoscopy: is it really more difficult for the novice? Surg Endosc. 2012;26:1231–7.
13. Santos BF, Enter D, Soper NJ, Hungness ES. Single-incision laparoscopic surgery (SILS™) versus standard laparoscopic surgery: a comparison of performance using a surgical simulator. Surg Endosc. 2011;25:483–90.
14. Kim IK, Kang J, Park YA, Kim NK, Sohn SK, Lee KY. Is prior laparoscopy experience required for adaptation to robotic rectal surgery?: Feasibility of one-step transition from open to robotic surgery. Int J Color Dis. 2014;29: 693–9.
15. Sng KK, Hara M, Shin JW, Yoo BE, Yang KS, Kim SH. The multiphasic learning curve for robot-assisted rectal surgery. Surg Endosc. 2013;27:3297–307.

7

Evaluation of serum prolidase activity and oxidative stress markers in men with BPH and prostate cancer

Faruk Kucukdurmaz[1*], Erkan Efe[1], Ahmet Çelik[2], Hasan Dagli[2], Metin Kılınc[2] and Sefa Resim[1]

Abstract

Background: Prostate cancer (PCa) and benign prostatic hyperplasia (BPH) are diseases of elderly men and are related to increased oxidative stress (OS). Although prolidase has a role in collagen metabolism, it is also used to evaluate OS in many diseases. However, there is a lack of data about serum prolidase activity (SPA) in prostate cancer. The aim of this study was to evaluate and compare SPA levels in males with BPH and PCa.

Methods: Evaluation was made of a total of 81 men who underwent transrectal ultrasound guided prostate biopsy for a definitive diagnosis due to high PSA levels. Patients were separated into 2 groups as BPH and PCa patients. Pre-biopsy malondialdehyde (MDA), superoxide dismutase (SOD), PSA levels and serum prolidase activities (SPA) were compared between the groups and the correlations of SPA with the other parameters were also investigated in both groups.

Results: BPH was diagnosed in 51 patients and PCa in 30. The mean age of patients was similar in both groups as 63.25 ± 5.81 years in the BPH group 65.30 ± 7.35 years in the PCa group(p:0.081). The median MDA and SOD levels were insignificantly increased in the PCa patients. SPA values were similar in BPH and PCa patients. SPA did not correlate with age, PSA, MDA or SOD levels in either group.

Conclusions: Our study results revealed that serum prolidase activity is similar in BPH and PCa cases and is not correlated with MDA, SOD or PSA levels.

Keywords: Prostate cancer, Benign prostatic hyperplasia, Prolidase, Oxidative stress

Background

Prostate cancer (PCa) is the most common non- skin cancer and one of the main reasons for cancer- specific deaths in men [1]. Prostate cancer is a major public health problem in western countries, especially in the elderly population. Since life expectancy and the prevalence of PCa have increased, there is also expected to be an increased economic burden of the disease [2].

Benign prostatic hyperplasia (BPH) is a progressive disorder that develops secondary to increased proliferation of stromal and glandular cells, with a predominance of mesencyhmal cells [3]. BPH is characterised by the proliferation of stromal cells and increased extracellular matrix (ECM) deposition involving collagens, glycoproteins and proteoglycans. Cellular proliferation in the prostate is mainly modulated by age- associated changes in endocrine factors, although the exact pathophysiological mechanisms of BPH are not yet fully understood [4, 5].

PCa and BPH are the leading urological problems of aging men and manifest with disturbing obstructive and irritative symptoms. In addition to androgen and age dependence, oxidative stress, infection and inflammation are the other accepted predisposing factors for BPH and PCa [6, 7].

Oxidative stress (OS) is defined as the imbalance between the production and detoxification of reactive oxygen species (ROS). Those species can be involved in tumorigenesis by inducing genomic damage, tumor angiogenesis and augmentation of tumor cell migration [8]. It

* Correspondence: drerkanefe@hotmail.com; farukdr@hotmail.com
[1]Department of Urology, Sutcu Imam University, Avsar Kampusu, 46100 Kahramanmaras, Turkey
Full list of author information is available at the end of the article

has also been reported that OS has a pivotal role in the aging process and disorders of aging males include BPH and PCa [9]. Malondialdehyde (MDA) is the principal end product of the lipid peroxidation pathway and is used as a marker to reflect oxidative status in normal subjects, BPH and PCa patients [5, 6, 9]. Superoxide dismutase (SOD) is the main endogenous antioxidant enzyme that counteracts the deleterious effects of ROS. Previous studies have reported that MDA levels are elevated and SOD activity is reduced in BPH and PCa patients compared to control groups [6, 9].

Matrix metalloproteinases (MMPs) are enzymes which are involved in in the degradation of ECM into proline and hydroxyproline [10]. Of these, prolidase is a manganese-dependent exopeptidase which cleaves to imidodipeptides and imidotripeptides with a C- terminal proline or hydroxyproline [11]. It is involved in the last stage of collagen turnover and, therefore, has a pivotal role in collagen metabolism, matrix remodelling and cell growth [10]. In addition, Yildiz et al. noted that serum prolidase activity (SPA) is directly correlated with oxidative stress and can be used as an OS marker [12]. Prolidase activity has been reported to be elevated in many tumor types including those in the kidney and bladder [13, 14]. Those studies also established that MDA levels were increased and SOD activities were reduced in men with bladder and kidney cancers. However, in both cancer types, prolidase activity was not found to be correlated with MDA concentrations and SOD activities.

Recently, prolidase activity has been investigated in men with BPH and has been reported to be significantly higher than that of control subjects [15]. However, there is a lack of data about SPA in PCa cases.

The objective of this reasearch was to compare MDA concentrations, SOD and prolidase activities of BPH and PCa patients. The associations between SPA, oxidative stress and antioxidant enzyme activities were also evaluated in both patient groups.

Methods

This study was conducted in Kahramanmaras Sutcu Imam University, Turkey. Informed consent was obtained from each participant and the study protocol was approved by the Clinical ResearchEthics Committee of Kahramanmaras Sutcu Imam University (2016/20–257). All procedures performed in the study were in accordance with the ethical standards of the institutional and/or national research committee and with the 1964 Helsinki declaration and its later amendments.

Subjects

The study population of this prospective research comprised patients who applied to our Urology Department between January 1 and June 1, 2017 with the complaint of lower urinary tract sypmtoms (LUTS). Participants were assessed using a comprehensive medical history and the International Prostate Symptom Score (IPSS) questionnaire to determine the symptom severity, measurement of peak urinary flow rate (Qmax; Aymed, Istanbul, Turkey) and digital rectal examination (DRE). Prostate specific antigen (PSA) testing was also performed for each patient. Patients who were over 40 years of age, with LUTS and a PSA value higher than the age-adjusted levels were enrolled in the study. This cohort comprised 130 males with PSA values higher than the age-adjusted levels and who underwent transrectal ultrasound (TRUS) guided prostate biopsy for a definitive diagnosis of either BPH or PCa. Exclusion criteria were determined as the presence of urinary tract infection, hematuria, previous medical or surgical intervention for prostate, history of previous prostate biopsy, diagnosis of any malignancy, renal and liver diseases, the use of antiinflammatory drugs, alcohol intake and antioxidant supplementation. When those criteria were applied, 49 patients were excluded and the study evaluation was made with a total of 81 subjects. At the beginning of the study, all cases were classified under two categories according to the pathology results as BPH or PCa. Patients diagnosed with PCa were also divided into subgroups according to the Gleason scores as Gleason = 6, Gleason = 7 and Gleason > 7. Prior to prostate biopsy, blood samples were obtained from each patient for SPA, MDA and SOD assays. These parameters were compared between the BPH and PCa subjects. Correlation of SPA with age, MDA, SOD and PSA was also investigated in both groups.

Laboratory analysis

The day before the prostate biopsy, blood samples were obtained between 09:00–11:00 a.m. from each patient following 12-h fasting. The venous blood samples were collected into heparinized tubes and centrifuged at 3000 rpm for 10 min. The separated serum samples were stored at −80 °C until the day of laboratory investigation of MDA, SOD and SPA.

Measurement of MDA

Plasma MDA levels were measured according to the Buege and Aust method [16]. MDA interacts with thiobarbiturate to give a red compound absorbing at 532 nm. The stock reagent (15% *w*/*v* trichloroacetic acid, 0.375% w/v thiobarbituric acid, 0.25 mol/l hydrochloric acid and 0.01% butylated hydroxytoluene) was thoroughly mixed with the sample and heated for 15 min in a boiling water bath. Then the sample was cooled and the precipitate was removed by centrifugation at 1000 x g for 10 min and the absorbance of the supernatant was determined at 532 nm against a blank containing all the reagents. The breakdown product of 1.1.3.3-tetraethoxypropane was used as the standard. MDA levels were calculated using $1.56 \times 10{-}5$ mol-1 cm-1 as the molar extinction coefficient. The results of the MDA measurements were given as nmol/ml.

Measurement of SOD activity

SOD activity was measured using the Fridovich method [17]. The principle is based on the inhibition of nitro blue tetrazolium chloride (NBT) reduction by the xanthine-xanthine oxidase system, which is a superoxide generator. Xanthine (Sigma-Aldrich) and xanthine oxidase (Sigma-Aldrich) generate superoxide radicals that interact with NBT (SigmaAldrich) to produce a red formazan dye. SOD activity is then measured according to the level of inhibition of this reaction. One unit of SOD was defined as the quantity of enzyme (mg) causing 50% inhibition in the NBT reduction rate. SOD activity was stated as U/ml.

Measurement of serum prolidase activity

Serum was diluted 40-fold with 2.5 mmol/L Mn2+ and 40 mmol/L Trizma HCl buffer (pH 8.0) and preincubated at +37 °C for 2 h. The resultant mixture which contained 30 mmol/L gly-pro, 40 mmol/L Trizma HCl buffer (pH 8.0), and 100 μL of preincubation serum in 1 mL was incubated at +37 °C for 30 min. The incubation reaction was stopped after the addition of 0.5 mL of 20% trichloroacetate solution. The supernatant was used for determination of proline with the Myara method which was modified from the Chinard technique [18]. All reagents were of analytical grade and purchased from Sigma (St. Louis, Missouri, USA) and Merck (Darmstadt, Germany). Intra and interassay precision performances of the assay were determined from a serum pool on 10 replicates in a single run and in 10 different runs, respectively, and yielded CV of 3.8 and 9.0%.The resultswere reported as U/L.

Statistical analysis

Analyses of the study data were performed using SPSS® 21.0 for Windows software.

The data were presented as mean ± standard deviation (SD), median, minimum and maximum values. Parametric continuous variables were compared using the Student's t test. Pearson's correlation test was used for correlation analyses. A value of $p < 0.05$ was accepted as statistically significant.

Results

Of the total 81 cases, BPH was diagnosed in 51 and PCa in 30 according to the pathology results of prostate biopsies. Of the 30 PCa patients, 12 were determined as Gleason = 6, 12 as Gleason = 7 and 6 as Gleason >7. The demographic and laboratory features of the groups are given in Table 1.

The mean age of the patients was similar in both groups as 63.25 ± 5.81 years in BPH group and 65.30 ± 7.35 years in PCa group (p:0.081). The mean body mass index (BMI) values were similar in both groups (22.57 ± 1.25 vs. 23.11 ± 1.84, p:0.752). No statistically significant difference was determined between BPH and PCa patients in respect of the mean IPSS values (17.54 ± 5.41 vs. 18.71 ± 6.04, p:0.124) and the Qmax values (9.84 ± 2.15 ml/s vs 10.21 ± 2.84 ml/s, p:0.232). PSA values were statistically significantly higher in the PCa cases (p = 0.025). The median MDA and SOD levels were increased in the PCa group but not to a statistically significant level. Serum prolidase activities were found to be similar in the BPH and PCa patients.

PSA, MDA, SOD levels and prolidase activities in BPH and subgroups of PCa are given in Table 2. PSA levels were not significantly different between the BPH, Gleason = 6 and Gleason = 7 PCa patients. PSA values of the PCa patients with Gleason score > 7 were significantly higher than those of the other groups. There were no statistically significant differences between the groups in terms of MDA and SOD levels. SPA was found to be similar among the study groups (Fig. 1).

The correlations of serum prolidase activities with age, PSA, MDA and SOD levels in males with BPH and PCa are presented in Table 3. In both groups, SPA did not show any correlation with age, PSA, MDA or SOD levels.

Discussion

In the present study, SPA, MDA and SOD levels in men with BPH and PCa have been evaluated. Also the correlation of SPA with age, PSA and other parameters was investigated. To the best of our knowledge, this is the first study to have compared SPA in BPH and PCa cases diagnosed from prostate biopsy due to high PSA levels.

Table 1 Demographic and laboratory parameters of the study population

	BPH (n = 51)	PCa (n = 30)	p value
Age	63.25 ± 5.81	65.30 ± 7.35	0.081
BMI (kg/m^2)	22.13 ± 1.28	22.74 ± 2.11	0.252
IPSS	17.21 ± 4.82	18.53 ± 5.12	0.121
PSA	6.20 (3.28–40.30)	13.24 (5.19–390.81)	0.025[a]
MDA	36.77(21.29-56.89)	38.7 (25.16–146.29)	0.075
SOD	19.44 (1.5–278.4)	40.42 (3.13–110.79)	0.512
SPA	1939 (1242–2722)	1845 (445–3244)	0.342

BMI Body mass index Hypertension, diabetes mellitus,*IPSS* International prostate symptom score, *PSA* Prostate specific antigen, *SOD* Superoxide dismutase, *MDA* Malondialdehyde, *SPA* Serum prolidase activity
Data were given as median (min-max) or mean ± standart deviation
[a]statistical significance

Table 2 Comparison of the age, oxidative stress, antioxidant enzyme and serum prolidase activity parameters according to pathology results of the patients

	BPH	Gleason = 6	Gleason = 7	Gleason > 7	P
SPA (IU)	1939 (1242–2722)	1872 (445–3244)	1548(864–2619)	1905(1512–2385)	0.330
PSA (ng/ml)	6.2(3.28–40.3)	9.3(6.6–38.0)	13.4(5.1–116.8)	55.3(6.4–390.8)	0.001[a]
MDA (nmol/ml)	36.76(21.2–56.8)	42.1(26.7–146.2)	38.7(25.1–53.0)	46.4(36.7–59.9)	0.078
SOD (u/ml)	19.43 (1.50–278.4)	37.3(3.1–84.4)	49.0(8.2–104.3)	39.2 (7.3–110.7)	0.647

Data were given as median (min-max), *SPA* Serum prolidase activity, *PSA* Prostate specific antigen, *MDA* Malondialdehyde, *SOD* Superoxide dismutase
[a]statistical significance

BPH and PCa are diseases of elderly males which both present with LUTS and the differential diagnosis for BPH and PCa is made by using PSA and DRE. Any suspicious lesion on DRE or a PSA value higher than the age-adjusted levels may necessitate the use of a TRUS-guided prostate biopsy for histopathological diagnosis.

The interactions between ECM components, cellular compartments and endocrine features render the role of ECM pivotal in the pathogenesis of epithelial abnormalities, including BPH and cancer [19]. Collagen is the main component of ECM in many tissues including prostate. Histochemical and morphometric analyses have established 3 major collagen types in human prostate as types I, III and IV. BPH is characterised by a change in collagen content (elevation of types I and IV, and a reduction in type III collagen) and an increase in ECM deposition [4]. The progression of cancer depends on the degradation of collagen and other ECM components which are mediated through proteolytic enzymes released from the cancer cells. MMPs are the enzymes necessary for the cleavage of ECM proteins which serve as a barrier to the invasion of tumor cells [20]. Prolidase, one of the MMP enzymes, is a homodimeric iminopeptidase which releases a carboxy-terminal proline or hydroxyproline from oligopeptides and is involved in collagen turnover and cell growth [11]. It regulates the last stage of the collagen breakdown. It has also been suggested to be the rate limiting factor of collagen metabolism. Since it has been suggested that the invasion and spread of cancer cells depend on the degradation of ECM, it can be hypothesized that prolidase activity can be associated with the invasiveness and aggressivity of the cancer [20]. Although serum prolidase activity has been well established in other cancer types including the kidney, bladder and ovaries [13, 14, 21], there are no data in literature about its activity in prostate cancer.

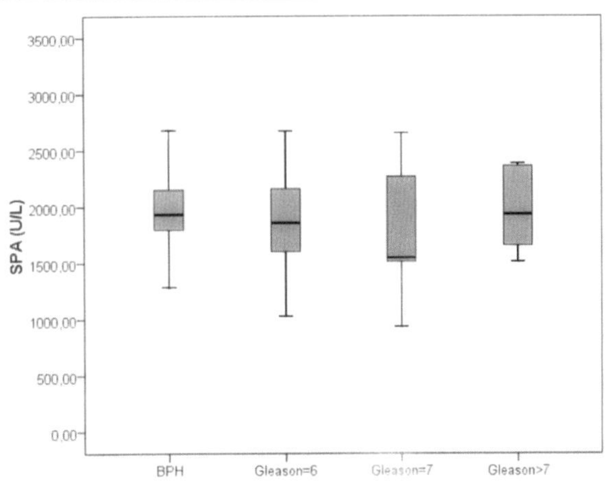

Fig. 1 Serum prolidase activities in men with BPH and prostate cancer

The results of the current study revealed that serum prolidase activity was reduced in PCa patients when compared to the BPH group, although the difference was not statistically significant. This may be due to the increased collagen turnover in patients with BPH as defined by Gecit et al. [15]. In addition, it was established that prolidase levels were not correlated with the PSA levels of PCa patients.

It has been reported that prolidase activity is elevated in bladder and kidney cancers. However, the findings obtained in the current study were similar to those of Palka et al., where prolidase levels were found to be lower in pancreatic cancer patients [22].

Oxidative stress, by way of ROS, may be associated with the production of DNA adducts indirectly by inducing autocatalytic lipid peroxidation which results in the formation of several degradation products such as malondialdehyde (MDA) and alkoxyl radicals. MDA, the final product of lipid peroxidation of polyunsaturated fatty acids, is used as a non-invasive biomarker of OS to evaluate radical-mediated pathophysiological conditions [23]. SOD, CAT and glutathione peroxidase (GPX) are the antioxidant enzymes involved in the endogenous

Table 3 Correlations of age, PSA, oxidant and antioxidant parameters with serum prolidase activity in men with benign prostatic hyperplasia and prostate cancer

	BPH	PCa		
	r	*p* value	r	*p* value
Age	−0.097	0.50	0.060	0.766
PSA	0.175	0.22	−0.045	0.825
MDA	−0.026	0.859	0.026	0.897
SOD	−0.108	0.45	−0.250	0.208

r Pearson correlation coefficient, *PSA* Prostate specific antigen, *MDA* Malondialdehyde, *SOD* Superoxide dismutase

defense mechanisms against increased ROS. Of these, SOD can be used to reflect the antioxidant activity in patients with BPH and/or PCa [6, 9]. Recently, prolidase has been shown to have a strong relationship with OS and is thought to be a novel marker to demonstrate the oxidative status of subjects in many disorders [24, 25].

Aging and subsequent OS are the common, recognized risk factors for BPH and PCa [7]. OS can produce vascular tissue damage, genomic damage and post-translational DNA alterations that are involved in DNA repair and apoptosis. Since the human prostate is subject to OS damage due to rapid cell turnover and fewer DNA repairing mechanisms, those events may result in point mutations, deletions or rearrangements which may lead to either benign hyperplasia or prostate cancer [26]. The relationship between OS, antioxidant enzymes and BPH has been evaluated in several reports with conflicting outcomes. Savas et al. reported no significant OS differences between men with BPH and a control group [27]. In contrast, Aydın et al. demonstrated increased MDA and a reduced antioxidant enzyme level in men with BPH [6]. More recently, Gecit et al. stated that men with BPH had higher OS when compared to control subjects [15]. It was also noted that prolidase activity was associated with increased OS parameters in BPH subjects.

Previous studies have shown that increased OS and reduced antioxidant enzyme levels were significant in PCa cases compared to BPH and control subjects [6, 9]. Since MDA is used to estimate OS in tissues, the use of MDA in the diagnosis of PCa has also become more prevalent. The MDA levels of PCa men have been reported to be significantly elevated when compared to BPH cases [9]. However, Dogru-Abbasoglu reported that serum lipid peroxide levels were not discriminative between BPH and PCa patients [28]. In the present study, it was determined that MDA concentrations were insignificantly increased in all PCa groups when compared to the BPH group and the differences in the MDA levels of the PCa patients were not correlated with the Gleason score.

Studies evaluating SOD enzyme activities in men with benign and malignant prostatic tissues have revealed that PCa patients had higher MDA and SOD levels compared to control subjects [29, 30]. In the present study, PCa patients had insignificantly higher SOD activities than BPH cases. Since the MDA levels were also insignificantly increased in men with PCa, it can be speculated that antioxidant enzymes might be increased in response to increased OS to nullify its deleterious effects.

Although it has been reported that prolidase activity is strongly related to OS, the results of the current study showed no associations between serum prolidase activity, MDA levels and SOD activities in BPH and PCa patients. In addition, prolidase activities were not correlated with the PSA values of the patients. This may have been due to the relatively small number of the patient population or the lack of knowledge about the factors related to the activity of prolidase in prostatic diseases. Therefore, further large scale studies are required to support these preliminary findings. In addition to the relatively small patient population, other limitations of the current study can be considered to be that MDA, SOD and serum prolidase activities in the prostatic tissues were not studied, other markers such as total antioxidant status (TAS), total oxidant status (TOS), NO level, vitamins (C and E), glutathione peroxidase (GPx), glutathione-S-transferase (GST) were not examined and metastatic evaluation of PCa patients was not performed.

Although prolidase has a pivotal role in collagen biosynthesis and has been suggested as a marker of OS, data about its activity in different cancer types and disorders known to be associated with increased OS have been conflicting. Therefore, prolidase should be combined with other biochemical markers in order to provide more accurate data to clinicians about the investigated disease activity.

Conclusions

BPH and PCa are diseases of aging men and are associated with increased OS. Although prolidase was thought to be a marker of OS in BPH, the results of this study failed to present any association between prolidase activity and OS in both patient groups. Prolidase activity was also not found to be related to PSA levels in either the BPH or PCa patients.

Abbreviations

BPH: Benign prostatic hyperplasia; DRE: Digital rectal examination; ECM: Extracellular matrix; LUTS: Lower urinary tract symptoms; MDA: Malondialdehyde; MMPs: Matrix metalloproteinase; OS: Oxidative stress; PCa: Prostate cancer; PSA: Prostate specific antigen; SOD: Superoxide dismutase; SPA: Serum prolidase activity

Acknowledgments

We would like to thank Dr. Mithat Temizer for the statistical analyses.

Funding

None.

Authors' contributions

FK designed the study protocol, performed the submission to the Ethics Committee, contributed to data collection and wrote the manuscript. EE contributed to data collection and interpretation of data. AC contributed to the design of the study protocol, data collection and statistical analyses. HD and MK performed the biochemical measurements and collected the data. SR supervised the study protocol and was involved in manuscript editing. All of the authors read and approved the final version of the manuscript.

Competing interests

The authors have no conflict of interests to declare.

Author details

[1]Department of Urology, Sutcu Imam University, Avsar Kampusu, 46100 Kahramanmaras, Turkey. [2]Department of Biochemistry, Sutcu Imam University, Kahramanmaras, Turkey.

References

1. Prostate Cancer FAQS. Prostate Cancer Foundation. https://www.pcf.org/faq_category/prostate-cancer-faqs/. Accessed 15 Apr 2016.
2. Luengo-Fernandez R, Leal J, Gray A, Sullivan R. Economic burden of cancer across the European Union: a population-based cost analysis. Lancet Oncol. 2013;14(12):1165–74.
3. Djavan B, Margreiter M, Dianat SS. An algorithm for medical management in male lower urinary tract symptoms. Curr Opin Urol. 2011;21(1):5–12.
4. Foster CS. Pathology of benign prostatic hyperplasia. Prostate. 2009;9:4–14.
5. Ahmad M, Suhail N, Mansoor T, Banu N, Ahmad S. Evaluation of oxidative stress and DNA damage in benign prostatic hyperplasia patients and comparison with controls. Indian J Clin Biochem. 2012;27(4):385–8.
6. Aydin A, Arsova-Sarafinovska Z, Sayal A, Eken A, Erdem O, Erten K, et al. Oxidative stress and antioxidant status in non-metastatic prostate cancer and benign prostatic hyperplasia. Clin Biochem. 2006;39(2):176–9.
7. Klein EA, Casey G, Silverman R. Genetic susceptibility and oxidative stress in prostate cancer: integrated model with implications for prevention. Urology. 2006;68(6):1145–51.
8. Nelson WG, DeMarzo AM, DeWeese TL. The molecular pathogenesis of prostate cancer: focus on the earliest steps. Eur Urol. 2001;39(Suppl 4):8–11.
9. Arsova-Sarafinovska Z, Eken A, Matevska N, Erdem O, Sayal A, Savaser A, et al. Increased oxidative/nitrosative stress and decreased antioxidant enzyme activities in prostate cancer. Clin Biochem. 2009;42(12):1228–35.
10. Surazynski A, Donald SP, Cooper SK, Whiteside MA, Salnikow K, Liu Y, et al. Extracellular matrix and HIF-1 signaling: the role of prolidase. Int J Cancer. 2008;122(6):1435–40.
11. Myara I, Charpentier C, Lemonnier A. Prolidase and prolidase deficiency. Life Sci. 1984;34(21):1985–98.
12. Yildiz A, Demirbag R, Yilmaz R, Gur M, Altiparmak IH, Akyol S, et al. The association of serum prolidase activity with the presence and severity of coronary artery disease. Coron Artery Dis. 2008;19(5):319–25.
13. Pirinççi N, Kaba M, Geçit I, Güneş M, Yüksel MB, Tanık S, et al. Serum prolidase activity, oxidative stress, and antioxidant enzyme levels in patients with renal cell carcinoma. Toxicol Ind Health. 2016;32(2):193–9.
14. Gecit I, Aslan M, Gunes M, Pirincci N, Esen R, Demir H, et al. Serum prolidase activity, oxidative stress, and nitric oxide levels in patients with bladder cancer. J Cancer Res Clin Oncol. 2012;138(5):739–43.
15. Gecit I, Meral I, Aslan M, Kocyigit A, Celik H, Taskın A, et al. Peripheral mononuclear leukocyte DNA damage, plasma prolidase activity, and oxidative status in patients with benign prostatic hyperplasia. Redox Rep. 2015;20(4):163–9.
16. Buege JA, Aust SD. Microsomal lipid peroxidation. Methods Enzymol. 1978; 52:302–10.
17. Fridovich I. Superoxide dismutase. Adv Enzymol. 1974;41:35–97.
18. Myara I, Myara A, Mangeot M, Fabre M, Charpentier C, Lemonnier A. Plasma prolidase activity: a possible index of collagen catabolism in chronic liver disease. Clin Chem. 1984;30(2):211–5.
19. Ewalt DH, Howard PS, Blyth B, Snyder HM 3rd, Duckett JW, Levin RM, et al. (1992) Is lamina propria matrix responsible for normal bladder compliance? J Urol 148(2 Pt 2):544–549.
20. Ilikhan SU, Bilici M, Sahin H, Akca AS, Can M, Oz II, et al. Assessment of the correlation between serum prolidase and alpha-fetoprotein levels in patients with hepatocellular carcinoma. World J Gastroenterol. 2015;21(22): 6999–7007.
21. Camuzcuoglu H, Arioz DT, Toy H, Kurt S, Celik H, Aksoy N. Assessment of preoperative serum prolidase activity in epithelial ovarian cancer. Eur J Obstet Gynecol Reprod Biol. 2009;147(1):97–100.
22. Palka J, Surazynski A, Karna E, Orlowski K, Puchalski Z, Pruszynski K, et al. Prolidase activity disregulation in chronic pancreatitis and pancreatic cancer. Hepato-Gastroenterology. 2002;49(48):1699–703.
23. Meagher EA, FitzGerald GA. (2000) Indices of lipid peroxidation in vivo: strengths and limitations. Free Radic biol med 15;28(12):1745-50.
24. Bozkurt M, Caglayan M, Oktayoglu P, Em S, Batmaz I, Sariyildiz MA, et al. Serum prolidase enzyme activity and oxidative status in patients with fibromyalgia. Redox Rep. 2014;19(4):148–53.
25. Duygu F, Koruk ST, Karsen H, Aksoy N, Taskin A, Hamidanoglu M. Prolidase and oxidative stress in chronic hepatitis C. J Clin Lab Anal. 2012;26(4):232–7.
26. Palapattu GS, Sutcliffe S, Bastian PJ, Platz EA, De Marzo AM, Isaacs WB, et al. Prostate carcinogenesis and inflammation: emerging insights. Carcinogenesis. 2005;26(7):1170–81.
27. Savas M, Verit A, Ciftci H, Yeni E, Aktan E, Topal U, et al. Oxidative stress in BPH. JNMA J Nepal Med Assoc. 2009;48(173):41–5.
28. Doğru-Abbasoğlu S, Aykaç-Toker G, Koçak T, Unlüer E, Uysal M. Antioxidant enzyme activities and lipid peroxides in the plasma of patients with benign prostatic hyperplasia or prostate cancer are not predictive. J Cancer Res Clin Oncol. 1999;125(7):402–4.
29. Battisti V, Maders LD, Bagatini MD, Reetz LG, Chiesa J, Battisti IE, et al. Oxidative stress and antioxidant status in prostate cancer patients: relation to Gleason score, treatment and bone metastasis. Biomed Pharmacother. 2011;65(7):516–24.
30. Surapaneni KM, Venkata GR. Lipid peroxidation and antioxidant status in patients with carcinoma of prostate. Indian J Physiol Pharmacol. 2006;50(4):350–4.

8

Can Randall's plug composed of calcium oxalate form via the free particle mechanism?

F. Grases[1*] and O. Söhnel[2]

Abstract

Background: The likelihood of a Randall's plug composed of calcium oxalate monohydrate (COM) forming by the free particle mechanism in a model of kidney with a structure recently described by Robertson was examined at the most favourable conditions for the considered mechanism.

Methods: The Robertson model of the kidney is used in the following development. The classical theory of crystallization was used for calculations.

Results: Initial COM nuclei were assumed to form at the beginning of the ascending loop of Henle where the supersaturation with respect to COM has been shown to reach the threshold level for spontaneous nucleation. Nucleation proceeds by a heterogeneous mechanism. The formed particles are transported in the nephron by a laminar flow of liquid with a parabolic velocity profile. Particles travel with a velocity dependent on their position in the cross-section of the nephron assumed to be straight tubule with smooth walls and without any sharp bends and kinks. These particles move faster with time as they grow as a result of being surrounded by the supersaturated liquid. Individual COM particles (crystals) can reach maximum diameter of 5.2×10^{-6} m, i.e. 5.2 μm, at the opening of the CD and would thus always be washed out of the CD into the calyx regardless of the orientation of the CD. Agglomeration of COM crystals forms a fractal object with an apparent density lower than the density of solid COM. The agglomerate that can block the beginning of the CD is composed of more crystals than are available even during crystaluria. Moreover the settling velocity of agglomerate blocking the opening of the CD is lower than the liquid flow and thus such agglomerate would be washed out even from upward-draining CD.

Conclusions: The free particle mechanism may be responsible for the formation of a Randall's plug composed by COM only in specific infrequent cases such as an abnormal structure of kidney. Majority of incidences of Randall's plug development by COM are caused by mechanism different from the free particle mechanism.

Keywords: Randall's Plug, Calcium oxalate monohydrate, Formation mechanism

Background

Renal papillary calcifications can be classified into two distinct groups [1]. One type results from a subepithelial calcification (hydroxyapatite) of the renal papillary tissue as a consequence of a previous injury. The disruption of the papillary epithelial layer by biological hydroxyapatite plaque becomes the nidus of a calcium oxalate monohydrate (COM) papillary calculus. The other type of papillary calcification results from occlusions of the openings of the ducts of Bellini by stone-forming crystals (so-called Randall's plugs). Randall's plugs are usually composed of calcium oxalate monohydrate and/or dihydrate (COD), biological hydroxyapatite and organic matter, and occur in the terminal collecting ducts. These Randall's plugs can be also related to COD calculi or COM papillary calculi formed on papillary tips.

Two mechanisms for blocking collecting ducts by solid concretions, i.e. Randall's plug, have been suggested, the free and fixed particle mechanisms [2]. The free particle mechanism assumes that during the residence time of

* Correspondence: fgrases@uib.es
[1]Laboratory of Renal Lithiasis Research, University Institute of Health Sciences Research(IUNICS), University of Balearic Islands, Palma of Mallorca, Spain
Full list of author information is available at the end of the article

urine in the nephron and collecting duct a spherical object that can obstruct the opening into the calyx develops as a result of growth of a single particle or by agglomeration of smaller particles. The fixed particle mechanism assumes that a large concretion develops on a solid nidus firmly attached to the collecting duct wall. A crystal of calcium oxalate (CaOx) formed in urine during its residence time in the nephron attached to a Bellini's duct or to subepithelial calcification (hydroxyapatite) of the renal papillary tissue followed by an injury can serve as such a solid nidus.

Formation of a Randall's plug by the free particle mechanism was generally considered to be highly improbable. Recently, Robertson implemented previously omitted hydrodynamic factors into the original free particle model and concluded that this mechanism can play a significant role in the formation of a Randall's plug [3, 4]. The additional hydrodynamic factors implemented were (i) the spatial velocity profile of a liquid flowing through a tube, (ii) the residence time of a particle in a tube as a function of its position, (iii) the drag effect of the tubular walls on the particle and (iv) the effect of gravity on crystals in upward-draining tubules. Implementation of these additional factors into the model of the free particle mechanism and the resulting conclusions were, however, only qualitatively described in the paper. The aim of the current work was to rigorously determine the feasibility of the free particle mechanism under the most favourable conditions for formation of a Randall's plug composed of COM when taking into consideration the hydrodynamic factors recently introduced by Robertson.

Methods

Kidney

Robertson model of the kidney [3] is used in the following calculations. This model describes the ascending Henle loop as a circular truncated cone with average length L_{HL} of 1.2×10^{-2} m and internal radius r_{LH} increasing from 1.12×10^{-5} to 1.20×10^{-5} m, the following distal tubule as a cone with a length L_D of 6×10^{-3} m and internal radius r_{DL} decreasing from 1.2×10^{-5} to 1×10^{-5} m, and the collecting duct (CD) as a cone with a length L_{CD} of 2.7×10^{-2} m and internal radius r_{CD} increasing from 1×10^{-5} to 4×10^{-5} m at its opening at the papilla. The number of CDs per kidney is 320 and the number of the nephrons per kidney is 1.31×10^6. Thus 4094 nephrons are attached to each CD in this model.

Urine

Liquid passing the ascending Henle loop and distal tubule is approximately ten times more diluted than the final urine leaving the collecting duct [3]; that is the volume of liquid passing though the Henle loop and distal tubule is ten times the volume of urine produced. A volume of 1.5×10^{-3} m^3 is considered to be an average diuresis per day of adults. The volume of urine produced between the morning and evening is two to four times that at night. The minimum night production of urine is thus 0.30×10^{-3} m^3 per 8 h by two kidneys [5, 6] and this value was used in calculations.

The density and dynamic viscosity of the liquid (i.e. ten-fold diluted urine) in the nephron used for calculations were taken as values for water at 37 °C, i.e. the density $\rho = 994$ kg m^{-3} and the dynamic viscosity $\mu = 6.91 \times 10^{-4}$ kg m^{-1} s^{-1}. The density of urine in the CD is 1015 kg m^{-3} at 37 °C [7] and the kinematic viscosity at 37 °C is $\nu = 0.829 \times 10^{-6}$ m^2 s^{-1} [8]. The dynamic viscosity of urine is $\mu = \nu \times \rho = 8.41 \times 10^{-4}$ kg m^{-1} s^{-1}.

Characteristics of liquid flow in tubules

The liquid flow in tubules at night was calculated from data in the Kidney section using expressions in Additional file 1, see Table 1.

The flow of liquid is purely laminar in the ascending Henle loop and distal tubule as indicated by the Reynolds number Re « 1 and laminar in the CD where the average Reynolds number is Re ~ 2. The parabolic velocity profile of liquid in laminar flow is described by

$$u(R) = 2\,u_{av}\left[1-(R/r)^2\right] \quad (1)$$

where r is the radius of the tubule and R is the distance from the tubule axis.

The hydrodynamics in the CD is rather complicated. Nearly all nephrons are connected to the CD at its upper section [9]. Assuming that all nephrons are connected to the CD in the first quarter of its length, then the area available for water absorption would be the inner surface of three quarters of the CD length. The finding of Robertson that concentration of solute in the liquid entering the CD is ten times less than that in the final urine [3] means that 90% of the liquid entering the CD must be reabsorbed in the CD and hence the volumetric liquid flow decreases along the CD, see Fig. 1.

The average volumetric flow rate is Ave[Q(L)] = 7.58×10^{-11} m^3 s^{-1}, the average linear velocity of liquid is 3.45×10^{-2} m s^{-1} and the transit time of liquid through CD is 0.8 s (Additional file 2).

Supersaturation

Supersaturation S of a liquid in the nephron with respect to COM that was used for the current study was derived from Fig. 1 in [4] using the highest reported level of plasma oxalate concentration 2.75×10^{-6} mol L^{-1}. Supersaturation in the ascending loop of Henle has been shown to linearly decrease from 14 to 7, to be 7 in the

Table 1 Characteristics of liquid flow in tubules at night

		Ascending Henle loop	Distal tubule	Collecting duct
Volume	V (m^3)	5.07×10^{-12}	2.29×10^{-12}	5.94×10^{-11}
Average radius	r (m)	1.16×10^{-5}	1.10×10^{-5}	2.65×10^{-4}
Volumetric flow	Q ($m^3\ s^{-1}$)	3.98×10^{-14}	3.98×10^{-14}	$1.63 \times 10^{-11\#}$
Average linear velocity	u_{av} ($m\ s^{-1}$)	9.42×10^{-5}	1.05×10^{-4}	$3.24 \times 10^{-3\#}$
Average transit time of liquid	t_{tr} (s)	127	57	0.8 (3.6*)
Reynolds number	Re (–)	3.2×10^{-3}	3.3×10^{-3}	2.1 (0.31#)

Value denoted by asterisk is the transit time if volumetric flow in the CD is equal to the flow rate at the opening, # value at the opening of the CD

distal tubule and to parabolically increase from 7 to 270 in the CD.

Nucleation

The onset of spontaneous nucleation of COM in an aqueous solution was shown to occur at a supersaturation 9 [10], 10 [11] and 14 [3]. Formation of primary particles of CaOx (by heterogeneous nucleation on present organic debris) with an initial diameter of 0.1×10^{-6} m [3, 12] was assumed to take place at the beginning of the ascending Henle loop (in accordance with Robertson model).

Crystal growth

The rate of crystal growth is usually expressed as the increase of radius or diameter D of a spherical particle with volume equal to volume of an average particle per unit of time. The growth rate equation of COM crystal was calculated using the equation [13]

$$dD/dt = 1.12x10^{-10}(S-1)^2 m\ s^{-1} \tag{2}$$

Results

Transit time and size of COM crystals

COM primary particles formed at the beginning of Henle loop are assumed to be uniformly distributed throughout the volume of the liquid. For simplicity let consider the flow to be like a set of thin concentric shells of fluid sliding over one another. The liquid flow in the tubule is laminar with parabolic velocity distribution, see eq.(1); the velocity of the fluid at the centre line being twice the average velocity of the fluid and the velocity being zero at the first shell adjoining the tubular wall. The thickness of shell was assumed to be the same as the size of primary particles - 0.1×10^{-6} m. Particles at different position in the cross-section of the tubule therefore move with different velocities and thus have different transit times through the tubule. Because of these different transit times crystals attain different sizes at the end of the tubule.

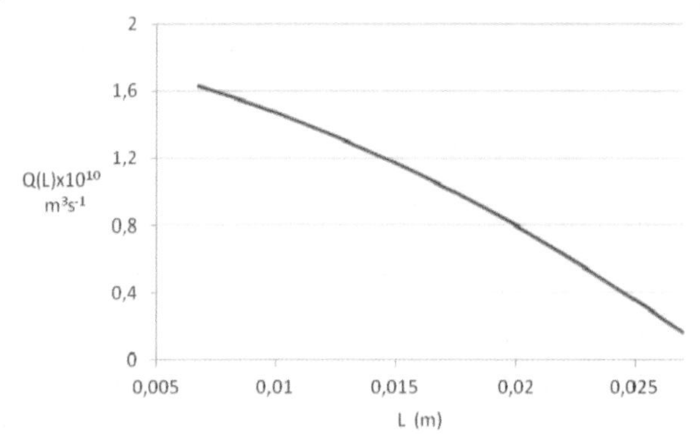

Fig. 1 The volumetric liquid flow through the CD as a function of distance, L, from its beginning

Liquid surrounding CaOx particles is supersaturated with respect to COM and hence particles increase in size by regular crystal growth. Particle in the first stagnant shell adjacent to the tubular wall does not move but grows. When increment of particle size is 0.1×10^{-6} m, particle extends to the adjoining shell and then moves with the velocity of the liquid in this shell. Particle travels certain distance until its size due to growth reaches into the next shell and starts moving with velocity of this shell. The transit time through the tubules of a particle initially situated near the wall was calculated using eq.(III.5) in Additional file 3.

Along the ascending loop of Henle supersaturation linearly decreases from 14 to 7, as shown Fig. 1 of [4]. The average value of the function $(S - 1)^2$ was calculated to be 94.33 (Additional file 1). The transit time of the slowest travelling spherical particle was calculated to be 358 s and during this time the particle was calculated to attain a diameter of 3.8×10^{-6} m. The transit time of a particle situated in the centre of the ascending Henle loop was calculated to be 64 s and during this time its diameter was calculated to increase to 0.7×10^{-6} m.

In the distal tubule supersaturation is 7 and thus a value of the function $(S - 1)^2$ is 36. The transit time of the slowest moving particle entering from the ascending loop of Henle to the distal tubule was calculated to be 72 s and during this time the diameter of the spherical particle increased to 4.1×10^{-6} m. The transit time of a particle situated in the centre of the distal tubule was calculated to be 28 s. The diameter of a spherical particle entering the distal tubule from the centre of the ascending loop of Henle and travelling in its centre was calculated to increase at its end to 1.0×10^{-6} m.

When supersaturation with respect to COM at the CD exceeds approximately 14, particles of solid phase are formed by spontaneous nucleation followed by their fast growth. As a result supersaturation rapidly falls close to the threshold value. Let assume that supersaturation along the CD is 15 and the transit time of liquid through the CD 49 s quoted in [4] is equal to the transit time of crystals though, in fact this transit time was calculated to be much shorter (0.8 s). The diameter of the slowest moving spherical particle entering the CD from the distal tubule was calculated to increase to 5.2×10^{-6} m while the diameter of the fastest moving spherical particle (situated in the tubule axis) would increase to 2.1×10^{-6} m.

Minimum and maximum transit times, through a nephron and CD, of a crystal nucleated at the beginning of the ascending loop of Henle were calculated to be 141 s (2.3 min) and 479 s (8 min), respectively. The maximum diameter of an individual COM crystal appearing in the CD opening was calculated to be 5.2×10^{-6} m. Hence the collecting duct cannot be blocked by an individual COM crystal formed in the nephron.

Agglomeration

Agglomerates are irregular spherical fractal objects as demonstrated in [14]. The apparent density of an irregular fractal agglomerate defined as the ratio of the mass of the agglomerate to the volume of a circumscribed sphere, i.e. occupied by agglomerate, decreases with its radius according to $\rho_{a'} \sim r_a^{Dm}$ where D_m represents the mass agglomerate fractal dimension [15]. The more D_m deviates from 3 (Euclidean objects), the higher the degree of object fractality, i.e. the object becomes less regular. The value of D_m for a three dimensional fractal agglomerate formed by the random motion of particles that irreversibly associate with a growing germ has been shown to be 2.5 [16]. The ratio of the apparent density of a fractal agglomerate to the density of a Euclidean object of the same radius is thus given by the equation

$$\rho_{a'}/\rho_s = 1/(r_a/r_{particle})^{0.5} \quad (3)$$

The apparent density of the agglomerate composed of COM spherical crystals with a diameter of 5.2×10^{-6} m (the density of COM is 2120 kg m^{-3} [http://www.chemicalbook.com/ChemicalProductProperty_EN_CB7154359.htm]) that can block the opening of the CD with a radius of 40×10^{-6} m was calculated to be $\rho_{a'} = 2120 / (40 / 2.7)^{0.5} = 551$ kg m^{-3}. Such an agglomerate has void spaces filled with air. The apparent density of the agglomerate that contains a gas or liquid in void spaces among crystals is

$$\rho_{a'} = F_s\rho_s + F_{g,1}\rho_{g,1} \quad (4)$$

where $F_{g,l}$ is the volume fraction of the agglomerate occupied by gas or liquid and $F_s + F_{g,l} = 1$. The volume fractions of COM agglomerate with radius of 40×10^{-6} m occupied by solid was calculated to be 0.260. The apparent density of the agglomerate with void space filled with liquid (i.e. when the agglomerate is submerged in urine) was then calculated to be 1302 kg m^{-3}. The apparent density of COM agglomerates was previously estimated to be 1500 kg m^{-3} [17].

Any agglomerate with a radius smaller than 40×10^{-6} m (the radius of the opening of the CD) would be washed away by a stream of urine from the downward-draining Bellini duct (see below). The mass of a Euclidean object of this size and with the above-described density would be 5.68×10^{-10} kg and hence the mass of the solid fraction of the agglomerate would be $5.68 \times 10^{-10} \times 0.260 = 1.48 \times 10^{-10}$ kg. Such an agglomerate would be composed of 948 crystals with a radius of 2.6×10^{-6} m. Assuming (the unrealistic case) that all of the crystals present in the Bellini's duct create this agglomerate, the number concentration of the constituting crystals would be $948 / 5.94 \times 10^{-11} = 1.6 \times 10^{13}$ m^{-3} of urine.

The number concentration of COM crystals present in urine during crystalluria has been shown to be 2.41×10^{10} m^{-3} [17], and this value hence indicates the number concentration of nuclei formed at the beginning of the ascending loop of Henle, that is the maximum number concentration of COM crystals in urine. Since this concentration is about three orders of magnitude lower than the concentration necessary for forming blocking agglomerate, the CD of any orientation cannot be blocked by agglomerates of COM crystals.

The half-time $\tau_{½}$ of agglomeration, i.e. the time necessary for halving the number of separate particles present in a unit volume of suspension, N_o, controlled by the laminar shear rate, is defined as [18]

$$\tau½ = 1/A\,N_o \quad (5)$$

with the A term given by

$$A = 2\,\alpha\,G\,r^3/3\,k_v \quad (6)$$

where r is the particle radius (m), α is the collision efficacy coefficient, k_v represents the volume shape factor and G is the shear rate (s^{-1}) defined as

$$G = 4\,Q/\pi r_{CD}{}^3 \quad (7)$$

where r_{CD} is a radius of the CD. For $Q = 1.63 \times 10^{-11}$ $m^3\,s^{-1}$ (Table 1) and $r_{CD} = 4 \times 10^{-5}$ m, the shear rate would be 324 s^{-1}. Taking $\alpha = 1$ (i.e. each collision is successful), r = 2.6 × 10^{-6} m, k_v = 4 π/3 and N_o = 1.63 × 10^{13} m^{-3} then the half time would be 527 s. The kinetics of agglomeration showed that formation of the blocking agglomerate in a suspension containing enough particles to form the agglomerate would be substantially longer than the transit time through the CD.

Concentration of COM particles in the CD and kinetics of their agglomeration showed that any agglomerate of COM crystals formed in the CD cannot acquire a large enough size to be retained and block the Bellini's duct.

Effect of gravity

Due to the changing position of the body, all of the CDs are not necessarily always downward-draining, and some can be in an upward-draining position. In such a case an agglomerate of a sufficient size can be retained in the collecting duct due to settling.

A solid particle cannot be conveyed upward when the terminal settling velocity of the particle exceeds the fluid velocity. The terminal velocity is the highest velocity attainable by an object as it falls through a fluid. The terminal settling velocity, u_{te}, of the particle in an unbounded fluid is given by the Stokes law if the Reynolds number of particle, $Re_p = u_{te} D \rho_s / \mu$, was considerably smaller than unity

$$u_{te} = g\left(\rho_s - \rho_l\right) D^2/18\,\mu \tag{8}$$

where g is the gravity acceleration 9.81 m s^{-2}. Re_p of a spherical COM particle with a diameter 5.2 × 10^{-6} m would be 2.5 × 10^{-3} for u_{te} = 1.94 × 10^{-5} m s^{-1} estimated from eq.(8). Because the requisite condition for use of eq.(8), i.e. $Re_p \ll 1$, is satisfied, the calculated value of u_{te} represents the terminal settling velocity of the considered particle. Liquid in a distance 5.2 × 10^{-6} m from the edge of the CD opening is moving with a linear velocity 1.6 × 10^{-3} m s^{-1} (eq.1). Since this fluid velocity exceeds by about two orders of magnitude the terminal settling velocity of the largest COM crystal that can develop in the nephron, all individual COM crystals are invariably washed away from the collecting duct.

The size of a COM agglomerate with a density 1500 kg m^{-3} and having the same settling velocity as the average linear velocity of the liquid at the CD opening was estimated using eq.(8) to be 1 × 10^{-4} m and its Re_p was estimated to be 0.58. Because the condition $Re_p \ll 1$ is not fulfilled, the terminal settling velocity of such an agglomerate has to be determined by iterations from the set of expressions

$$\begin{aligned} Re_p &= u_{te} D' \rho_s/\mu \\ D &= 3\,u_{te}^2 c_D\,\rho_l/\left[4\left(\rho_s - \rho_l\right) g\right] \\ c_D &= 24/Re_p + 4/\sqrt{Re_p} + 0.4 \end{aligned} \tag{9}$$

where c_D is the drag coefficient [19]. The diameter of a spherical agglomerate of COM crystals with a density 1500 kg m^{-3} that can be retained in an upward-draining CD, i.e. having a settling velocity equal to or higher than the average linear velocity of the liquid at the CD opening, was calculated to be 8.86 × 10^{-5} m and Re_p was calculated to be 0.51. The size of this agglomerate exceeds the size of the CD opening. Therefore, any agglomerate of COM crystals formed in the CD has a sedimentation velocity lower than the velocity of liquid flow and would therefore be washed out into the calyx even from an upward-draining CD. Performed calculations thus indicate that CDs in any orientation cannot be blocked by any an agglomerate of COM crystals.

Wall effect

The influence of walls on a settling particle, known as the wall effect, leads to an increase in the drag force exerted on a falling particle that results in a retarding effect on the terminal velocity of settling [20, 21]. The wall effect becomes important when the diameter of the particle becomes fairly noticeable with respect to the diameter of the tubule. In these cases the settling velocity calculated for an unbounded medium from eqs. (8,9) has to be corrected using the expression [22]

$$u_{te}(\text{corr}) = u_{te}(\text{eqs.7, 8})/\left[1 - (D/2r)^{1.5}\right] \tag{10}$$

The settling velocity of larger particles is in fact lower than those previously calculated without considering the influence of the wall effect. This fact further diminishes the likelihood of a Randall's plug forming by the free particle mechanism.

Discussion

Formation of a Randall's plug in the Bellini's duct by the free particle mechanism assumes that a particle of sufficient size, be it a single crystal or agglomerate of smaller crystals, is retained in the duct and develops into the full-sized Randall's plug. The feasibility of this mechanism was evaluated for a model kidney with a structure as described recently by Robertson. The composition of Randall's plug consisting of COM crystals considered in the present analysis is identical with the composition considered in the analysis Robertson even though the plug can also contain or be composed of COD crystals [23]. The conditions prevailing in the nephron considered in the current analysis – the highest reported supersaturation with respect to COM, the lowest liquid flow, absence of inhibitors of COM crystallization, all crystals present in the CD having the same maximum achievable size and fast agglomeration of crystals into single particle – are all the most favourable for formation of Randall's plug by the free particle mechanism.

Hydrodynamic conditions prevailing in the loop of Henle and distal tubule calculated above are in satisfactory agreement with the results of the Robertson model [3, 4]. The substantial discrepancy in the calculated transit time of liquid through the CD (4 s versus 50 s) is difficult to explain because the details of the Robertson model have not been published. However, the volumetric flow rate and the linear velocity of liquid at the opening of the CD derived from basic data - diuresis and number of CDs per kidney - are correct and hence were used in all calculations.

COM nuclei originating at the beginning of the ascending loop of Henle where the supersaturation with respect to COM attains value of 14 are expected to be formed by heterogeneous nucleation. This means that the number of formed primary particles is largely governed by the number of effective heteronuclei (organic debri) present in the liquid. A uniform spatial distribution of COM primary particles can be expected. Individual particles thus move with different velocities with a parabolic velocity profile according to their distance from the tubule wall. The velocity of particles increases from zero for particles close to the wall to double the average linear velocity of the liquid for particles in the centre of tubule. Particles close to the wall do not move, but grow because they are surrounded by moving supersaturated liquid of the adjoining shell. When the particle grows to the point at which it extends into the adjoining 2nd shell it starts moving with the velocity of this shell. This process repeats until the particle leaves the nephron and is washed out into the calyx. Maximum attainable size of COM individual particle at the opening of the CD travelling in the vicinity of tubule wall was calculated to be about five micrometers and its total transit time was calculated to be about 18 min assuming a constant flow of liquid. The settling velocity of particle was not considered in these calculations because it is negligible compared to the velocity of the liquid flow. The final size of the particle and its transit time through the nephron depend on the prevailing level of supersaturation. At higher supersaturation the final particle size is larger and the transit times shorter whereas at lower values it is vice versa. Even in specific cases, such as dramatically decreased production of urine when the transit time would be much longer, the size of individual COM particles would still be far smaller than the size necessary for blocking the CD. Experimental study of growth of CaOx crystals in urine-like solution led to similar conclusion [24].

The final size of COM particle depends on prevailing level of supersaturation and duration of its contact with supersaturated liquid, i.e. on its transit time through the nephron. Particle is carried by the liquid in assumed pure laminar flow. Pure laminar flow in the nephron is, to some extent, disturbed at sharp bends of tubule, in the vicinity of kinks present in the nephron and at termination of the nephron at the collecting duct. Impact of these irregularities influencing laminar flow on the transit time of particle is difficult to estimate because quantitative data describing these irregularities are not available. Moreover, it is doubtful that the chemical engineering treatment of these disturbances suitable for tubes of larger diameter is applicable for capillaries (nephron).

Isolated buoyant spheroidal particle in a uniform simple laminar shear flow at low Reynolds number does not move along the straight line but moves in closed orbits. The centre of the particle moves with the velocity of the undisturbed fluid at that point. Particle also tends to drift to the centre of a capillary [25]. Therefore a spheroidal primary particle initially situated in the close vicinity of tubular wall gradually drifts away from the wall and thus crosses over to the adjoining shell of faster moving liquid sooner than is expected in the used model based on the regular crystal growth. On the other hand, friction between particle and the tubular wall slows down the velocity of particle movement compared to the velocity of the respective liquid shell. Because no quantitative data are available, it was assumed that opposite effect of these two factors is roughly equal and negligibly influence calculated particle transit time through the nephron and hence the determined final particle size.

Flat prismatic COM particles predominantly appearing in urine tend to align with the laminar flow direction. But in regions where some turbulence appears, flat particles tend to adopt position perpendicular to the flow [26]. Particles aligned with the laminar flow move slower than model in Additional file 3 predicts, but particles perpendicular to the flow move faster than calculated. Based on the current knowledge it is impossible to estimate duration of each orientation during transit time of particles through the nephron. Effect of periodic changes in particle orientation on transit time was assumed to be balanced by assumption of spherical shape of particle used in calculations.

The growth rate of COM particles expressed by eq. (2) and used in the current analysis describes uninhibited growth that is when inhibitors of growth, such as citrate, magnesium, phytate, zinc, low-molecular weight peptides, certain amino acids etc. are absent. Since these inhibitory substances are actually always present in urine, though in individually different concentrations, the actual growth of COM particles in urine is generally lower than that given by eq.(2) and hence the real size of COM particles in the CD is smaller than those indicated by the above calculations.

Any single particle of COM formed in the nephron and CD at night, and during other situations when production of urine is low, cannot attain the size that can block the CD. An alternative mechanism in which a blocking object is formed by the agglomeration of COM particles in the CD was considered. Here, since the orientation of the kidney and hence of the CD frequently varies with the changing position of the human body two separate cases were examined: downward- and upward-draining positions of the CD.

CD in the downward-draining position can be blocked only if the blocking object was formed during the transit time of the liquid through the CD. An agglomerate with a radius 4×10^{-5} m can be theoretically retained at the beginning of CD and block it. Such an agglomerate cannot develop in the CD since it would consist of significantly more particles than the maximum possible number of particles present in the CD. Even if the required number of particles were present in the CD, the formation of an agglomerate of such size would be impossible within the given time frame from view-point of agglomeration kinetics. Smaller agglomerates originating in the CD cannot be retained in the Bellini's duct and are without exception washed out into the calyx. A Randall's plug thus cannot develop in downward-draining CDs by the free particle mechanism.

The settling velocity of particles must be considered in the upward-draining CDs because it diminishes the capability of a liquid stream to wash them out into the calyx. An individual COM particle cannot attain during transit through nephron diameter 6.7×10^{-5} m at which its settling velocity equals velocity of liquid stream at the opening of CD. An agglomerate would need to have a diameter of 8.86×10^{-4} m to display a terminal settling velocity equal to the linear velocity of a liquid at the CD opening, even without considering the retarding effect of the tubule wall on the settling velocity. Such a diameter does exceed the dimensions of the CD opening in the used kidney model. Moreover, number of crystals needed to form such a large agglomerate is about three orders of magnitude greater than maximum number present in the CD during the transit time. Therefore any agglomerate formed in the CD is smaller than the size of a blocking agglomerate and would be washed out of the CD regardless of its orientation. Transporting solid particles in vertical pipelines requires the bulk fluid velocity to be greater than twice the particle settling velocity [27] and this condition was fulfilled in our case.

Calculations showed that any COM particle that can be formed in the nephron, be it a single crystal or agglomerate, was too small to be retained unbounded in the CD of any orientation. The Randall's plug thus cannot originate in the kidney with parameters corresponding to the used kidney model by the free particle mechanism even during period of decreased urine production such as at night.

All mammals display a peristaltic movement of renal calyces [28]. During a period of compression the CD experiences a contraction, which is periodically repeated, as a wave. As a result of this movement the papillae, and consequently the CD, are evidently subjected to some regular squeezing, to facilitate the expulsion of liquid and present solid objects. These features further support that a mechanism other than the free particle mechanism is responsible for the formation of the Randall's plug.

The detail structure of the kidney has been observed to vary quite considerably from one individual to the next. The number of CDs per kidney has been observed to vary from 50 to 1120, and the diameter of the CD at its beginning and opening to vary from 2×10^{-5} to 3×10^{-5} m and from 8×10^{-5} to 2×10^{-4} m respectively [2]. The most favourable combination of kidney parameters for forming a Randall's plug by the free particle mechanism would include 1120 CDs, a CD diameter of 2×10^{-4} m at its opening and a low urine production of 0.30×10^{-3} m^3 per 8 h. This case corresponds to a volumetric flow rate of 4.65×10^{-12} m^3 s^{-1} and a linear flow velocity of urine at the CD opening of 1.48×10^{-4} m s^{-1}. The terminal settling velocity of a crystal with diameter 8×10^{-6} m located in the vicinity of wall would be equal to the linear flow velocity of fluid and would be retained in the upward-draining CD. Under favourable conditions - deficiency of inhibitors of crystal growth and presence of agglomeration promoters – such crystals by growth and fast agglomeration could form a blocking concretion before the position of the CD is changed from upward to downward pointing as a result of natural body movements.

The free particle mechanism may be responsible for the formation of a Randall's plug in infrequent specific cases. However, the majority of incidences of renal papillary calcifications are caused by a different mechanism such as the fixed particle mechanism. A similar conclusion was reached by Finlayson and Reid [2] who analyzed the formation of the Randall's plug using a probabilistic approach applied on a slightly different model of the kidney.

Conclusions

Formation of a Randall's plug composed of COM in the Bellini's duct of kidney with structure described recently by Robertson by the free particle mechanism is rather improbable even under the most favourable conditions prevailing in the nephron – the highest reported supersaturation, the lowest typical urine production, absence of inhibitors of COM crystallization, maximum size of crystals present in the CD and fast agglomeration of crystals into one particle. The free particle mechanism may be responsible for the formation of a Randall's plug composed of COM only in infrequent specific cases characterized namely by abnormal structure of kidney, dramatically decreased urine production, deficiency of inhibitors of crystal growth combined with the presence of agglomeration promoters and long-term upward-draining position of the CD. Majority of incidences of renal papillary calcifications are caused by other mechanisms such as the fixed particle mechanism.

Abbreviations

A: Area (m^2); c_D: Drag coefficient; D: Diameter of particle (m); D_m: Mass agglomerate fractal dimension (–); F: Volume fraction (–); g: Gravity acceleration ($m\ s^{-2}$); G: Shear rate (s^{-1}); k_g: Growth rate constant; k_v: Volume shape factor (–); L: Length (m); N_o: Number of separate particles present in a unit volume of suspension (m^{-3}); Q: Volumetric flow rate, i.e. volume of liquid passing tubule per second ($m^3\ s^{-1}$); R: Distance from the tubule axis (m); r: Radius of tubule (m); Re_p: Reynolds number of particle (–); Re: Reynolds number (–); S: Supersaturation (–); t: Time (s); t_{tr}: Transit time (s); u: Linear velocity of liquid ($m\ s^{-1}$); u_{te}: Terminal settling velocity of particle ($m\ s^{-1}$); V: Volume of tubule (m^3)**Greek symbols**

τ: Time (s).; α: Collision efficacy coefficient (–).; ρ: Density ($kg\ m^{-3}$).; μ: Dynamic viscosity ($kg\ m^{-1}\ s^{-1}$).; $\tau_{½}$: Half time of agglomeration.; ρ_a: Apparent density of agglomerate - the ratio of mass of agglomerate to volume of Circumscribed sphere ($kg\ m^{-3}$).**Subscripts**

a: Agglomerate; av: Average; g: Gas; l: Liquid**Abbreviations**

Ave: Average value of a function; CaOx: Calcium oxalate; CD: Collecting duct; COD: Calcium oxalate dihydrate; COM: Calcium oxalate monohydrate

Acknowledgements

None.

Funding

Not applicable.

Authors' contributions

FG contributed in the design of the work and in the discussion of the results. OS developed the theoretical calculations and contributed in the discussion. Both authors read and approved the final manuscript.

Competing interest

The authors declare that they have no competing interests.

Author details

[1]Laboratory of Renal Lithiasis Research, University Institute of Health Sciences Research(IUNICS), University of Balearic Islands, Palma of Mallorca, Spain. [2]University of J.E. Purkyně, Faculty of Environmental Studies, Ústí n.L, Czech Republic.

References

1. Khan SR, Canales BK. Unified theory on the pathogenesis of Randall's plaques and plugs. Urolithiasis. 2015;43(Suppl 1):S109–23.
2. Finlayson B, Reid F. The expectation of free and fixed particles in urinary stone disease. Investig Urol. 1978;15:442–8.
3. Robertson WG. Kidney models of calcium oxalate stone formation. Nephron Physiol. 2004;98:21–30.
4. Robertson WG. Potential role of fluctuations in the composition of renal tubular fluid through the nephron in the initiation of Randall's plugs and calcium oxalate crystalluria in a computer model of renal fiction. Urolithiasis. 2015;43(Suppl 1):S93–S107.
5. Le Vay D, Mitchell GAG, James Scott Robson JS. Renal system, anatomy. https://www.britannica.com/science/human-renal-system/Human-excretion. Accessed 7 Sept 2017.
6. Coe F (2016). Why 24 hour urine: supersaturation. Univ. Chicago Kidney stone evaluation and treatment program. Kidneystones.uchicago.edu/why-24-hour-urines/.
7. Lee M (2009) Basic skills in interpreting laboratory data. Ch 7. The kidneys. Amer Soc Health-System Pharm Inc. ISBN 978-1-58528-180-0. p.173.
8. Inman BA, Etienne W, Rubin R, Owusu RA, Oliveira TR, Rodriques DB, Maccarini PF, Stauffer PR, Mashal A, Dewhirst MW. The impact of temperature and urinary constituents on urine viscosity and its relevance to bladder hyperthermia treatment. Int J Hyperth. 2013;29:206–10. doi: 10.3109/02656736.2013.775355.
9. Madsen KM, Tisher CC. Structural-functional relationships along the distal nephron. American Journal of Physiology-Renal Physiology. 1986; 250(1):F1–F15.
10. Petrova V, Gvozdev NV, Rashkovich LN. Growth and dissolution of calcium oxalate monohydrate (com) crystals. J Optoelectronics and Advanced Materials. 2004;6(1):261–8.
11. Robertson WG, Peacock M, Nordin EC. Activity prducts in stone-forming and non-stone forming urine. Clin Sci. 1968;34:579–94.
12. Grohe B, Rogers KA, Goldberg HA, Hunter GK. Crystallization kinetics of calcium oxalate hydrates studied by scanning confocal interference microscopy. J Cryst Growth. 2006;295:148–57.
13. Nielsen AE. Theory of electrolyte crystal growth. p. 35-44. In: Jancic SJ, de Jong EJ, editors. Industrial crystallization 81. Amsterdam: North Holland Publ Comp; 1981. ISBN 0-444-86402-4.
14. Grases F, Millan A, Söhnel O. Role of agglomeration in calcium oxalate monohydrate urolith development. Nephron. 1992;61:145–50.
15. Pabst W, Gregorová E. Characterization of particles and particle systems. Prague: ICT; 2007 p.7.
16. Stoll S, Diez S. Fractal structures and mechanisms in coagulation/flocculation processes in environmental systems: the theoretical aspects. In: Senesi N, Wilkinson KJ, editors. Biophysical chemistry of fractal structures and processes in environmental systems, vol. Vol. 11. London: J Wiley and Sons Ltd; 2008. p. 111–49. ISBN 978-0-470-01474-5.
17. Kok DJ, Khan SR. Calcium oxalate nephrolithiasis: a free or fixed particle diseases. Kidney Int. 1994;46:847–54.
18. von Smoluchowski MV. Mathematical theory of the kinetics of coagulation of colloidal solutions. Z Phys Chem. 1917;92:129–68.
19. Weber M. Liquid-solid flow. Thermopedia. doi: 10.1615/AtoZ.l.liquid-solid_flow. http://www.thermopedia.com/content/51/.
20. Song D, Gupta RK, Chhabra RP. Wall effects on the terminal velocity of spherical particles in Newtonian and non-Newtonian fluids. Boston: Comsol conference proceedings; 2011.
21. Mingzhong L, Guodong Z, Jianquan X, Yanchao L, Shukai T (2014). Prediction of the wall factor of arbitrary particle settling through various fluid media in a cylindrical tube using artificial intelligence. Sci World J, vol. 2014, Article ID 438782, 10 pages. doi: 10.1155/2014/438782.
22. Fidleris V, Whitmore RL. Experimental determination of wall effect for spheres falling axially in cylindrical vessels. British J of Appl Phys. 1961; 12:490–4.
23. Grases F, Söhnel O, Costa-Bauzá A, Servera A, Benejam J (2016). A case of Randall's plugs associated to calcium oxalate Dihydrate calculi. Urol Case Rep, Jul 6;7:37-38. doi: 10.1016/j.eucr.2016.04.003. Epub 2016 Dec 6.
24. Miller JD, Randolph AD, Drach GW. Observations upon calcium oxalate crystallization kinetics in simulated urine. J Urol. 1977;117(3):342–5.
25. Jeffery GB. The motion of ellipsoidal particles immersed in a viscous fluid. Proceedings of the Royal Society A. 1922;102(715):161–79. doi: 10.1098/rspa.1922.0078. http://rspa.royalsocietypublishing.org.
26. Trebbin M, Steinhauser D, Perlich J, Buffet A, Roth SV, Zimmermann W, Thiele J, Förster S. Anisotropic particles align perpendicular to the flow direction in narrow microchannels. Proc Natl Acad Sci U S A. 2013;110(17): 6706–11. doi: 10.1073/pnas.1219340110.
27. Govier GW, Aziz K. The flow of complex mixtures in pipes. New York-London: Van Nostrand Reinhold Comp; 1972. p. 468.
28. Schmidt-Nielsen B, Schmidt-Nielsen B. On the function of the mammalian renal papilla and the peristalsis of the surrounding pelvis. Acta Physiol. 2011;202:379–85.

Expression of micro-RNAs and genes related to angiogenesis in ccRCC and associations with tumor characteristics

Rita de Cássia Oliveira[1], Renato Fidelis Ivanovic[1], Katia Ramos Moreira Leite[1], Nayara Izabel Viana[1], Ruan César Aparecido Pimenta[1], José Pontes Junior[1,2], Vanessa Ribeiro Guimarães[1], Denis Reis Morais[1], Daniel Kanda Abe[1], Adriano João Nesrallah[2], Miguel Srougi[1], William Nahas[2] and Sabrina Thalita Reis[1*]

Abstract

Background: Clear cell renal cell carcinoma (ccRCC) is the third most common urological cancer in adults. Our aim is to evaluate genes and miRNAs expression profiles involved with angiogenesis and tumor characteristics in ccRCC.

Methods: The expression levels of miRNAs miR-99a, 99b, 100; 199a; 106a; 106b; 29a; 29b; 29c; 126; 200a, 200b and their respective target genes: mTOR, HIF1-α, VHL, PDGF, VEGF, VEGFR1 and VEGFR2 were analyzed using qRT-PCR in tumor tissue samples from 56 patients with ccRCC. Five samples of benign renal tissue were utilized as control. The expression levels of miRNAs and genes were related to tumor size, Fuhrman nuclear grade and microvascular invasion.

Results: miR99a was overexpressed in most samples and its target gene mTOR was underexpressed, this also occurs for miRNAs 106a, 106b, and their target gene VHL. An increase in miR-200b was correlated with high-risk tumors ($p = 0.01$) while miR-126 overexpression was associated with Fuhrman's low grade ($p = 0.03$).

Conclusions: Our results show that in ccRCC there are changes in miRNAs expression affecting gene expression that could be important in determining the aggressiveness of this lethal neoplasia.

Keywords: Angiogenesis, Genes, microRNAs, Renal cell carcinoma clear cell type

Background

Clear cell renal cell carcinoma (ccRCC) is the third most common urological cancer after prostate and bladder cancer and represents approximately 3% of cancers in adults as well as 85% of primary malignant kidney tumors [1]. Early detection and correct follow-up of the patients may influence the prognosis of the disease. Therefore, to improve our understanding of ccRCC pathogenesis, is necessary to identify new biomarkers enabling prediction of early metastasis after nephrectomy, and develop new targeted therapies [2].

MicroRNAs (miRNAs) are a class of small noncoding RNA with approximately 22 nucleotides and has critical roles in a many biological processes through translational repression or degradation of target messenger RNAs (mRNAs). Dysregulation of miRNAs has been shown to result in gene expression alteration and contributes to invasion and metastasis of many human tumors [3]. Prior studies indicated that miRNAs are also involved in other processes like tumor angiogenesis [4, 5]. Particularly, many urologic tumors have altered levels of numerous miRNAs [6]. Thus, changed expression of miRNAs may be useful for diagnosis, prediction of prognosis and treatment selection in patients with certain urologic cancers [7, 8]. Remarkably, targeted disruption of angiogenesis-related miRNAs may be a potential target treatment for RCC and other cancers [9].

ccRCC is characteristically highly vascularized and related to a germinative mutation of the von Hipple-Lindau (VHL) gene. Under adequate oxygen conditions, the VHL protein controls the expression of HIF-1α leading to its ubiquitination and degradation by the proteasome. In the absence of the VHL protein, due to gene

* Correspondence: sasareis@gmail.com
[1]Laboratory of Medical Investigation (LIM55), Urology Department, University of Sao Paulo Medical School, Av. Dr. Arnaldo 455, 2° floor, room 2145, Sao Paulo 01246-903, Brazil
Full list of author information is available at the end of the article

mutation and or deletion, even during normal oxygen conditions HIF1-α will bind to the constitutively expressed HIF1, thus forming a heterodimer (HIF-1) activating transcription of genes related to angiogenesis and cell survival as VEGF, EGFR, PDGF, TGF-α, erythropoietin [10] ERK and mTOR. The discovery of the VHL-HIF1 pathway was responsible for the developing of target drugs represented by monoclonal antibodies and molecules responsible for tyrosine kinase inhibition action [11].

Some microRNAs have been called angiomirs because they regulate the angiogenesis process [12]. miR-126 [13]; miR-100, [14], miR-200 [15] and miR-26a [16] are some examples of this group of miRNAs.

Few studies have evaluated the presence of angiomirs in tumor development in urology, specially in ccRCC [17, 18]. Our aim is to evaluate genes and miRNAs expression profiles involved with angiogenesis and tumor characteristics in ccRCC.

Clinical significance

The association between these biomarkers and ccRCC may contribute to the development of alternative tools that can facilitate the early detection and prognosis of this disease.

Methods

Patients

The study comprised the analysis of specimens from 56 patients diagnosed with ccRCC who were surgically treated by radical or partial nephrectomy at Hospital das Clinicas of University of Sao Paulo Medical School between January/2008 and March/2012 (Table 1). Final pathological status, tumor size, Fuhrman's nuclear grade and micro vascular invasion were retrospectively reviewed. Patients were grouped according to a prognosis classification described by Dall'Oglio et al. into high, intermediate and low risk tumors [19]. The control group was composed of normal kidney tissues from patients with ureteropelvic junction obstruction.

The expression levels of the following miRNAs (miR-99a, 99b, 100; 199th; 106a; 106b; 29a; 29b; 126; 200b) and their target genes (mTOR, HIF1-α, VHL, PDGF-β, VEGFA, VEGFR2) were correlated to ccRCC prognostic factors. Follow-up was 12 months at least and all samples had their confidentiality guaranteed.

Subjects provided written informed consent to participate the study and allowed their biological samples to be genetically analyzed. Approval for the study was given by the Institutional Board of Ethics (CAPPesq – Comissão de Ética para Análise de Projetos de Pesquisa) under the number 352891.

Storage of samples

The surgical specimens were collected immediately after surgery. Tumor fragments with almost 1cm^2 were placed into RNA later (Sigma-Aldrich, St. Louis, MO, USA) and stored at −80 °C. The samples were used for the analysis of miRNAs and target genes expression. We analyzed miR-99a, 99b, 100; 199th; 106a; 106b; 29a; 29b; 126 and 200b and their target genes mTOR, HIF1-α, VHL, PDGF-β, VEGFA and VEGFR2.

Table 1 Pathological and Clinical characteristics of the patients

Age (years)	
Average	63.2
Median	51
Gender	
Male	37 (66.0%)
Female	19 (33.9%)
Parcial Nephrectomy	16 (28.6%)
Radical Nephrectomy	40 (71.4%)
Fuhrman's Grade	
1–2	32 (57.2%)
3–4	24 (42.8%)
Microvascular Invasion	
Absent	44 (78.6%)
Present	12 (21.4%)
Pathological Stage (T)	
pT1-T2	26 (46.4%)
pT3-T4	30 (53.6%)
Pathological Stage (N)	
N0	54 (96.4%)
N1	02 (3.6%)
Pathological Stage (M)	
MO	48 (85.7%)
M1	08 (14.3%)

miRNA isolation of RNA and cDNA synthesis

We used the mirVana kit (Ambion, Austin, TX) for RNA and miRNA extraction, and cDNA was obtained using the TaqMan miRNA Reverse Transcription kit (Applied Biosystems, Foster City, CA) for miRNA and the High-Capacity cDNA Reverse Transcription kit for RNA according to the manufacturer's recommendations. A quantity of 10 ng miRNA was subjected to miRNAs of interest sequence-specific primer stem-loop reverse transcription. The PCR reaction for obtaining cDNA from miRNA was performed using Veriti equipment (Applied Biosystem, Foster City, CA) according to the following parameters: 30 min at 16 °C, 30 min at 42 °C, and 5 min at 85 °C. The same equipment was used to obtain cDNA from RNA with the following parameters: 10 min at 25 °C, 120 min at 37 °C, and 5 min at 85 °C.

cDNA synthesis

Complementary DNA (cDNA) was obtained using miRNA TaqMan®miRNA Reverse Transcription Kit (Applied Biosystems, Foster City, CA) with the following quantities: A quantity of 200 ng/l miRNA was diluted in 20 μL of water. 3uL of this volume was subjected to reverse transcription, which was added 7 μL mix containing the kit reagents: 0,15 μl DNTP mix 0,5 μl the enzyme reverse transcriptase, the enzyme 1,5 μl buffer of 0,19 μl RNAse inhibitor, 3,66 μl nuclease of free water and 1 μl of primer with stem-loop sequence to specific miRNA totaling 10 μl cDNA. The PCR reaction for obtaining cDNA from miRNA was performed using Veriti equipment (Applied Biosystem, Foster City, CA) according to the following parameters: 30 min at 16 °C, 30 min at 42 °C, and 5 min at 85 °C.

The same equipment was used to obtain cDNA from RNA with the following parameters: 10 min at 25 °C, 120 min at 37 °C, and 5 min at 85 °C. The RNA cDNA synthesis was performed using the High-Capacity cDNA Reverse Transcription® kit (Applied Biosystems) using reverse transcriptase and random primers Multiscribe™. The total RNA was diluted in nuclease-free H2O to a final volume of 20 μl and concentration of 500 μL/ng. In this volume were added 4 μl of random oligonucleotides (10X), 1,6 μl dNTP mix (25X), 4 μl of enzyme buffer (10X) 2 μl of the enzyme reverse transcriptase and 8,4 μl nuclease-free water. The solution was then subjected to temperature cycling (25 °C for 10 min, 37 °C for 120 min and 85 °C for 5 min) in Veriti® thermocycler (Applied Biosystems). At the end of both cDNA reactions were stored at −20 °C until use.

Analysis of miRNA and RNA expression

The miRNA and RNA expression levels were analyzed by qRT-PCR using an ABI 7500 Fast Real-Time PCR System (Applied Biosystems). The target sequences were amplified in a 10 μl reaction containing 5 μl TaqMan Universal PCR Master Mix, 0.5 μl TaqMan Gene Expression Assays, 1 μl cDNA, and 3.5 μl DNase-free water. The PCR cycling conditions were 2 min at 50 °C, 10 min at 95 °C, and 40 cycles of 15 s at 95 °C and 1 min at 60 ° C. All reactions were performed in duplicate, and TaqMan B2M and RNU 43 were utilized as the endogenous controls for gene and microRNA expression, respectively.

We used the CT method to calculate the relative expression of the microRNA and target genes using the formula CT = (CT target gene, ccRCC sample - CT endogenous control, ccRCC sample) – (CT target gene, Control sample - CT endogenous control, Control sample). The fold change in gene expression was calculated as 2^{-CT}.

Statistical analysis

Statistical analyzes were performed using SPSS 19.0 software for Windows (SPSS Inc., Chicago, USA). T student test or Mann-Whitney tests were used to compare the expression of miRNAs miR-99a, 99b, 100; 199th; 106a; 106b; 29a; 29b; 29c; 126; 200a, 200b with their target genes and ccRCC size, clinical stage and Fuhrman's grade nuclear. A p value ≤0.05 was considered statistically significant for all calculations.

Results

ccRCC angiogenesis gene and miRNA expression profile

The genes with the highest overexpression were VEGFA (84%) and PDGF (86%) while mTOR (88%) and VHL (86%) presented the lowest expressions (Table 2). Genes with moderate expression included: VEGFR1 (59%), VGFR2 (55%) and HIF1-α (57%) (Fig. 1). The miRNAs which were overexpressed were: miR-99a (80.0%), miR-99b (94.0%), miR-200b (95%), miR-106a (100%) and miR-106b (97%). miRNAs 126 and 100 appeared underexpressed in 81.0% and 67.0% of patients, respectively. miRNAs 199a, 29a and 29b presented a very heterogeneous expression (Fig. 2).

ccRCC angiogenesis gene and miRNA expression profile and prognostic factor

We studied the correlation between the ccRCC angiogenesis miRNAs and gene expressions with the prognostic factors. Considering gene expression, although not statistically significant we observed an increased of HIF1-α gene expression in patients with micro vascular invasion ($p = 0.08$). An increase in miR-200b correlated with high-risk tumors ($p = 0.01$) while miR-126 overexpression was associated with Fuhrman's low grade ($p = 0.03$) (Tables 3 and 4).

Univariate analysis revealed that pathological stage, tumor size, Fuhrman's nuclear grade and micro vascular invasion were significantly different in patients with high-risk tumors ($p = 0.000$; $p = 0.000$; $p = 0.000$; $p = 0.000$, respectively). To determine statistically significant clinical variables related to prognosis classification we used multivariate analysis to identify the importance of the isolated factors. Results showed that tumor size (0.475, 95% CI 0.436–0.777, $p = 0.000$), High Fuhrman's nuclear grade (0.492, 95% CI 0.479–0.780, $p = 0.000$), micro vascular invasion present (0.332, 95% CI 0.378–0.730, $p = 0.000$) and miR-200b greater than 13.06 (vs 13.06 or more) (0.159, 95% CI 0.076–0.331, $p = 0.003$) were independently related to the high-risk tumors.

ccRCC miRNA expression profile and target genes

A possible regulatory effect could be speculated for miR-99a overexpression (86%) and a mTOR underexpression (71.6%), A similar result was observed between VEGFA

Table 2 Gene expression and prognostic factors of ccRCC

	mTOR	VEGFR1	VEGFR2	VEGFA	HIF1A	PDGF	VHL
Low (*n* = 18)	0.63(1.32)	1.96(2.10)	3.17(6.12)	11.87 (16.14)	1.56 (2.27)	5.91 (11.18)	0.29 (1.04)
Intermediate (*n* = 29)	1.32 (5.43)	1.84(4.85)	1.11(1.38)	7.10 (4.47)	1.05 (1.29)	4.27 (9.39)	18.28 (87.65)
High *n* = 9	0.55 (0.63)	4.48(6.10)	1.51(2.26)	4.20 (4.58)	3.12 (5.58)	7.05 (9.53)	5.18 (6.73)
p	0.82[b]	0.37[b]	0.89[b]	0.18[b]	0.43[b]	0.76[b]	0.67[b]
Size ≥7 cm (*n* = 30)	0.52 (1.11)	1.74 (2.06)	2.41 (5.14)	10.33 (13,53)	1.27 (1.97)	6.62 (12.76)	0.39 (1.20)
Size <7 cm (*n* = 26)	1.54 (5.84)	2.69 (5.81)	1.31 (1.72)	6.32 (4.45)	1.74 (3.10)	3.56 (5.17)	18.84 (85.70)
p	0.97[a]	0.59[a]	0.87[a]	0.17[a]	0.50[a]	0.97[a]	0.12[a]
MVI absent (*n* = 44)	0.45 (0.95)	2.03(4.11)	2.08 (4.27)	9.77 (11.28)	1.10(1.63)	5.24(10.57)	12.54(72.60)
MVI present (*n* = 12)	3.39 (9.18)	2.75(4.76)	1.10 (1.71)	3.61(3.57)	2.91(4.36)	4.89(7.41)	3.66(5.73)
p	0.25[a]	0.61[a]	0.46[a]	0.57[a]	0.08[a]	0.91[a]	0.68[a]
Fuhrman's Grade I e II (*n* = 32)	1.43 (5.32)	1.57 (1.79)	2.43 (4.97)	9.86 (13.09)	1.54 (2.11)	4.39 (9.21)	0.19 (0.84)
Fuhrman's Grade III e IV (*n* = 24)	0.40 (0.52)	3.00 (6.10)	1.19 (1.68)	6.57 (4.81)	1.45 (3.06)	6.17 (10.97)	20.65 (89.28)
p	0.81[a]	0.45[a]	0.56[a]	0.26[a]	0.89[a]	0.51[a]	0.13[a]
Metastasis Absent (*n* = 48)	0.46(0.93)	1.81 (2.86)	1.96 (4.14)	8.53 (11.20)	1.54(2.76)	5.59 (10.78)	1.18 (3.44)
Metastasis Present (*n* = 8)	3.64(9.71)	4.03 (8.24)	1.41 (2.10)	7.98(4.54)	1.27(1.20)	3.05(3.04)	54.33(151.70)
p	0.82[a]	0.49[a]	0.71[a]	0.89[a]	0.77[a]	0.49[a]	0.79[a]
pT1–2 (*n* = 26)	0.51 (1.16)	1.33 (1.74)	2.47 (5.31)	10.12 (14.05)	1.47 (2.13)	7.07 (13.16)	0.20 (0.86)
pT3–4 (*n* = 30)	1.48 (5.62)	3.03 (5.63)	1.33 (1.72)	6.83 (4.67)	1.53 (2.95)	3.34 (4.95)	19.00 (85.67)
p	0.38[a]	0.51[a]	0.97[a]	0.26[a]	0.80[a]	0.16[a]	0.18[a]

[a]Mann-Whitney test [b] Kruskall-Wallis Test

(77% overexpressed) and miR-126 (78% under expressed) and miR-106a (100%) and 106b (97%), both overexpressed; with VHL gene underexpression (86%) (Figs. 1 and 2).

Discussion

ccRCC is considered the sixth leading cause of cancer deaths in Western countries. The incidence of this neoplasia is steadily increasing in the last years, each year; around 200,000 patients are diagnose with this disease resulting in approximately 100,000 deaths [20, 21]. The angiogenesis, process of development of capillaries from preexisting blood vessels, is essential for the growth of malignant tumors [22]. The VEGFA pathway plays an important role in regulating the process of angiogenesis, and von Hippel Lindau (VHL) gene loss or the hypoxia may explain the increased expression of this gene. In both situations, the HIF1-α gene moves to the cell nucleus, promoting VEGFA and PDGFa transcription [10, 23], As a result many drugs targeting angiogenesis have been developed and are currently being used to treat metastatic disease [24–26].

The importance of angiogenesis regulatory genes is not restricted to targeted therapy. Djordjevic et al. demonstrated that overexpression VEGFA gene was

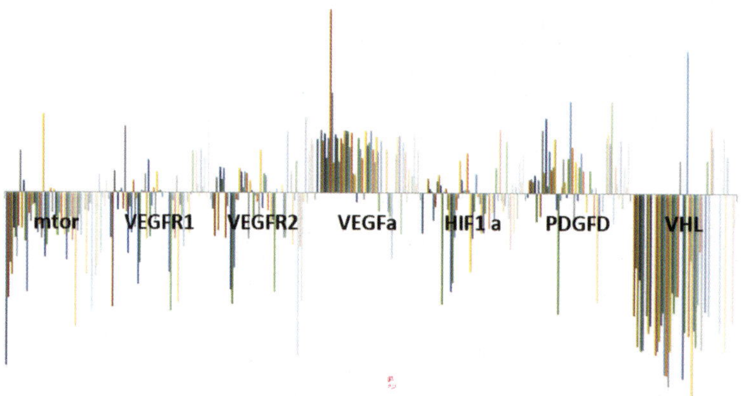

Fig. 1 Graphical representation of the expression levels of genes related to angiogenesis in ccRCC tissue compared with control

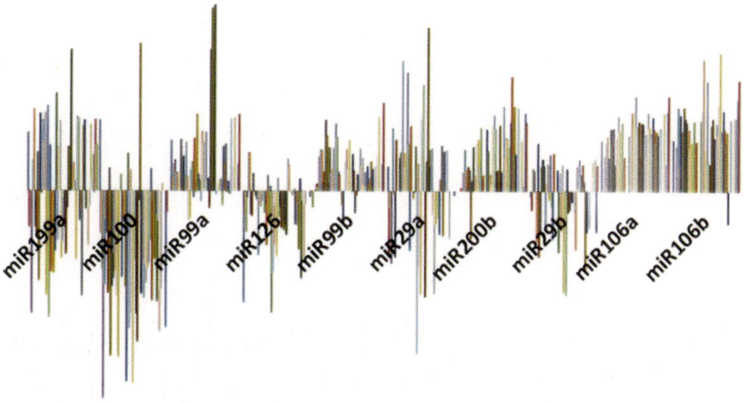

Fig. 2 Graphical representation of the expression levels of miRNAs related to angiogenesis in ccRCC tissue compared with control

associated with high Fuhrman's grade [27]. Also, Burgesser et al. correlated the expression of VEGFA, HIF1a, CD34 and Ki67 with most important prognostic factors in RCC in 83 patients. VEGFA expression was related to shorter survival rate after nephrectomy.

Our study is consistent with previous findings since we have found VEGFA overexpression that could be related to VHL under expression. It may be possible that in our cohort the mechanism involved in tumor development was VHL gene loss. However, we did not see HIF1-α overexpression in our cohort. On the contrary, HIF1-α was under expressed in 57% of our cases. However, when microvascular invasion was present, HIF1-α had higher expression compared to patients without microvascular invasion (no statistical significance).

Maybe, HIF1-α could be a marker of micro vascular invasion. Berghoffet. al. observed HIF1-α levels in brain metastasis samples from RCC, melanoma, breast, lung and colorectal cancer by immunohistochemistry. Increased HIF1-α levels were found in brain metastases from the RCC patients, and these had major effects on angiogenesis when compared to other tumors [28].

Table 3 miRNA expression and prognostic factors of ccRCC

	miR-199a	miR-100	miR-99a	miR-99b	miR-126	miR-29a	miR-29b
Low (*n* = 18)	60.12(104.18)	0.51(1.34)	17.89(34.38)	22.01(37.5)	2.10(4.1)	19.25(28.23)	3.94(7.35)
Intermediate (*n* = 29)	59.99(159.22)	5.62(25.37)	22.18 (49.15)	13.07(31.1)	0.96(2.9)	10.90(28.49)	2.72(2.89)
High *n* = 9	48.64(85.19)	0.77(1.75)	44.44(75.01)	65.13(159.)	0.37(0.3)	7.05(9.72)	5.30(2.91)
P	0.65[b]	0.63[b]	0.50[b]	0.17[b]	0.29[b]	0.57[b]	0.47[b]
Size ≥7 cm (*n* = 30)	61.13(91.26)	5.69(26.31)	19.77(39.93)	22.79(42.3)	1.57(3.6)	13.80(24.88)	3.48(6.21)
Size <7 cm (*n* = 26)	55.80(166.90)	0.90(2.77)	27.68(56.40)	23.59(84.3)	1.02(2.1)	12.62(28.97)	3.29(2.90)
P	0.88[a]	0.36[a]	0.57[a]	0.96[a]	0.49[a]	0.88[a]	0.12[a]
MVI absent (*n* = 44)	63.00(145.83)	3.90(20.87)	15.77(34.2)	17.73(35.1)	1.55(3.2)	15.24(29.69)	3.19(5.13)
MVI present (*n* = 12)	43.28(73.27)	0.88(1.80)	51.97(76.99)	43.48(127.)	0.36(0.3)	5.37(7.45)	4.30(3.50)
P	0.65[a]	0.63[a]	0.05[a]	0.72[a]	0,43[a]	0.33[a]	0.54[a]
Fuhrman's Grade I e II (*n* = 32)	39.95(87.23)	0.49(1.32)	23.61(45.13)	17.40(31.4)	1.92(3.7)	19.08(34.41)	3.63(6.04)
Fuhrman's Grade III e IV (*n* = 24)	79.35(169.23)	6.35(26.88)	23.28(52.73)	29.41(88.9)	0.55(1.2)	5.70(7.80)	3.11(3.06)
p	0.28[a]	0.33[a]	0.98[a]	0.51[a]	**0.03[a]**	0.10[a]	0,71[a]
pT1–2 (*n* = 26)	50.88(82.18)	6.36(27.40)	22.79(42.04)	23.35(43.8)	1.19(2.7)	14.85(25.19)	3.86(6.32)
pT3–4 (*n* = 30)	65.37(166.50)	0.69(2.59)	24.12(53.93)	23.01(81.1)	1.41(3.1)	11.84(28.52)	2.96(3.03)
P	0.69[a]	0.28[a]	0.92[a]	0.98[a]	0.78[a]	0.71[a]	0.51[a]
Metastasis Absent (*n* = 48)	49.76(84.62)	3.46(19.85)	19.01(39.85)	25.78(69.88)	1.17(2.54)	12.23(26.81)	3.61(418.33)
Metastasis Present (*n* = 8)	107.88(286.69)	1.89(4.94)	48.92(81.75)	6.41(6.35)	2.20(5.18)	18.95(28.74)	2.24(3.24)
p	0.25[a]	0.83[a]	0.12[a]	0.47[a]	0.39[a]	0.57[a]	0.46[a]

[a]Mann-Whitney test [b] Anova [b] Kruskall-Wallis Test
significant *p*-value are highlighted in bold

Table 4 Continuation of the miRNA expression and prognostic factors of ccRCC

	miR-200b	miR-106a	miR-106b
Low ($n = 18$)	43.39(89.17)	65.14(65.16)	159.44(171.94)
Intermediate ($n = 29$)	58.51(98.63)	110.15(141.57)	90.68(85.67)
High $n = 9$	563.01(1128.21)	202.94(270.20)	123.81(100.46)
P	**0.01[b]**	0.23[b]	0.31[b]
Size ≥7 cm ($n = 30$)	57.91(97.01)	79.23(68.51)	125.34(140.61)
Size <7 cm ($n = 26$)	162.81(545.59)	139.51(196.72)	102.81(92.03)
P	0.36[a]	0.766	0.58[a]
MVI absent ($n = 44$)	55.97(95.09)	93.38(127.07)	119.47(126.44)
MVI present ($n = 12$)	355.35(899.73)	173.31(213.58)	94.63(90.02)
p	0.53[a]	0.17[a]	0.17[a]
Fuhrman's Grade I e II ($n = 32$)	56.44(99.57)	103.91(158.18)	135.37(152.50)
Fuhrman's Grade III e IV ($n = 24$)	169.48(557.25)	113.84(143.83)	101.01(92.55)
P	0.33[a]	0.83[a]	0.40[a]
pT1–2 ($n = 26$)	48.99(94.76)	67.86(60.49)	115.03(103.12)
pT3–4 ($n = 30$)	161.87(521.68)	143.33(187.99)	115.59(136.84)
P	0.33[a]	0.11[a]	0.98[a]
Metastasis Absent ($n = 48$)	119.99(0.47)	117.25(5.12)	109.83(122.37)
Metastasis Present ($n = 8$)	50.56(114.07)	54.21(43.87)	149.38(113.15)
p	0.66[a]	0.38[a]	0.50[a]

[a]Mann-Whitney test [b]Anova [b] Kruskall-Wallis Test
significant *p*-value are highlighted in bold

In the present study, a moderate PDGF gene expression (63%) could be seen. Wang et al. through microarray tests on 174 patients studied the role of PDGF-B and its receptor (PDGFR-β) in RCC progression. As PDGF-B expression increased among the samples a significant reduction in risk of death was found. In addition, PDGF-B induction in xenograft mice models could inhibit tumor growth and reduce cell proliferation [29].

In our study, mTOR was under expressed in 88% of patients, but it was increased in patients with adverse prognostic factors such as micro vascular invasion and metastatic disease, although not statistically significant. Similarly, Haddad et al. proved that mTOR, expression was inversely correlated to bad prognostic factors like high grade tumors and presence of necrosis in patients with ccRCC treated by nephrectomy [30].

Many papers reported changes in gene expression as prognostic markers. However they cannot be applied yet into clinical practice due to inaccuracy in comparison to known classical factors [31]. Thus, the investigation of new molecular markers cannot be considered finished.

At this point miRNA expression profile in ccRCC is not limited to determine new prognostic factors but also to explain molecular mechanisms related to its development and progression.

As previously mentioned, MicroRNAs are small non-coding RNAs that regulate the expression of target genes by translation repression or transcriptional regulation, so playing a role in many biological pathways [2, 7]. miRNAs have been classified as tumor suppressor or oncogenes [2]. Actually, miRNAs are estimated to regulate 30% of all gene transcripts, it is highly possible that their aberrant expression will contribute to ccRCC formation by altering the balance between oncogenes and tumor suppressor genes. When oncogenic miRNAs are overexpress in tumors, tumor suppressor genes are downregulated [6, 32].

Genes previously studied may be controlled by one or more microRNAs. miR-126 was under expressed in 78% of cases and has VEGFA gene as target that was overexpressed in 77% of the cases. Similar results were described by Khella et al. in a study where the opposite expression of miR-126 and VEGFA was identified [33]. In addition, in this paper, we provide important evidence in supporting of miR-126 functioning as a tumor suppressor in ccRCC, because miR-126 underexpression was associated with higher histological grade. miR-126 is considered a highly conserved miRNA with increased expression in vascularized tissues [34]. This miRNA has been reported to be associated with tumorigenesis of many types of cancer [35]. Wong et al. [36] showed that lower level of miR-126 represents tumor recurrence and poor survival in the HCC patients who received liver transplant surgery confirming our data in ccRCC.

VEGFA receptors can be controlled by miR-200b [37]. In our study, miR-200b was overexpressed while VEGFA receptors were moderately under expressed. While VEGFR1 and 2 genes were not correlated with any of the prognostic factors, miR-200b had a positive correlation with high risk neoplasms according to the pathological triad [19]. This is the first study to report miR-200b as a prognostic factor in ccRCC. Also, in prostate cancer our group demonstrated that overexpression of miR-200b correlated with localized tumors while its low expression was associated with locally advanced tumors (pT3), Gleason > 8 and shorter free biochemical recurrence survival [38].

Another inverse correlation, which suggests a regulatory mechanism is the VHL gene underexpression (86%) and its regulatory miRNAs overexpression: miR-106a (100%) and miR-106b (97%). The posttranscriptional inhibition performed by miR-106a and miR-106b may represent another mechanism other than gene mutation or even increase the effects of the mutation nullifying the intact allele. This is supported by experiments, which have silenced the VHL gene, leading to an increased in HIF1 and VEGFA expression [39]. These miRNAs have been described as prognostic factors in RCC but we were unable to demonstrate any association [40].

Finally, we demonstrated that miR-99a was overexpressed in 80% of the samples whereas mTOR was decreased in 88%. Cui et al. studied the effects of miR-99a over mTOR gene by miR-99a transfection in cell lines and RCC xenograft models. The miR-99a acts by inhibiting mTOR gene expression in both cell lines and in experimental models. It was confirmed that the high expression of miR-99a interfered with the G-1 phase of the cell cycle and delayed cell proliferation, decreasing tumor progression in vivo [41]. miR-99a did not correlate with clinical or pathological characteristics in our study, but the antagonist relationship with mTOR gene corroborates with the study by Cui et al. [41].

Some limitations of our study should be mentioned. This is a retrospective study and the number of patients is low in the control group and would be interesting to validate the results with a larger number of controls and cases enrolled prospectively. In a prospective study, it becomes easier to add behavioral characteristics of patients, like smoking and obesity that all may potentially interfere with analysis of recurrence, which was not possible in our work because we did not have this information. Moreover, the validation of these results in serum sample and functional studies in RCC cell line can improve the quality of our study and the clinical applicability of the results.

Conclusion

In conclusion, we can postulate the role of miR-200b and miR-126 in the prognosis of this neoplasia. Our results support that in ccRCC there is an unbalance in the expression of genes and miRNAs related to process as angiogenesis, cell proliferation and survival. These finding besides helping us to understand the molecular mechanism of ccRCC gives us a reason to further investigate miR-126 and miR-200b as a potential biomarker and therapeutic target for this neoplasia.

Abbreviations

ccRCC: Clear cell renal cell carcinoma; cDNA: Complementary DNA; miRNAs: MicroRNAs; mRNAs: Messenger RNAs; VHL: Von Hipple-Lindau

Acknowledgements

CNPq 440564/2014-1.

Funding

This study was supported by CNPq (Conselho Nacional de desenvolvimento científico e tecnológico) under protocol number 440564/2014–1.

Authors' contributions

Study concept and design: STR, KRML, RCO. Acquisition of data: DKA, AJN, MS, WN. Analysis and interpretation of data: NIV, RCAP, RFI, VRG, DRM. Drafting of the manuscript: STR, RCO, RFI. Funding acquisition: NIV, RCAP. Critical revision of the manuscript for important intellectual content: STR, KRML, MS. All authors read and approved the final manuscript.

Competing interests

The authors declare that they have no competing interests.

Author details

[1]Laboratory of Medical Investigation (LIM55), Urology Department, University of Sao Paulo Medical School, Av. Dr. Arnaldo 455, 2° floor, room 2145, Sao Paulo 01246-903, Brazil. [2]Uro-Oncology Group, Urology Department, University of Sao Paulo Medical School and Institute of Cancer Estate of Sao Paulo (ICESP), Sao Paulo, Brazil.

References

1. Bukowski RM. Prognostic factors for survival in metastatic renal cell carcinoma: update 2008. Cancer. 2009;115(10 Suppl):2273–81.
2. Schaefer A, Stephan C, Busch J, Yousef GM, Jung K. Diagnostic, prognostic and therapeutic implications of microRNAs in urologic tumors. *Nature reviews Urology*. 2010;7(5):286–97.
3. Adams BD, Kasinski AL, Slack FJ. Aberrant regulation and function of microRNAs in cancer. Current biology : CB. 2014;24(16):R762–76.
4. Suarez Y, Sessa WC. MicroRNAs as novel regulators of angiogenesis. Circ Res. 2009;104(4):442–54.
5. Bridge G, Monteiro R, Henderson S, Emuss V, Lagos D, Georgopoulou D, Patient R, Boshoff C. The microRNA-30 family targets DLL4 to modulate endothelial cell behavior during angiogenesis. Blood. 2012;120(25):5063–72.
6. Catto JW, Alcaraz A, Bjartell AS, De Vere White R, Evans CP, Fussel S, Hamdy FC, Kallioniemi O, Mengual L, Schlomm T, et al. MicroRNA in prostate, bladder, and kidney cancer: a systematic review. Eur Urol. 2011;59(5):671–81.
7. Schaefer A, Jung M, Kristiansen G, Lein M, Schrader M, Miller K, Stephan C, Jung K. MicroRNAs and cancer: current state and future perspectives in urologic oncology. Urol Oncol. 2010;28(1):4–13.
8. Ru Y, Dancik GM, Theodorescu D. Biomarkers for prognosis and treatment selection in advanced bladder cancer patients. Curr Opin Urol. 2011;21(5): 420–7.

9. Fendler A, Stephan C, Yousef GM, Jung K. MicroRNAs as regulators of signal transduction in urological tumors. Clin Chem. 2011;57(7):954–68.
10. Longo R, D'Andrea MR, Sarmiento R, Salerno F, Gasparini G. Integrated therapy of kidney cancer. *Annals of oncology : official journal of the European Society for Medical Oncology / ESMO.* 2007;6(18 Suppl):vi141–8.
11. Smaldone MC, Maranchie JK. Clinical implications of hypoxia inducible factor in renal cell carcinoma. Urol Oncol. 2009;27(3):238–45.
12. Zhang C. MicroRNAs in vascular biology and vascular disease. J Cardiovasc Transl Res. 2010;3(3):235–40.
13. van Solingen C, Seghers L, Bijkerk R, Duijs JM, Roeten MK, van Oeveren-Rietdijk AM, Baelde HJ, Monge M, Vos JB, de Boer HC, et al. Antagomir-mediated silencing of endothelial cell specific microRNA-126 impairs ischemia-induced angiogenesis. J Cell Mol Med. 2009;13(8A):1577–85.
14. Grundmann S, Hans FP, Kinniry S, Heinke J, Helbing T, Bluhm F, Sluijter JP, Hoefer I, Pasterkamp G, Bode C, et al. MicroRNA-100 regulates neovascularization by suppression of mammalian target of rapamycin in endothelial and vascular smooth muscle cells. Circulation. 2011;123(9):999–1009.
15. Roy S, Sen CK: miRNA in wound inflammation and angiogenesis. *Microcirculation (New York, NY : 1994)* 2012, 19(3):224–232.
16. Li Y, Fan L, Liu S, Liu W, Zhang H, Zhou T, Wu D, Yang P, Shen L, Chen J, et al. The promotion of bone regeneration through positive regulation of angiogenic-osteogenic coupling using microRNA-26a. Biomaterials. 2013; 34(21):5048–58.
17. Zaravinos A, Radojicic J, Lambrou GI, Volanis D, Delakas D, Stathopoulos EN, Spandidos DA. Expression of miRNAs involved in angiogenesis, tumor cell proliferation, tumor suppressor inhibition, epithelial-mesenchymal transition and activation of metastasis in bladder cancer. J Urol. 2012;188(2):615–23.
18. Yuan HX, Zhang JP, Kong WT, Liu YJ, Lin ZM, Wang WP, Guo JM. Elevated microRNA-185 is associated with high vascular endothelial growth factor receptor 2 expression levels and high microvessel density in clear cell renal cell carcinoma. Tumour Biol. 2014;35(12):12757–63.
19. Dall'Oglio MF, Antunes AA, Sarkis AS, Crippa A, Leite KR, Lucon AM, Srougi M. Microvascular tumour invasion in renal cell carcinoma: the most important prognostic factor. BJU Int. 2007;100(3):552–5.
20. Miyamoto H, Miller JS, Fajardo DA, Lee TK, Netto GJ, Epstein JI. Non-invasive papillary urothelial neoplasms: the 2004 WHO/ISUP classification system. Pathol Int. 2010;60(1):1–8.
21. Montironi R, Santinelli A, Pomante R, Mazzucchelli R, Colanzi P, Filho AL, Scarpelli M. Morphometric index of adult renal cell carcinoma. Comparison with the Fuhrman grading system. Virchows Archiv : an international journal of pathology. 2000;437(1):82–9.
22. Eklund L, Bry M, Alitalo K. Mouse models for studying angiogenesis and lymphangiogenesis in cancer. Mol Oncol. 2013;7(2):259–82.
23. Ebbinghaus SW, Gordon MS. Renal cell carcinoma: rationale and development of therapeutic inhibitors of angiogenesis. Hematol Oncol Clin North Am. 2004;18(5):1143–59. ix-x
24. Choueiri TK, Bukowski RM, Rini BI. The current role of angiogenesis inhibitors in the treatment of renal cell carcinoma. Semin Oncol. 2006;33(5): 596–606.
25. Ljungberg BJ, Jacobsen J, Rudolfsson SH, Lindh G, Grankvist K, Rasmuson T. Different vascular endothelial growth factor (VEGF), VEGF-receptor 1 and −2 mRNA expression profiles between clear cell and papillary renal cell carcinoma. BJU Int. 2006;98(3):661–7.
26. Posadas EM, Limvorasak S, Sharma S, Figlin RA. Targeting angiogenesis in renal cell carcinoma. Expert Opin Pharmacother. 2013;14(16):2221–36.
27. Djordjevic G, Mozetic V, Mozetic DV, Licul V, Ilijas KM, Mustac E, Oguic R, Fuckar Z, Jonjic N. Prognostic significance of vascular endothelial growth factor expression in clear cell renal cell carcinoma. Pathol Res Pract. 2007; 203(2):99–106.
28. Berghoff AS, Ilhan-Mutlu A, Dinhof C, Magerle M, Hackl M, Widhalm G, Hainfellner JA, Dieckmann K, Pichler J, Hutterer M, et al. Differential role of angiogenesis and tumour cell proliferation in brain metastases according to primary tumour type: analysis of 639 cases. Neuropathol Appl Neurobiol. 2015;41(2):e41–55.
29. Wang W, Qi L, Tan M, Zhang Z, Du J, Wei X, Yao X. Effect of platelet-derived growth factor-B on renal cell carcinoma growth and progression. *Urologic oncology.* 2015;33(4):168.e117–27.
30. Haddad AQ, Kapur P, Singla N, Raman JD, Then MT, Nuhn P, Buchner A, Bastian P, Seitz C, Shariat SF, et al. Validation of mammalian target of rapamycin biomarker panel in patients with clear cell renal cell carcinoma. Cancer. 2015;121(1):43–50.
31. Bui MH, Zisman A, Pantuck AJ, Han KR, Wieder J, Belldegrun AS. Prognostic factors and molecular markers for renal cell carcinoma. Expert Rev Anticancer Ther. 2001;1(4):565–75.
32. Chow TF, Youssef YM, Lianidou E, Romaschin AD, Honey RJ, Stewart R, Pace KT, Yousef GM. Differential expression profiling of microRNAs and their potential involvement in renal cell carcinoma pathogenesis. Clin Biochem. 2010;43(1–2):150–8.
33. Khella HW, White NM, Faragalla H, Gabril M, Boazak M, Dorian D, Khalil B, Antonios H, Bao TT, Pasic MD, et al. Exploring the role of miRNAs in renal cell carcinoma progression and metastasis through bioinformatic and experimental analyses. Tumour Biol. 2012;33(1):131–40.
34. Nikolic I, Plate KH, Schmidt MH. EGFL7 meets miRNA-126: an angiogenesis alliance. J Angiogenes Res. 2010;2(1):9.
35. Harris TA, Yamakuchi M, Ferlito M, Mendell JT, Lowenstein CJ. MicroRNA-126 regulates endothelial expression of vascular cell adhesion molecule 1. Proc Natl Acad Sci U S A. 2008;105(5):1516–21.
36. Wong QW, Lung RW, Law PT, Lai PB, Chan KY, To KF, Wong N. MicroRNA-223 is commonly repressed in hepatocellular carcinoma and potentiates expression of Stathmin1. Gastroenterology. 2008;135(1):257–69.
37. Silva-Santos RM, Costa-Pinheiro P, Luis A, Antunes L, Lobo F, Oliveira J, Henrique R, Jeronimo C. MicroRNA profile: a promising ancillary tool for accurate renal cell tumour diagnosis. Br J Cancer. 2013;109(10):2646–53.
38. Katz B, Reis ST, Viana NI, Morais DR, Moura CM, Dip N, Silva IA, Iscaife A, Srougi M, Leite KR. Comprehensive study of gene and microRNA expression related to epithelial-mesenchymal transition in prostate cancer. PLoS One. 2014;9(11):e113700.
39. Zhang T, Niu X, Liao L, Cho EA, Yang H. The contributions of HIF-target genes to tumor growth in RCC. PLoS One. 2013;8(11):e80544.
40. Slaby O, Jancovicova J, Lakomy R, Svoboda M, Poprach A, Fabian P, Kren L, Michalek J, Vyzula R. Expression of miRNA-106b in conventional renal cell carcinoma is a potential marker for prediction of early metastasis after nephrectomy. Journal of experimental & clinical cancer research : CR. 2010; 29:90.
41. Cui L, Zhou H, Zhao H, Zhou Y, Xu R, Xu X, Zheng L, Xue Z, Xia W, Zhang B, et al. MicroRNA-99a induces G1-phase cell cycle arrest and suppresses tumorigenicity in renal cell carcinoma. BMC Cancer. 2012;12:546.

Positive surgical margins and biochemical recurrence following minimally-invasive radical prostatectomy – An analysis of outcomes from a UK tertiary referral centre

Ashwin Sachdeva[1,2], Rajan Veeratterapillay[1], Antonia Voysey[1], Katherine Kelly[1], Mark I. Johnson[1], Jonathan Aning[1] and Naeem A. Soomro[1,2*]

Abstract

Background: Positive surgical margins are a strong prognostic marker of disease outcome following radical prostatectomy, though prior evidence is largely from a PSA-screened population. We therefore aim to evaluate the biochemical recurrence in men with positive surgical margins (PSM) after minimally-invasive radical prostatectomy (MIRP) in a UK tertiary centre.

Methods: Retrospective study of men undergoing laparoscopic or robotic-assisted radical prostatectomy between 2002 and 2014. Men with positive surgical margins (PSM) were identified and their biochemical recurrence (BCR) rate compared with men without PSM. The primary outcome measures were BCR rates and time to BCR. Cox regression was used to estimate adjusted hazard ratios for biochemical recurrence rate (BCR), accounting for potential confounders.

Results: Five hundred ninety-two men were included for analysis. Pre-operative D'Amico risk stratification showed 37.5%, 53.3% and 9.3% of patients in the low, intermediate and high-risk groups, respectively. On final pathological analysis, the proportion of patients with local staging pT2, pT3a and pT3b was 68.8%, 25.2% and 6.1% respectively. Overall positive margin rate was 30.6%. On multivariate analysis, the only pre-operative factor associated with PSM was age >65years. Patients with PSM were more likely to have higher tumour volume and more advanced pathological local stage. The BCR rate was 10.7% in margin-positive patients and 5.1% in margin-negative patients, at median 4.4-year follow-up. Upon multivariate analysis, high pre-operative PSA and high Gleason group were the only significant predictors of BCR (P<0.05).

Conclusions: In comparison to patients with negative surgical margins, those with PSM do not translate into worse medium-term oncological outcomes in the majority of cases amongst our cohort. We found that high pre-operative PSA and high Gleason group were the only significant predictors of BCR.

Background

Surgical margin status at pathological analysis after radical prostatectomy for prostate cancer is a key metric to define the oncological adequacy of prostate resection [1]. With active surveillance considered the primary management option for low-risk prostate cancer, radical prostatectomy (RP) is increasingly being used for intermediate or high-risk patients, as part of multi-modal therapy [2]. Positive surgical margin (PSM) rates have been associated with RP for higher-risk disease with reported incidence between 11-48% [1–3]. PSM has been highlighted as a risk factor for disease progression after surgery and, as such, margin status has been incorporated as a component of multiple prostate cancer outcome prediction models [4–6].

* Correspondence: naeem.soomro@nuth.nhs.uk
[1]Department of Urology, Freeman Hospital, Newcastle-upon-Tyne Hospitals NHS Foundation Trust, Newcastle-upon-Tyne, UK
[2]Northern Institute for Cancer Research, Newcastle University, Newcastle-upon-Tyne, UK

In contemporary practice, patients with the finding of PSM alone at RP can be managed with PSA surveillance, adjuvant or salvage radiotherapy [7] or entered into clinical trials (for example RADICALS) [1, 4]. For patients with biochemical relapse (BCR) following RP, the European Association of Urology advises the use of salvage radiotherapy with at least 66Gy at a PSA level of < 0.5ng/ml [8].

In a recent report regarding contemporary MIRP in the UK, the authors reported a trend towards increasing use of MIRP amongst patients with high risk disease, but with a high positive surgical margin rate of 33.6% amongst patients with pT3 disease [9]. However, longer-term oncological outcome data following MIRP in the UK are lacking. Furthermore, only a small percentage of patients in the UK are diagnosed with prostate cancer by PSA screening [10], in comparison to the widespread adoption of routine PSA screening in USA and some European countries [11]. Therefore, oncological outcomes of RP in a relatively unscreened UK population may be hypothesised to vary from those previously reported for screened cohorts.

In this report we describe the PSM rates in a consecutive series of patients undergoing minimally invasive radical prostatectomy at a large UK tertiary referral centre. We explore the factors predicting PSM and assess the medium term oncological outcomes as regards to biochemical recurrence rates.

Methods

Study population

Following approval by the local audit and research department, consecutive patients undergoing minimally invasive radical prostatectomy (MIRP - laparoscopic or robotic assisted) at our institution (between January 2002 and April 2014) were identified from a departmental database. Excised specimens underwent centralised pathological review. Patients undergoing open radical prostatectomy during this period were excluded. Retrospective review of their medical electronic records, histopathology data and biochemistry investigations was conducted. Data extracted included pre-operative parameters (demographics, PSA, prostate biopsy Gleason score, clinical stage), operative details (technique and whether lymphadenectomy was performed) and postoperative radical prostatectomy pathology (presence of positive surgical, tumour Gleason score, tumour stage, tumour volume). Patients who had detectable PSA (ie >0.1ng/mol) 12 weeks post-operatively, less than 12 months of follow-up or those for whom PSA follow-up data were unavailable, were excluded from this study.

Follow-up and biochemical recurrence

PSA follow-up data were captured. BCR was defined as undetectable PSA post radical prostatectomy, which subsequently rose to ≥ 0.2ng/mol. For patients with biochemical recurrence, the need and timing of adjuvant therapy (if any) was recorded.

Statistical analysis

Patient and disease characteristics between patients stratified by incidence of surgical margins and biochemical recurrence were compared using the Chi square test. Student's T test was used to compare means and Mann-Whitney U test was used to compare medians. Potential co-variates including age, pre-operative PSA, Gleason score, and tumour volume, were included in a Cox regression model to estimate adjusted hazard ratios for positive surgical margins and biochemical recurrence. Kaplan-Meier survival curves were built using the time of biochemical recurrence as a failure event. A false discovery rate adjustment was applied for multiple comparisons. Results were deemed to be statistically significant if p value was less than 0.05.

Results

The overall positive surgical margin rate was 30.6%

In total 592 men underwent minimally invasive radical prostatectomy (MIRP) between 2002 and 2012. Median age at MIRP was 63 years (IQR 58-67 years). Median PSA at diagnosis was 7.9ng/ml (IQR 5.7-11.8ng/ml) and median follow-up was 52.8 months (IQR 25.0-73.6 months). Demographic data is summarised in Table 1. Pre-operative D'Amico risk stratification noted 37.5% of patients in the low-risk group, 53.3% in the intermediate-risk group and 9.3% in the high-risk group. 393 patients underwent laparoscopic RP (LRP) and 199 underwent robotic-assisted RP (RARP). On final pathological analysis, the proportion of patients with local staging pT2, pT3a and pT3b was 68.8%, 25.2% and 6.1% respectively. Lymph node sampling was performed on 41.7% patients (247 of 592), of whom 19 patients (8.0%) had evidence of lymph node involvement. Positive surgical margins (PSM) were identified in 181/592 (30.6%) excised pathological specimens.

PSM was associated with older age but not biopsy Gleason score

On univariate analysis (Table 1), the only preoperative factors associated with PSM were patient age >65years and PSA >10ng/ml. Patients with PSM were also more likely to have higher Gleason score on final pathology, higher tumour volume and more advanced pathological local stage. The overall PSM was marginally higher following RARP, as compared to LRP (36.2% vs 27.7%, p = 0.05). There was no significant change in PSM over time (LRP: p = 0.5; RARP: p = 0.4).

On multivariate logistic regression (Table 2), key factors predictive of PSM were patient age >65 years (OR 2.11, 95% CI 1.41-3.15), higher pT stage (pT3a OR

Table 1 Patient & disease characteristics overall, stratified by surgical margin status

Variable	Patients with positive margins	Patients with negative margins	Overall	*p* value
N (%)	181 (30.6)	411 (69.4)	592	
Patient age at time of surgery				
Under 65 years	82 (45.3)	252 (61.3)	334 (56.4)	0.009
65 years and above	99 (54.7)	159 (38.7)	258 (43.6)	
Pre-op PSA				
0.0-9.9	103 (57.9)	276 (68.3)	379 (65.1)	0.03
10.0-19.9	58 (32.6)	110 (27.2)	168 (28.9)	
20.0 and above	17 (9.6)	19 (4.5)	35 (6.0)	
Missing	2	7	9	
Gleason score on biopsy				
Group 1 (GS 2-6)	81 (44.8)	191 (46.5)	272 (46.0)	0.5
Group 2 (GS 3+4)	74 (40.9)	165 (40.2)	239 (40.4)	
Group 3 (GS 4+3)	20 (11.0)	35 (8.5)	55 (9.3)	
Group 4 (GS 8)	3 (1.7)	16 (3.9)	19 (3.2)	
Group 5 (GS 9-10)	3 (1.7)	4 (1.0)	7 (1.2)	
Pathological Gleason score				
Group 1 (GS 2-6)	26 (14.4)	117 (28.5)	143 (24.2)	<0.001
Group 2 (GS 3+4)	92 (50.8)	218 (54.0)	310 (52.4)	
Group 3 (GS 4+3)	33 (18.2)	40 (9.7)	73 (12.3)	
Group 4 (GS 8)	20 (11.1)	31 (7.5)	51 (8.6)	
Group 5 (GS 9-10)	10 (5.5)	5 (1.2)	15 (2.5)	
Pathological tumour stage				
pT2	89 (49.2)	318 (77.4)	407 (68.8)	<0.001
pT3a	68 (37.6)	81 (19.7)	149 (25.2)	
pT3b	24 (13.3)	12 (2.9)	36 (6.1)	
Lymph node involvement	10 (11.8)	7 (4.6)	17 (7.2)	0.06
Tumour volume of excised specimen				
Median (IQR)	3.9 (1.8-6.7)	2.02 (0.81-4.0)	2.4 (1.0-5.1)	<0.001
Surgical approach				
LRP	109 (60.2)	284 (69.1)	393 (66.4)	0.05
RARP	72 (39.8)	157 (30.9)	199 (33.6)	
Post-operative PSA*				
Biochemical recurrence (%)	15/140 (10.7)	18 of 350 (5.1)	33 of 490 (6.7)	0.045
Median time to BCR (in months, IQR)*	10.9 (3.7-24.5)	13.1 (4.9-37.7)	12.1 (4.9-31.4)	0.5

*PSA data available for 532 of 592 patients. 490 patients had undetectable PSA post-operatively

2.69, 95% CI 1.73-4.18; pT3b OR 6.35, 95% CI 2.77-14.57), larger tumour volume (OR 1.09, 95% CI 1.03-1.16), and the use of a robotic-approach (OR 2.52, 95% CI 1.18-5.37).

The biochemical recurrence rate in PSM was 10.7%

PSA follow up data were available for 532 patients (89.9% of the cohort, Fig. 1) at a median follow-up of 30.3 months (16.0 - 52.7). Of these, 42 patients had detectable PSA post-operatively and were therefore excluded. In comparison to patients with undetectable PSA, these 42 patients tended to have more aggressive disease (Additional file 1: Table S1).

The overall biochemical recurrence rate (BCR) was 6.7% with a median time to BCR of 13.3 (11.6-33.5) months. Comparing PSM and NSM, the BCR at median follow-up of 52.8 months (IQR 25.0-73.6 months) was 10.7% and 5.1% respectively (p 0.026, Fig. 2). There was no difference in time to BCR between patients with PSM and NSM with a median time to

Table 2 Logistic regression results with 95% CI & p values (what factors predict PSM)

	Univariate analysis			Multivariate analysis		
Variable	OR	95% CI	*p* value	OR	95% CI	*p* value
Year of procedure						
2002-2009	1.00	-	-	1.00	-	-
2010-2012	1.15	0.76-1.73	0.5	0.72	0.43-1.19	0.2
2013-2014	1.25	0.79-1.96	0.4	0.37	0.15-0.93	0.03
Patient age at time of surgery						
Under 65 years	1.00	-	-	1.00	-	-
65 years & above	1.89	1.33-2.70	<0.001	2.11	1.41-3.15	<0.001
Pre-op PSA						
0.0-9.9	1.00	-	-	1.00	-	-
10.0-19.9	1.41	0.96-2.09	0.2	1.05	0.67-1.65	0.8
20.0 and above	2.53	1.26-5.10	0.02	1.30	0.56-3.00	0.5
Gleason score on biopsy						
Group 1 (GS 2-6)	1.00	-	-	1.00	-	-
Group 2 (GS 3+4)	1.06	0.72-1.54	0.8	0.75	0.48-1.17	0.2
Group 3 (GS 4+3)	1.35	0.73-2.47	0.4	0.86	0.43-1.69	0.6
Group 4 (GS 8)	0.44	0.13-1.56	0.3	0.22	0.05-0.90	0.04
Group 5 (GS 9-10)	1.77	0.39-8.08	0.6	0.86	0.15-4.89	0.9
Pathological tumour stage						
pT2	1.00	-	-	1.00	-	-
pT3a	3.00	2.01-4.47	<0.001	2.69	1.73-4.18	<0.001
pT3b	7.15	3.44-14.85	<0.001	6.35	2.77-14.57	<0.001
Median tumour volume of excised specimen	1.16	1.10-1.22	<0.001	1.09	1.03-1.16	0.005
Surgical modality						
LRP	1.00	-	-	1.00	-	-
RARP	1.48	1.03-2.13	0.08	2.52	1.18-5.37	0.02

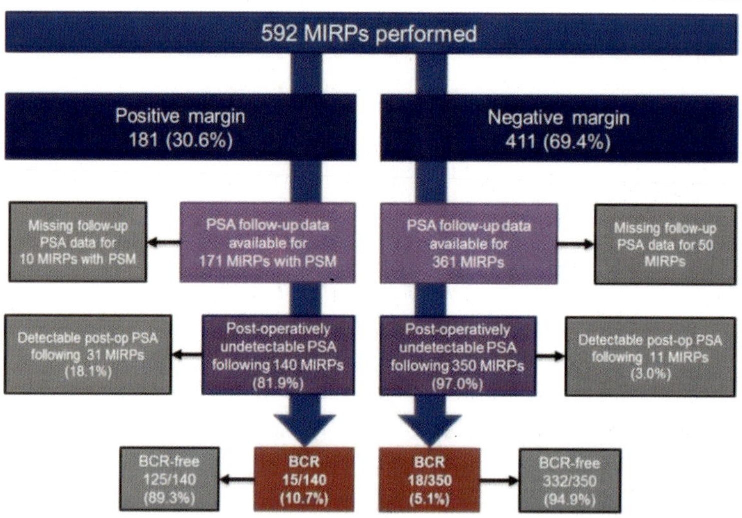

Fig. 1 Flow diagram of study population

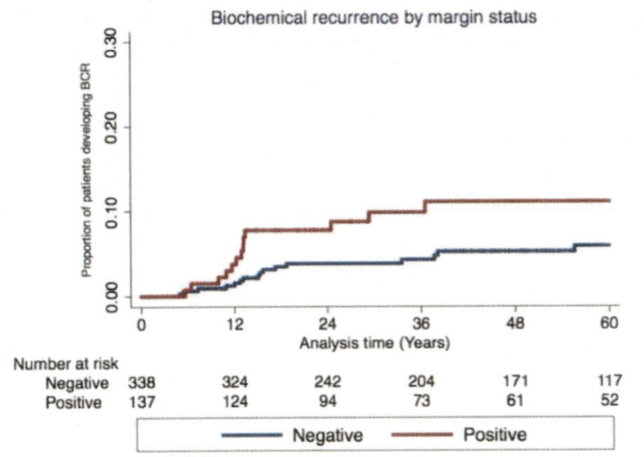

Fig. 2 Kaplan Meier survival analysis of time to biochemical recurrence stratified by margin status

BCR of 13.1 (10.8-29.3) months and 15.5 (12.0-37.7) respectively (p 0.49).

Upon univariate analysis, pre-operative PSA greater than 10ng/ml, larger tumour volume and PSM were associated with BCR (Table 3). However, upon multivariate Cox regression analysis to adjust for potential confounders, higher pre-operative PSA and higher Gleason group disease were associated with BCR (Additional file 1: Table S2). Of note, margin status was not associated with development of BCR.

Discussion

This is the largest reported single-centre UK series of oncological outcomes, including biochemical recurrence rates, following MIRP. The overall PSM in this cohort of 592 patients was 30.6%. Upon adjustment for potential confounders, the only variables associated with greater incidence of PSM were older age at time of surgery, pT3 stage disease, higher tumour volume, and use of a RARP approach.

Comparative data indicate that the incidence of positive margins is equivalent among the open, laparoscopic, and RARP approaches [12]. A recent meta-analysis reported a 15% mean rate of PSMs in RARP series published between 2008 and 2011, with a range of 6.5–32% [3]. PSM rates in contemporary series range between 10.4 to 31.1%. The largest report, by Wright et al, was based on a database study of 65,633 patients having radical prostatectomy. PSMs were reported in 21.2% of cases and were more common in pT3a than pT2 tumours (44% vs 18%, p <0.001) and higher grade tumours (28% vs 18%, p <0.001) [13]. Reported RARP series have noted a PSM rate of 15.7-29.5% [9, 14–18]. Preoperative PSA, prostate volume on trans-rectal ultrasound, clinical T (cT) stage, and pathological stage (pT2 vs pT3) have been reported as independent predictors of the presence of any PSM, while cT stage and biopsy Gleason score have been reported as predictors of posterolateral PSM [14, 15].

From a UK perspective, of all 2,163 radical prostatectomies (54.6% laparoscopic and 19.6% RARP) entered in the British Association of Urological Surgeons database in 2011, the overall PSM was 42.3% with no difference between laparoscopic (26.6%) and robotic (22.5%) cases [19]. Our findings of PSM rates are comparable to published reports on minimally invasive prostatectomy. We do note however a higher PSM rate in patients undergoing robotic surgery (36.2%) in our cohort and this may be representative of a learning curve effect. It is worth noting an increasing proportion of patients being offered surgery for high-risk disease. A recent study of robotic RP in this group was reported by Kang et al who reported a 25.1% PSM rate, and that higher tumour stage and volume were associated with PSM [20]. Furthermore, a recent UK series reported that accumulated experience with robotic RP was associated with a temporal decrease in PSM rate (22.5% in 2005-2008 vs 19.8% in 2013-15), despite an increase in the proportion of patients having surgery for higher risk disease [9].

In our study, patients with PSM were more likely to develop biochemical recurrence (10.7%) versus those with negative margins (5.1%). The median time to BCR for patients with PSM was 13.1 months. On multivariate analysis, factors predicting biochemical failure were high pre-operative PSA and higher pathological Gleason group at MIRP. The oncological implications of a positive surgical margin at radical prostatectomy are difficult to predict [1]. Nine large contemporary studies have investigated the impact of PSMs on biochemical recurrence rates, metastatic progression and prostate-cancer mortality (Table 4). Whilst all studies found PSMs to be associated with a higher risk of BCR, data on time to metastatic progression and death were less clear. Increased risk of PCa death was noted in men with positive compared with negative surgical margins, at 4.2 year [13] and 10 year follow-up [21]. However, this impact was fairly marginal relative to the impact of Gleason score and tumour stage on pathological assessment of the excised prostate [21]. From the literature, it is apparent that PSM increases the risk of disease recurrence but the range of risk and the time to event (death from prostate cancer) are very wide, depending mostly on the presence or absence of other risk modifiers. Even if the risk is real, competing causes of mortality may obscure the predictive value of PSMs for death due to PCa [1].

Biochemical recurrence is a marker of disease progression and associated with poor prognosis. Previous reports of BCR in patients with PSM are variable due to differing lengths of follow-up and surgical approach. Studies with patients predominantly undergoing open RP have reported a BCR rate of 26.7% at 6 years [22] to

Table 3 Patient & disease characteristics of patients with PSM, stratified by biochemical recurrence at end of study period

Variable	BCR-free	BCR	All PSMs	*p* value
N (%)	125 (89.3)	15 (10.7)	140	
Patient age at time of surgery				
Under 65 years	60 (48.0)	7 (46.7)	67 (47.9)	0.4
65 years and above	65 (52.0)	8 (53.3)	73 (52.1)	
Pre-op PSA				
0.0-9.9	81 (64.8)	4 (26.7)	85 (60.7)	0.003
10.0-19.9	38 (30.4)	7 (46.7)	45 (32.1)	
20.0 and above	6 (4.8)	4 (26.7)	10 (7.2)	
Pathological Gleason score				
Group 1 (GS 2-6)	20 (16.0)	0	20 (14.3)	0.4
Group 2 (GS 3+4)	59 (55.2)	8 (53.3)	77 (55.0)	
Group 3 (GS 4+3)	18 (14.4)	5 (33.3)	23 (16.4)	
Group 4 (GS 8)	13 (10.4)	2 (13.3)	15 (10.7)	
Group 5 (GS 9-10)	5 (4.0)	0	5 (3.6)	
Surgical approach				
LRP	75 (60.0)	10 (66.7)	85 (60.7)	0.6
RARP	50 (40.0)	5 (33.3)	55 (39.3)	
Tumour volume of excised specimen				
Median (IQR)	3.7 (1.7-6.6)	5.1 (2.5-10.2)	3.8 (1.8-6.7)	<0.001
Pathological tumour stage				
pT2	67 (53.6)	5 (33.3)	72 (51.4)	0.4
pT3a	44 (35.2)	6 (40.0)	50 (35.7)	
pT3b	14 (11.2)	4 (26.7)	18 (12.9)	
Lymph node involvement	7 (13.5)	0 (0.0)	0 (11.5)	0.4
Margin location				
Apex	33 (26.4)	4 (26.7)	37 (26.4)	0.4
Base	23 (18.4)	1 (6.7)	24 (17.1)	
Multifocal	19 (15.2)	5 (33.3)	24 (17.1)	
Other	50 (40.0)	5 (33.3)	55 (39.3)	
Adjuvant therapy				
Salvage radiotherapy	12 of 41 (29.3)	10 of 14 (64.1)	22 of 55 (40.0)	
Radiotherapy & hormones	0	1 of 14 (7.2)	1 of 55 (1.8)	
Missing	84	1	85	

Note: Patients with detectable PSA or missing PSA data post-operatively were excluded

54.3% at 10 years [21]. In contrast, shorter follow-up data is available for patients with PSM following MIRP, with a BCR rate ranging from 6.2% at 1 year [14] to 29.0% at 6.3 years [23]. A recent multi-institutional study reported outcomes of over 5000 patients following RARP and reported BCR rates of 14.1% at a median follow-up of 4.2 years [18]. Our results are within this range and, based upon previous data, it is likely that additional patients may go on to develop BCR at longer follow-up.

The choice of therapeutic strategy for patients with PSM remains controversial. Recent evidence suggests that adjuvant radiotherapy may lead to a 50–60% reduction in the risk of PSA progression in men with pathologically advanced prostate cancer [24, 25]. However, not all men with PSMs are destined to have treatment failure and indeed the majority of men with isolated PSMs, with or without extra-prostatic extension, are cured after RP alone [1, 3]. Therefore, recommending adjuvant radiotherapy to all men with

Table 4 Comparison of PSM & BCR with previously published data

		Ref	Study period	Total number of patients	Pre-operative PSA mean (median) in ng/mL	Median tumour vol. (cc)	Surgical approach			PSM rate (%)	Stratified by pathological stage			% BCR	Stratified by margin status		Median follow-up
							% LRP	% Open	% RARP		pT2	pT3a	pT3b		PSM	NSM	
This study	Freeman Hospital, UK	-	2002-2014	592	3.65 (2.4)	PSM 3.9 NSM 2.0	66.4%	-	33.6%	30.6%	21.9%	45.6%	66.7%	6.7%	10.7%	5.1%	4.4 years
Wright et al.	SEER, USA	[13]	1998-2006	65,633	-	-	-	-	-	21.2%	17.7%	43.8%	-	-	-	-	N/A
Mauermann et al.	Quebec, Canada	[22]	1987-2010	1,712	8.5 (6.8)	-	10.6%	89.4%	-	34.5%	27.6%	54.1%	49.5%*	16.4%	26.7%	10.9%	6 years
Ficarra et al.	Padua, Italy	[14]	2005-2008	322	-	-	-	-	100.0%	29.5%	10.6%	57.5%	72.2%	3.2%	6.2%	1.8%	1 year
Patel et al.	Multi-institution	[15]	2002-2009	8,418	-	-	-	-	100.0%	15.7%	9.5%	33.2%	48.2%	-	-	-	N/A
Boorjian et al.	Mayo Clinic, USA	[32]	1990-2006	11,729**	PSM (5.9) NSM (8.1)	PSM 3.3 NSM 1.1	-	100.0%	-	31.1%	23.4%	52.9%	55.4%	25.6%	44.0%	23.0%	8.2 years
Chalfin et al.	John Hopkins, USA	[21]	1982-2011	4,461	6.8 (5.4)	-	-	100.0%	-	10.4%	14.6%	22.2%	31.5%	16.7%	54.5%	12.3%	10 years
Sooriakumaran et al.	Stockholm	[16]	2002-2006	944	6.4	-	-	-	100.0%	21.6%	16.0%	33.3%	57.9%	15.2%	29.0%	12.0%	6.3 years
Evans et al.	Victoria, Australia	[33]	2008-2012	2219	-	-	8.1%	53.0%	38.8%	27.2%	16.1%	50.7%		-	-	-	N/A
Sukumar et al.	Detroit, USA	[17]	2001-2010	4803	6.1	Mean 7.5	-	-	100.0%	24.7%	11.2%	50.5%		9.8%	-	-	2.2 years
Abdollah et al.	Multi-institution	[18]	2001-2010	5670	6.4 (5.2)	-			100.0%	24.0%		34.3%***		14.1%	-	-	4.2 years
Gnanapragasam et al.	Cambridge, UK	[9]	2005-2015	1500	8.5 (7.3)	-			100.0%	21.5%	9.1%	29.6%	53.6%	-	-	-	N/A
Range										10.4-34.5%	9.1-27.6%	22.2-57.4%	31.5-72.2%	3.2-25.6%	6.2-54.5%	1.8-23.0%	1-10 years

*Includes pT4 (2002 TNM staging, changed to pT3b in 2010); **Patients with N1 disease excluded (PSM rate 295/484 = 61%); ***High-risk D'Amico group

isolated PSMs should be done with caution especially when factoring in the added morbidity associated with radiotherapy treatment.

Detectable PSA following radical prostatectomy is often considered treatment failure. In our cohort, 7.9% had detectable PSA post-operatively, and were excluded from subsequent analyses. These patients tended to have more aggressive disease and were more likely to have had positive surgical margins (73.8% in patients with detectable PSA, vs 28.6% in patients with undetectable PSA post-operatively, p<0.001, Additional file 1: Table S1). Similarly, Koulikov et al reported similar findings, whereby patients with low-detectable PSA (>0.03 and <0.2ng/ml) and PSA velocity >0.05ng/year, were more likely to have positive surgical margins and an increased incidence of biochemical recurrence [26]. These data suggest that men with low-detectable PSA post-prostatectomy may be divided into two groups based upon PSA velocity, those with stable PSA who do not often develop biochemical recurrence and those with unstable PSA who go on to develop biochemical recurrence. There is some evidence to suggest that this subgroup of patients may benefit from adjuvant radiotherapy [27].

There are some limitations to this study due to retrospective design and lack of PSA follow-up data for all patients. This is due to patients moving to their local units for follow-up. While previous reports and ours have predominantly focussed on reviewing the influence of pre-operative and surgical factors on long-term outcome, it is prudent to also note the potential impact of pathological features at the tumour margin. Pathological data regarding length of positive margin and grade pattern at the margin have previously been reported to predict BCR [28]. However, such data were not available for inclusion in our study. Moreover, molecular and biochemical features at tumour margins [29, 30] may also impact long term oncological outcomes, and subtyping positive margins based upon such features may provide a more effective method of identifying patients with PSM likely to benefit from personalised adjuvant therapies, as has been proposed for resection of other malignancies [31]. Lastly, this is a consecutive series of patients with an increasing volume of MIRPs performed each year. Therefore, it is difficult to accurately control for the effect of the learning curve. However, we adjusted for year of procedure, which may help adjust for this potential confounder to some degree. Interestingly, our data compares well to other series though we await the long-term maturation of this cohort.

Conclusion

In comparison to patients with negative surgical margins, those with PSM do not translate into worse medium-term oncological outcomes in the majority of cases amongst our cohort. We found that high pre-operative PSA and Gleason grade group were the only robust predictors of BCR.

Abbreviations

BCR: Biochemical recurrence; LRP: Laparoscopic radical prostatectomy; MIRP: Minimally-invasive radical prostatectomy; NSM: Negative surgical margin; PSA: Prostate specific antigen; PSM: Positive surgical margin; RARP: Robotic-assisted radical prostatectomy

Acknowledgements

None.

Funding

AS is funded by a National Institute of Health Research Academic Clinical Fellowship. RV, AV, KK, MIJ, JA and NAS do not report any external funding.

Authors' contributions

AS, RV, AV and KK collected and analysed the data. AS, RV and JA wrote the paper. MIJ, NAS and JA were involved in study design and reviewed the final manuscript.

Competing interests

AS reports research grants from the National Institute of Health Research Academic Clinical Fellowship, Cancer Research UK and The Urology Foundation, for an unrelated project. RV, AV, KK, MIJ, JA and NAS have disclosed no conflicts of interest.

References

1. Yossepowitch O, Briganti A, Eastham JA, Epstein J, Graefen M, Montironi R, Touijer K. Positive surgical margins after radical prostatectomy: a systematic review and contemporary update. Eur Urol. 2014;65(2):303–13.
2. Touijer K, Secin FP, Cronin AM, Katz D, Bianco F, Vora K, Reuter V, Vickers AJ, Guillonneau B. Oncologic outcome after laparoscopic radical prostatectomy: 10 years of experience. Eur Urol. 2009;55(5):1014–9.
3. Novara G, Ficarra V, Mocellin S, Ahlering TE, Carroll PR, Graefen M, Guazzoni G, Menon M, Patel VR, Shariat SF, et al. Systematic review and meta-analysis of studies reporting oncologic outcome after robot-assisted radical prostatectomy. Eur Urol. 2012;62(3):382–404.
4. Mann MJ, DeCastro GJ, Desai M, Benson MC, McKiernan JM. Predictive significance of surgical margin status after prostatectomy for prostate cancer during PSA era. Urology. 2008;72(6):1203–7.
5. Pfitzenmaier J, Pahernik S, Tremmel T, Haferkamp A, Buse S, Hohenfellner M. Positive surgical margins after radical prostatectomy: do they have an impact on biochemical or clinical progression? BJU Int. 2008;102(10):1413–8.
6. Swindle P, Eastham JA, Ohori M, Kattan MW, Wheeler T, Maru N, Slawin K, Scardino PT. Do margins matter? The prognostic significance of positive surgical margins in radical prostatectomy specimens. J Urol. 2005;174(3):903–7.
7. Bolla M, van Poppel H, Tombal B, Vekemans K, Da Pozzo L, de Reijke TM, Verbaeys A, Bosset JF, van Velthoven R, Colombel M, et al. Postoperative radiotherapy after radical prostatectomy for high-risk prostate cancer: long-term results of a randomised controlled trial (EORTC trial 22911). Lancet. 2012;380(9858):2018–27.
8. Cornford P, Bellmunt J, Bolla M, Briers E, De Santis M, Gross T, Henry AM, Joniau S, Lam TB, Mason MD, van der Poel HG, van der Kwast TH, Rouvière O, Wiegel T, Mottet N. EAU-ESTRO-SIOG Guidelines on Prostate Cancer. Part II: Treatment of Relapsing, Metastatic, and Castration-Resistant Prostate Cancer. Eur Urol. 2017;71(4):630–42.
9. Gnanapragasam VJ, Thurtle D, Srinivasan A, Volanis D, George A, Lophatananon A, Stearn S, Warren AY, Lamb AD, Shaw G, et al. Evolution and oncological outcomes of a contemporary radical prostatectomy

practice in a UK regional tertiary referral centre. BJU Int. 2016;118(5):779–84.

10. Melia J, Moss S, Johns L. Contributors in the participating I: Rates of prostate-specific antigen testing in general practice in England and Wales in asymptomatic and symptomatic patients: a cross-sectional study. BJU Int. 2004;94(1):51–6.
11. Jemal A, Fedewa SA, Ma JM, Siegel R, Lin CC, Brawley O, Ward EM. Prostate Cancer Incidence and PSA Testing Patterns in Relation to USPSTF Screening Recommendations. Jama-J Am Med Assoc. 2015;314(19):2054–61.
12. Tewari A, Sooriakumaran P, Bloch DA, Seshadri-Kreaden U, Hebert AE, Wiklund P. Positive surgical margin and perioperative complication rates of primary surgical treatments for prostate cancer: a systematic review and meta-analysis comparing retropubic, laparoscopic, and robotic prostatectomy. Eur Urol. 2012;62(1):1–15.
13. Wright JL, Dalkin BL, True LD, Ellis WJ, Stanford JL, Lange PH, Lin DW. Positive surgical margins at radical prostatectomy predict prostate cancer specific mortality. J Urol. 2010;183(6):2213–8.
14. Ficarra V, Novara G, Secco S, D'Elia C, Boscolo-Berto R, Gardiman M, Cavalleri S, Artibani W. Predictors of positive surgical margins after laparoscopic robot assisted radical prostatectomy. J Urol. 2009;182(6):2682–8.
15. Patel VR, Coelho RF, Rocco B, Orvieto M, Sivaraman A, Palmer KJ, Kameh D, Santoro L, Coughlin GD, Liss M, et al. Positive surgical margins after robotic assisted radical prostatectomy: a multi-institutional study. J Urol. 2011;186(2):511–6.
16. Sooriakumaran P, Haendler L, Nyberg T, Gronberg H, Nilsson A, Carlsson S, Hosseini A, Adding C, Jonsson M, Ploumidis A, et al. Biochemical recurrence after robot-assisted radical prostatectomy in a European single-centre cohort with a minimum follow-up time of 5 years. Eur Urol. 2012;62(5):768–74.
17. Sukumar S, Rogers CG, Trinh QD, Sammon J, Sood A, Stricker H, Peabody JO, Menon M, Diaz-Insua M. Oncological outcomes after robot-assisted radical prostatectomy: long-term follow-up in 4803 patients. BJU Int. 2014; 114(6):824–31.
18. Abdollah F, Dalela D, Sood A, Sammon J, Jeong W, Beyer B, Fossati N, Rogers CG, Diaz-Insua M, Peabody J, et al. Intermediate-term cancer control outcomes in prostate cancer patients treated with robotic-assisted laparoscopic radical prostatectomy: a multi-institutional analysis. World J Urol. 2016;
19. Laird A, Fowler S, Good DW, Stewart GD, Srinivasan V, Cahill D, Brewster SF, McNeill SA. British Association of Urological S: Contemporary practice and technique-related outcomes for radical prostatectomy in the UK: a report of national outcomes. BJU Int. 2015;115(5):753–63.
20. Dev HS, Wiklund P, Patel V, Parashar D, Palmer K, Nyberg T, Skarecky D, Neal DE, Ahlering T, Sooriakumaran P. Surgical margin length and location affect recurrence rates after robotic prostatectomy. Urol Oncol. 2015;33(3):109 e107–13.
21. Chalfin HJ, Dinizo M, Trock BJ, Feng Z, Partin AW, Walsh PC, Humphreys E, Han M. Impact of surgical margin status on prostate-cancer-specific mortality. BJU Int. 2012;110(11):1684–9.
22. Mauermann J, Fradet V, Lacombe L, Dujardin T, Tiguert R, Tetu B, Fradet Y. The impact of solitary and multiple positive surgical margins on hard clinical end points in 1712 adjuvant treatment-naive pT2-4 N0 radical prostatectomy patients. Eur Urol. 2013;64(1):19–25.
23. Sooriakumaran P, Srivastava A, Shariat SF, Stricker PD, Ahlering T, Eden CG, Wiklund PN, Sanchez-Salas R, Mottrie A, Lee D, et al. A multinational, multi-institutional study comparing positive surgical margin rates among 22393 open, laparoscopic, and robot-assisted radical prostatectomy patients. Eur Urol. 2014;66(3):450–6.
24. Kang SG, Schatloff O, Haidar AM, Samavedi S, Palmer KJ, Cheon J, Patel VR. Overall rate, location, and predictive factors for positive surgical margins after robot-assisted laparoscopic radical prostatectomy for high-risk prostate cancer. Asian J Androl. 2016;18(1):123-8. doi: 10.4103/1008-682X.148723.
25. Wiegel T, Bottke D, Steiner U, Siegmann A, Golz R, Storkel S, Willich N, Semjonow A, Souchon R, Stockle M, et al. Phase III postoperative adjuvant radiotherapy after radical prostatectomy compared with radical prostatectomy alone in pT3 prostate cancer with postoperative undetectable prostate-specific antigen: ARO 96-02/AUO AP 09/95. J Clin Oncol. 2009;27(18):2924–30.
26. Koulikov D, Mohler MC, Mehedint DC, Attwood K, Wilding GE, Mohler JL. Low detectable prostate specific antigen after radical prostatectomy–treat or watch? J Urol. 2014;192(5):1390–6.
27. Swanson GP, Hussey MA, Tangen CM, Chin J, Messing E, Canby-Hagino E, Forman JD, Thompson IM, Crawford ED. Swog: Predominant treatment failure in postprostatectomy patients is local: analysis of patterns of treatment failure in SWOG 8794. J Clin Oncol. 2007;25(16):2225–9.
28. Savdie R, Horvath LG, Benito RP, Rasiah KK, Haynes AM, Chatfield M, Stricker PD, Turner JJ, Delprado W, Henshall SM, et al. High Gleason grade carcinoma at a positive surgical margin predicts biochemical failure after radical prostatectomy and may guide adjuvant radiotherapy. BJU Int. 2012;109(12):1794–800.
29. Straub B, Muller M, Krause H, Goessl C, Schrader M, Heicappell R, Miller K. Molecular staging of surgical margins after radical prostatectomy by detection of telomerase activity. Prostate. 2001;49(2):140–4.
30. Theodorescu D, Frierson HF Jr, Sikes RA. Molecular determination of surgical margins using fossa biopsies at radical prostatectomy. J Urol. 1999;161(5):1442–8.
31. Mao L, Clark D. Molecular margin of surgical resections–where do we go from here? Cancer-Am Cancer Soc. 2015;121(12):1914–6.
32. Boorjian SA, Karnes RJ, Crispen PL, Carlson RE, Rangel LJ, Bergstralh EJ, Blute ML. The impact of positive surgical margins on mortality following radical prostatectomy during the prostate specific antigen era. J Urol. 2010;183(3):1003–9.
33. Evans SM, Millar JL, Frydenberg M, Murphy DG, Davis ID, Spelman T, Bolton DM, Giles GG, Dean J, Costello AJ, et al. Positive surgical margins: rate, contributing factors and impact on further treatment: findings from the Prostate Cancer Registry. BJU Int. 2014;114(5):680–90.

When to perform bone scintigraphy in patients with newly diagnosed prostate cancer? a retrospective study

Yiwei Lin, Qiqi Mao, Bin Chen, Liujiang Wang, Ben Liu, Xiangyi Zheng and Liping Xie*

Abstract

Background: To determine when a bone scintigraphy investigation is appropriate in patients with newly diagnosed prostate cancer (PCa).

Methods: We retrospectively reviewed 703 newly diagnosed PCa patients who were referred for bone scintigraphy. The association between age, prostate specific antigen (PSA), Gleason score (GS) and bone scintigraphy result were investigated by series of crude or stratified analysis.

Results: Overall, 15.08% (106/703) patients had bone metastases. PSA and GS between positive bone scan group and negative bone scan group were significantly different, while age was not. The incidence of bone metastasis in patient with PSA < 20 ng/ml or GS < 8 was less than 10%, but increased dramatically with rising PSA and upgrading GS. In multivariate analysis, PSA ≥ 20 ng/ml (OR = 5.10, 95%CI (2.12-12.27)) and GS ≥ 8 (OR = 3.61, 95%CI (1.55-8.41)) were independently predictive of positive bone scan.

Conclusions: Patients with PSA ≥ 20 ng/ml or GS ≥ 8 were in higher risk of bone metastasis, bone scintigraphy was recommended. But a bone scintigraphy is of limited value in PCa patients with PSA ≤ 20 ng/ml and GS ≤ 7.

Keywords: Prostate cancer, Prostate specific antigen, Gleason score, Bone scintigraphy

Background

Prostate cancer (PCa) is one of the leading malignant diseases in male in Western countries but it is relatively uncommon in China. However, recent widespread use of serum prostate-specific antigen (PSA) made PCa a growing health problem in China, with a bulky increase in incidence [1]. Early detection of bone metastases will be of great importance, as it can alert the clinician to the possible complications inherent in skeletetal destruction and reduce morbidity. Bone scintigraphy remains the most sensitive modality for detection of bone metastases, being superior to clinical evaluation, bone radiographs, serum alkaline phospatase measurement and prostatic acid phosphatase (PAP) determination [2].

However, routine use of bone scintigraphy staging is controversial. Subgroups of PCa patients with minimal risk for bone metastases can be safely excluded from bone scintigraphy. Numerous studies have demonstrated serum PSA, Gleason score (GS) and clinical tumor stage can be successfully used as indicators to predict which patients required bone scintigraphy for bone metastasis. According to a novel risk stratification tool proposed by Briganti et al.[3], bone scintigraphy might be considered only for patients with a biopsy GS > 7 or with PSA > 10 ng/ml and cT2/T3 disease prior to treatment. Ritenour et al. [4] recommend using GS as primary threshold to enhance predictability of positive bone scan in newly diagnosed patient with PCa. Bone scans should be done for patients with GS ≤ 7 when PSA ≥ 30 ng/ml, and for patients with GS > 7 when PSA ≥ 10 ng/ml. However, the criteria varied from different regions. Zaman et al. [5] found that there was an overall increased incidence of bone metastasis in newly diagnosed patients with PCa and even at PSA ≤20 ng/ml and GS ≤ 7 in Asian males, while other studies [6–8] indicated that bone scan can be eliminated for PCa patients with PSA < 10 ng/ml. Currently,

* Correspondence: xielp@zjuem.zju.edu.cn; xielp@zju.edu.cn
Department of Urology, The First Affiliated Hospital, School of Medicine, Zhejiang University, Qingchun Road 79, Hangzhou 310003, Zhejiang Province, China

limited data [9, 10] was available to strengthen which recommendation was more suitable for Chinese patients. Thus, we conducted a retrospective study in order to determine the diagnostic correlation among PSA, GS, clinical tumor stage and bone metastasis in newly diagnosed PCa patients in local population in China.

Methods

The current study was approved by ethics committee at our hospital. It included newly diagnosed PCa patients from January 2011 to December 2014 in the Department of Urology at the First Affiliated Hospital of Zhejiang University in China. The consecutive 703 records of the patients were reviewed retrospectively for bone scan images, PSA levels and GS in biopsy, after excluding those with prior 5-alpha reductase inhibitors medication or surgical treatment for benign prostatic hyperplasia. All the bone scans were carried out as a routine clinical evaluation to further stage the prostate cancer prior to prostatectomy, radiotherapy or androgen deprivation therapy. The PSA tests were within 30 days of bone scan, and the most recent bone scan results after prostate biopsy were included in the study to avoid bias caused by delayed diagnosis of bone metastases during tumor progession.

The primary outcome measured was the presence of bone metastasis on bone scintigraphy. Whole body bone scintigraphy was performed using Tc-99-methylenediphosphonate (Tc 99 m MDP) and reviewed by 2 certified nuclear medicine physicians with extensive experience. The skeletal metastasis on bone scintigraphy was defined as either solitary or multiple asymmetric areas of increased tracer uptake presence, excluding tracer accumulations related to previous trauma and degenerative bone disease [11]. Patients equivocal bone scan findings (298 cases) also underwent computed tomography (98 cases), magnetic resonance imaging (MRI) (198 cases) and/or subsequent bone scan (2 cases) to confirm the bone scintigraphy findings. Conflicting evaluations were resolved by discussion. When needed, the consult from senior physician was sought.

The association between age, PSA, GS and bone scintigraphy result were investigated by series of crude or stratified analysis. Chi-square test was used for the comparison of proportions. Multivariate logistic regression analysis was used to compare the association between the independent variables (PSA and GS) and bone scan findings. To counter the skewness of the PSA values, a natural logarithm of PSA, lnPSA was used to generate a receiver operating characteristic (ROC) curve. All statistical analyses were performed using STATA, version 11.0 (StataCorp LP, College Station, TX, USA) and the outcome was considered significant only when the p value <0.05.

Results

We identified 703 men who had been diagnosed with PCa and fulfilled our inclusion criteria. The mean age of included 703 patients was 69.9 years. The biopsy GS ranged from 6 to 10 with a mean value of 7.4, and the median PSA value was 22.1 ng/ml (interquartile range, 55.8 ng/ml). The proportion of patients with highly suspicious findings of bone metastases based on bone scan in our cohort was 15.08% (106/703). The comparative baseline characteristics of the two groups with different bone metastasis status were listed in Table 1. In the two groups, no difference between age was detected (for mean age, $p = 0.13$; for stratified subgroups, $p = 0.96$). However, there was a significant difference in PSA and GS between two groups ($p < 0.05$).

Moreover, we evulated the predictivity of PSA and GS on bone metastasis. Logistic regression with bony metastasis as the dependent variable and lnPSA and GS as independent variables was carried out to determine whether PSA and Gleason scores were additive. Both ln PSA and GS were statistically significant predictors of bone metastasis. However, receiver operating characteristic (ROC) curve for accuracy of ln PSA on bone metastasis has an area under curve (AUC) 0.829, which was superior over GS (AUC = 0.698) (Fig. 1). The multivariable model combing lnPSA and GS presented with AUC of 0.835 (Fig. 2), which was non-significant comparing with lnPSA alone ($p = 0.21$). The sensitivity and specificity of PSA at a cut-off (88 ng/ml) with maximal Youden's index was 67.9% and 89.1% respectively, while GS at a cut-off (≥8) was a little bit more sensitive (69.81%) and less specific (68.01%) for diagnosing bone metastasis.

Table 1 Patients' baseline characteristics, $N = 703$

	All Patients	without bone metastasis (%)	with bone metastasis (%)	p value
Age, yr				
≤ 60	87	73 (12.2)	14 (13.2)	0.96
60-70	255	217 (36.3)	38 (35.8)	
≥ 70	361	307 (51.4)	54 (50.9)	
mean	69.7	69.9	68.7	0.13
PSA, ng/ml				
≤ 10	150	144 (24.1)	6 (5.7)	<0.05
10-20	184	175 (29.3)	9 (8.5)	
≥ 20	369	278 (46.6)	91 (85.8)	
mean	110.4	48.5	361.7	<0.05
GS				
< 7	132	125 (20.9)	7 (6.6)	<0.05
= 7	306	281 (47.1)	25 (23.6)	
> 7	265	191 (32.0)	74 (69.8)	
mean	7.5	7.3	7.9	<0.05

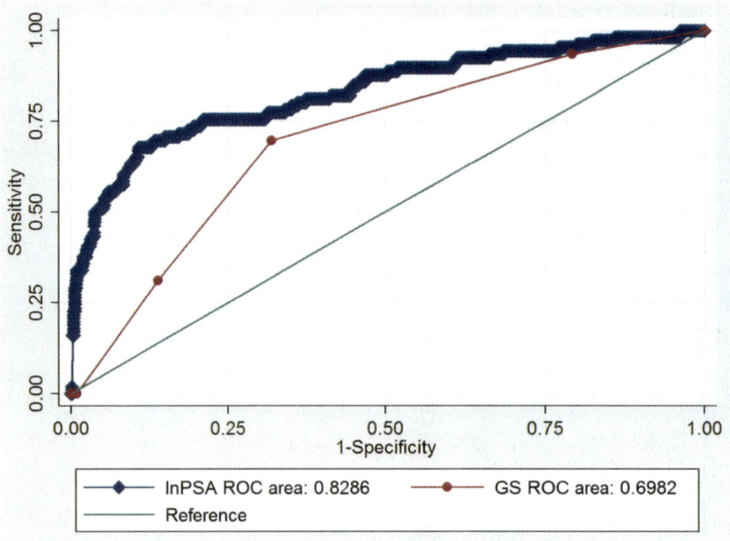

Fig. 1 ROC curve analysis of lnPSA and GS for predicting bone metastasis

We further stratified the PSA into 3 groups: ≤10 ng/ml, 10-20 ng/ml, and ≥20 ng/ml. The prevalence of bone metastases increased progressively with PSA level. Bone metastasis was detected in 6 (6/150, 4.00%) patients with PSA below 10 ng/ml, and 9 (9/184, 4.89%) with PSA between 10 and 20 ng/ml. For the patients with PSA above 20 ng/ml, there was a dramatic increase in bone metastasis proportion (91/369, 24.66%). Correspondingly, multivariate analysis revealed higher risk (OR = 5.10, 95%CI (2.12-12.27)) of bone metastasis in patient with PSA > 20 ng/ml (Table 2).

For GS, larger proportion of bone metastasis was presented in patients with higher GS. 5.30% (7/132), 8.17% (25/306) and 27.92% (74/265) patients were found with bone metastasis in GS < 7, =7 and >7 respectively (Table 1). In multivariate analysis, GS (>7) was proven to be independently predictive of positive bone scan (OR = 3.61, 95%CI (1.55-8.41)) (Table 2).

Discussion

Numerous studies have been conducted to find out proper criteria for ruling out bone metastases in patients

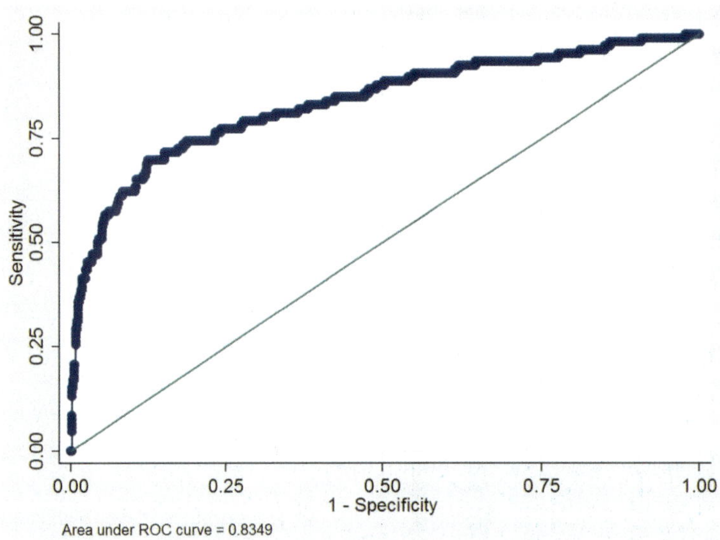

Fig. 2 ROC curve analysis of combing lnPSA and GS for predicting bone metastasis

Table 2 Predictors of positivity of bone scintigraphy using multivariate analysis

	OR (95% CI)	*p* Value
PSA, ng/ml		
≤ 10	*Reference*	
10-20	1.11(0.38-3.22)	0.85
≥ 20	5.10(2.12-12.27)	<0.05
GS		
< 7	*Reference*	
= 7	1.15 (0.47-2.76)	0.78
> 7	3.61 (1.55-8.41)	<0.05

with low risk of bone metastasis. PSA and biopsy GS were the most common parameters for assessing the bone metastasis risk. Oesterling et al. [12] were the first to address the possibility of serum PSA levels being able to predict bone scan results. They concluded that omitting bone scan for PSA less than 10 ng/ml is safe. The studies in some region of Asia also demonstrated that in well differentiated tumor, 10 ng/ml was the optimal cut-off PSA value for reserving bone scintigraphy [7, 8, 13]. However, American Urological Association (AUA) and the European Association of Urology (EAU) recommended that bone scan could be omitted in asymptomatic patients with well-differentiated tumor with PSA less than 20 ng/ml. The variation in criteria for bone scan recommendation was because of tremendous difference in incidence and stage pattern in different region worldwide [14]. In Asia, more aggressive and poorly differentiated PCa was presented, since twice as many Asian men had a GS of 8 or greater, the worst stage at presentation while comparing with non-Asian men [15]. Therefore, Zaman et al. [5] suggested that we must be careful in adopting current guidelines.

In China, the incidence of PCa is rapidly increasing, ranking eighth among the most common cancers in the male population in 2008 [1]. Although the reported incidence and mortality of PCa was much lower in China compared to Western countries, the mortality-to-incidence rate ratio (MR/IR) of PCa in China was found to be much higher [16]. These data suggest that higher proportion of advanced disease at the time of diagnosis, and that patient had a shorter survival time thereafter. Thus, precise staging for newly diagnosed PCa patient is of great importance, especially for bone metastasis staging, which has a profound influence on prognosis. Currently, bone scintigraphy is still regarded as the gold standard for detecting skeletal metastases in patients with newly diagnosed PCa. However, there was ongoing debate that whether we should propose bone scintigraphy as a routine staging modality for all patients, since the overuse of bone scan will result in unnecessary patient anxiety, radiation exposure, time consumption, and significant financial burden for both patients and healthcare system. In China, a clear PSA-driven cancer stage migration was presented after the initialization of PSA screening in some regions and more early stage disease was presented [17]. Thus, we believed the criteria for omitting bone scan in newly diagnosed case should be validated for Chinese patients.

Several studies have been conducted to search for the optimal bone scan indications for Chinese PCa patients, but with heterogeneous results [9, 10, 18]. Our current study revealed a similar trend that high PSA (>20 ng/ml) or poorly differentiated (GS > 7) were associated with increased bone metastasis risk in newly diagnosed PCa patients. PSA and GS could predict bone metastasis. In our cohort, only 3.76% (10/266) bone metastatic disease were with PSA < 20 ng/ml and GS < 8, which was almost negligible. Even more, we identified that PSA alone was powerful enough to predict bone metastasis, since the multivariable model combing lnPSA and GS did not significantly enhance the predictivity of lnPSA. For the predictability of GS, one issue still should be addressed when interpreting our results. The biopsy GS can probably bias surgical specimens, since GS upgrading between biopsy and surgical pathological specimens occurs 30–50% [19]. The accurate prediction of final GS largely depends on prostate biopsy schemes [20] and prostate size [19]. Thus, we speculated that the predictability of GS was weaker than PSA.

Meanwhile, several other issues still should be addressed when interpreting our results. Firstly, the follow-up time is short, which would prevent delayed diagnosis of bone metastatases. Then, metastatic lesions detected by bone scan were not histologically confirmed, thus the inconsistence between bone scan and histology would biased our results.

Conclusion

Based on our findings, patients with PSA ≥ 20 ng/ml or GS > 7 were in higher risk of bone metastasis, and bone scintigraphy was strongly recommended for these patients. For the patients with PSA < 20 ng/ml or GS < 8, bone scintigraphy is of limited value unless a curative treatment is contemplated. On the other hand, considering the presence of metastatic disease in these low risk patients, a more precise stratification tool should be established to safely eliminate bone scintigraphy.

Abbreviations

CI: Confidence interval; GS: Gleason score; OR: Odds ratio; PCa: Prostate cancer; PSA: Prostate specific antigen

Funding

This study was supported by a grant from national key clinical specialty construction project of China & health sector scientific research special project (Grant No. 201002010).

Authors' contributions

YWL and QQM drafted the manuscript. BC and LJW performed the statistical analysis. BL and XYZ collected the clinical data. LPX made the literatures review and revised the manuscript. All authors have read and approved the final manuscript.

Competing interests

The authors declare that they have no competing interests.

References

1. Peng P, Gong YM, Bao PP, Ke JZ, Xiang YM, Zhang ML, Zheng Y. Estimates and prediction of prostate cancer incidence, mortality and prevalence in China, 2008. Zhonghua Liu Xing Bing Xue Za Zhi. 2012;33(10):1056–9.
2. McGregor B, Tulloch AG, Quinlan MF, Lovegrove F. The role of bone scanning in the assessment of prostatic carcinoma. Br J Urol. 1978;50(3):178–81.
3. Briganti A, Passoni N, Ferrari M, Capitanio U, Suardi N, Gallina A, Da Pozzo LF, Picchio M, Di Girolamo V, Salonia A, et al. When to perform bone scan in patients with newly diagnosed prostate cancer: external validation of the currently available guidelines and proposal of a novel risk stratification tool. Eur Urol. 2010;57(4):551–8.
4. Ritenour CW, Abbott JT, Goodman M, Alazraki N, Marshall FF, Issa MM. The utilization of Gleason grade as the primary criterion for ordering nuclear bone scan in newly diagnosed prostate cancer patients. ScientificWorldJournal. 2009;9:1040–5.
5. Zaman MU, Fatima N, Sajjad Z. Metastasis on bone scan with low prostate specific antigen (</=20 ng/ml) and Gleason's score (<8) in newly diagnosed Pakistani males with prostate cancer: should we follow Western guidelines? Asian Pac J Cancer Prev. 2011;12(6):1529–32.
6. Lai MH, Luk WH, Chan JC. Predicting bone scan findings using sPSA in patients newly diagnosed of prostate cancer: feasibility in Asian population. Urol Oncol. 2011;29(3):275–9.
7. Hirobe M, Takahashi A, Hisasue S, Kitamura H, Kunishima Y, Masumori N, Iwasawa A, Fujimori K, Hasegawa T, Tsukamoto T. Bone scanning–who needs it among patients with newly diagnosed prostate cancer? Jpn J Clin Oncol. 2007;37(10):788–92.
8. Lee SH, Chung MS, Park KK, Yom CD, Lee DH, Chung BH. Is it suitable to eliminate bone scan for prostate cancer patients with PSA </= 20 ng/mL? World J Urol. 2012;30(2):265–9.
9. Wang TY, Chen XP, Li XS, Jia Y, Cheng J, Zhang JH, Cai L, Zhang Z, Gong K, He ZS, et al. Predictive value of prostate-specific antigen and Gleason sum for results of radionuclide bone scintigraphy in patients with prostate cancer. Beijing Da Xue Xue Bao. 2012;44(4):528–34.
10. Zhou JQ, Zhu Y, Yao XD, Zhang SL, Dai B, Zhang HL, Ye DW. Necessity analysis of bone scan in patients with newly diagnosed prostate cancer. Zhonghua Yi Xue Za Zhi. 2013;93(4):248–51.
11. Hricak H, Choyke PL, Eberhardt SC, Leibel SA, Scardino PT. Imaging prostate cancer: a multidisciplinary perspective. Radiology. 2007;243(1):28–53.
12. Oesterling JE, Martin SK, Bergstralh EJ, Lowe FC. The use of prostate-specific antigen in staging patients with newly diagnosed prostate cancer. JAMA. 1993;269(1):57–60.
13. Yang G, Zuo S, Ma C, Liu B, Wang G, Wang X, Wu H. The diagnostic correlations of bone scintigraphy, pathological grade and PSA for metastatic prostate cancers. Chin-Ger J Clin Oncol. 2009;8(12):702–4.
14. Quinn M, Babb P. Patterns and trends in prostate cancer incidence, survival, prevalence and mortality. Part I: international comparisons. BJU Int. 2002;90(2):162–73.
15. Man A, Pickles T, Chi KN. Asian race and impact on outcomes after radical radiotherapy for localized prostate cancer. J Urol. 2003;170(3):901–4.
16. Zhang L, Wu S, Guo LR, Zhao XJ. Diagnostic strategies and the incidence of prostate cancer: reasons for the low reported incidence of prostate cancer in China. Asian J Androl. 2009;11(1):9–13.
17. Cullen J, Elsamanoudi S, Brassell SA, Chen Y, Colombo M, Srivastava A, McLeod DG. The burden of prostate cancer in Asian nations. J Carcinog. 2012;11:7.
18. Wang Y, Guo J, Xu L, Zhao N, Xu Z, Wang H, Zhu Y, Jiang S, Yang N, Yang Y, et al. Should Bone Scan be Performed in Chinese Prostate Cancer Patients at the Time of Diagnosis? Urol Int. 2013;91(2):160–4.
19. Davies JD, Aghazadeh MA, Phillips S, Salem S, Chang SS, Clark PE, Cookson MS, Davis R, Herrell SD, Penson DF, et al. Prostate size as a predictor of Gleason score upgrading in patients with low risk prostate cancer. J Urol. 2011;186(6):2221–7.
20. Mian BM, Lehr DJ, Moore CK, Fisher HA, Kaufman Jr RP, Ross JS, Jennings TA, Nazeer T. Role of prostate biopsy schemes in accurate prediction of Gleason scores. Urology. 2006;67(2):379–83.

Increased expression of neuregulin 1 in the urothelium of rat bladder with partial bladder outlet obstruction

Seung Woo Yang[1], Seong Woo Jeong[2] and Ki Hak Song[1*]

Abstract

Background: This study determined whether changes in the expression of neuregulin (NRG) 1, erbB2 tyrosine kinase (ErbB2) and the M2 muscarinic receptor in the urothelium and detrusor muscle of the rat bladder were associated with partial bladder outlet obstruction (PBOO).

Methods: Male Sprague-Dawley rats (body weight 250–300 g) were used and subdivided into control ($n = 10$) and PBOO groups ($n = 20$). PBOO was induced for 21 days, and the expression of NRG1, ErbB2 and M2 muscarinic receptor mRNA and protein was evaluated using reverse transcriptase-polymerase chain reaction (RT-PCR) and western blotting, respectively.

Results: In the urothelium of rat bladder samples, protein expression and mRNA expression of NRG1, ErbB2 and M2 muscarinic receptor were significantly increased in the PBOO group compared to the control group ($p < 0.05$). Only mRNA expression levels of NRG1/ ErbB2 were higher in the detrusor muscle of the PBOO group compared to the control group ($p < 0.05$).

Conclusions: Our study demonstrated remarkable changes in the expression of NRG1/ErbB2 receptor mRNA and protein in the urothelium and muscle layer. These results suggest that NRG1 overexpression plays some kind of role against the PBOO-induced upregulated muscarinic receptors in detrusor overactivity.

Keywords: Neuregulin-1, Receptor, ErbB-2, Outlet obstruction, Bladder, Rats

Background

Bladder outlet obstruction (BOO) is caused by common disorders that result from congenital anomalies, such as bladder neck sclerosis, posterior urethral valve, urethral stricture and benign prostatic hyperplasia (BPH) [1, 2]. BOO may lead to detrusor overactivity via cholinergic denervation of the detrusor muscle and subsequent acetylcholine hypersensitivity [3]. Overactive bladder (OAB) induced by partial BOO (PBOO) is derived from an aberration in the micturition reflex, which leads to involuntary detrusor contraction of either myogenic or neurologic origin [4]. Several studies demonstrated that the urothelium of bladder is more than a simple barrier because it actively contributes to bladder function [4–7]. The urothelium may play a role in the mechanosensory transduction during voiding via its ability to release many substances in response to stretch during filling, including ATP [8, 9], prostaglandins [9], nitric oxide [10], acetylcholine [11] and nerve growth factor [12], which affect nerve, smooth muscle, interstitial and immune cells.

Neuregulin (NRG) 1 is a trophic factor in the family of growth factors, and it contains an epidermal growth factor (EGF)-like domain. The roles of NRG1 in synaptic plasticity, neuronal and glial development and cardiomyocyte regeneration after heart injury were investigated extensively [13, 14]. Multiple binding profiles and various G-coupled protein receptors modulate NRG1/ErbB signalling, and we reported previously that NRG1/ErbB signalling was associated with inflammatory states of the rat bladder, such as interstitial cystitis [15]. NRG1-mediated ErbB activation modulates interneuron function.

* Correspondence: urosong@cnu.ac.kr
[1]Department of Urology, School of Medicine, Chungnam National University Hospital, Chungnam National University, 282 Monwha-ro, Jung-gu, Daejeon, Republic of Korea35015
Full list of author information is available at the end of the article

However, the roles of NRG1/ErbB signalling in the regulation of PBOO-induced OAB are not known.

The present study evaluated changes in the expression and distribution of NRG1/ErbB2 and M2 muscarinic receptors in the urothelium and detrusor muscle of rat bladders subjected to PBOO and determined whether these changes were associated with PBOO-induced OAB.

Methods

Experimental animals and PBOO surgery

Male Sprague-Dawley rats (250–300 g, Daehan Biolink Co. Ltd., Daejeon, Korea) were used in this study, and all experiment animals followed a protocol approved by the Ethics Committee on Animal Research at Chungnam National University, Daejeon, Korea (CNU-00261). Animals were raised in pairs in a cage covered with sawdust. Water and food were provided ad libitum. The temperature was controlled at 25 °C ± 1 °C, and the humidity was maintained at 55% ± 5%. Illumination varied in 12-h intervals. Thirty rats were used in this study, and rats were randomly divided into two groups (20 in the PBOO group and 10 in the control group). Each rat was anaesthetized using intramuscular ketamine (15 mg/kg) and rompun (5 mg/kg). A lower midline abdominal incision was made and deepened into the pelvic cavity to expose the bladder and urethra. A 3–0 silk ligature was placed around the urethra, and a 24-gage angio needle sheath was used to create a partial BOO in the PBOO group. The sheath was removed, and the incision was closed. PBOO was created using previously reported methods [16]. A sham operation was performed in the control group under same circumstances as the PBOO group.

Tissue preparation for analyses

Rats were anaesthetized 21 days after PBOO induction in the same manner described above, and cystectomy was performed through an abdominal incision at the level of the ureteric orifices. The rats were sacrificed by carbon dioxide inhalation. Specimens were divided vertically into two portions (one half for RT-PCR and one half for western blotting). The divided bladder tissue was placed into a dish containing a phosphate-buffered saline solution. The urothelium and detrusor muscle were separated using microscissors and microforceps under the direct vision of a phase-contrast microscope.

Total RNA extraction

Total RNA was extracted from the urothelium and detrusor muscle of control and PBOO rats. Tissue was homogenized in a 5-mL glass tube containing 0.8 mL of TRIzol (Invitrogen, Carlsbad, CA, USA) for 5 min at room temperature. The homogenate was transferred to a 1-mL tube, mixed with 160 μL of chloroform for 5 min at 4 °C, and centrifuged for 10 min at 13,200×g at 4 °C. The supernatant was transferred to another tube, and 1 mL of isopropyl alcohol (Sigma-Aldrich Co., St. Louis, MO, USA) was added. This solution was incubated for 30 min at 4 °C and centrifuged for 8 min at 13,200×g at 4 °C. The pellet was mixed with 500 μL of 75% ethanol and centrifuged for 10 min at 13,200×g at 4 °C. The supernatant was discarded, and the pellet was dried in room air for 5 min. The pellet was dissolved in 50 μL of diethylpyrocarbonate (DEPC, Sigma-Aldrich Co.) water and stored at −75 °C. Electrophoresis using an agarose gel and ethidium bromide staining was performed to confirm the RNA quality and integrity.

Reverse transcriptase- polymerase chain reaction (RT-PCR)

Total RNA was extracted from the urothelium and detrusor muscle tissues of rat bladders of the PBOO group and controls using TRIzol reagent and the chloroform method. Complementary DNA was synthesized using the First Strand cDNA Synthesis Kit (Fermentas Inc., Glen Burnie, MD, USA) with oligo-dT as the primer. Primers F-5′-CCCGCCGGCTATTGGTGACTT-3′ and R-5′-ATGA CCACCCCGGCT CGTATGT-3′ were used to amplify NRG1 (358-bp). ErbB2 (483-bp) cDNA was synthesized using F-5′-AGCCCCCAGCCC GAGTATGTGAAC-3′ and R-5′-GAGCCGTCTGCCCTGGAT-GTAATG-3′. Oligomers F-5′-TCTCGAGCCAGCAAGAGCAGGAT-3′ and R-5′-GCCAGCAGAATAGCCAAGATT-3′ were used to synthesize cDNA of the M2 muscarinic receptor (557-bp). Primers F-5′-GATGGCATGGACTGTGGTCA-3′ and R-5′-GTCATCATCTCCGCCCCTTC-3′ were used to produce cDNA of glyceraldehyde 3–phosphate dehydrogenase (GAPDH, 189-bp). PCR reactions were performed and programmed in three steps as follows: 94 °C for 5 min, 35 cycles of 94 °C for 30 s/58 °C for 40 s/72 °C for 30 s, and 72 °C for 5 min. PCR product sizes were analysed using electrophoresis on 2% agarose gels. GAPDH was used as a housekeeping gene.

Protein extraction and western blotting

Frozen tissue of the urothelium and detrusor muscle obtained from cystectomy was ground with a mortar and pestle and homogenized at 4 °C in 1× radioimmunoprecipitation assay buffer (Sigma-Aldrich®, St. Louis, MO, USA, ready-to-use solution containing 150 mM of NaCl, 1.0% IGEPAL® CA-630, 0.5% sodium deoxycholate, 0.1% SDS, 50 mM Tris, pH 8.0.). Homogenates were transferred to Eppendorf tubes on ice, incubated for 5 min and centrifuged at 13,000 g for 20 min at 4 °C. The supernatant was transferred to newly labelled Eppendorf tubes, and total protein content was measured using a Bradford assay kit (Thermo scientific, Pittsburgh, PA, USA), according to the manufacturer's instructions. The samples were mixed with lysis buffer, boiled at 95 °C for 5 min, and cooled. A sample containing 50 μg of total protein was loaded onto a 12% sodium dodecyl sulphate polyacrylamide gel, and proteins were separated using electrophoresis for 2 h. Proteins were transferred to polyvinylidene fluoride membranes (Dyneon, 3 M, St. Paul, MN, USA) using a trans-blot semidry transfer cell (Mini-Protean® TetraCell, Bio-Rad, Hercules, CA, USA) for 1 h at 15 V. The membrane was washed with Tris-buffered saline Tween-20 and incubated with 5% skimmed milk for 1 h to block non-specific binding. Membranes were incubated with the following primary antibodies overnight at 4 °C: NRG1 monoclonal mouse antibody (1:200, Abcam, Cambridge, MA, USA), ErbB2 polyclonal rabbit antibody (1:200, Abcam), and M2 muscarinic receptor polyclonal goat antibody (1:200, Santa Cruz Biotechnology, Inc., Dallas, TX, USA). Membranes were washed with PBS 3 times, and the antibody binding was detected using goat anti-mouse antibodies for NRG1 (1:200, Abcam), goat anti-rabbit antibodies for ErbB2 (1:200, Abcam) and donkey anti-goat antibodies for M2 muscarinic receptor (1:2000, Santa Cruz Biotechnology) conjugated to horseradish peroxidase. The secondary antibodies were incubated at room temperature for 1 h. Bands were visualized using enhanced chemiluminescence (Vilber Lourmat, Marne La Vallée, France).

Statistical analysis

Data were analysed using the Mann-Whitney test for comparisons between two groups. A p-value <0.05 was considered statistically significant. All data are presented as the means ± standard deviation. All calculations were performed using IBM SPSS Statistics ver. 20.0 (IBM Co., Armonk, NY, USA).

Results

Western blot assay of NRG1, ErbB2 and M2 muscarinic receptors

We investigated the expression of M2 muscarinic receptor (75 kDa), NRG1 (44 kDa) and ErbB2 (185 kDa) receptor using western blot analysis in the urothelium and detrusor muscle of bladders from PBOO-induced OAB and control rats (Fig. 1a). The relative intensities and distributions of NRG1, the ErbB2 receptor and M2 muscarinic receptor in the urothelium were approximately 1.6-, 1.5-, and 1.4-fold higher, respectively, in the PBOO group than the control group (1.80 ± 0.15 vs. 1.10 ± 0.15, 1.24 ± 0.28 vs. 0.82 ± 0.15, and 1.25 ± 0.25 vs. 0.90 ± 0.11, $P < 0.05$) (Fig. 1b, c, d). The relative intensities and distributions of NRG1, the ErbB2 receptor and M2 muscarinic receptor in detrusor muscle were approximately, 1.2-, 1.3-, and 1.4- fold higher, respectively, in the PBOO group than the control group (1.86 ± 0.36 vs. 1.60 ± 0.17, 1.23 ± 0.27 vs. 0.93 ± 0.18, and 1.20 ± 0.30 vs. 0.89 ± 0.15, $P > 0.05$) (Fig. 1b, c, d).

mRNA expression of NRG1, ErbB2 receptor, and M2 muscarinic receptor

We evaluated the mRNA expression levels of NRG1 (358 bp), ErbB2 (483 bp) and M2 muscarinic receptor (557 bp) in the urothelium and detrusor muscle of bladders from PBOO-induced OAB and control groups using RT-PCR. The mRNA expression level of NRG1 was higher in the urothelium and detrusor muscle of rat bladders with PBOO-induced OAB than control rats (Fig. 2a, b) ($P < 0.05$). The mRNA expression of ErbB2 exhibited a similar pattern to NRG1; however, the PBOO group exhibited significantly higher levels of ErbB2 in the urothelium and detrusor muscle (Fig. 2a, c) ($P < 0.05$). There was no significant difference in the mRNA expression level of M2 muscarinic receptors in the detrusor muscle of rat bladder ($P > 0.05$). A significant difference was observed in the mRNA expression levels of M2 muscarinic receptors in the urothelium of rat bladder between the PBOO group and control (Fig. 2a, d) ($P < 0.05$).

Discussion

BOO produces significant alterations in bladder structure, such as detrusor hypertrophy, and function, including elevated detrusor pressure during contraction and detrusor instability, which lead to impairment in the storage and emptying of the bladder and morphological and physiological transformations of the urothelium, suburothelium and detrusor muscle [17, 18]. The urothelium affects nerve activity, contraction of the detrusor muscle and bladder function by evoking the release of various mediators in response to the sensing of mechanical and chemical stimuli [6]. A recent human study demonstrated urothelium dysfunction, increased suburothelial inflammation and apoptosis, and altered sensory protein expression in the mucosa of bladders in patients with BOO [18].

Muscarinic receptors may be an important factor in the voiding reflex of bladders. Activation of muscarinic receptors is one of the mechanisms driving detrusor muscle contractions. Five different subtypes of muscarinic receptor are expressed in the urothelium of mouse bladder [19], and the M2 muscarinic receptor favourably couples to the inhibition of adenylyl cyclase via the Gi subunit [20]. The density of M2 muscarinic receptors is greater than the density of M3 muscarinic receptors in the bladder and other smooth muscles, but subtype-selective muscarinic receptor antagonists demonstrated that M3 muscarinic receptors exhibit higher affinity than M2 muscarinic receptors under normal bladder conditions [21]. An increase in total and M2 muscarinic receptor density is observed in certain pathological

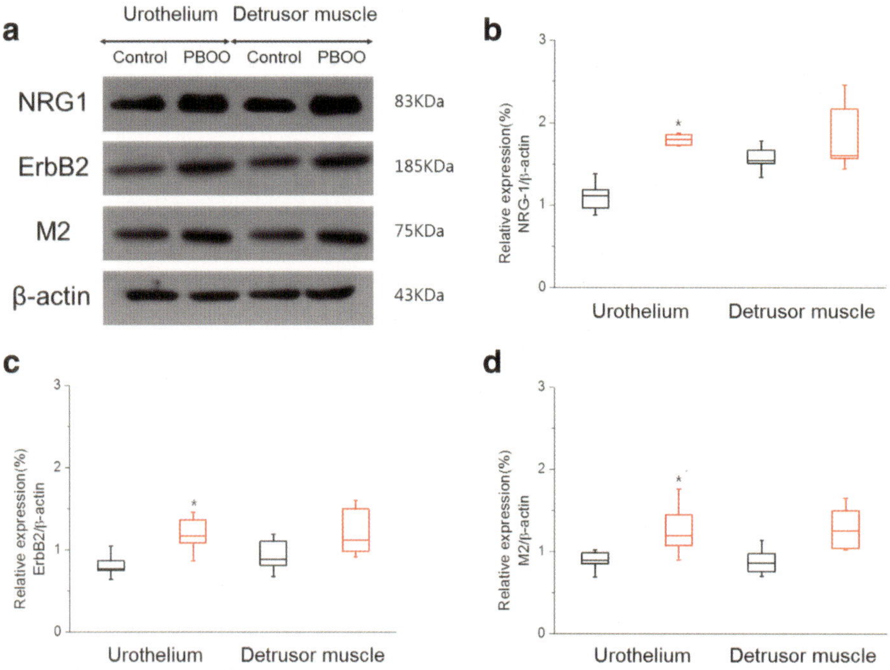

Fig. 1 Representative immunoblots (**a**) and comparison of relative expression of NRG-1 (**b**), ErbB2 (**c**) and M2 muscarinic receptor (**d**) protein expression in urothelium and detrusor muscle between control (black plot) and PBOO group (red plot). β-actin was used as the loading control. Values of NRG-1, ErbB2 and M2 muscarinic receptor expression are normalized relative to β-actin expression. The asterisk indicates a significant difference (Mann Whitney test $p < 0.05$)

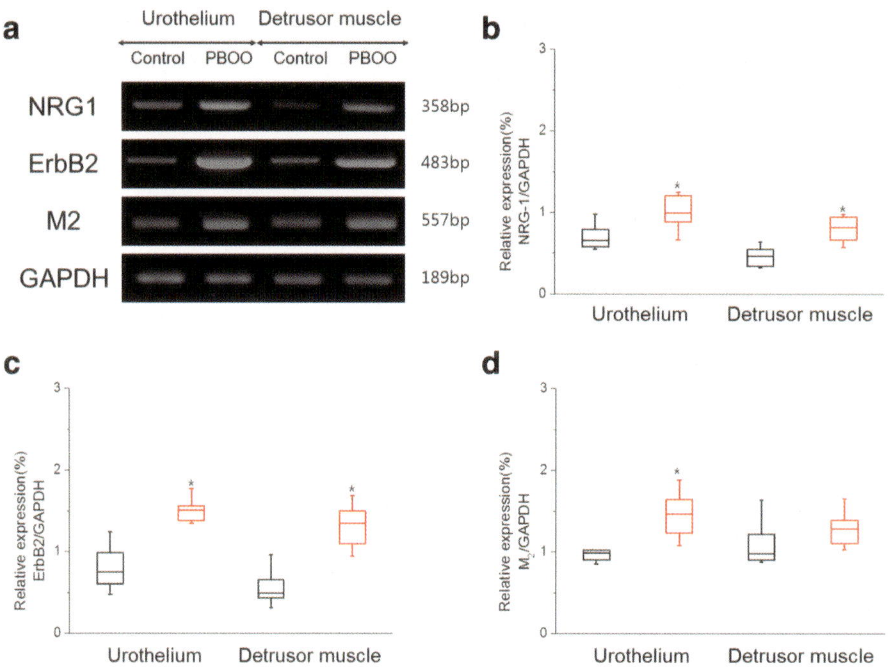

Fig. 2 Representative RT-PCR expression (**a**) and comparison of relative expression of NRG-1 (**b**), ErbB2 (**c**) and M2 muscarinic receptor (**d**) mRNA expression in urothelium and detrusor muscle between control (black plot) and PBOO group (red plot). GAPDH was used as the loading control. Values of NRG-1, ErbB2 and M2 muscarinic receptor expression are normalized relative to GAPDH expression. The asterisk indicates a significant difference (Mann Whitney test $p < 0.05$)

conditions, especially in hypertrophied bladders following spinal cord injury and denervation. The pathophysiology of BOO-induced OAB includes mediation of bladder afferent neural transduction via overexpression of M2 and M3 muscarinic, P2X3 [22] and TRPV4 [23] receptors in the urothelium. However, the expression of M2 and M3 muscarinic receptors in BOO-induced urothelium is controversial. Bschleipfer [24] et al. reported that BOO did not induce significant alterations in the human urothelial non-neuronal cholinergic system at the mRNA level. However, Jiang [18] et al. noted that patients with BOO exhibited increased P2X3 and M2 muscarinic receptor expression but lower M3 muscarinic receptor expression in the bladder mucosa. Braverman and Ruggieri [25] reported that rat bladder hypertrophy induced by BOO, independent of bladder denervation, shifted the muscarinic receptor subtype mediating bladder contraction from M3 towards M2 muscarinic receptors. Kim [22] et al. reported overexpression of M2 and M3 muscarinic and P2X3 receptors in the urothelium of the BOO group, and overexpression of M3 muscarinic receptors in the muscle layer of the BOO group was also noted. However, our study demonstrated no significant difference in the immunoreactivity of M2 muscarinic receptors in the detrusor muscle, but the PBOO group exhibited increased M2 muscarinic receptor expression in the urothelium. This evidence supports the significant roles of M2 muscarinic receptors in BOO-induced bladder dysfunction.

There are few reports on NRG1 in the urinary bladder, but research on NRG1 in the heart is very active. NRG1 is a member of the EGF family, and NRG1/ErbB signalling may function in many tissues to create, and perhaps repair, tissue architecture via accommodation of cell-to-cell interactions in some organs, such as breast and heart [26]. Okoshi et al. demonstrated that NRG1 produced a negative inotropic effect via activation of the muscarinic response in cultured cardiomyocytes [27]. Activation of muscarinic receptors may lead to improved fractional shortening via modulation of the inotropic response to beta-adrenergic stimulation [28]. Another role of NRG1 in the heart was regenerative activity following focal ischaemia. Bersell [14] et al. demonstrated that NRG1/ErbB4 signalling induced mononucleated cardiomyocytes to proliferate, which resulted in the cardiac repair mechanisms in old myocardial infarction without influencing the level of apoptosis. NRG1/ErbB signalling is likely an important paracrine mediator of cell-to-cell interactions that exerts a negative inotropic effect via activation of the muscarinic response and helps regenerate cardiomyocytes following cardiac ischaemia via an NRG1-mediated ErbB2/ErbB4 signalling pathway.

Yamaguchi [29] et al. reported that BOO-produced bladder ischaemia resulted in urothelial damage via activation of hypoxia-inducible factor pathways and further oxidative stress and denervation disturbed urothelial homeostasis. They suggested that the extent of bladder dysfunction in chronic bladder ischaemia depended on the duration and degree of ischaemia. A moderate degree of bladder ischaemia may result in detrusor overactivity and storage symptoms via a post-junctional hypersensitivity because of partial denervation of the detrusor muscle and sensitization of afferent pathways. The progression from moderate to severe bladder ischaemia increases damage to the detrusor muscle and the progression of denervation, which may result in detrusor underactivity and voiding symptoms. The results of the present study demonstrated increased protein and mRNA expression levels of NRG1/ErbB2 in the urothelium, but not the muscle layer. Our findings suggest that upregulated NRG1/ErbB receptors may exert a functional role via receptors located in the urothelium as a result of muscarinic receptor activation and NRG1/ErbB may be associated with detrusor smooth muscle proliferation against chronic bladder ischaemia. Arrighi [30] et al. reported that M2 and M3 muscarinic receptors mediated human detrusor smooth muscle contraction and proliferation via Akt/PI3K and MAP kinases. We previously reported the effects of NRG1 on the expression of nicotinic acetylcholine receptors via the ErbB2/ErbB3-PI3K-MAPK signalling cascade in major pelvic ganglion [31]. Upregulated NRG1 may play a role in detrusor muscle proliferation using the PI3K-MAPK signalling cascade via upregulated M2 muscarinic receptors.

Conclusions

We found remarkable changes in muscarinic and NRG1/ErbB receptors in PBOO-induced OAB. These results suggest that the overexpression of muscarinic and NRG1/ErbB2 receptors in the bladder, especially the urothelium, play a potential role in the afferent sensory responses of the urinary bladder. The NRG1 may be up-regulated by activation of the muscarinic receptors through PI3K/MAPK signaling cascades which is 10 multiple binding profiles to affect the ErbB2 receptor and protects the bladder against bladder ischemia by BOO. However, comprehension about muscarinic and neuregulin/ErbB receptors is limited, and further research about agonists, antagonists and knock-out mice should be performed. The results of these studies would increase our understanding of the development OAB induced by BOO and contribute to improved treatments for overactive bladder.

Abbreviations

BOO: Bladder outlet obstruction; BPH: Benign prostatic hyperplasia; OAB: Overactive bladder; PBOO: Partial BOO

Acknowledgements

The authors acknowledges the members of the department of Urology, Chungnam National University.

Funding

This work was supported by research fund of Chungnam National University.

Authors' contributions

SWY and KHS were involved in protocol, project development, data collection and management, data analysis, and manuscript writing and editing; SWJ was involved in data collection and management and data analysis. All authors read and approved the final manuscript.

Competing interests

The authors declare that they have no competing interests.

Author details

[1]Department of Urology, School of Medicine, Chungnam National University Hospital, Chungnam National University, 282 Monwha-ro, Jung-gu, Daejeon, Republic of Korea35015. [2]Department of Physiology, Yonsei University Wonju College of Medicine, Wonju, Republic of Korea.

References

1. Mostwin JL. Pathophysiology: the varieties of bladder overactivity. Urology 2002;60(5 Suppl 1):22–26; discussion 27.
2. Pontes-Junior J, Nunes RL. Dos reis ST, de Oliveira LC, Viana N, Leite KR, et al. adhesion molecules of detrusor muscle cells are influenced by a hypercholesterolemic diet or bladder outlet obstruction in a Wistar rat model. BMC Urol. 2013;13:50.
3. Banakhar MA, Al-Shaiji TF, Hassouna MM. Pathophysiology of overactive bladder. Int Urogynecol J. 2012;23:975–82.
4. Tyagi P. Pathophysiology of the urothelium and detrusor. Can Urol Asso J. 2011;5:S128–30.
5. Birder LA. More than just a barrier: urothelium as a drug target for urinary bladder pain. Am J Physiol Renal Physiol. 2005;289:F489–95.
6. Birder LA. Urothelial signaling. Auton Neurosci. 2010;153:33–40.
7. Kanai A, Andersson KE. Bladder afferent signaling: recent findings. J Urol. 2010;183(4):1288–95.
8. Ferguson DR, Kennedy I, Burton TJ. ATP is released from rabbit urinary bladder epithelial cells by hydrostatic pressure changes–a possible sensory mechanism? J Physiol. 1997;505(Pt 2):503–11.
9. Sui G, Fry CH, Montgomery B, Roberts M, Wu R, Wu C. Purinergic and muscarinic modulation of ATP release from the urothelium and its paracrine actions. Am J Physiol Renal Physiol. 2014;306(3):F286–98.
10. Birder LA, Apodaca G, De Groat WC, Kanai AJ. Adrenergic- and capsaicin-evoked nitric oxide release from urothelium and afferent nerves in urinary bladder. Am J Phys. 1998;275(2 Pt 2):F226–9.
11. Beckel JM, Kanai A, Lee SJ, de Groat WC, Birder LA. Expression of functional nicotinic acetylcholine receptors in rat urinary bladder epithelial cells. Am J Physiol Renal Physiol. 2006;290(1):F103–10.
12. Steers WD, Tuttle JB. Mechanisms of disease: the role of nerve growth factor in the pathophysiology of bladder disorders. Nat Clin Prac Urol. 2006;3(2):101–10.
13. Mei L, Xiong WC. Neuregulin 1 in neural development, synaptic plasticity and schizophrenia. Nat Rev Neurosci. 2008;9(6):437–52.
14. Bersell K, Arab S, Haring B, Kuhn B. Neuregulin1/ErbB4 signaling induces cardiomyocyte proliferation and repair of heart injury. Cell. 2009;138(2):257–70.
15. Song KH, Youn CS, Lee CL, Yang SW, Chang YS, Jeong SW, et al. Increased expression of Neuregulin 1 and erbB2 tyrosine kinase in the bladder of rats with cyclophosphamide-induced interstitial cystitis. Int Neurourol J. 2015;19(3):158–63.
16. Melman A, Tar M, Boczko J, Christ G, Leung AC, Zhao W, et al. Evaluation of two techniques of partial urethral obstruction in the male rat model of bladder outlet obstruction. Urol. 2005;66(5):1127–33.
17. Andersson KE, Arner A. Urinary bladder contraction and relaxation: physiology and pathophysiology. Physiol Rev. 2004;84(3):935–86.
18. Jiang YH, Lee CL, Kuo HC. Urothelial dysfunction, suburothelial inflammation and altered sensory protein expression in men with bladder outlet obstruction and various bladder dysfunctions: correlation with Urodynamics. J Urol. 2016;196(3):831–7.
19. Zarghooni S, Wunsch J, Bodenbenner M, Bruggmann D, Grando SA, Schwantes U, et al. Expression of muscarinic and nicotinic acetylcholine receptors in the mouse urothelium. Life Sci. 2007;80(24–25):2308–13.
20. Caulfield MP, Birdsall NJ. International Union of Pharmacology. XVII. Classification of muscarinic acetylcholine receptors. Pharmacol Rev. 1998; 50(2):279–90.
21. Eglen RM, Hegde SS, Watson N. Muscarinic receptor subtypes and smooth muscle function. Pharmacol Rev. 1996;48(4):531–65.
22. Kim JC, Yoo JS, Park EY, Hong SH, Seo SI, Hwang TK. Muscarinic and purinergic receptor expression in the urothelium of rats with detrusor overactivity induced by bladder outlet obstruction. BJU Int. 2008;101(3):371–5.
23. Cho KJ, Park EY, Kim HS, Koh JS, Kim JC. Expression of transient receptor potential vanilloid 4 and effects of ruthenium red on detrusor overactivity associated with bladder outlet obstruction in rats. World J Urol. 2014;32(3):677–82.
24. Bschleipfer T, Weidner W, Kummer W, Lips KS. Does bladder outlet obstruction alter the non-neuronal cholinergic system of the human urothelium? Life Sci. 2012;91(21–22):1082–6.
25. Braverman AS, Ruggieri MR. Hypertrophy changes the muscarinic receptor subtype mediating bladder contraction from M3 toward M2. Am J Phys. 2003;285(3):R701–8.
26. Talmage DA. Mechanisms of neuregulin action. Novartis Found Symp. 2008;289:74–84. discussion 84-93
27. Okoshi K, Nakayama M, Yan X, Okoshi MP, Schuldt AJ, Marchionni MA, et al. Neuregulins regulate cardiac parasympathetic activity: muscarinic modulation of beta-adrenergic activity in myocytes from mice with neuregulin-1 gene deletion. Circulation. 2004;110(6):713–7.
28. Vasti C, Hertig CM. Neuregulin-1/erbB activities with focus on the susceptibility of the heart to anthracyclines. W. J Cardiol. 2014;6(7):653–62.
29. Yamaguchi O, Nomiya M, Andersson KE. Functional consequences of chronic bladder ischemia. Neurourol Urodyn. 2014;33(1):54–8.
30. Arrighi N, Bodei S, Zani D, Michel MC, Simeone C, Cosciani Cunico S, et al. Different muscarinic receptor subtypes modulate proliferation of primary human detrusor smooth muscle cells via Akt/PI3K and map kinases. Pharmacol Res. 2013;74:1–6.
31. Kim HG, Lee CK, Cho SM, Whang K, Cha BH, Shin JH, et al. Neuregulin 1 up-regulates the expression of nicotinic acetylcholine receptors through the ErbB2/ErbB3-PI3K-MAPK signaling cascade in adult autonomic ganglion neurons. J Neurochem. 2013;124(4):502–13.

Predictive value of C-reactive protein in patients treated with sunitinib for metastatic clear cell renal cell carcinoma

Martin Pilskog[1,2], Christian Beisland[3,5], Lars A. Akslen[1,4], Leif Bostad[4], Åse Haug[2], Daniel Heinrich[6], Karin M. Hjelle[3,5] and Oddbjørn Straume[1,2*]

Abstract

Background: Sunitinib has become mainstay first line treatment for patients with metastatic renal clear cell carcinoma (mRCC). Still, useful predictive markers of response are lacking and urgently needed for clinical decision making.

Methods: In the present study we investigated the predictive value of standard serum markers as well as clinical markers, including C-reactive protein (CRP), Neutrophil to Lymphocyte ratio (NLR) and early hypertension (eHTN) in an unselected prospective patient population treated with sunitinib for mRCC. Forty-six patients were enrolled in a prospective single-arm study of predictive markers for sunitinib response. Response rates according to RECIST 1.1 were used as primary end-point. Secondary objectives were to evaluate prognostic value of the candidate markers with regard to progression free survival (PFS) and overall survival (OS). In addition, toxicity rates and quality of life was recorded.

Results: Median PFS and OS was 9.1 months and 15.0 months, respectively. Of 38 patients evaluable for response, 1 patient had complete response (CR), 7 had partial response (PR), 18 had stable disease (SD) and 12 had progressive disease (PD). Normal CRP at baseline was significantly associated with objective response (CR + PR) ($p = 0.01$). Normal CRP was also significantly associated with improved PFS and OS (Log rank, $p = 0.05$ and <0.01, respectively). Early hypertension, NLR and IMDC risk score were not significantly associated with response rates or survival.

Conclusion: Baseline CRP was a significant predictive factor of sunitinib response *and* a prognostic factor of survival. Baseline CRP might be a useful biomarker in the treatment planning of mRCC. Due to the relatively small sample size, our results need to be confirmed in larger studies.

Background

The frequent inactivation of the Von Hippel Lindau (*VHL*) gene in clear cell renal cell carcinoma, leading to increased levels of hypoxia inducible factor 1 (HIF1) and vascular endothelial growth factor (VEGF), provides the rationale for treatment with antiangiogenic receptor tyrosine kinase (rTKI) inhibitors. Since the reporting of the first positive clinical trial [1], showing an overall survival benefit from a rTKI, sunitinib has become mainstay first line treatment for patients with metastatic renal cell carcinoma (mRCC). Although objective response rates are reported for around 50% of the patients, development of resistance to the treatment is a major problem [2]. Clearly, a subset of patients does not benefit from treatment with sunitinib, and side effects are frequent. Interestingly, hypertension is a common side effect of angiogenesis inhibitors and has been associated with improved treatment response [3]. In the research community, considerable effort has been made to identify and validate predictive biomarkers of response to sunitinib treatment, but so far, no biomarkers have been established as useful in clinical decision making and treatment planning.

There is increasing evidence to support an important role of systemic inflammation in development and progression

* Correspondence: Oddbjorn.straume@helse-bergen.no
[1]Centre for Cancer Biomarkers CCBIO, University of Bergen, Bergen, Norway
[2]Department of Oncology, Haukeland University Hospital, 5021 Bergen, Norway
Full list of author information is available at the end of the article

of RCC [4], as recently substantiated by positive results from a clinical trial with the PD-1 inhibitor nivolumab in mRCC [5]. VEGF does not only stimulate tumor associated angiogenesis, but also plays an important role in the local immune response in wounds (physiologic) and tumors (pathologic) by inducing accumulation of immature dendritic cells, myeloid-derived suppressor cells, regulatory T cells, as well as by inhibiting the migration of T lymphocytes to the tumor [6]. Thus, it is relevant to also explore biomarkers primarily associated with inflammatory responses in the search for predictive markers for response to anti-VEGF therapy.

C-reactive protein (CRP) is an established biomarker for systemic inflammation, available in most clinical datasets, and provides prognostic information in several cancers including RCC [7]. Another biomarker of inflammation, neutrophil-to-lymphocyte ratio (NLR), adds prognostic information in RCC, and was recently suggested as a predictive marker of response to sunitinib in mRCC [8]. In the present trial we investigated the predictive value of serum markers, including CRP and NLR, in an unselected prospective patient population treated with sunitinib for mRCC. In addition, we report on toxicity and health related quality of life (HRQoL) data.

Methods

Patients and treatment

Between October 2007 and October 2014, a regional cohort of 77 patients with mRCC was screened for inclusion in this prospective study at Haukeland University Hospital, Bergen, Norway. Forty-six patients were enrolled after signing the informed consent sheet (CONSORT Flow Diagram, Additional file 1: Fig. S1). Inclusion criteria included: previously untreated metastatic or non-resectable clear cell RCC, WHO performance state 0–2, no known brain metastases, evaluable tumor lesions according to RECIST (version 1.1) and no significant comorbidity or laboratory abnormalities. See Additional file 2: Table S1 for all inclusion criteria. Sunitinib was administered 50 mg/day on schedule 4 weeks on/ two weeks off. Patients continued on treatment until disease progression, significant toxicity or consent withdrawal. Data was collected from the hospital records and included demographics, treatment modifications, adverse events, radiologic response data and survival. Data cut-off date was July 31 2015.

The main objective of this study was to identify and evaluate the predictive value of candidate markers readily available in a standard clinical setting, in mRCC patients treated with sunitinib. Candidate markers included early hypertension (eHTN), IMDC risk groups, baseline neutrophil to lymphocyte ratio (NLR), baseline CRP and baseline EORTC QoL symptom scale. Response rates according to RECIST 1.1 were used as primary endpoint. Secondary objectives were to evaluate prognostic value of the candidate markers with regard to progression free survival (PFS) and overall survival (OS). In addition, toxicity rates and HRQoL was recorded.

Assessment of response, adverse events and quality of life

The primary endpoint was objective response (OR) defined as complete response (CR) or partial response (PR) according to RECIST v.1.1 as well as clinical benefit (CB) defined as CR + PR and including stable disease (SD) for more than 6 months. Disease stabilization is considered beneficial to patients experiencing progression at the time of inclusion and CB is frequently included as an additional statistical endpoint in trials investigating antiangiogenic drugs in which therapeutic activity and clinical benefit are present, even in the absence of radiological tumor shrinkage [9]. Importantly, all patients were in clinical and/or radiological progression at the time of inclusion. OR and CB were calculated on the basis of investigator assessment. Response evaluation by CT-scan or MRI was performed every 12 weeks. Patients with clinically evident disease progression or death due to mRCC before first radiological progression were recorded as progressive disease (PD). Best overall response (BOR), recorded as change in size of target lesion, was not available in these patients. PFS was defined as the time from treatment initiation until disease progression according to RECIST v.1.1. OS was defined as the time from enrollment until death of any cause.

Standard blood samples, including CRP and neutrophil/lymphocyte counts, were taken at treatment initiation and every 6 weeks during treatment. Adverse events were graded according to the National Cancer Institute Common Terminology Criteria for Adverse events, version 3.0 (CTCAE v.3.0), and were recorded at each 6-week cycle. Early hypertension (eHTN) was particularly evaluated for its potential role as a predictive marker for treatment response. We recorded eHTN in two different ways. First, we defined eHTN as either maximum post-baseline systolic blood pressure (SBP) $\geq$140 mmHg or maximum post-baseline diastolic blood pressure (DBP) $\geq$90 mmHg recorded at week 6 and week 12 [3]. Second, we recorded eHTN as HTN $\geq$ grade 1 defined by CTCAE v.3.0 at week 6 and week 12. All other adverse events were recorded every six weeks throughout the entire treatment period. Patients that stopped treatment due to toxicity before 1st tumor response evaluation at week 12 were not included in the analyses of response rates or PFS, but were included in the analyses of OS.

HRQoL was assessed by a validated Norwegian version of the questionnaire of the European Organization for Research and Treatment of Cancer (EORTC QLQ-C30 v.3.0) at baseline and every 12 weeks during treatment.

The QLQ-C30 contains a global health/QoL scale, five functional scales (physical, role, cognitive, emotional, and social), three symptom scales (fatigue, pain, and nausea/vomiting) and six single items (dyspnoea, insomnia, anorexia, constipation, diarrhoea, and financial difficulties). The answers are given according to a 4-point Likert format, with the exception of questions about general health and quality of life, which are given according to a 7-point Likert format. Scores was calculated as described in the EORTC QLQ-C30 Scoring manual (3rd edition) [10]. The C 30 functional scales and the global scale were transformed so that 100% indicates best function and 0% least function of the individual QoL index, whereas the C30 symptom scales were transformed so that 0% indicates the least and 100% the most symptoms. We compared the upper quartile with the lower 3 quartiles for the symptom sum score and the lower quartile with the upper 3 quartiles for the functional sum score and global health/QoL score.

Statistical analyses

The Mann-Whitney U test was used to compare the distribution of continuous variables between two groups such as responders and non-responders. Comparisons between categorical variables were performed by using the Fisher's exact test. Spearman's rank correlation coefficient was used to test correlations between variables of interest. Logistic regression analysis was used to test the relative importance of predictive factors for sunitinib response. Cronbach's α was used to estimate the reliability of the global health score and the functional/symptomatic scores made up of more than one question. Kaplan-Meier estimates were applied for time-to-event endpoints such as PFS and OS, and log rank-test was applied for testing of differences between groups. Sample size calculations were based on a difference in response rate of 40% (i.e. 10% and 50%) between groups identified by the candidate markers. Thirty-eight patients were needed to achieve a power of 80% with an α-value of 0.05. All p-values are two-sided. Statistical investigation were done using IBM SPSS Statistics version 22.

Results

Patient population and treatment efficacy

The characteristics of the 46 patients enrolled in the study are presented in Table 1. In our cohort the median age was 63.1 (range 41.1–84.0). By July 31st, 2015 the median follow up time was 13.8 months (range 1.8–83.9). Twenty-six patients had prior removal of the primary tumor, twenty-four by radical and 2 by partial nephrectomy. Six patients had resection of bone metastasis, eight patients had resection of other metastasis, one patient had gamma knife radiosurgery of brain metastasis and two patients had radiation therapy against bone metastasis prior to sunitinib treatment. Median time on treatment was 5.7 months (range 0.5–63.0). Median time from first diagnosis of renal cell carcinoma to treatment was 3.2 months (range 0.3–124). Median time to treatment from diagnosis of metastasis was 1.4 months (range 0.3–66.5).

Table 1 Baseline Patients Characteristics

	Study cohort (n = 46)
Age, years	
Median	63.1
Range	41.1–84.0
Sex - No. (%)	
Male	29 (63.0)
Female	17 (37.0)
WHO performance status - No. (%)	
0	30 (65.2)
1	16 (34.8)
2	0 (0.0)
Site of metastases - No. (%)	
Brain	1 (2.2)
Lung	35 (76.1)
Pleura	3 (6.5)
Liver	4 (8.7)
Bone	16 (34.8)
Lymph nodes	28 (60.9)
Number of disease sites - No. (%)	
1	10 (21.7)
2	11 (23.9)
≥ 3	25 (54.3)
Hypertension before treatment - No. (%)	
Yes	24 (52.2)
No	22 (47.8)
IMDC risk score – No. (%)	
Good	7 (15.2)
Intermediate	16 (34.8)
Poor	21 (45.7)
Missing	*2 (4.3)*
Time from initial diagnosis - No. (%)	
≤ 12 months	33 (71.7)
> 12 months	13 (28.3)
Prior removal of primary tumor - No. (%)	
Radical nephrectomy	24 (52.2)
Partial nephrectomy	2 (4.3)
No	20 (43.5)

Abbreviations: *WHO* World Health Organisation, *IMDC* International Metastatic Renal Cell Carcinoma Database Consortium

By July 31 2015, median progression free survival (PFS) was 9.1 months (range 0.5–57.3) and median overall survival (OS) was 15.4 months (range 1.8–83.9). At data cut-off, 9 patients were still alive, and six patients were still on sunitinib treatment without signs of progression. Twenty-three patients started second line systemic treatment. We observed 1 complete response (CR), 7 partial responses (PR) and 18 patients had stable disease (SD) ≥ 6 months. Twelve patients showed progressive disease (PD), of which 10 were confirmed by radiology and 2 were confirmed by clinical progress before week 12. Eight patients stopped treatment before week 12 and were recorded as non-evaluable for response rates and PFS. Of these, six were due to toxicity without evidence of disease progression, one patient due to appendicitis and one protocol violation. Of interest, seven of these eight patients were females.

Predictive value of pre-treatment clinical and biochemical markers and survival analyses

The correlations between clinical, as well as biochemical markers assessed ahead of treatment initiation and sunitinib response are given in Table 2. The association between clinical, as well as biochemical markers assessed ahead of treatment initiation, PSF and OS is given in Table 3.

C-reactive protein (CRP)

Median CRP at baseline was 17.0 mg/L, range 0–235 mg/L. Seventeen of 37 patients evaluated for overall response had normal CRP (≤10 mg/L). Normal CRP at baseline was significantly associated with OR (CR + PR) (Fisher's exact test, $p = 0.01$) (Fig. 1). Seven/17 (41%) of patients with normal CRP had an objective response to sunitinib, compared with 1/20 (5%) patients with elevated CRP had an objective response. Logistic regression analysis was used to test the relative importance of the candidate predictive factors for sunitinib response(eHTN, IMDC risk groups, baseline NLR, baseline CRP, baseline EORTC QoL symptom scale). Only CRP level at baseline was an independent predictive variable of response, with an odds ratio of 14.3 ($p = 0.02$) of not having an objective response if CRP was above normal (10 mg/L). CRP at baseline was significantly correlated with several other variables including age, function sum score, symptom sum score, performance status and tumor load (Additional file 3: Table S2). Median PFS was significantly longer among patients with normal CRP at baseline (median 14.7 vs 5.3 months, log rank $p = 0.05$). Similarly, an improved OS was found in patients with normal CRP at baseline (median 26.0 vs 12.1 months, log-rank $p < 0.01$) (Fig. 2 a, b).

Neutrophil to lymphocyte ratio (NLR)

Twenty-two of 34 (64%) patients evaluated for response and available NLR, had NLR ≤3 at baseline (median = 2.7, range 1.0–7.9) and NLR at baseline was not significantly correlated with OR or CB. Eighty-three % of patients evaluated for response had NLR ≤3 at week 6 (median = 1.6, range 0.4–5.9) and this was not significantly correlated to OR or CB. A shift from NLR >3 at baseline to ≤3 at week 6 ($n = 10$) was not significantly associated with OR or CB. Median PFS among patients with baseline NLR ≤3 was significantly better than patients with baseline NLR >3 (median 14.7 vs 6.7 months, log rank $p = 0.05$). A borderline association was present between baseline NLR ≤3 and OS (median 25.2 vs 13.2 months, log-rank $p = 0.06$). High NLR at baseline was significantly correlated with increased tumor load ($r = 0.43$, $p = 0.005$, Spearman).

Treatment induced early hypertension (eHTN)

Applying the first definition of eHTN (SBP ≥140 or DBP ≥90 mmHg at week 6 and week 12) seventeen of 32 patients (53%) evaluated for response had eHTN after week 6. Median SBP over DBP was 145 (range: 120–170) mmHg over 89 (range: 60–170) mmHg, and was not significantly associated to OR or CB. Using the same definition at week 12, fifteen of 19 patients (79%) had eHTN. Median SBP over DBP was 142 (range: 120–170) mmHg over 88 (range: 65–107) mmHg, and was significantly associated with improved CB, but not OR (Fischer's exact test $p = 0.04$ and $p = 0.53$, respectively) (Table 2). The second definition (based on CTCAE v 3.0) of eHTN was not significantly associated OR or CB (data not presented). eHTN at week 12 was associated with improved PFS and OS (Table 3). All seven patients with increased blood pressure during the two first cycles used anti-hypertensive drug(s) at baseline.

Risk scores

The distribution of IMDC risk score [11] is given in Table 1. IMDC risk score was not significantly associated with OR or CB. Good IMDC risk score versus intermediate and poor was not significantly correlated to PFS (median 20.4 vs 9.1 vs 8.4 months, log-rank $p = 0.10$), but was significantly associated with OS (median 67.9 vs 12.7 vs 13.7 months, log-rank $p = <0.01$). We found similar results for MSKCC risk score and WHO performance status (PS) (data not presented).

Metastatic sites

The distribution of metastatic sites is given in Table 1. There was no significant association between metastatic site and response rates. Although present in only 3 patients, pleura metastasis was significantly associated with reduced PFS (median 2.6 vs 9.1 months, log rank

Table 2 Univariate analyses of clinical and biochemical markers in relation to response to sunitinib

Variable	Best overall tumor response (RECIST ver. 1.1)					
	OR[1] n(%)	SD[2]+PD[3] n(%)	*p* value[4]	CB[5] n(%)	PD[3] n(%)	*p* value
Total	8(21)	30(79)		26(68)	12(32)	
Age			0.69			0.73
< 63.1	4(17)	19(83)		15(65)	8(35)	
≥ 63.1	4(27)	11(73)		11(73)	4(27)	
Sex			0.17			0.45
Female	4(40)	6(60)		8(80)	2(20)	
Male	4(14)	24(86)		18(64)	10(36)	
Number of disease sites			0.71			0.31
≤ 2	3(18)	14(82)		10(59)	7(41)	
> 2	5(24)	16(76)		16(76)	5(24)	
Prior nephrectomy			0.26			0.73
Yes	6(29)	15(71)		15(71)	6(29)	
No	2(12)	15(88)		11(65)	6(35)	
Pretreatment hypertension[6]			0.70			0.30
Yes	5(26)	14(74)		15(79)	4(21)	
No	3(16)	16(84)		11(58)	8(42)	
Treatment induced eHTN[7] ≤ week 6			1.00			0.70
Yes	4(23)	13(77)		13(76)	4(24)	
No	4(27)	11(73)		10(67)	5(33)	
Treatment induced eHTN[8] ≤ week 12			0.53			0.04
Yes	5(33)	10(67)		13(87)	2(13)	
No	0(0)	4(100)		1(25)	3(75)	
IMDC risk			0.77			0.46
Good	2(29)	5(71)		6(86)	1(14)	
Intermediate	3(25)	9(75)		9(75)	3(25)	
Poor	3(18)	14(82)		10(59)	7(41)	
NLR baseline ≤3			1.00			0.46
Yes	5(23)	17(77)		16(73)	6(27)	
No	3(25)	9(75)		7(58)	5(42)	
NLR week 6 ≤ 3			0.32			0.15
≤ 3	7(23)	23(77)		22(73)	8(27)	
> 3	0(0)	6(100)		2(33)	4(67)	
NLR shifted from >3 to ≤3 at week 6			1.00			0.06
Yes	2(25)	6(75)		6(75)	2(25)	
No	0(0)	3(100)		0(100)	3(100)	
NLR shifted from ≤3 to >3 at week 6			1.00			0.50
Yes	0(0)	2(100)		1(50)	1(50)	
No	5(26)	14(74)		14(74)	5(26)	
CRP ≤10 (mg/L)			0.01			0.09
Yes	7(41)	10(59)		14(82)	3(18)	
No	1(5)	19(95)		11(55)	9(45)	

Table 2 Univariate analyses of clinical and biochemical markers in relation to response to sunitinib *(Continued)*

EORTC QoL symptom scale at BL[9]			0.31			0.02
Upper quartile	0(0)	7(100)		2(29)	5(71)	
Lower 3 quartiles	8(27)	22(73)		24(80)	6(20)	

Abbreviations: *IMDC* International Metastatic Renal Cell Carcinoma Database Consortium, *LDH* Lactate dehydrogenase, *ULN* Upper limit of normal, *LLN* lower limit of normal, *NLR* neutrophil/lymphocyte ratio, *CRP* C-reactive protein, *BL* baseline

[1]Objective response (Complete + Partial response)

[2]Stable disease

[3]Progressive disease

[4]Fisher's exact test

[5]Clinical benefit (OR + SD)

[6]Defined as on anti-hypertensive treatment before initiation of sunitinib

[7]Defined as systolic blood pressure(SBP) $\geq$140 mmHg or diastolic blood pressure (DBP) $\geq$90 mmHg $\leq$ week 6

[8]Defined as $\geq$140 mmHg or diastolic blood pressure (DBP) $\geq$90 mmHg $\leq$ week 12

[9]Quality of Life

p = 0.05) and OS (median 10.8 vs 17.5 months, log-rank p = 0.04). Presence of lung metastasis was significantly associated with reduced OS (median 13.2 vs 48.2 months, log-rank p = 0.04). Other metastatic sites (brain, bone, liver or lymph nodes) were not significantly associated with PFS or OS.

Toxicity

Adverse events occurring during treatment with sunitinib according to CTCAE v.3.0 are summarized in Additional file 4: Table S3. The most common adverse effects of lower grade (1 + 2) were nausea (52.2%), anemia (47.8%), fatigue (45.7%) and diarrhea (39.1%). The most common severe adverse effects (grade 3 + 4) were hypertension (19.6%), fatigue (15.2%), low serum platelets (15.2%), hand-foot skin reaction (10.9%) and diarrhea (10.9%). We observed one grade 5 adverse effect (death due to appendicitis) probably not related to sunitinib treatment.

Health related quality of life

The results of the HRQoL questionnaires at baseline (n = 45) and at the first treatment evaluation (n = 28, after 12 weeks) are presented in Additional file 5: Table S4. Only for "Fatigue", there was a statistically significant increase in the score during treatment compared with the baseline value (p=0.041, Wilcoxon ranked signed test). The Cronbach- α of the indices derived by more than one question showed acceptable/good values (0.74-0.89), except for "cognitive function" (0.30) and "social functioning" (0.56). The Cronbach- α of the sum scores of functional indexes (0.80) and symptom indexes (0.79) were acceptable/good. In contrast to Global health status/QoL and Functional scale, a Symptom sum score below median was significantly associated to improved CB (Fisher's exact test, p = 0.02, Table 2). Investigating symptom sum scores indicated that the upper quartile had significantly worse OS (median 12.7 vs 25.2 months, log-rank p = 0.01) and PFS (median 2.9 vs 14.7 months, log-rank p = <0.01). No such difference could be demonstrated for global health/QoL status or functional sum score (data not shown).

Discussion

Until recently, palliative surgery, radiation therapy and chemotherapy were the only treatment options for metastatic RCC (mRCC), and primary therapy resistance, reduced quality of life and short survival were major challenges in this patient group. Currently, three major categories of systemic treatment exist for the largest subgroup of mRCC, the clear cell carcinomas: cytokines and immune checkpoint inhibitors, anti VEGF targeted drugs and mTOR inhibitors [12]. The two latter of these new treatment options have emerged based on recent knowledge of the pathogenesis of clear cell renal cancer. The von Hippel-Lindau (VHL) tumor suppressor gene is lost or mutated in 60–90% in sporadic cases [13] and is a major contributor to development of this cancer. Loss of VHL leads to a chronic stress response state in the cells trough high levels of HIF1-α, a transcription factor for a number of stress response proteins, including vascular endothelial growth factor (VEGF). In addition to being a potent angiogenic growth factor, VEGF plays a role in the local immune response in wounds and tumors by inducing accumulation of immature dendritic cells, myeloid-derived suppressor cells, regulatory T cells, as well as by inhibiting the migration of T lymphocytes to the tumor [6]. Renal cell cancer is regarded as highly immunogenic and angiogenic tumors, supporting VEGF as a promising target for treatment. The VEGF receptor inhibitor Sunitinib is currently first line treatment for mRCC [12], but a significant portion of the patients do not respond, and the search for good predictive markers of response has been disappointing so far. Whereas most focus in the search for predictive markers has been on angiogenesis, less focus has been on markers of immune responses. In the current study, we evaluated readily available clinical and biochemical markers, associated with systemic inflammation, for their association with response to sunitinib.

Table 3 Survival analyses according to clinical and biochemical variables

Variable	PFS[1]			OS[2]		
	Median	95% CI[3]	*p*-value[4]	Median	95% CI	*p*-value
Age			0.29			0.47
< 63.1	8.7	6.2–11.2		17.5	5.5–29.4	
≥ 63.1	20.4	3.2–37.7		15.0	12.4–17.6	
Sex			0.03			0.87
Female	NR	-		12.7	7.3–18.2	
Male	8.7	6.6–10.7		18.0	10.5–25.4	
Number of disease sites			0.80			0.52
≤ 2	12.9	2.1–23.7		17.5	11.3–23.7	
> 2	9.1	8.3–9.8		13.9	10.2–17.6	
Prior nephrectomy			0.07			<0.01
Yes	14.7	5.9–23.5		26.0	20.1–31.8	
No	8.7	3.1–14.3		10.8	4.5–17.0	
Pretreatment hypertension			0.42			0.79
Yes	17.0	6.2–27.7		18.0	9.4–26.5	
No	8.4	3.7–13.1		11.6	5.3–17.9	
Treatment induced early hypertension[5] at week 6			0.68			0.85
Yes	14.7	9.6–19.8		18.0	3.5–32.5	
No	8.7	3.9–13.5		12.1	3.8–20.4	
Treatment induced early hypertension[5] at week 12			<0.01			<0.01
Yes	14.7	10.1–19.3		26.0	24.1–27.9	
No	2.6	1.9–3.3		7.7	4.4–11.0	
IMDC risk score			0.10			<0.01
Good	20.4	13.1–27.7		67.9	38.4–97.5	
Intermediate	9.1	6.0–12.2		12.7	10.6–14.9	
Poor	8.4	0–17.7		13.7	5.4–22.1	
NLR baseline ≤3			0.05			0.06
Yes	14.7	8.8–20.6		25.2	10.6–39.8	
No	6.7	2.0–11.4		13.2	10.3–16.1	
NLR week 6 ≤ 3			0.09			<0.01
Yes	10.8	6.0–15.7		25.2	13.7–36.7	
No	1.8	0.2–3.5		3.8	3.3–4.3	
NLR shifted from >3 to ≤3 week 6			<0.01			<0.01
Yes	8.4	6.0–10.7		13.2	7.0–19.4	
No	1.3	0.9–1.7		3.6	0.8–6.4	
NLR shifted from ≤3 to >3 at week 6			0.75			0.16
Yes	NR	-		4.0	2.3–5.7	
No	14.7	9.2–20.3		26.0	24.2–27.7	
CRP			0.05			<0.01
≤ 10 (mg/L)	14.7	2.5–26.9		26.0	0.6–51.4	
> 10 (mg/L)	5.3	0.9–9.8		12.1	8.8–15.5	
EORTC QoL symptom scale at BL			<0.01			0.01
Upper quartile	2.8	2.2–3.5		12.7	4.8–20.7	
Lower 3 quartiles	14.7	4.6–24.8		25.2	12.7–37.7	

Abbreviations: *IMDC* International Metastatic Renal Cell Carcinoma Database Consortium, *LDH* Lactate dehydrogenase, *ULN* Upper limit of normal, *LLN* lower limit of normal, *NLR* neutrophil/lymphocyte ratio, *CRP* C-reactive protein, *NR* Not reached, *BL* Baseline

[1]Progression free survival

[2]Overall survival

[3]Confidence interval

[4]Log rank test

[5]Defined as systolic blood pressure(SBP) ≥140 mmHg or diastolic blood pressure (DBP) ≥90 mmHg

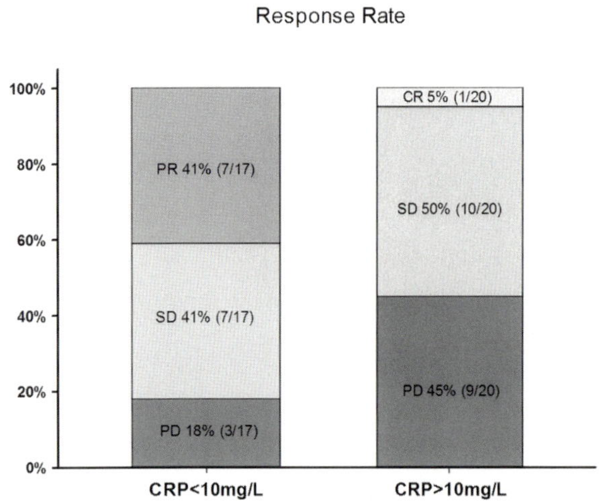

Fig. 1 Response rates as a function of baseline CRP levels. Patients with a baseline CRP ≤ 10 mg/L (normal) showed an objective response rate (CR + PR) of 41% whereas patients with elevated CRP showed an objective response rate of 5%. CR, complete response; PR, partial response; SD, stable disease; PD, progressive disease

C-reactive protein (CRP) is an acute-phase protein that increases rapidly following interleukin-6 secretion by macrophages and T cells following infection, inflammation and cancer [14]. CRP is a negative prognostic marker in most cancers. In the present study we found normal CRP to be a possible predictive factor of response. Whereas 41% of the patients with normal CRP at baseline experienced an objective response, this was the case for only 5% of patients with CRP levels at baseline above normal. CRP was also associated with PFS and OS supporting its role as a prognostic marker as well, and this is in line with previous reports [15–17]. Our finding supports the results of a recent study by Fujita et al. where normal level of CRP at baseline was an independent predictive marker of response by multivariate analysis [15]. In a retrospective study of 200 patients treated with sunitinib 61% of patients with normal CRP responded vs 32% of patients with elevated CRP [18]. In our trial, CRP was correlated to several factors including other markers of systemic inflammation such as high platelet counts, anemia as well as tumor load and performance status. Thus, CRP might represent a marker of disease burden identifying a patient subpopulation with poor prognosis, less likely to respond. Nevertheless, the significant association with response rates suggests that CRP might be a useful marker, in addition to other clinical and biochemical features to consider prior to initiation of systemic treatment. IL-6 is an important tumor-promoting protein associated with stress responses, inflammation and angiogenesis [19]. Through its major downstream target STAT3 several tumor promoting pathways are activated, including HIF1-α and VEGF [19]. Moreover, IL6 have direct stimulating effect on endothelial cells, and has been implicated in resistance to anti-VEGF therapy [20]. Being closely correlated to IL6 expression, increased CRP levels might therefore be a surrogate marker of IL6 driven disease, again being associated with expression of multiple angiogenic factors [21], thus less responsive to specific anti-VEGF treatment like sunitinib. Our results indicate that an inflammatory response, defined by high CRP is associated with poor response to sunitinib and poor prognosis in these patients. The effect of sunitinib on inhibiting the angiogenesis supporting and immunosuppressive effect of VEGF, thus seem to be more pronounced in patients with a non-inflammatory state defined by normal CRP.

The neutrophil-to-lymphocyte ratio (NLR) is also a marker of systemic inflammation in cancer patients and was found to add prognostic [22] and predictive [8] information in RCC in retrospective studies. Like CRP, NLR is readily available in standard blood samples in a regular clinical setting. Our NLR counts were comparable to what has been reported in other clinical datasets.

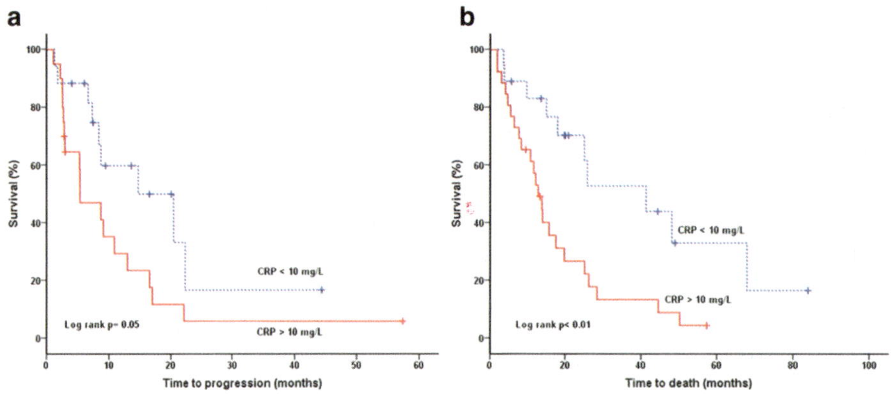

Fig. 2 Kaplan-meier estimates of **a**) progression free survival (PFS) and **b**) overall survival (OS) grouped by CRP level. The normal CRP (≤ 10 mg/L) cohort showed significantly improved PFS and OS compared with patients with elevated CRP

Although significantly associated with CRP, we did not find a statistically significant association with sunitinib response or survival. The significant correlation with performance status and tumor load suggests that NLR is a nonspecific marker of disease burden. Still, due to relatively small sample size and low statistical power, our data must be interpreted carefully.

Treatment induced early hypertension (eHTN) was not significantly associated with treatment response in our dataset. In our patient population, the baseline blood pressure was slightly higher when compared with the clinical trial population studied by Rini et al. [3], and 52% of our patients were hypertensive at baseline. Still, the number of patients recorded as having sunitinib induced eHTN after cycle 1 and 2, using the same criteria, was nearly the same (~80%). eHTN at week 12 was associated with improved survival, but this is most likely due to the fact that the responders in the study stayed on treatment long enough to develop hypertension. Even if pharmacodynamically interesting, as eHTN occurs *after* sunitinib initiation it is not going to be an applicable predictive marker in the clinic.

Our finding that higher baseline HRQoL symptoms score is prognostic for PFS and OS in treatment with Sunitinib is in line with the earlier report by Cella et al. [23]. In that report, however, a different QoL tool was used. Herrmann et al. demonstrated by using EORTC QLQ-C30, that "global QoL" was prognostic for PFS [24]. Our study did not confirm this finding. In general, there were only small changes in HRQoL scores form baseline to 12 weeks. Herrmann et al. also showed a relatively small change in the different HRQoL scales after 12 weeks [24]. This could be due to the administration of Sunitinib (4 weeks on/ 2 weeks off), with subsequent remission of eventual treatment induced symptoms. There are indications that long-term survivors might retain a good HRQoL over years, as described by Carmichael et al. [25].

A major challenge in studies exploring predictive markers of treatment response in clinical data-sets is the fact that most of the candidate predictive markers are prognostic as well, thus significantly correlated with PFS and OS independent of the treatment given. Combined predictive and prognostic markers are best evaluated in two-arm trials. In single arm trials such as ours, response rates according to RECIST are superior to PFS and OS as primary end-point when assessing predictive markers of treatment response. Many biomarker studies in mRCC have been performed retrospectively in data-sets from large clinical trials, and these patients are frequently positively selected and do not optimally reflect the normal patient population. The strength of our study is the prospective design and the "Real-World" patient population enrolled, reflecting a normal clinical setting. When compared with large retrospective multicenter studies as well as smaller single-center studies, the majority of our patients were in the poor risk group according to IMDC criteria. Whereas the portion of poor-risk patients varies between 18 and 33% in comparable studies [8, 11, 15], 46% of our patients belonged to this group. In addition, all patients were in confirmed clinical and/or radiological progression at the time of inclusion. Accordingly, patients with very slow progression or stable metastases were observed without systemic treatment and screened for inclusion in the study only after confirmed disease progression. In comparison with clinical phase III trials, PFS and OS were lower in our patients. Compared with the adverse events reported in clinical trials [26], the frequency of toxicity from sunitinib in metastatic renal cell cancer recorded in our study was similar, or somewhat less frequent. Especially, the hematological toxicity including anemia, neutropenia, thrombocytopenia and lymphopenia was less frequent in our trial, although using the same criteria (CTCAE v. 3.0). The most likely explanation for this discrepancy is that we assessed adverse events, including laboratory, every 6 weeks, where most of the patients were off the drug in the 4 + 2 weeks cycle.

In addition to the lack of a control group, our study has some weaknesses. First, the number of patients included is low and thereby the study lacks the significant power to detect minor differences in response rates between groups based on the biomarkers under investigation. Thus, our finding should be validated in an independent and larger cohort of patients. Second, CRP and NLR are non-specific markers of inflammation and angiogenesis, and further studies are required to identify the key regulators controlling the systemic responses to metastatic disease. In this report, we focused on biomarkers available in standard clinical blood samples routinely used in the clinic. Further studies of candidate biomarkers in serum and plasma, such as IL6 and IL8 are ongoing.

Conclusion

In conclusion, in this prospective study of sunitinib in patients with mRCC we found that normal level of s-CRP at baseline is significantly associated with improved response rates and might serve as guidance in the selection of optimal treatment. Still, due to the relatively small sample size and low statistical power, our results need to be confirmed in larger studies.

Abbreviations

IMDC: International Metastatic Renal Cell Carcinoma Database Consortium; MSKCC: Memorial Sloan Kettering Cancer Center

Funding

The study was supported by grants from The Norwegian Research Council, The Norwegian Cancer Society as well an unrestricted grant from Pfizer Norway. The authors alone are responsible for the content and writing of the paper. This work was partly supported by the Research Council of Norway through its Centres of Excellence funding scheme, project number 223250.

Authors' contributions

MP, CB, LAA, OS: Conception and design, acquisition of data, analysis and interpretation of data, project funding, and were major contributors in writing the manuscript. LB performed the histological examination of the H&E stained tumor biopsies, and was a major contributor in writing the manuscript. ÅH, DH and KMH collected the clinical data including the QoL data, and were major contributors in writing the manuscript. All authors have read and approved the final version of the manuscript.

Competing interests

The authors declare that they have no competing interests.

Author details

[1]Centre for Cancer Biomarkers CCBIO, University of Bergen, Bergen, Norway. [2]Department of Oncology, Haukeland University Hospital, 5021 Bergen, Norway. [3]Department of Urology, Haukeland University Hospital, 5021 Bergen, Norway. [4]Department of Pathology, Haukeland University Hospital, 5021 Bergen, Norway. [5]Department of Clinical Medicine, University of Bergen, Bergen, Norway. [6]Department of Oncology, Akershus University Hospital, 1478 Lørenskog, Norway.

References

1. Motzer RJ, Hutson TE, Tomczak P, Michaelson MD, Bukowski RM, Oudard S, Negrier S, Szczylik C, Pili R, Bjarnason GA, et al. Overall survival and updated results for sunitinib compared with interferon alfa in patients with metastatic renal cell carcinoma. J Clin Oncol. 2009;27(22):3584–90.
2. Rini BI, Atkins MB. Resistance to targeted therapy in renal-cell carcinoma. Lancet Oncol. 2009;10(10):992–1000.
3. Rini BI, Cohen DP, DR L, Chen I, Hariharan S, Gore ME, Figlin RA, Baum MS, Motzer RJ. Hypertension as a biomarker of efficacy in patients with metastatic renal cell carcinoma treated with sunitinib. J Natl Cancer Inst. 2011;103(9):763–73.
4. Mantovani A, Allavena P, Sica A, Balkwill F. Cancer-related inflammation. Nature. 2008;454(7203):436–44.
5. Motzer RJ, Escudier B, McDermott DF, George S, Hammers HJ, Srinivas S, Tykodi SS, Sosman JA, Procopio G, Plimack ER, et al. Nivolumab versus Everolimus in advanced renal-cell carcinoma. N Engl J Med. 2015;
6. Voron T, Marcheteau E, Pernot S, Colussi O, Tartour E, Taieb J, Terme M. Control of the immune response by pro-angiogenic factors. Front Oncol. 2014;4:70.
7. Casamassima A, Picciariello M, Quaranta M, Berardino R, Ranieri C, Paradiso A, Lorusso V, Guida M. C-reactive protein: a biomarker of survival in patients with metastatic renal cell carcinoma treated with subcutaneous interleukin-2 based immunotherapy. J Urol. 2005;173(1):52–5.
8. Keizman D, Ish-Shalom M, Huang P, Eisenberger MA, Pili R, Hammers H, Carducci MA. The association of pre-treatment neutrophil to lymphocyte ratio with response rate, progression free survival and overall survival of patients treated with sunitinib for metastatic renal cell carcinoma. Eur J Cancer. 2012;48(2):202–8.
9. Ratain MJ, Eckhardt SG. Phase II studies of modern drugs directed against new targets: if you are fazed, too, then resist RECIST. J Clin Oncol. 2004;22(22):4442–5.
10. Fayers P, Aaronson N, Bjordal K, Groenvold M, Curran D, Bottomley A, Group obotEQoL: The EORTC QLQ-C30 scoring manual (3rd edition). In. Brussels: the European organisation for research and treatment of Cancer; 2001.
11. Heng DY, Xie W, Regan MM, Harshman LC, Bjarnason GA, Vaishampayan UN, Mackenzie M, Wood L, Donskov F, Tan MH, et al. External validation and comparison with other models of the international metastatic renal-cell carcinoma database consortium prognostic model: a population-based study. Lancet Oncol. 2013;14(2):141–8.
12. Jonasch E, Gao J, Rathmell WK. Renal cell carcinoma. BMJ. 2014;349:g4797.
13. Kaelin WG Jr. The von Hippel-Lindau tumor suppressor protein and clear cell renal carcinoma. Clin Cancer Res. 2007;13(2 Pt 2):680s–4s.
14. Ljungberg B, Grankvist K, Rasmuson T. Serum interleukin-6 in relation to acute-phase reactants and survival in patients with renal cell carcinoma. Eur J Cancer. 1997;33(11):1794 8.
15. Fujita T, Iwamura M, Ishii D, Tabata K, Matsumoto K, Yoshida K, Baba S. C-reactive protein as a prognostic marker for advanced renal cell carcinoma treated with sunitinib. International journal of urology : official journal of the Japanese Urological Association. 2012;19(10):908–13.
16. Kawai Y, Osawa T, Kobayashi K, Inoue R, Yamamoto Y, Matsumoto H, Nagao K, Hara T, Sakano S, Nagamori S, et al. Factors prognostic for survival in Japanese patients treated with Sunitinib as first-line therapy for metastatic clear cell renal cell cancer. Asian Pacific journal of cancer prevention: APJCP. 2015;16(14):5687–90.
17. Teishima J, Kobatake K, Kitano H, Nagamatsu H, Sadahide K, Hieda K, Shinmei S, Shoji K, Inoue S, Hayashi T, et al. The impact of change in serum C-reactive protein level on the prediction of effects of molecular targeted therapy in patients with metastatic renal cell carcinoma. BJU Int. 2016; 117(6B):E67–74.
18. Beuselinck B, Vano YA, Oudard S, Wolter P, De Smet R, Depoorter L, Teghom C, Karadimou A, Zucman-Rossi J, Debruyne PR, et al. Prognostic impact of baseline serum C-reactive protein in patients with metastatic renal cell carcinoma (RCC) treated with sunitinib. BJU Int. 2014;114(1):81–9.
19. Middleton K, Jones J, Lwin Z, Coward JI. Interleukin-6: an angiogenic target in solid tumours. Crit Rev Oncol Hematol. 2014;89(1):129–39.
20. Kwon KA, Kim SH, SY O, Lee S, Han JY, Kim KH, Goh RY, Choi HJ, Park KJ, Roh MS, et al. Clinical significance of preoperative serum vascular endothelial growth factor, interleukin-6, and C-reactive protein level in colorectal cancer. BMC Cancer. 2010;10:203.
21. Gopinathan G, Milagre C, Pearce OM, Reynolds LE, Hodivala-Dilke K, Leinster DA, Zhong H, Hollingsworth RE, Thompson R, Whiteford JR, et al. Interleukin-6 stimulates defective angiogenesis. Cancer Res. 2015; 75(15):3098–107.
22. Ohno Y, Nakashima J, Ohori M, Hatano T, Tachibana M. Pretreatment neutrophil-to-lymphocyte ratio as an independent predictor of recurrence in patients with nonmetastatic renal cell carcinoma. J Urol. 2010;184(3):873–8.
23. Cella D, Bushmakin AG, Cappelleri JC, Charbonneau C, Michaelson MD, Motzer RJ. Baseline quality of life as a prognostic survival tool in patients receiving sunitinib for metastatic renal cell carcinoma. Br J Cancer. 2012; 106(4):646–50.
24. Herrmann E, Gerss J, Bierer S, Kopke T, Bolenz C, Hertle L, Wulfing C. Pre-treatment global quality of health predicts progression free survival in metastatic kidney cancer patients treated with sorafenib or sunitinib. J Cancer Res Clin Oncol. 2009;135(1):61–7.
25. Carmichael C, Yuh BE, Sun V, Lau C, Hsu J, Saikia J, Liu X, Wilson T, Ferrell B, Pal SK. Quality of life in patients with metastatic renal cell carcinoma: assessment of long-term survivors. Clin Genitourin Cancer. 2013;11(2):149–54.
26. Motzer RJ, Hutson TE, Cella D, Reeves J, Hawkins R, Guo J, Nathan P, Staehler M, de Souza P, Merchan JR, et al. Pazopanib versus sunitinib in metastatic renal-cell carcinoma. N Engl J Med. 2013;369(8):722–31.

14

Expression and function of phosphodiesterases (PDEs) in the rat urinary bladder

Xiaofei Zhu[1†], Kui Zhai[2*†], Yue Mi[3†] and Guangju Ji[2*]

Abstract

Background: It has been shown that hosphodiesterases (PDEs) play an important role in mediating the smooth muscle tone of rat urinary bladder. However, the gene expression profiles of them were still unknown.

Methods: Urinary bladder Strips were obtained from both neonatal and adult Sprague-Dawley rats. RT-PCR/western blot and organ bath were used to measure the expression and function of PDEs.

Results: Adult rat urinary bladder expressed various PDE mRNA with the following rank order: PDE5A ≈ PDE9A ≈ PDE10A > PDE2A ≈ PDE4A ≈ PDE4D > PDE4B ≈ PDE3B ≈ PDE8B ≈ PDE7A ≈ PDE7B > PDE1A. PDE1B, PDE1C, PDE3A, PDE4C, PDE8A, and PDE11A were not detected. Of interest, the mRNA and protein of PDE3A were significantly decreased in adult rat urinary bladder compared to neonatal rat urinary bladder. Cilostamide, a specific inhibitor for PDE3, significantly inhibited the amplitude and frequency of carbachol-enhanced phasic contractions of neonatal rat bladder strips by 38.8% and 12.1%, respectively. Compared to the neonatal rat bladder, the effect of cilostamide was significantly blunted in adult rat urinary bladder: the amplitude and frequency of carbachol-enhanced phasic contractions were decreased by 13.4% ($P < 0.01$ vs neonatal rat bladder) and 4.4%, respectively. However, the mRNA and the protein levels of PDE3B were similar between neonatal and adult rat bladder.

Conclusion: We found that several PDE isoforms were expressed in the rat urinary bladder with distinct levels. Moreover, we showed that the function of PDE3 was blunted in adult rat bladder likely due to the decreased expression of PDE3A.

Keywords: Gene expression, Phasic contraction, Phosphodiesterases, Rat urinary bladder

Background

Through mediating cAMP and/or cGMP levels, phosphodiesterases (PDEs) are involved in several physiological processes of urinary bladder. Artim et al. showed that PDE5 mediated the phasic contractions of neonatal rat bladder through nitric oxide-cGMP- protein kinase G pathway [1]. Our previous study found that PDE3 and PDE4 regulated the phasic contractions of neonatal rat bladder through PKG and PKA pathways, respectively [2]. To date, 11 PDE families have been identified [3]: 3 families (PDEs 4, 7, and 8) selectively hydrolyze cAMP, 3 families selectively hydrolyze cGMP (PDEs 5, 6, and 9), and 5 families (PDEs 1, 2, 3, 10, and 11) hydrolyze both cyclic nucleotides with varying efficacies. As some of these PDE families consist of more than one gene and some genes are alternatively spliced, 21 different isoforms and more than 50 variants have been identified [4].

The urinary bladder is the organ that collects urine excreted from kidneys before disposal by urination. One of the most important features of the urinary detrusor smooth muscle is its ability to generate considerable phasic contractions [1, 2, 5]. These spontaneous phasic contractions change markedly with age [5]: during the first 2–3 weeks of life, they are characterized by high-amplitude low-frequency spontaneous contractions; then, they turn into low-amplitude high-frequency pattern characteristic of normal adult rat. The spontaneous

* Correspondence: zhaikui@ibp.ac.cn; gj28@ibp.ac.cn
†Equal contributors
[2]National Laboratory of Biomacromolecules, Institute of Biophysics, Chinese Academy of Sciences, 15 Datun Road, Beijing 100101, China
Full list of author information is available at the end of the article

activities in neonatal rat bladder are likely to be myogenic [6] and can also be modulated by the interstitial cell network [7–9].

In this study, we tested the expression profiles of all PDEs families except PDE6 (its expression is restricted to the retina) in adult rat urinary bladder with RT-PCR techniques. Moreover, we evaluated the functional role of PDE3 in mediating the phasic contraction of neonatal and adult rat bladder strips through pharmacological method.

Methods

Animals and regents

Neonatal (10-day old) and adult (90-day old) Sprague-Dawley rats were purchased from Vital River Laboratories (Beijing, China). All animal procedures described in this study were performed according to the Guide for the Care and Use of Laboratory Animals published by the US National Institutes of Health (NIH Publication No. 85–23, revised 1996), and with approval from the Institute of Biophysics Committee on Animal Care. The rat was anesthetized by 5% chloral hydrate and the whole bladder was removed, placed into cold Tyrode solution composed of (mM): 137 NaCl, 5.4 KCl, 1.8 $CaCl_2$, 1.0 $MgCl_2$, 10 glucose, 10 HEPES, (pH 7.4). After the cleaning of the fat tissues, the bladder was cut into two longitudinal pieces by using a fine dissecting scissors along the axis from the neck to the fundus.

Cilostamide (Cil) was from Tocris Bioscience (Bristol, UK). All other reagents were from Sigma Aldrich unless mentioned.

Polymerase chain reaction (PCR)

Reverse transcriptional-PCR were performed as previously reported [2, 10]. Standard PCR was performed using GoldStar Taq DNA Polymerase (CWBIO, Beijing, China) according to the manufacturer's instructions. The primers sequences were shown in Table 1. PCR conditions were set up as follows: 94 °C for 2 min, then the following three steps for 34 cycles (94 °C for 30 s, 55 °C for 30 s, 72 °C for 1 min), and a final step of cooling to 4 °C. PCR products were run on a 1.7% agarose gel and visualized under UV light using ethidium bromide staining. qRT-PCR was performed on a Corbett Rotor-Gene 6600 QPCR system machine using TransScript™ Green qRT-PCR SuperMix (TRANSGENE BIOTECH, Beijing, China) according to manufacturer's instructions. The sequences of gene-specific primers were 5′TCACAGGGCCTTAACTTACAC3′ (forward) and 5′GGAGCAAGAATTGGTTTGTCC3′ (reverse) for PDE3A, and 5′GCAAGAGAGAGGCCCTCAG3′ (forward) and 5′TGTGAGGGAGATGCTCAGTG3′ (reverse) for GAPDH. Amplifications were performed with a 10 min template denaturation step at 95 °C, followed by three steps for 35 cycles (denaturation at 95 °C for 30 s, annealing at 58 °C for 30 s, and extension at 72 °C for 30 s). All samples were amplified in triplicate and the mean was obtained for further calculations. The comparative $2^{-\Delta\Delta Ct}$ method was used to analyze mRNA fold changes between neonatal and

Table 1 The primer sequences of PDE isoforms

Name	Sequences
PDE1A (Forward, F)	5′CCACTTTGTGATCGGAAGTC3′
PDE1A (Reverse, R)	5′TTCTGCTGAATGATGTCCACC3′
PDE1B (F)	5′CAGGGTGACAAGGAGGCAGAG3′
PDE1B (R)	5′GACATCTGGTTGGTGATGCC3′
PDE1C (F)	5′TCTCAAAGGATGACTGGAGG3′
PDE1C (R)	5′GCTTCTCTGTCACCCTGTC3′
PDE2A (F)	5′CCTCCTGTGACCTCTCTGACC3′
PDE2A (R)	5′TGAACTTGTGGGACACCTTGG3′
PDE3A (F)	5′TCACAGGGCCTTAACTTACAC3′
PDE3A (R)	5′GGAGCAAGAATTGGTTTGTCC3′
PDE3B (F)	5′CCTCAGGCAGTTTTATACAATG3′
PDE3B (R)	5′TGCTTCTTCATCTCCCTGCTC3′
PDE4A (F)	5′GTGGAGAAGTCTCAGGTGGG3′
PDE4A (R)	5′TGGAACTTGTCAGGCAGGG3′
PDE4B (F)	5′TAGAAGATAACAGGAACTGG3′
PDE4B (R)	5′GCAATGTCTATGTCAGTCTC3′
PDE4C (F)	5′ACGTGGCGTACCACAACAGC3′
PDE4C (R)	5′TACCGCGAGGTGATGGTTCTC3′
PDE4D (F)	5′GGATAATGGAGGAGTTCTTCC3′
PDE4D (R)	5′CGATTGTCCTCCAAAGTGTCC3′
PDE5A (F)	5′CCCTGGCCTATTCAACAACGG3′
PDE5A (R)	5′GTGGGTCAGGGCCTCATACAG3′
PDE7A (F)	5′TGGACAAGCCAAGTGTATGCTG3′
PDE7A (R)	5′TTTAAGTAACAGTGCATGGCC3′
PDE7B (F)	5′AAAGCCCAGTGGAAGAGC3′
PDE7B (R)	5′CGAAGGGAGGTGGTAAATG3′
PDE8A (F)	5′CAACAAGCCTCTGAAAGC3′
PDE8A (R)	5′TCGGTCTGGGAGAAATAC3′
PDE8B (F)	5′ACCACAACTCCACCCATG3′
PDE8B (R)	5′AGAGGCTTGTTGATGCTG3′
PDE9A (F)	5′TGGGTGGACTGTTTACTGG3′
PDE9A (R)	5′CGGTCTTCATTGTCTTTCG3′
PDE10A (F)	5′TGCTTGGTGGCGTTTGTTAG3′
PDE10A (R)	5′TTCTCTGATGCCTGGGATGTAC3′
PDE11A (F)	5′TTTAGCGGTGATTGTGGG3′
PDE11A (R)	5′TCTCGAAGTACAGCGTGAGG3′
GAPDH (F)	5′CAAGTTCAACGGCACAGTCAAG3′
GAPDH (R)	5′GCACCAGTGGATGCAGGGAT3′

adult rat. Then the calculated $2^{-\Delta\Delta Ct}$ was transformed into a percentage using the control as 100% to show the mRNA expression difference.

Western blots

Western blots were performed as previously described [2]. In brief, 10 μg protein of each sample was separated by SDS-polyacrylamide gel electrophoresis using 12% gels. The resolved proteins were transferred to PVDF membranes (Millipore) at 300 mA for 45 min or 1 h. The membranes were blocked for 1 h with Tris-buffered saline-Tween 20 (TBST) containing 5% BSA at room temperature with slow shaking. The blocked membranes were probed with polyclonal anti-PDE3A antibody (Santa Cruz Biotechnology, California, USA, 1:1000), polyclonal anti-PDE3B antibody (Santa Cruz Biotechnology, California, USA, 1:3000), and monoclonal anti-GAPDH antibody (Sigma-Aldrich, St. Louis, MO, 1:10,000) at 4 °C overnight. After washing, the membrane was incubated with peroxidase-conjugated IgG (ZSJQ-BIO, Beijing, China, 1:10,000) for 1 h at room temperature. Final detection was performed using enhanced chemiluminescence detection solution 1 and 2 (1:1) (ECL, Millipore, Billerica, MA). Densitometry was used to measure the expression of PDE3A and PDE3B relative to GAPDH or α-actin with ImageJ (NIH).

Contractile measurement of rat bladder strips

Contractile measurement of rat bladder strips was performed as previously reported [2]. The bladder strips (with intact mucosa) were tied up and mounted in a classical isolated organ bath (coupled the model BL-420F acquisition system, Chengdu TME Technology Co, Ltd., Sichuan, China) to measure isometric tension. The bladder strips were allowed to equilibrate in physiological salt solution [in mM: NaCl 119, KCl 4.7, $CaCl_2$ 2.5, $MgSO_4$ 1.17, KH_2PO_4 1.18, glucose 11, $NaHCO_3$ 25] for 1.5 h before drug testing. After equilibration, 100 nM carbachol was applied to enhance the amplitude and frequency of phasic contractions, without significantly changing the baseline tension, as previously described [1]. The effects of the PDE3 inhibitors, Cil (1 μM), were studied on the carbachol-enhanced phasic contraction. In experiments performed in the presence of pharmacological reagents diluted in dimethylsulfoxide (DMSO), control bladder strips were treated in the presence of the equivalent concentration of DMSO (<0.1%). The mean amplitude and frequency of carbachol-enhanced phasic contractions were during 5 min before or 5 min after application of Cil or DMSO (<0.1%). The effect of Cil on both parameters was expressed in percentage of the amplitude and frequency of carbachol-enhanced phasic contractions measured before drug application. Baseline tone was not appreciably changed by various treatments and therefore was not subjected to detailed analysis.

Data analysis

Data were represented as mean ± SEM of *n* strips in organ bath experiments or *N* rats in RT-PCR/western blotting experiments. Significant differences were determined by Student's t-test. Only results with values of $P < 0.05$ were considered significant.

Results

Using RT-PCR technique, we determined the mRNA levels of 18 different PDE isoforms in adult rat urinary bladder. As shown in Fig. 1 and Table 2, PDE5A, PDE9A and PDE10A were most highly expressed; PDE2A, PDE4A, PDE4B, PDE4D, and PDE8B were moderately detected; PDE3B, PDE7A, and PDE7B were slightly found; while PDE1B, PDE1C, PDE3A, PDE4C, PDE8A, and PDE11A were absent in all samples tested. Taken together, the mRNA of several PDE isoforms were expressed in rat urinary bladder with distinct levels.

In contrast to our previous finding that PDE3A was highly expressed in neonatal rat bladder [2], PDE3A mRNA was not detected in adult rat urinary bladder. To further verify this, we took qRT-PCR on mRNA from both neonatal and adult rat urinary bladder. As shown in Fig. 2a, the mRNA levels of PDE3A was about 60%

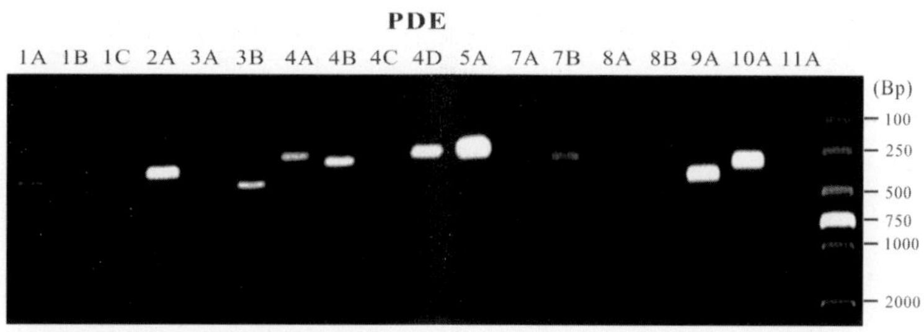

Fig. 1 Expression of the mRNA for different PDE isoforms in adult rat urinary bladder. RT-PCR was performed on mRNA extracted from the whole bladder tissues in the presence of primers for PDE1A, PDE1B, PDE1C, PDE2A, PDE3A, PDE3B, PDE4A, PDE4B, PDE4C, PDE4D, PDE5A, PDE7A, PDE7B, PDE8A, PDE8B, PDE9A, PDE10A, PDE11A, and GAPDH. PCR products were resolved by electrophoresis on a 1.7% agarose gel. The representative gels stained with ethidium bromide was shown. *Position* of molecular weight markers is indicated in base pairs (Bp)

Table 2 The expression levels of PDE isoforms in adult rat urinary bladder

	PDE																	
	1A	1B	1C	2A	3A	3B	4A	4B	4C	4D	5A	7A	7B	8A	8B	9A	10A	11A
1	+	-	-	++	-	+	++	++	-	++	+++	+	+	-	+	+++	+++	-
2	+	-	-	++	-	+	++	++	-	++	+++	+	+	-	+	+++	+++	-
3	+	-	-	++	-	+	++	++	-	++	+++	+	+	-	+	+++	+++	-

+++ indicates high expression; ++ indicates medium expression; + indicates low expression; – indicates no detection

decreased in adult rat urinary bladder compared to neonatal rat urinary bladder ($p < 0.01$). Next, we measured its protein levels by using a specific PDE3A antibody. We found that the PDE3A protein was also significantly lowered in adult rat urinary bladder than in neonatal rat urinary bladder (Fig. 2b-c). Our results indicated that PDE3A expression was significantly lower in adult rat urinary bladder than in neonatal rat urinary bladder.

Next, we test the functional roles of PDE3 in the phasic contractions of adult rat urinary bladder smooth muscle. We found that Cil (1 μM), a specific PDE3 inhibitor, significantly decreased the amplitude of carbachol-enhanced contractions of adult rat bladder strips by 13.4 ± 4.0% ($P < 0.05$), and slightly, although not significantly, reduced their frequency by 4.4 ± 4.9%. When comparing to the neonatal bladder smooth muscle strips, Cil-mediated effects on the phasic contractions of smooth muscle strips were much smaller in adult rat urinary bladder. In detail, the effects of Cil were decreased by 2.5 fold (from 38.8% to 13.4%, $p < 0.01$) in amplitude without a significant decrease (12.1% to 4.4%, $p > 0.05$) in frequency. These results suggested that PDE3-mediated functional role was blunted in adult rat urinary bladder.

There are two subfamilies of PDE3, PDE3A and PDE3B [11]. They are encoded by different genes and participate in different cellular processes. Is there any relationship between the PDE3B expression and the blunted effects of Cil in adult rat bladder? To answer this question, we tested PDE3B mRNA and protein levels in neonatal and adult rat urinary bladder. As shown in Fig. 3a, PDE3B mRNA was detected in both neonatal ($N = 4$) and adult ($N = 3$) rat urinary bladders. However, the expression level was not significantly different between those two groups (Fig. 3a). Moreover, PDE3B protein expression in neonatal and adult urinary bladders was not different ($N = 3$ each; Fig. 3b). Taken together, PDE3B was not altered between neonatal and adult rat urinary bladder, suggesting that it is not involved in the blunted effects of Cil in adult rat bladder.

Discussion

Cyclic nucleotide PDEs carry out essential roles in signal transduction by modulating cAMP and cGMP levels and have been recognized as potential targets of several bladder diseases such as overactive bladder. The presence and activities of PDE1–5 have been tested and confirmed in the rodent, rabbit, guinea pig, and human urinary bladder by pharmacological, biochemical, immunohistochemical and molecular methods [12–16]. By using qPCR technique, Lakics et al. have shown that several PDE isoform of PDE7–10 were expressed in the human urinary bladder [16]. Moreover, the expression of PDE5 in different cell types of urinary bladder such as the urothelium, suburothelial interstitial cells and bladder blood smooth muscle cells has been determined in the guinea pig [17]. However, the molecular levels of the whole PDEs family in the rodent urinary bladder are still unknown. Here, we established the mRNA expression levels of 18 different PDE isoforms in rat urinary bladder by RT-PCR. Our results indicated that PDE5 is one of the major isoform expressed in rat urinary bladder,

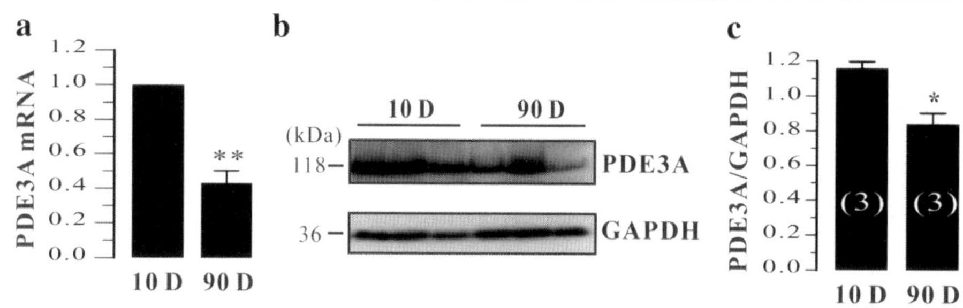

Fig. 2 PDE3A expression was determined by qRT-PCR and western blotting in neonatal and adult rat urinary bladder, respectively. **a** Summary data of qRT-PCR from neonatal ($N = 3$) and adult ($N = 3$) rat bladder. **b-c** The representative blots and the summary data of these blots are shown. Position of molecular weight markers is indicated in kDa. Data are Mean ± SEM of N independent rat bladders. *$P < 0.05$ and **$P < 0.01$ are neonatal versus adult

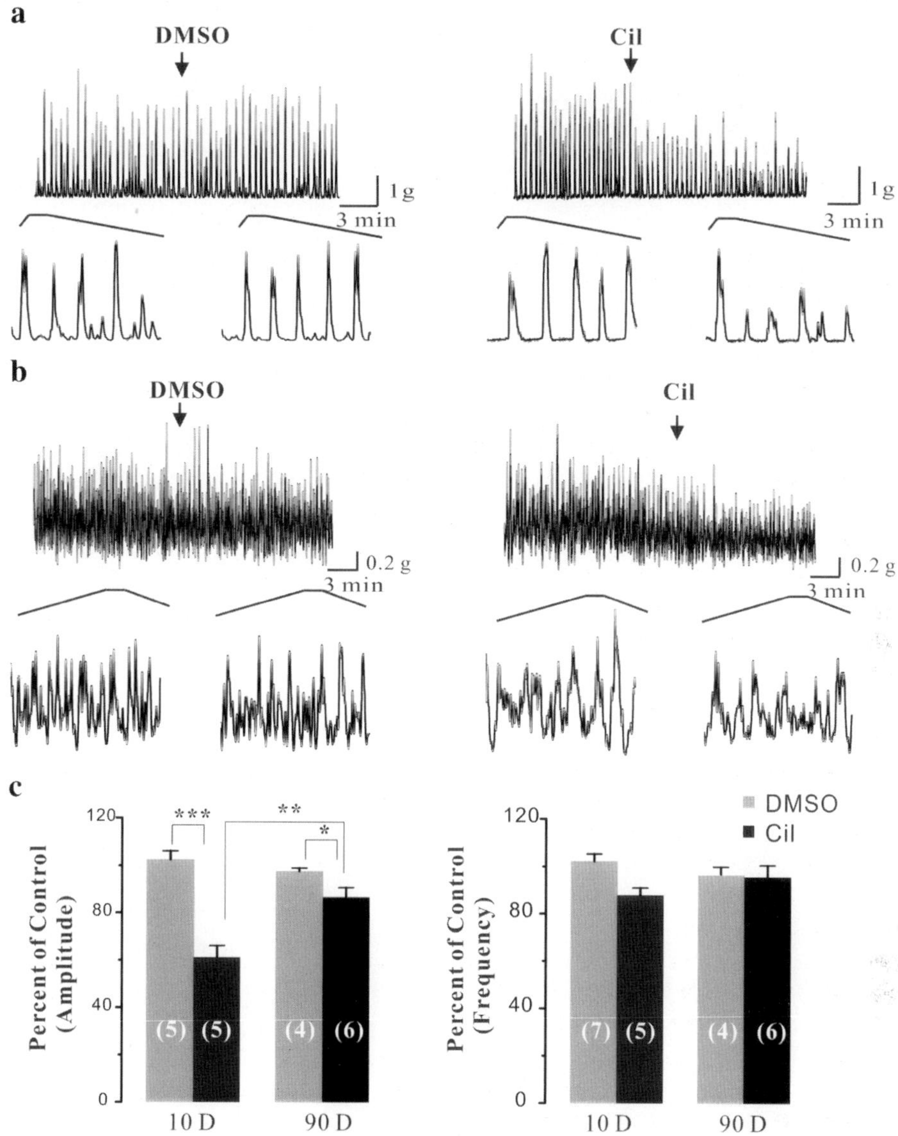

Fig. 3 Effects of Cil on the carbachol-enhanced phasic contractions of neonatal and adult rat urinary bladder strips. **a** Original traces of carbachol-enhanced phasic contractions in neonatal rat bladder strips before and after the application of DMSO (<0.1%) and the PDE3 inhibitor Cil (1 μM). **b** Original traces of carbachol-enhanced phasic contractions in adult rat bladder strips before and after the application of DMSO (<0.1%) and the PDE3 inhibitor Cil (1 μM). The *arrows* indicate the times of drugs application. **c** Summary data showing the average effect of DMSO (vehicle) and Cil on the carbachol-enhanced phasic contractions amplitude and frequency. Data are expressed as mean ± SEM of n independent bladder strips as indicated in *brackets*. $^{*}P < 0.05$ $^{**}P < 0.01$ and $^{***}P < 0.001$ as indicated

corresponding with its important role in the urinary bladder [15, 17]. In consistent with the finding in human urinary bladder [14], PDE9A gene was shown to be highly expressed in rat urinary bladder. Meanwhile, Nagasaki et al. showed that PDE9 protein was widely distributed in the urothelial epithelium of the human lower urinary tract including the bladder [18]. Thus, it would be of interest to test its functional roles in the bladder. Although PDE10A gene was abundantly expressed, little is known about its role in the rat and human urinary bladder. It has been well known that PDE1 was a major isoform expressed the in human urinary bladder [14]. However, the function of PDE1 in the rat urinary bladder was still controversial. Qiu et al. showed that PDE1 inhibitor had a strong relaxant effect on pre-contracted bladder strips [12]. Our previous study found that PDE1 inhibitor had no effect on spontaneous phasic contraction of bladder strips [2]. One possibility is that the PDE1 inhibitor vinpocetine used in Qiu's study is not specific to PDE1. It can inhibit voltage-sensitive sodium channels and cause a dose-dependent decrease in extracellular calcium [19].

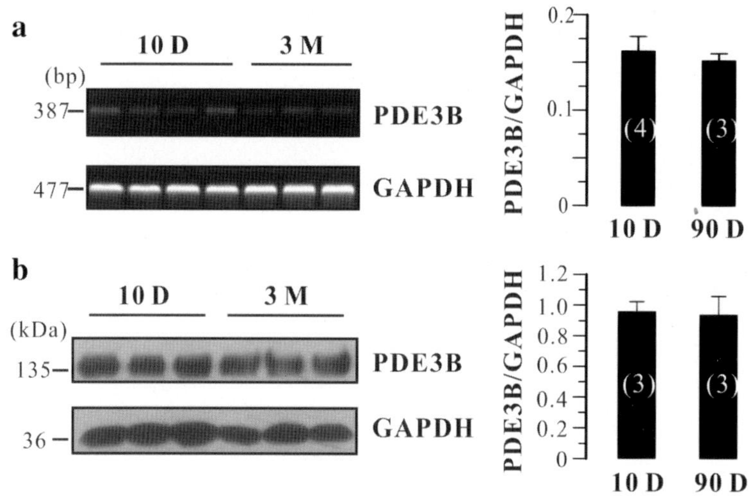

Fig. 4 PDE3B expression was determined by RT-PCR and western blotting in neonatal and adult rat urinary bladder, respectively. **a** The representative gels and summary data of RT-PCR were shown. **b** The representative blots and summary data of western blotting were shown. Position of molecular weight markers is indicated in Bp or kDa, respectively. Data are Mean ± SEM of *N* independent rat bladders as indicated in *brackets*

Moreover, our results indicated that only PDE1A was slightly expressed while both PDE1B and PDE1C were not detected, suggesting that PDE1 expression is varied among species. This difference might partially explain that PDE1 inhibitors exhibit effects in human [20–22] but not in rat bladder [2].

The PDE3 family contains two subfamilies, PDE3A and PDE3B, which are encoded by distinct but related genes [11]. PDE3A and PDE3B isoforms are widely expressed but also exhibit tissue-specific patterns. For example, PDE3A is highly expressed in cardiovascular system, platelets, and oocytes, while PDE3B is mainly expressed in adipocytes, hepatocytes, and pancreatic β-cells [11]. In the present study, we found that both mRNA and protein of PDE3A were dramatically decreased in adult rat urinary bladder (Fig. 2), whereas PDE3B was not altered (Fig. 3). Although the physiological significance underlying in this process are unknown, we speculated that PDE3A might play an important role in the development of rat urinary bladder. It has been established that PDE3A is involved in smooth muscle phenotype switch [23–25] and regulates VSMC cycle progression through controlling cAMP pools [26]. In addition, neonatal urinary bladder is much more proliferative than adult urinary bladder [27]. Thus, it is not surprised that PDE3A would be an important regulator in the development of urinary bladder. However, this possibility should be further tested.

There is evidence that the characteristics of bladder spontaneous activity are age-dependent [28], and are related to changes in expression of several proteins such as large conductance Ca^{2+}-activated K^{+} channels [5] and connexin [29]. Our results showed that Cil-mediated effects on the phasic contractions were blunted in adult rat bladder strips (Fig. 4) likely due to decreased PDE3A expression. Although PDE3B was consistently expressed throughout the development (Fig. 3), it could not compensate for the PDE3A-mediated effects. These results suggest that PDE3A and PDE3B may take different roles in mediating urinary bladder smooth muscle tone. Nevertheless, these results supported that the notion that PDE3A and PDE3B exhibit distinct functional roles.

Conclusion

In conclusion, our results for the first time provided a comprehensive view of the gene expression profiles of PDE isoforms in rat urinary bladder. We also found that the function of PDE3 was blunted in adult rat bladder likely due to the decreased expression of PDE3A but not PDE3B, suggesting that PDE3A and PDE3B might play different roles in the urinary bladder.

Abbreviations

Cil: Cilostamide; DMSO: Dimethylsulfoxide; PCR: Polymerase chain reaction; PDE: Phosphodiesterase

Acknowledgements

Not applicable.

Funding

This work was supported by a grant from the National Science Foundation of China (Grant No. 31300956) and the Beijing Nature Science Foundation (Grant No. 7172133).

Authors' contributions

Conceived and designed the experiments: KZ GJ. Performed the experiments: XZ, KZ, YM. Analyzed the data: KZ. Wrote the paper: KZ, GJ. All the authors have read and approved the final version of the manuscript.

Authors' information
Not applicable.

Competing interests
The authors declare that they have no competing interests.

Author details
[1]Department of Urology, Beijing Jishuitan Hospital, Beijing, China. [2]National Laboratory of Biomacromolecules, Institute of Biophysics, Chinese Academy of Sciences, 15 Datun Road, Beijing 100101, China. [3]Department of Urology, Peking University First Hospital, Beijing, China.

References

1. Artim DE, Kullmann FA, Daugherty SL, Wu HY, de Groat WC. Activation of the nitric oxide-cGMP pathway reduces phasic contractions in neonatal rat bladder strips via protein kinase G. Am J Physiol Renal Physiol. 2009;297(2): F333–40.
2. Zhai K, Chang Y, Wei B, Liu Q, Leblais V, Fischmeister R, Ji G. Phosphodiesterase types 3 and 4 regulate the phasic contraction of neonatal rat bladder smooth myocytes via distinct mechanisms. Cell Signal. 2014;26(5):1001–10.
3. Lugnier C. Cyclic nucleotide phosphodiesterase (PDE) superfamily: a new target for the development of specific therapeutic agents. Pharmacol Ther. 2006;109:366–98.
4. Bender AT, Beavo JA. Cyclic nucleotide phosphodiesterases: molecular regulation to clinical use. Pharmacol Rev. 2006;58(3):488–520.
5. Ng YK, de Groat WC, Wu HY. Smooth muscle and neural mechanisms contributing to the downregulation of neonatal rat spontaneous bladder contractions during postnatal development. Am J Physiol Regul Integr Comp Physiol. 2007;292(5):R2100–12.
6. Szell EA, Somogyi GT, de Groat WC, Szigeti GP. Developmental changes in spontaneous smooth muscle activity in the neonatal rat urinary bladder. Am J Physiol Regul Integr Comp Physiol. 2003;285(4):R809–16.
7. Gillespie JI, Markerink-van Ittersum M, de Vente J. cGMP-generating cells in the bladder wall: identification of distinct networks of interstitial cells. BJU Int. 2004;94(7):1114–24.
8. Rahnama'i MS, van Koeveringe GA, van Kerrebroeck PE, de Wachter SG. The effect of indomethacin on the muscarinic induced contractions in the isolated normal guinea pig urinary bladder. BMC Urol. 2013;13:8.
9. Finney SM, Stewart LH, Gillespie JI. Cholinergic activation of phasic activity in the isolated bladder: possible evidence for M3- and M2-dependent components of a motor/sensory system. BJU Int. 2007;100(3):668–78.
10. Zhai K, Hubert F, Nicolas V, Ji G, Fischmeister R, Leblais V. Beta-adrenergic cAMP signals are predominantly regulated by phosphodiesterase type 4 in cultured adult rat aortic smooth muscle cells. PLoS One. 2012;7(10):e47826.
11. Ahmad F, Degerman E, Manganiello VC. Cyclic nucleotide phosphodiesterase 3 signaling complexes. Horm Metab Res. 2012;44(10):776–85.
12. Qiu Y, Kraft P, Craig EC, Liu X, Haynes-Johnson D. Identification and functional study of phosphodiesterases in rat urinary bladder. Urol Res. 2001;29(6):388–92.
13. Qiu Y, Kraft P, Craig EC, Liu X, Haynes-Johnson D. Cyclic nucleotide phosphodiesterases in rabbit detrusor smooth muscle. Urology. 2002;59(1):145–9.
14. Lakics V, Karran EH, Boess FG. Quantitative comparison of phosphodiesterase mRNA distribution in human brain and peripheral tissues. Neuropharmacology. 2010;59(6):367–74.
15. Rahnama'i MS, Uckert S, Hohnen R, van Koeveringe GA. The role of phosphodiesterases in bladder pathophysiology. Nat Rev Urol. 2013;10(7):414–24.
16. Rahnama'i MS, Hohnen R, Van Kerrebroeck PE, van Koeveringe GA. Phosphodiesterase type 2 distribution in the guinea pig urinary bladder. World J Urol. 2015;33(10):1623–33.
17. Rahnama'i MS, van Koeveringe GA, Hohnen R, Ona S, van Kerrebroeck PE, de Wachter SG. Distribution of phosphodiesterase type 5 (PDE5) in the lateral wall of the guinea pig urinary bladder. BJU Int. 2013;112(2):246–57.
18. Nagasaki S, Nakano Y, Masuda M, Ono K, Miki Y, Shibahara Y, Sasano H. Phosphodiesterase type 9 (PDE9) in the human lower urinary tract: an immunohistochemical study. BJU Int. 2012;109(6):934–40.
19. Sitges M, Galvan E, Nekrassov V. Vinpocetine blockade of sodium channels inhibits the rise in sodium and calcium induced by 4-aminopyridine in synaptosomes. Neurochem Int. 2005;46(7):533–40.
20. Uckert S, Stief CG, Odenthal KP, Becker AJ, Truss MC, Jonas U. Comparison of the effects of various spasmolytic drugs on isolated human and porcine detrusor smooth muscle. Arzneimittelforschung. 1998;48(8):836–9.
21. Truss MC, Uckert S, Stief CG, Kuczyk M, Jonas U. Cyclic nucleotide phosphodiesterase (PDE) isoenzymes in the human detrusor smooth muscle. I. Identification and characterization. Urol Res. 1996;24(3):123–8.
22. Truss MC, Uckert S, Stief CG, Forssmann WG, Jonas U. Cyclic nucleotide phosphodiesterase (PDE) isoenzymes in the human detrusor smooth muscle. II. Effect of various PDE inhibitors on smooth muscle tone and cyclic nucleotide levels in vitro. Urol Res. 1996;24(3):129–34.
23. Tilley DG, Maurice DH. Vascular smooth muscle cell phosphodiesterase (PDE) 3 and PDE4 activities and levels are regulated by cyclic AMP in vivo. Mol Pharmacol. 2002;62(3):497–506.
24. Dunkerley HA, Tilley DG, Palmer D, Liu H, Jimmo SL, Maurice DH. Reduced phosphodiesterase 3 activity and phosphodiesterase 3A level in synthetic vascular smooth muscle cells: implications for use of phosphodiesterase 3 inhibitors in cardiovascular tissues. Mol Pharmacol. 2002;61(5):1033–40.
25. Palmer D, Maurice DH. Dual expression and differential regulation of phosphodiesterase 3A and phosphodiesterase 3B in human vascular smooth muscle: implications for phosphodiesterase 3 inhibition in human cardiovascular tissues. Mol Pharmacol. 2000;58:247–52.
26. Begum N, Hockman S, Manganiello VC. Phosphodiesterase 3A (PDE3A) deletion suppresses proliferation of cultured murine vascular smooth muscle cells (VSMCS) via inhibition of mitogen activated protein kinase (MAPK) signaling and alterations in critical cell cycle regulatory proteins. J Biol Chem. 2011;286(29):26238–49.
27. Jost SP. Cell cycle of normal bladder urothelium in developing and adult mice. Virchows Arch B Cell Pathol Incl Mol Pathol. 1989;57(1):27–36.
28. Szigeti GP, Somogyi GT, Csernoch L, Szell EA. Age-dependence of the spontaneous activity of the rat urinary bladder. J Muscle Res Cell Motil. 2005;26(1):23–9.
29. Ikeda Y, Fry C, Hayashi F, Stolz D, Griffiths D, Kanai A. Role of gap junctions in spontaneous activity of the rat bladder. Am J Physiol Renal Physiol. 2007; 293(4):F1018–25.

A *Drosophila* genetic model of nephrolithiasis: transcriptional changes in response to diet induced stone formation

Vera Y. Chung* and Benjamin W. Turney

Abstract

Background: Urolithiasis is a significant healthcare issue but the pathophysiology of stone disease remains poorly understood. *Drosophila* Malpighian tubules were known to share similar physiological function to human renal tubules. We have used *Drosophila* as a genetic model to study the transcriptional response to stone formation secondary to dietary manipulation.

Methods: Wild-type male flies were raised on standard medium supplemented with lithogenic agents: control, sodium oxalate (NaOx) and ethylene glycol (EG). At 2 weeks, Malpighian tubules were dissected under polarized microscope to visualize crystals. The parallel group was dissected for RNA extraction and subsequent next-generation RNA sequencing.

Results: Crystal formation was visualized in 20%(±2.2) of flies on control diet, 73%(±3.6) on NaOx diet and 84%(±2.2) on EG diet. Differentially expressed genes were identified in flies fed with NaOx and EG diet comparing with the control group. Fifty-eight genes were differentially expressed (FDR <0.05, $p < 0.05$) in NaOx diet and 20 genes in EG diet. The molecular function of differentially expressed genes were assessed. Among these, Nervana 3, Eaat1 (Excitatory amino acid transporter 1), CG7912, CG5404, CG3036 worked as ion transmembrane transporters, which were possibly involved in stone pathogenesis.

Conclusions: We have shown that by dietary modification, stone formation can be manipulated and visualized in *Drosophila* Malpighian tubules. This genetic model could be potentially used to identify the candidate genes that influence stone risk hence providing more insight to the pathogenesis of human stone disease.

Background

Urolithiasis is a major healthcare problem accounting for over 83,000 hospital attendances in the UK each year [1]. There is a high (around 10%) lifetime prevalence of stone disease as well as recurrence rate worldwide [2]. In the last two decades, significant advance was made in the minimal invasive surgical treatment of stone disease. Effective medical therapies for prevention and treatment of stone disease are still lacking because little is known about the molecular pathophysiology of kidney stone disease.

Kidney stone is thought to be related to interaction of genetic factors and environment. In human renal stone disease, there are clear environmental influences including diet rich in animal protein, high salt intake, dehydration and obesity. Genetic predisposition to stone disease is also well recognized. Approximately 25% of stone formers have a positive family history [3] but only a small minority have a monogenic cause such as cystinuria, Dent's disease or primary hyperoxaluria.

Overall, calcium oxalate (CaOx) stones constitute the most common (~80%) stone type and are currently regarded as idiopathic in etiology. A systematic genetic study of CaOx stones excluded monogenetic inheritance but twin studies have estimated the heritability of kidney stones to be 56% [4].

In order to study the pathogenesis of human CaOx stone disease, various animal models have been established. Amongst these, *Drosophila melanogaster* has been proposed as a powerful translational model of human nephrolithiasis [5]. The advantages include similarity between *Drosophila* Malpighian tubule and human renal tubule, cost-effectiveness, convenience to observe crystals and relative ease to perform genetic manipulation. The

* Correspondence: chungyeungvera@gmail.com
Oxford Stone Group, Department of Urology, Nuffield Department of Surgical Sciences, University of Oxford, Oxford, UK

Drosophila Malpighian tubules share similar features with human renal tubules in terms of physiological function, anatomical structure and genetic activity [5]. Flies are an unprotected species and can be acquired and maintained at low cost. Their short life cycle allows rapid observation of the effects of environmental alternation. *Drosophila* has been shown to readily form CaOx stones with dietary supplement of lithogenic agents within days [6]. Furthermore, the *Drosophila* genome is highly conserved and fully characterized. Extensive genomic tools are readily available to facilitate genetic manipulation in this versatile model organism. As such, we have used *Drosophila* as a genetic model to try to better understand the molecular pathophysiology of stone disease.

Methods

Drosophila stocks

Wild-type *Drosophila melanogaster* (Canton S strain) were raised in standard fly medium (composition: 72.3% water, 18.6% maize, 3.8% yeast, 2.2% soya, 3.1% agar) in a 25 °C, 50–60% humidity incubator. Only male flies were selected for the experiment.

Lithogenic diets

Three experimental diets were prepared: control group with standard fly medium, 0.05% Sodium oxalate (NaOx) added to standard fly medium and 0.5% ethylene glycol (EG) added to standard fly medium. Biological triplicates were prepared in each group.

Fly lifespan study

New emergents were isolated on day 3 after eclosion under light anesthesia. They were randomly divided into 3 treatment groups. The starting population for each condition was 100. The maintenance density was 25 flies per vial. Every 3 days the flies were transferred to fresh medium and numbers of dead flies were counted. Lifespan was recorded and subjected to survival analysis.

Malpighian tubules preparation

After 2 weeks of feeding on three different diets, the flies were killed on CO_2 pad. The Malpighian tubules and hindgut were extracted in physiological medium (Schneider's drosophila medium.

Fifteen flies were dissected for each biological triplicate. Freshly dissected tubules and hindgut were prepared for polarized light microscopy examination. Parallel groups were dissected and processed for RNA extraction.

Birefringence microscopy

Malpighian tubules and hindgut were prepared fresh and observed under normal and polarized white light with an Olympus BX60 microscope. The percentage of crystal formation were documented and tubules were photographed. The tubules with crystal formation were photographed and scaled.

RNA extraction and quality control

Total RNA was extracted from Malpighian tubules and hindgut of 15 flies in each biological replicate.

Qiagen MiRNeasy Mini Kit was used for RNA extraction.

RNA integrity was verified with Agilent 2100 Bioanalyzer (RNA 6000 Pico kit). Next generation RNA sequencing was performed and sequencing data was analyzed in collaboration with the Computational Biology Research Group using STAR (Spliced Transcripts Alignment to a Reference) and edgeR software.

Statistics

Statistical analyses were carried out with Prism biostatistical software (Graphpad, San Diego, CA).

Results

Effect on lifespan

The lifespan was significantly reduced by food enriched with 0.05% NaOx and 0.5% EG ($p < 0.0001$) (Fig. 1). The administration of EG had a more pronounced impact on the lifespan compared with NaOx ($p < 0.0001$). The median and maximum lifespan in the control group was 43 and 64 days, 40 and 55 days in the NaOx diet, 31 and 52 days in the EG diet respectively.

Inducing crystallization in Malpighian tubules

The normal anatomy of Malpighian tubules is shown in Fig. 2. There are two pairs of Malpighian tubules in *Drosophila*: anterior and posterior pair. The two tubules joins into the ureter which then empties into the midgut

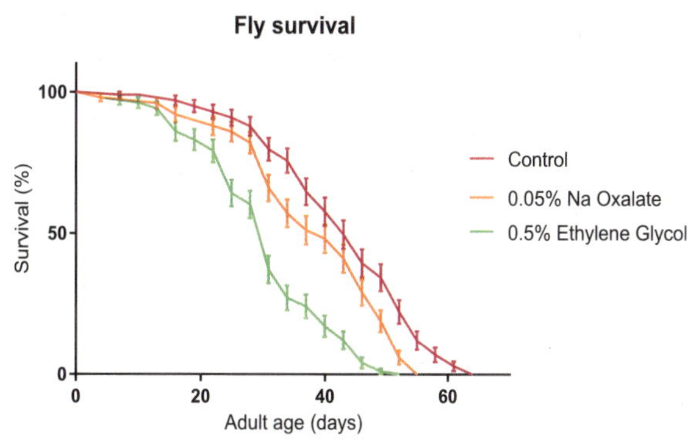

Fig. 1 Drosophila survivorship in response to administration of lithogenic agents (0.05% NaOx, 0.5% EG) compared with control group. The lifespan was significantly reduced by food enriched with 0.05% NaOx ($p < 0.0001$) and 0.5% EG ($p < 0.0001$) compared with control group. EG had a more pronounced impact on the lifespan compared with NaOx ($p < 0.0001$). Log rank test was used to for comparison of survival curves

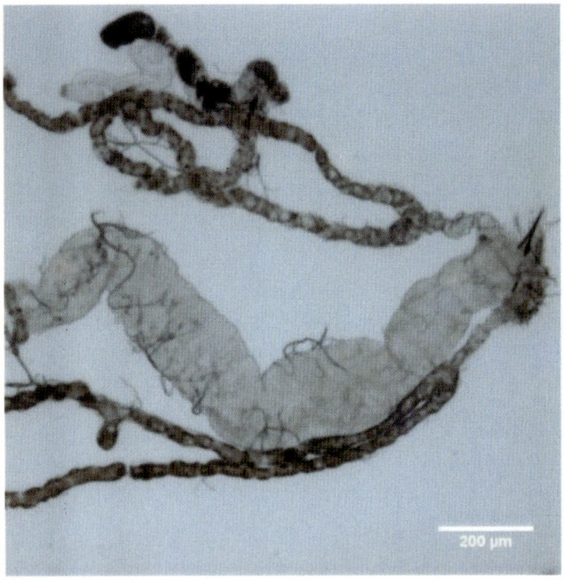

Fig. 2 Photograph of Malpighian tubules under 10× s magnification. Two pairs of Malpighian tubules coalesce into a common ureter which empty into the junction of midgut and hindgut

and hindgut junction. One Malpighian tubule measures about 2 mm long, with the inner diameter measuring about 50 um. Urine was generated via transport of ions, solutes followed by water across the tubular lumen, and sequentially excreted to the hindgut [5].

The concentration of lithogenic agents (0.05% for NaOx and 0.5% for EG) was selected following optimization studies to adequately induce crystallization without leading to excessive premature death [6].

Crystal formation was detected as early as 1 week after initiation ingestion of lithogenic diets. Degree of crystallization was given a visual scale of 0, 1+, 2+, and 3+ in each condition (Fig. 3) [6]. All scoring was performed by a single observer.

The birefringent crystals were most commonly visualized in the distal tubules. There were no crystals observed in the hindgut.. It was noticed that the crystal morphology in the NaOx group was small and extensive, in contrast to the more sizable and polyangular shape in the EG diet.

There was significantly ($p < 0.003$ by chi-square test) higher rate of stone formation in the NaOx and EG diets (Table 1). Flies on control diet had a mean incidence of 20% stone formation whereas the incidence was 73% and 84% in NaOx and EG diets respectively. The incidence of crystal formation subcategorized to mild (1+), moderate (2+) and strong degrees (3+) was illustrated in Fig. 4.

RNA sequencing and quality control

The parallel group of experimental flies was dissected after 2 weeks on lithogenic diets. Malpighian tubules were processed for total RNA extraction. Quality of extracted RNA was verified by Nanodrop and Agilent 2100 Bioanalyzer. The electrophoretic ribosomal RNA (rRNA) profile of insects was different from the standard rRNA integrity benchmark. It was common to observe single rRNA peak in insect RNA which does not represent degradation [7]. The electrophoretic profile in Drosophila RNA could be explained by the fact that the 28 s rRNA was processed into two fragments that co-migrate with the 18 s rRNA. The RNA integrity in our samples was shown to be satisfactory with tight banding and no evidence of degradation (Fig. 5).

After verification of RNA integrity, next generation RNA sequencing was performed to sequence the whole transcriptome of 9 samples. The mRNA was extracted from the total RNA and subsequently converted to cDNA. Second strand cDNA synthesis incorporated dUTP. The cDNA was end-repaired, A-tailed and adapter-ligated. Samples underwent uridine digestion and then amplification. The prepared libraries were size selected, multiplexed before paired end sequencing over one lane of a flow cell.

Sequenced genes and possible candidate genes

Library preparations were analyzed by the Computational Biology Research Group, University of Oxford, UK. Differentially expressed genes with FDR (false detection rate) < 0.05 and p-value <0.05 in all three biological triplicates were listed (Table 2). There were a total 58 genes identified in NaOx diet and 20 genes in EG diet. The mean expression level, Log Fold Change and p-Value of differentially expressed genes compared with control were displayed as smear plots and volcano plots (Fig. 6). Their molecular functions were matched in Flybase database and categorized (Fig. 7). Although there was no overlap between the differentially expressed genes in both treatment groups, their biological functions were very similar.

We identified those genes which function as transmembrane ion transporter that may be actively involved in in crystal formation. These potential candidate genes and their specific molecular functions were displayed in Table 3.

Discussion

The formation of kidney stones is likely the result of complicated interactions of multiple genetic factors in addition to environmental influence. In this model we have successfully induced CaOx crystals in *Drosophila* Malpighian tubules by diets enriched with lithogenic agents. Our study is the first to try to elucidate transcriptive changes in response to stone formation in the *Drosophila* model.

A previous pilot study on the experimental induction of lithogenic agents in *Drosophila* has shown that such diets had a negative impact on *Drosophila* survival in a dose dependent manner [6]. The crystal composition was analyzed by energy-disperse X-ray spectroscopy and

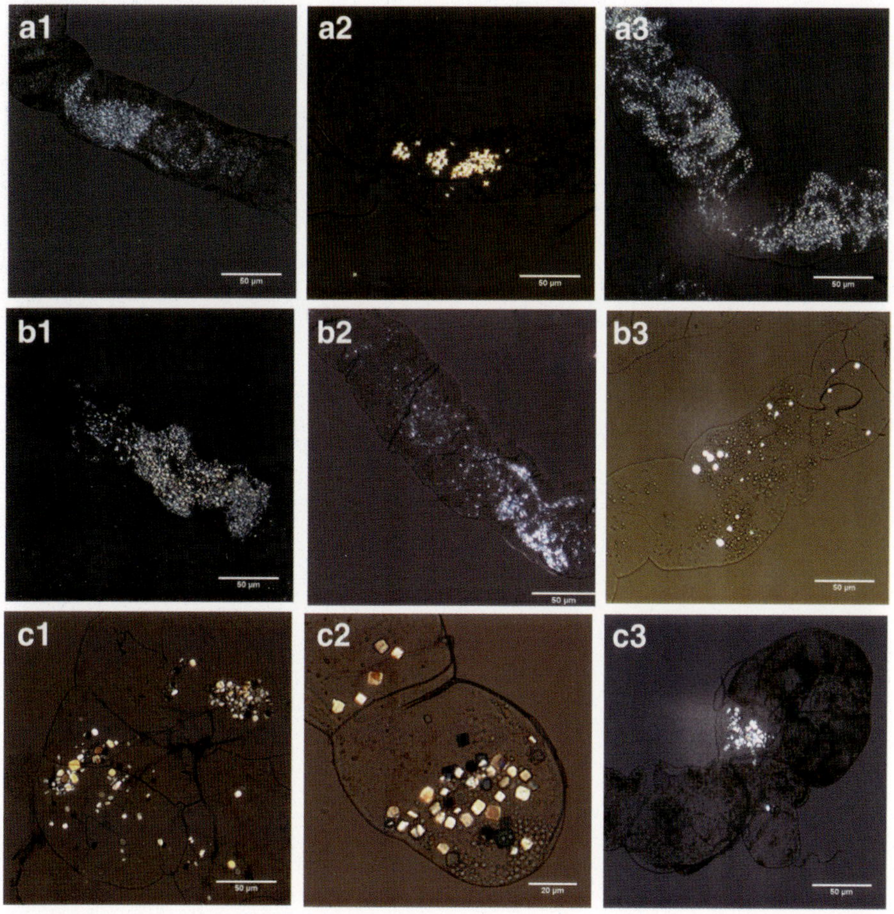

Fig. 3 Degree of crystal formation in Malpighian tubules by visual scale, 20× s magnification. 0: no stone formation, +: mild, 2+: moderate, 3+ strong crystal formation

scanning electron microscopy, which revealed predominantly CaOx monohydrate or CaOx dihydrate [6, 8].

Our survival study demonstrated in similar fashion that *Drosophila's* lifespan was significantly reduced by food enriched with 0.05% NaOx and 0.5% EG. The overall incidence crystal formation in control flies in our experiment was higher (20% vs 6.6%) but slightly lower in the lithogenic diets (84% vs 94%) compared with the pilot study.

Unlike the mammalian species, the Malpighian tubule in insects is the only organ for excreting solutes and water to the tubular lumen, as there is no glomerulus [9]. The distal segment of Malpighian tubules secretes

Table 1 Incidence of stone formation in Drosophila Malpighian tubules in 3 experimental conditions

Drosophila diet	Overall incidence of crystal formation (%)
control	20 ± 2.2
0.05% sodium oxalate	73 ± 3.6
0.5% ethylene glycol	84 ± 2.2

Values were expressed as means ± standard error of mean

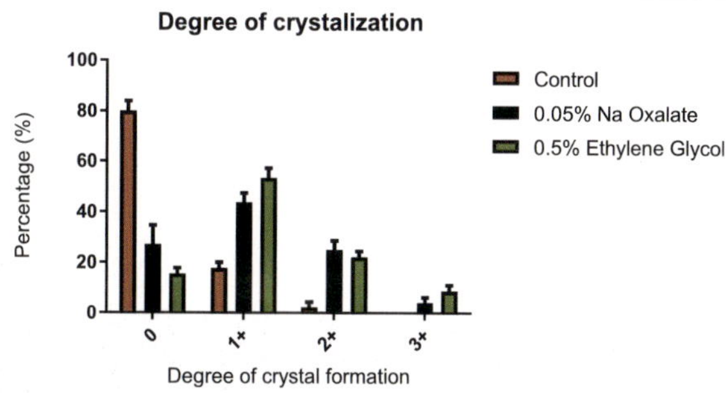

Fig. 4 Incidence of crystal formation according to degree of crystallization. The degree of crystallization was given a visual scale of 0, 1+, 2+ and 3+ by a single observer. The incidence of crystal formation of the control group was 80%(0), 17.8% (1+) and 2.2% (2+) respectively. The incidence of crystal formation in flies fed on NaOx diet was 27% (0), 43.8% (1+), 25% (2+) and 4.2% (3+). In the EG cohort, the incidence was 15.6% (0), 53.3% (1+), 22.2% (2+), 8.9% (3+) respectively

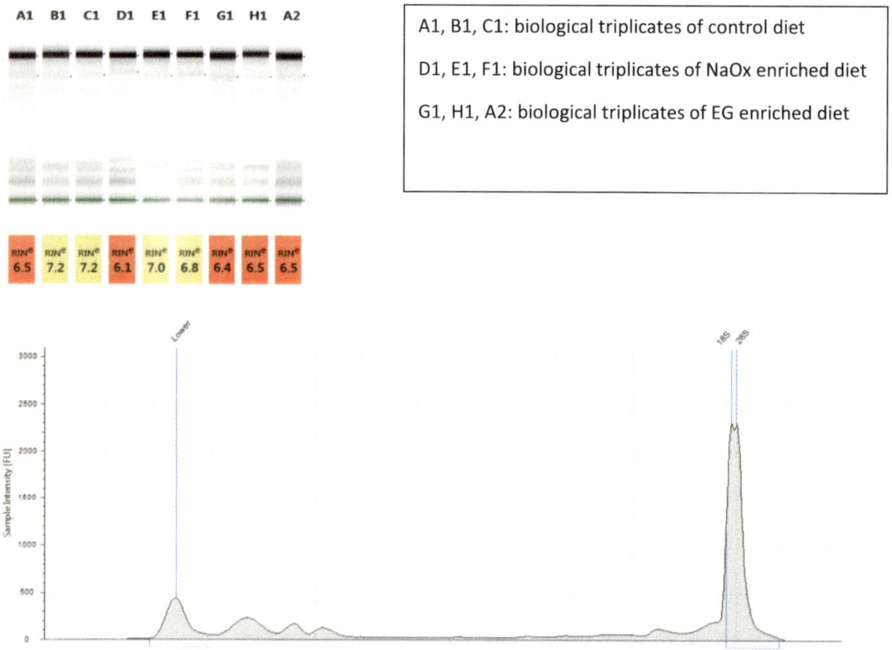

Fig. 5 RNA quality verification by Agilent 2100 Bio-analyzer. Gel image and electrophoretic profile of *Drosophila* Malpighian tubules RNA samples showed high quality RNA extraction. The electrophoretic ribosomal RNA profile of insects has single 28S peak which is commonly seen in insect RNA

electrolytes, organic solutes and water, and the proximal segments function as solute and water reabsorption [10]. The body calcium levels was regulated by Malpighian tubules by excretion through secretion into the lumen [11]. Administration of NaOx provides additional dietary supplement of oxalate, little evidence is available on how EG was metabolized in *Drosophila* however. Inferred from the metabolic pathway in the mammals, EG is degraded into four components: glycoaldehyde, glycolic acid, glyoxylic acid and oxalic acid. Excessive oxalic acid precipitates as CaOx stone in the tubules as a result [12]. The survival study demonstrated that the crystal accumulation in Malpighian tubules has a negative impact on the *Drosophila* lifespan, probably as a result of obstruction to the excretory organs and subsequent inability to maintain body hemostasis. EG induced a more profound negative impact on the lifespan, which could be related to associated metabolic acidosis [12] due to accumulated glycolic acid in addition to crystal formation.

Among the 58 differentially expressed genes in NaOx treatment group and 20 in EG group, we narrowed down the potential candidate genes by a number of criteria: molecular function, biological process and Log Fold changes compared with expression levels in the control group. There were no functionally significant overlapping genes between the two treatment groups, probably due to the fact that different biological pathways were involved in NaOx and EG diets. Genes that functions as transmembrane ion transporters had been singled out, namely Nervana 3, CG7912 and Eaat 1 in NaOx group; CG3036 and CG5404 in EG group. Crystallin coding for calcium ion binding protein and Dh44 which functions a diuretic hormone involved in body fluid secretion might also be of interest.

Nervana 3 codes for β subunit of Na+/K+ transporting ATPase, which catalyzes the hydrolysis of ATP coupled with the exchange of Na + and K+ ions across the plasma membrane. The β subunit regulates the transportation of sodium pumps to the plasma membrane [13]. Na + and K+ transport has been implicated in Ca2+ ion across renal tubules and homeostasis [14]. Though there was no previous work to elucidate the role of Na+/K+ pump in the Malpighian tubule, it was shown in rat and rabbit model that the basal-lateral plasma membrane contain Na+/Ca2+ exchange system which mediates the counter-transport of Ca2+ and Na + across the basal cell border [15, 16]. A protein which functioned as Na+/Ca2 +/K+ exchanger has been described in Drosophila to promote Ca2+ extrusion from cells [17].

CG7912 is predicted to have the molecular function of high-affinity sulfate transmembrane transporter. Its function in *Drosophila* was inferred from homology to mammalian transporters. Presumably, it catalyzes the high affinity transfer of sulfate across the plasma membrane up its

Table 2 Differentially expressed genes in NaOx and EG group compared with control

	Gene ID	Log Fold Change	*P* value	FDR
Sodium oxalate group (58 genes)	ymp	4.10	2.46E-04	4.27E-02
	CG4907	3.95	3.08E-04	4.99E-02
	CG13806	3.03	2.97E-04	4.99E-02
	CG15086	3.02	1.10E-05	4.69E-03
	CG43755	2.80	1.79E-04	3.30E-02
	w-cup	2.65	5.88E-05	1.67E-02
	CG3124	2.63	8.60E-06	4.04E-03
	CG9975	2.59	1.60E-04	3.07E-02
	CG9411	2.50	3.06E-04	4.99E-02
	S-Lap7	2.28	2.21E-04	3.92E-02
	CG4836	2.10	2.04E-04	3.68E-02
	Muc68Ca	1.59	1.62E-05	6.09E-03
	Drs	1.40	1.20E-04	2.50E-02
	CG10383	1.35	3.85E-08	5.17E-05
	Drsl2	1.35	1.09E-05	4.69E-03
	CG12896	1.33	6.96E-05	1.77E-02
	CG14695	1.17	2.29E-05	7.95E-03
	CG6967	1.06	7.99E-05	1.92E-02
	Cry	0.95	8.28E-06	4.04E-03
	CG13075	0.85	1.63E-04	3.07E-02
	CG8678	0.84	6.20E-06	3.24E-03
	CG5953	0.73	2.58E-04	4.40E-02
	l(1)G0148	−0.79	6.09E-05	1.68E-02
	Slif	−0.94	1.85E-05	6.67E-03
	Eaat1	−0.94	7.78E-05	1.92E-02
	Cyp28d1	−0.94	6.84E-05	1.77E-02
	CG4783	−0.95	1.07E-04	2.29E-02
	CG9238	−0.99	3.32E-05	1.01E-02
	Jon74E	−1.03	9.67E-05	2.11E-02
	CG2781	−1.05	1.54E-04	3.07E-02
	CG1946	−1.06	1.57E-04	3.07E-02
	CG8083	−1.07	5.32E-08	6.24E-05
	mag	−1.11	4.66E-05	1.37E-02
	zetaTry	−1.15	8.53E-05	1.99E-02
	Npc2d	−1.19	6.69E-09	1.05E-05
	CG42492	−1.21	8.67E-05	1.99E-02
	CG7912	−1.25	2.44E-05	8.12E-03
	Bace	−1.30	6.24E-07	6.51E-04
	nrv3	−1.30	2.79E-06	2.09E-03
	CG10592	−1.34	3.06E-11	7.20E-08
	CG5150	−1.37	1.16E-11	3.64E-08
	CG32483	−1.41	9.60E-07	9.01E-04
	TotM	−1.42	9.48E-05	2.11E-02
	CG15822	−1.43	1.36E-04	2.79E-02
	TotA	−1.46	4.46E-06	2.79E-03
	Diedel3	−1.52	5.61E-10	1.05E-06
	CG12057	−1.52	4.76E-06	2.79E-03
	CG18607	−1.60	1.50E-05	5.89E-03
	CG6012	−1.64	3.45E-06	2.31E-03
	CG7781	−1.68	5.05E-06	2.79E-03
	TotC	−1.70	2.89E-06	2.09E-03
	CG9134	−1.95	6.57E-05	1.76E-02
	CG6639	−2.64	1.50E-05	5.89E-03
	CG12374	−2.94	5.04E-30	4.73E-26
	CG34462	−3.00	3.27E-05	1.01E-02
	CG4830	−3.05	1.47E-06	1.26E-03
	CG34109	−3.09	2.51E-05	8.12E-03
	Obp56d	−3.90	1.61E-13	7.56E-10
Ethylene glycol group (20 genes)	Hr38	2.46	3.68E-05	2.22E-02
	Dh44	2.38	4.49E-05	2.46E-02
	CG12057	1.84	1.12E-06	1.49E-03
	CG17192	1.73	2.04E-07	9.48E-04
	CR43314	1.49	3.53E-05	2.22E-02
	Ets21C	1.37	8.96E-05	4.30E-02
	CG8299	1.36	2.72E-05	2.15E-02
	CG18744	1.35	7.85E-07	1.36E-03
	CG3036	1.25	8.81E-07	1.36E-03
	CG1718	1.21	3.01E-05	2.15E-02
	CG5404	1.20	4.35E-07	1.35E-03
	CG31324	1.16	8.84E-05	4.30E-02
	CG5151	1.09	3.80E-06	4.42E-03
	W	1.03	9.25E-05	4.30E-02
	Jon66Ci	−1.19	2.92E-05	2.15E-02
	Jon66Cii	−1.38	7.94E-08	7.38E-04
	IM2	−1.41	8.36E-06	8.64E-03
	CG5770	−1.54	7.97E-07	1.36E-03
	Cpr49Ae	−2.94	3.83E-05	2.22E-02
	LysP	−3.63	1.05E-05	9.78E-03

Positive log FC (Fold changes) denoted up regulation of genes whereas negative Log FC denoted down regulation
FDR False detection Rate

concentration gradient ([18] Flybase). In the murine model, targeted disruption of renal sulfate transporter genes NaS1 and Sat1 leads to hyposulfatemia and hypersulfaturia. Loss of Sat1 leads to hyperoxaluria, hyperoxalemia and calcium oxalate urolithiasis [19, 20]. These data suggest that sulfate transporters play an essential role for sulfate and oxalate homeostasis.

Similarly, the function of excitatory amino acid transporter (Eaat 1) as a sodium dicarboxylate symporter is inferred from homology to mammalian transporters. Its coding protein is an integral component of membrane which mediates concomitant uptake of sodium and dicarboxylate [21]. The rat ortholog of sodium dicarboxylate transporter (NaDC) was reported to mediate citrate uptake from renal proximal tubule. Citrate is an important inhibitor of calcium-stone formation and most of the citrate reabsorption is thought to occur via a sodium dicarboxylate transporter (NaDC1) located in the apical membrane. NaDC1 has been localized in opossum kidney proximal tubule cells and was responsible for calcium regulated citrate reabsorption in proximal tubules [22]. In the rat model, increased NaDC1 expression on the renal proximal tubule epithelial cells was associated with a decline in urinary citrate excretion, suggesting this transporter could play an important role in nephrolithiasis development [23]. In our study, Eaat1 demonstrated decreased expression in sodium oxalate diets compared with control, suggesting a protective effect to tubular stone formation.

The other candidate gene, Crystallin encodes a calcium ion binding protein [24] and is a major structural constituent of eye lens [25]. The implication of this gene in the biological process of stone formation is yet to be elucidated.

Similarly, in the EG treatment group, the protein products of gene CG3036 and CG5404 work as transmembrane transporter i.e. sodium-phosphate symporter and

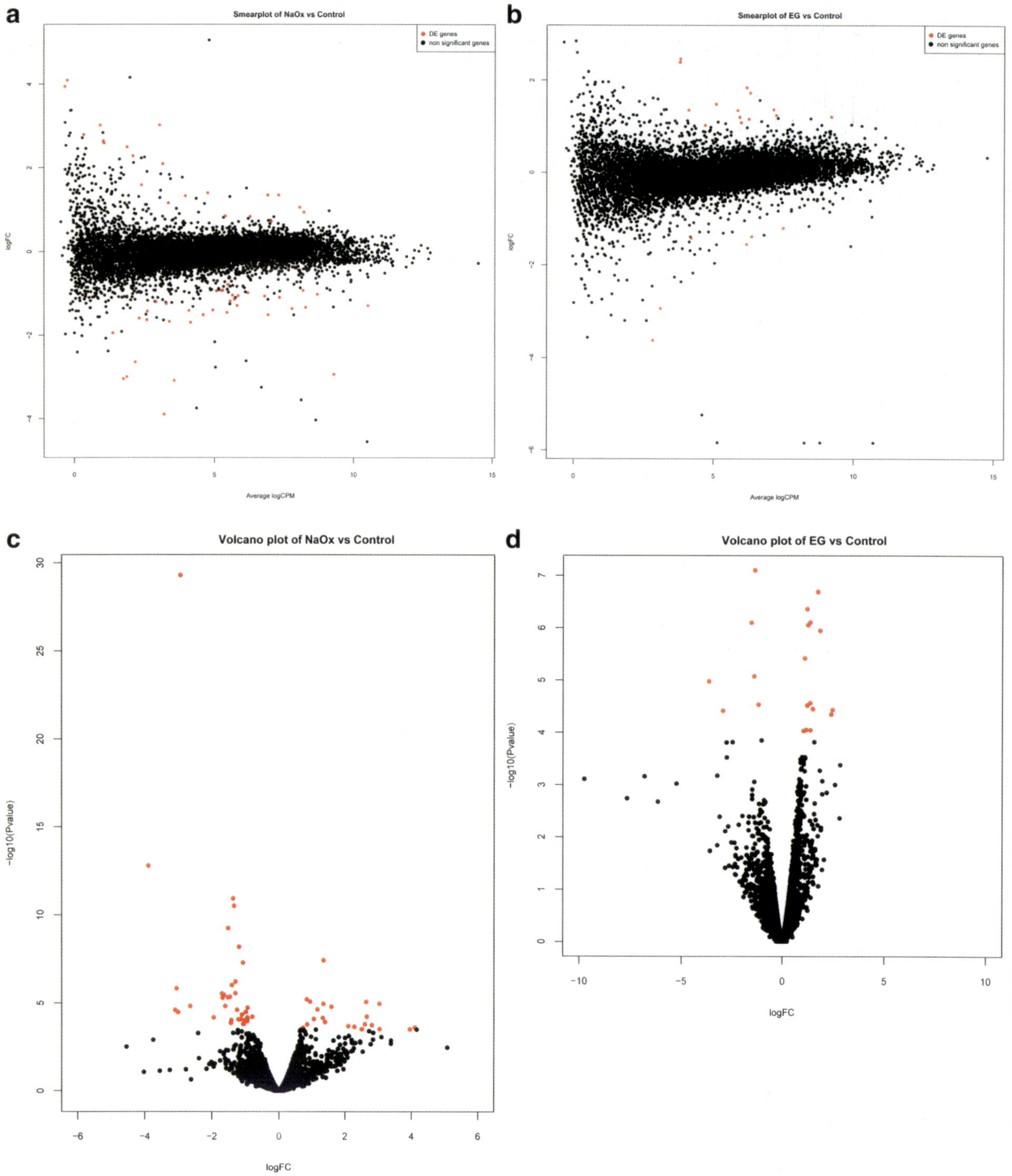

Fig. 6 Smear plots and volcano plots of differentially expressed genes in NaOx and EG groups. Differentially expressed genes (FDR <0.05, $p < 0.05$) compared with control were labelled as red points whereas insignificant genes were labelled as black. The mean expression level, Log Fold Change and *p*-Value of differentially expressed genes were displayed as smear plots and volcano plots. **a** Smear plot of NaOx group compared with control. **b** Smear plot of EG group compared with control. **c** Volcano plot of NaOx group compared with control. **d** Volcano plot of EG group compared with control

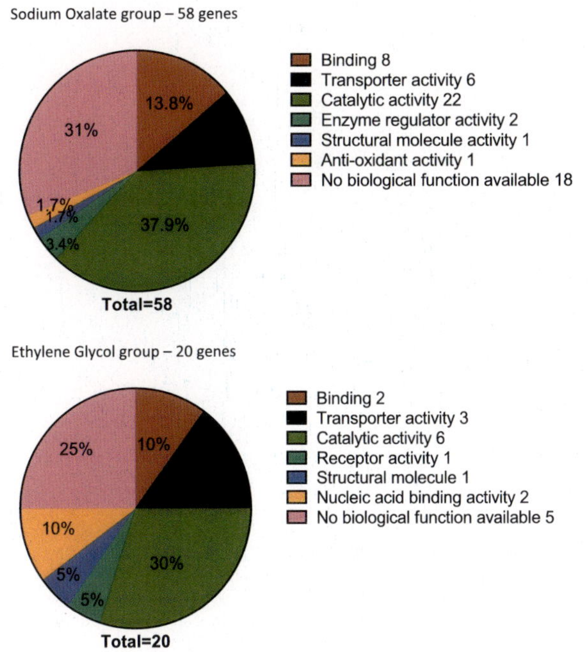

Fig. 7 Molecular functions of differentially expressed genes

high affinity sulfate transmembrane transporter, despite that the function of these gene products has not been directly measured Sodium phosphate co-transporter (Npt2a) null mice are shown to have hypercalciuria and hyperphosphaturia, and develop tubular and interstitial Ca phosphate deposits [26]. Crystals of CaOx may result for nucleation surrounding the Ca phosphate crystal [27] In human, hypophosphatemic hypercalciuric nephrolithiasis associated with rickets is the related to mutations in the type 2c sodium-phosphate co-transporter [28]. The up regulation of CG3036 in Drosophila might be a counteractive response to lower down tubular Ca level to reduce CaOx stone formation.

Dh44 is a gene that encodes a corticotrophin releasing factor (CRF) like peptide with 44 amino acids. Functional studies showed that the protein product stimulated fluid production, and this effect was mediated by cyclic AMP in principal cells only [29]. The significant up regulation of this diuretic hormone in Malpighian tubules could be a direct protective effect of body fluid secretion in response to crystal formation.

These differentially expressed genes could play a role in the biological pathway of calcium oxalate stone formation or could be a regulated response to the obstructive uropathy, metabolic acidosis and failure to maintain electrolyte or acid-base balance in *Drosophila* Malpighian tubules. We made the hypothesis that genes encoding transmembrane ion transporter or diuretic hormone might be more critical in these processes but other genes might also be relevant. Molecular function of many differentially expressed genes remained unknown, so that further investigations will be required to elucidate the exact roles of these genes and how they function as a whole in the process of CaOx crystal formation.

Despite the high incidence of crystal formation in flies fed with lithogenic agents, we do not know if there was any difference in the transcriptive changes in stone formers and non-stone former. Experiments designed to study the difference of stone-formers and non-stone formers might provide further insight in the pathogenesis.

In this experiment of environmentally induced stone formation, we have successfully used the drosophila as a model to demonstrate transcriptional changes in a number of genes that may play a role in the pathogenesis of stone formation. To evaluate the contribution of these genes to stone formation, RNAi could be used to preform tissue-specific knockdown or overexpression studies to modify stone formation, using the extensive collection of genetic reagents available in *Drosophila*. Downstream proteomic analysis could further provide information of the function of possible candidate genes.

Conclusions

Our results suggest that drosophila proved to be a powerful experimental organism for studying nephrolithiasis. The transcriptome secondary to crystal formation could provide useful insight into the pathophysiology of stone formation and potential therapeutic target for the treatment of nephrolithiasis.

Table 3 Candidate genes which function as transmembrane ion transporter, Ca ion binder or diuretic hormone that may play a role in crystal formation

	Gene name	GO Molecular function	Log FC
Sodium oxalate group	nervana 3	plasma membrane Na:K- exchanging ATPase activity	−1.29
	Excitatory amino acid transporter 1	Na: dicarboxylate symporter activity; Na:glutamate symporter activity	−0.93
	CG7912	High affinity Sulfate transmembrane transporter	−1.25
	Crystallin	Ca ion binding	0.945
Ethylene Glycol group	CG3036	Na: phosphate symporter activity	1.24
	CG5404	high affinity sulfate transmembrane transporter	1.2
	Dh44	Diuretic hormone activity	2.38

Abbreviations

CaOx: Calcium oxalate; EG: Ethylene glycol; FC: Fold changes; FDR: False discovery rate; mRNA: Messenger RNA; NaOx: Sodium oxalate; rRNA: Ribosomal RNA

Acknowledgements

We appreciate the help of Dr. Markus Toegel, Dr. Tudor Fulga from Weatherall Institute of Molecular Medicine, University of Oxford for the generous support during the experiments. We thank the High-Throughput Genomics Group at the Wellcome Trust Centre for Human Genetics (funded by Wellcome Trust grant reference 090532/Z/09/Z and MRC Hub grant G0900747 91070) for the generation of the sequencing data. We also appreciate the help of Mr. Mark Sullivan and Dr. Rebecca Konietzny for reviewing the manuscript.

Funding

Not applicable.

Authors' contributions

VC prepared the experiment samples, participated in the RNA sequencing, carried out data analysis and drafted the manuscript. BT designed the study, participated in data analysis and manuscript revision. Both authors read and approved the final manuscript.

Competing interests

The authors declare that they have no competing interests.

References

1. Turney BW, Reynard JM, Noble JG, Keoghane SR. Trends in urological stone disease. BJU Int. 2012;109(7):1082–7.
2. Scales CD Jr, Smith AC, Hanley JM, Saigal CS. Prevalence of kidney stones in the United States. Eur Urol. 2012;62(1):160–5.
3. Curhan GC, Willett WC, Rimm EB, Stampfer MJ. A prospective study of dietary calcium and other nutrients and the risk of symptomatic kidney stones. N Engl J Med. 1993;328(12):833–8.
4. Resnick M, Pridgen DB, Goodman HO. Genetic predisposition to formation of calcium oxalate renal calculi. N Engl J Med. 1968;278(24):1313–8.
5. Miller J, Chi T, Kapahi P, Kahn AJ, Kim MS, Hirata T, et al. Drosophila Melanogaster as an emerging translational model of human nephrolithiasis. J Urol. 2013;190(5):1648–56.
6. Chen YH, Liu HP, Chen HY, Tsai FJ, Chang CH, Lee YJ, et al. Ethylene glycol induces calcium oxalate crystal deposition in Malpighian tubules: a drosophila model for nephrolithiasis/urolithiasis. Kidney Int. 2011;80(4):369–77.
7. Winnebeck EC, Millar CD, Warman GR. Why does insect RNA look degraded? J Insect Sci. 2010;10:159.
8. Hirata T, Cabrero P, Berkholz DS, Bondeson DP, Ritman EL, Thompson JR, et al. In vivo Drosophilia genetic model for calcium oxalate nephrolithiasis. Am J Physiol Renal Physiol. 2012;303(11):F1555–62.
9. Dow JA, Romero MF. Drosophila provides rapid modeling of renal development, function, and disease. Am J Physiol Renal Physiol. 2010;299(6):F1237–44.
10. Beyenbach KW. Transport mechanisms of diuresis in Malpighian tubules of insects. J Exp Biol. 2003;206(Pt 21):3845–56.
11. Wessing A, Zierold K. The formation of type-I concretions in drosophila Malpighian tubules studied by electron microscopy and X-ray microanalysis. J Insect Physiol. 1999;45(1):39–44.
12. Leth PM, Gregersen M. Ethylene glycol poisoning. Forensic Sci Int. 2005; 155(2–3):179–84.
13. Sun B, Wang W, Salvaterra PM. Functional analysis and tissue-specific expression of Drosophila Na+,K+–ATPase subunits. J Neurochem. 1998;71(1):142–51.
14. Friedman PA. Codependence of renal calcium and sodium transport. Annu Rev Physiol. 1998;60:179–97.
15. Gmaj P, Murer H, Kinne R. Calcium ion transport across plasma membranes isolated from rat kidney cortex. Biochem J. 1979;178(3):549–57.
16. Friedman PA, Figueiredo JF, Maack T, Windhager EE. Sodium-calcium interactions in the renal proximal convoluted tubule of the rabbit. Am J Phys. 1981;240(6):F558–68.
17. Winkfein RJ, Pearson B, Ward R, Szerencsei RT, Colley NJ, Schnetkamp PP. Molecular characterization, functional expression and tissue distribution of a second NCKX Na+/Ca2+ –K+ exchanger from drosophila. Cell Calcium. 2004;36(2):147–55.
18. dos Santos G, Schroeder AJ, Goodman JL, Strelets VB, Crosby MA, Thurmond J, et al. FlyBase: introduction of the Drosophila Melanogaster release 6 reference genome assembly and large-scale migration of genome annotations. Nucleic Acids Res. 2015;43(Database issue):D690–7.
19. Markovich D. Physiological roles of mammalian sulfate transporters NaS1 and Sat1. Arch Immunol Ther Exp. 2011;59(2):113–6.
20. Dawson PA, Russell CS, Lee S, McLeay SC, van Dongen JM, Cowley DM, et al. Urolithiasis and hepatotoxicity are linked to the anion transporter Sat1 in mice. J Clin Invest. 2010;120(3):706–12.
21. Reizer J, Reizer A, Saier MH Jr. A functional superfamily of sodium/solute symporters. Biochim Biophys Acta. 1994;1197(2):133–66.
22. Hering-Smith KS, Mao W, Schiro FR, Coleman-Barnett J, Pajor AM, Hamm LL. Localization of the calcium-regulated citrate transport process in proximal tubule cells. Urolithiasis. 2014;42(3):209–19.
23. He Y, Chen X, Yu Z, Wu D, Lv Y, Shi S, et al. Sodium dicarboxylate cotransporter-1 expression in renal tissues and its role in rat experimental nephrolithiasis. J Nephrol. 2004;17(1):34–42.
24. Srivastava SS, Mishra A, Krishnan B, Sharma Y. Ca2+–binding motif of betagamma-crystallins. J Biol Chem. 2014;289(16):10958–66.
25. Jobby MK, Sharma Y. Calcium-binding to lens betaB2- and betaA3-crystallins suggests that all beta-crystallins are calcium-binding proteins. FEBS J. 2007;274(16):4135–47.
26. Khan SR, Canales BK. Ultrastructural investigation of crystal deposits in Npt2a knockout mice: are they similar to human Randall's plaques? J Urol. 2011;186(3):1107–13.
27. Tiselius HG. A hypothesis of calcium stone formation: an interpretation of stone research during the past decades. Urol Res. 2011;39(4):231–43.
28. Stechman MJ, Loh NY, Thakker RV. Genetic causes of hypercalciuric nephrolithiasis. Pediatr Nephrol. 2009;24(12):2321–32.
29. Cabrero P, Radford JC, Broderick KE, Costes L, Veenstra JA, Spana EP, et al. The Dh gene of Drosophila Melanogaster encodes a diuretic peptide that acts through cyclic AMP. J Exp Biol. 2002;205(Pt 24):3799–807.

16

Patient driven care in the management of prostate cancer: analysis of the United States military healthcare system

Muhammad Ali Chaudhary[1*], Jeffrey J. Leow[1], Matthew Mossanen[2], Ritam Chowdhury[1], Wei Jiang[1], Peter A. Learn[3], Joel S. Weissman[1] and Steven L. Chang[2]

Abstract

Background: Patient preferences are assumed to impact healthcare resource utilization, especially treatment options. There is limited data exploring this phenomenon. We sought to identify factors associated with patients transferring care for prostatectomy, from military to civilian facilities, and the receipt of minimally invasive radical prostatectomy (MIRP).

Methods: Retrospective review of 2006-2010 TRICARE data identified men diagnosed with prostate cancer (ICD-9 185) receiving open radical prostatectomy (ORP; ICD-9: 60.5) or MIRP (ICD-9 60.5 + 54.21/17.42). Patients diagnosed at military facilities but underwent surgery at civilian facilities were defined as "transferring care". Logistic regression models identified predictors of transferring care for patients diagnosed at military facilities. A secondary analysis identified the predictors of MIRP receipt at civilian facilities.

Results: Of 1420 patients, 247 (17.4%) transferred care. These patients were more likely to undergo MIRP (OR = 7.83, $p < 0.01$), and get diagnosed at low-volume military facilities (OR = 6.10, $p < 0.01$). Our secondary analysis demonstrated that transferring care was strongly associated with undergoing MIRP (OR = 1.51, $p = 0.04$).

Conclusions: Patient preferences induced a demand for greater utilization of MIRP and civilian facilities. Further work exploring factors driving these preferences and interventions tailoring them, based on evidence and cost considerations, is required.

Keywords: TRICARE, Robotic surgery, Prostatectomy, Patient preference

Background

The modern healthcare sector is complex, with supply and demand operating at patient, provider, and facility levels. Different factors play a vital role in creating and increasing the demand for utilization of certain healthcare services [1–4]. Among them the effects of hospital and provider level factors have been well described in the literature. Delamater and colleagues have shown that the hospitalization rate in a particular geographical area is directly related to the number of hospital beds available [1], pointing towards the role of hospitals in creating a demand for healthcare services. Weeks et al. demonstrate that healthcare providers can induce a demand for greater utilization of healthcare resources [2].

There are limited studies, however, that have explored the role of patient preferences on the utilization of healthcare resources. For instance, Tak et al. demonstrated that patients who are more engaged in their care are associated with increased healthcare utilization among hospitalized patients [3]. While these findings are provocative, there remains a poor understanding regarding the true impact of patient preferences on utilization of certain treatment options.

The surgical management of localized prostate cancer provides a pertinent preference-specific procedure to study patient demand for utilization of healthcare resources. The popularity of minimally invasive radical prostatectomy (MIRP) over open radical prostatectomy

* Correspondence: mchaudhary@bwh.harvard.edu
[1]Center for Surgery and Public Health, Department of Surgery, Brigham and Women's Hospital, Harvard Medical School, Harvard T H Chan School of Public Health, Boston, MA, USA
Full list of author information is available at the end of the article

(ORP), particularly with the robotic surgical platform, has been anecdotally associated with direct-to-consumer advertising and market forces [5] rather than definitive clinical benefit [6–9]. Our recent work demonstrates heterogeneous dissemination of MIRP, with MIRP becoming the predominant form of surgery among civilian hospitals while ORP remains the most common surgical procedure in military institutions [10]. This dichotomy in the surgical approach for radical prostatectomy provides a unique opportunity to evaluate the presence of "patient-induced demand" for MIRP by examining a contemporary cohort of men in TRICARE, a health care program of the United States Department of Defense (DOD) that allows men with prostate cancer to receive care in either military or civilian facilities.

Methods

Aims

The aims of this study were to determine the predictors of the transference of care from one healthcare system to another and the receipt of MIRP.

Data

The study utilized TRICARE insurance claims data (2006-2010) from the Military Health System Data Repository (MDR). TRICARE is the healthcare insurance program for uniformed service personnel, retirees and their dependents in the United States. TRICARE Prime beneficiaries receive comprehensive medical coverage through either the Direct Care System (DCS) at military facilities, or the Purchased Care System (PCS) at civilian facilities. Healthcare providers at the military facilities are salaried employees while those within the civilian facilities work at a mix of for-profit and non-profit civilian hospitals. Longitudinal follow up is available for patients while they are covered by TRICARE. We limited our analysis to TRICARE Prime for two reasons. First, TRICARE Prime enrollees are assigned a primary care manager (PCM), who manages their healthcare. Thus, they are less likely to receive care that is not in the purview of TRICARE coverage and the care provided would be better documented. Second, these plans have a low to no enrollment fee, no copayments and deductibles if care is provided within a military facility or if the patient was referred out through the military facilities or for those living outside a defined geographic catchment area of a military facility. Thus patients could opt for either a civilian or a military facility without cost being a barrier.

TRICARE is neither used to treat soldiers in combat zones nor provide care administered though Veterans Administration (VA) facilities. The TRICARE database, population being treated, mode of healthcare delivery and validation of the data elements have been described in prior literature [11–13].

Study cohort, outcomes and covariates

We identified 5082 men diagnosed with prostate cancer (*International Classification of Disease, 9th Revision* [ICD-9]: 185) who underwent radical prostatectomy (RP; ICD-9: 60.5) from 2006 to 2010. Patients were dichotomized by the type of RP as ORP (ICD-9 60.5 only) or MIRP (ICD-9 60.5 + 54.21 and/or 17.42). Information was abstracted for the institution where a TRICARE beneficiary received his diagnosis of prostate cancer and subsequent surgery.

Men diagnosed at a military facility but who later underwent RP at a civilian facility were defined as having "transferred care". Transference of care and receipt of MIRP were outcomes of interest in the primary and secondary analysis, respectively.

Demographics, Medicare eligibility, income (based on rank), comorbid condition and procedure type (MRP vs. ORP) were taken as patient level covariates while prostatectomy volume and availability of MIRP were taken as hospital level covariates.

Primary analysis

For our primary analysis, we sought to determine the predictors for transferring care for surgery from a military to a civilian facility. We restricted our patient cohort to men residing within 40 miles of a military facility performing RP because those who live farther away can seek care at civilian facilities at little or no out of pocket costs. Therefore, our analytic cohort was comprised of patients who were arguably financially incentivized to remain within a military facility for the treatment. The adjusted model incorporated demographic information, including age, self-reported race/ethnicity, marital status, and military rank. To account for patient health status, we utilized the Centers for Medicare and Medicaid Services-Hierarchical Condition Category (CMS-HCC) model [14]. We also included the year of procedure to assess for differences across the study period. Hospitals were segregated by surgical volume into low (<24 RP annually) and high (≥24 RP annually) based on an a priori assumption that high volume centers perform at least two RP per month.

Secondary analysis

To further evaluate whether the type of surgery (MIRP vs. ORP) may have influenced the decision to transfer health care systems, we created a second cohort comprised of TRICARE beneficiaries with prostate cancer specifically undergoing RP at a civilian facility representing 1026 men. This cohort was dichotomized into men who received their diagnosis and treatment at a civilian facility and those who received their diagnosis at a military facility and then transferred care to a civilian facility for the treatment, to determine if transferring care from military to civilian facilities was associated with a receipt of MIRP. Our adjusted model included the same clinical, demographic and hospital variables as in the primary analysis.

Statistical analysis

We summarized patient and surgical characteristics for patients who underwent RP with descriptive statistics and multivariable logistic regression, comparing those who transferred care with those who did not transfer care (primary analysis) and comparing those who underwent ORP vs. MIRP at civilian facilities (secondary analysis). Chi square tests were used to compare categorical variables and ANOVA was used for continuous variables. We accounted for inter-hospital variations by clustering at the hospital level. Statistical analyses were performed using SAS 9.3 (SAS Institute, NC). All tests were two-sided and a *p*-value of <0.05 was considered statistically significant. The study protocol was reviewed and approved by our institutional review board. Permission to access data within MDR was obtained by a data use agreement between our institute and the Uniformed Services University of Health Sciences.

Results

Among the 1420 men in the primary analysis focused on men diagnosed with prostate cancer at military facilities, 247 (17.4%) transferred care from military to civilian facilities for their treatment (Table 1). Men who transferred care tended to be slightly younger (median age 57.8 vs. 59 years, $p = 0.01$), had a higher median HCC (0.39 vs. 0.37, $p < 0.01$), and were more likely Black when compared to men did not transfer (31.2% vs. 25.2% $p < 0.01$). Among men who transferred care to a civilian facility, 45.3% underwent MIRP, while among men who remained at military facilities, 13.7% underwent MIRP ($p < 0.01$). Significant differences were also noted by year with proportion of patients transferring care increasing from 15.6% in 2006 to 25.4% in 2010 ($p < 0.01$) (Fig. 1).

In adjusted analysis, men who transferred their care had higher adjusted odds of identifying with a minority (non-White) race [odds ratio (OR): 1.96, 95% Confidence Interval (95% CI): 1.34-2.87, $p < 0.01$], undergoing MIRP (OR: 7.83, 95% CI: 3.30-18.62, $p < 0.01$), and being diagnosed at a low volume center for RP (<24 RP annually) (OR: 6.10, 95% CI: 2.20-16.95, $p < 0.01$). (Table 2) Less healthy individuals were also more likely to seek care at civilian institutions [HCC: (OR: 2.88 95% CI: 1.38-5.98, $p < 0.01$)]. In contrast, active duty status was associated with lower likelihood of transferring care (OR: 0.54, 95% CI: 0.32-0.90, $p = 0.05$).

Table 1 Demographic and clinical characteristics of TRICARE beneficiaries in the United States who, after diagnosis of prostate cancer at a military facilities, transferred their care to a civilian facilities to undergo radical prostatectomy, compared to those who did not transfer care

Characteristic	Non-Transferers	Transferers	*p*-value
n (%)	1173 (82.6%)	247 (17.4%)	
Median Age at Procedure	59	57.8	
Mean Age at Procedure	58.48 (8.1)	57.11 (7.6)	0.01
Race			<0.01
White	754 (64.3%)	122 (49.4%)	
Black	295 (25.2%)	77 (31.2%)	
American Indian/Asian/Other	124 (10.6%)	13 (5.3%)	
Unknown	0 (0.0%)	35 (14.2%)	
Marital Status			0.09
Married	971 (82.8%)	191 (77.3%)	
Single	119 (10.1%)	36 (14.6%)	
Unknown	83 (7.1%)	20 (8.1%)	
Beneficiary category			0.98
Active duty	164 (14.0%)	35 (14.2%)	
Non-active duty	1009 (86.0%)	212 (85.8%)	
Medicare eligibility			0.06
Eligible	216 (18.4%)	33 (13.4%)	
Not eligible	957 (81.6%)	214 (86.6%)	
Sponsor rank			0.80
Enlisted	693 (59.1%)	139 (56.3%)	
Officer	388 (33.1%)	84 (34.0%)	
Unknown	92 (7.8%)	24 (9.7%)	
Procedure Type			<0.01
Open	1012 (82.3%)	135 (54.7%)	
Minimally Invasive	161 (13.7%)	112 (45.3%)	
Mean HCC	0.37 0.24	0.40 0.23	<0.01

In the secondary analysis, among the 1026 TRICARE beneficiaries who underwent surgery in a civilian facility, 247 (24.1%) transferred care from a military facility. Compared to patients initially diagnosed at civilian facilities, transferers from military facilities were more likely to be non-White as (49.4% versus 38.6%, $p < 0.01$) and less healthy [median HCC:(0.39 versus 0.33, $p < 0.01$)] (Appendix 1).

The independent predictors of undergoing MIRP in the secondary analysis are presented in Table 3. Patients undergoing MIRP had higher risk adjusted odds of being transfers from a military facility (OR: 1.51, 95% CI: 1.03-2.22, $p = 0.04$). The odds of undergoing MIRP were also inversely associated with increasing HCC (OR: 0.28, 95%

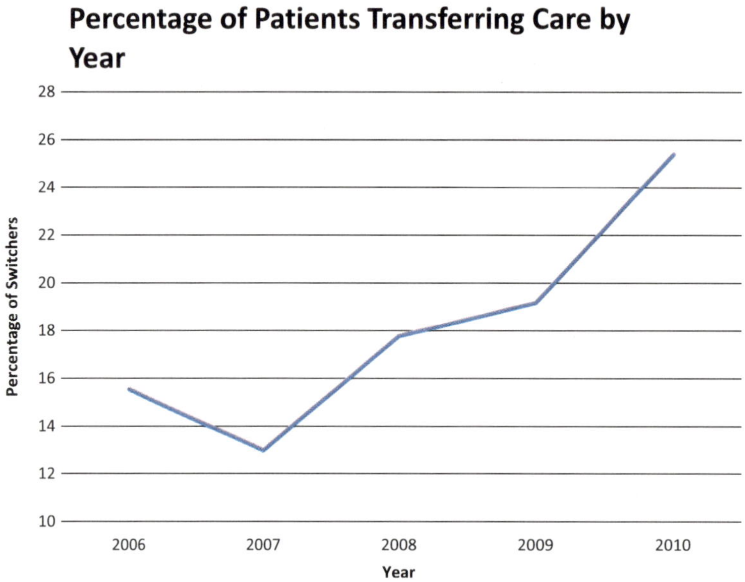

Fig. 1 Proportion of TRICARE beneficiaries in the United States who, after diagnosis of prostate cancer at a military facility, transferred care to a civilian facility to undergo radical prostatectomy ($p < 0.01$)

CI: 0.09-0.83] per 1.0 unit increase, $p = 0.02$). MIRP was also more likely to be performed in 2010 compared to 2006 (OR: 33.33, 95% CI: 20.00-50.00, $p < 0.01$).

Discussion

In this study of TRICARE beneficiaries diagnosed with prostate cancer who have access to care at military and civilian facilities, we found evidence supporting the premise that "patient-induced demand" drives the utilization of MIRP. Our study shows that a substantial proportion of patients (17.4%) transferred care from military to civilian facilities in order to undergo RP, despite logistic incentives for staying within the military healthcare system for treatment. Both analyses demonstrate that the men who transferred care were most strongly associated with undergoing MIRP. These findings support the hypothesis that patient preferences may represent an important factor for inducing the demand for utilization of healthcare services for surgical intervention.

The main strength of this study is the uniqueness of the patient population. TRICARE patients are universally insured under the same TRICARE Prime benefit plan. This minimizes the possibility of confounding by insurance status and different types of insurance coverage. Secondly, these patients not only had the logistical advantage of living close to a military facility (within 40 miles) that offered radical prostatectomy but also the financial incentive of receiving care completely free of charge by remaining at the military facility. Despite these benefits, a sizable proportion (nearly one-fifth) of these patients chose to transfer care to civilian facilities. Since out-of-pocket costs at civilian facilities would act as a deterrent for transferring care, this is further evidence in support of the relationship between patient preferences and the demand for healthcare utilization.

To the best of our knowledge, this is the first study to investigate the impact of prostate cancer patient preferences as the driving force for the utilization of a specific surgical intervention. The possibility for patient-induced demand for MIRP among men with prostate cancer was previously implied by Chang et al. [15] and Makarov et al. [16] who reported that the availability of robotic technology increased the volume of RP for individual surgeons and hospitals, respectively. Previous studies among men with prostate cancer have demonstrated patient preferences for various treatment options for prostate cancer (e.g. active surveillance, surgery, radiation, or hormonal therapy) [17–19], cosmetic results of different types of prostatectomies [20] and on functional outcomes (erectile function and continence) [21]. Our results expand on this pre-existing body of work, and demonstrate that patient preferences indeed induce a demand for greater utilization of healthcare services, which could feasibly impact the overall burden of disease.

Our secondary analysis studied civilian facilities to which TRICARE beneficiaries with prostate cancer transferred care from a military facility, to identify possible motivations for transferring care. We found that transferring care from a military facility was strongly associated with undergoing MIRP. These findings suggest that even within the civilian facilities, patients transferring care are more likely to undergo MIRP compared to patients who were initially diagnosed at and remained at the civilian facilities for surgery. This may imply that

Table 2 Risk-adjusted predictors of transferring care from a military to a civilian facility among TRICARE beneficiaries in the United States

Predictors	OR	95%CI		*p*-value
Age at procedure	0.98	0.94	1.01	0.11
Race				
White	Reference			
Non-white race	1.96	1.34	2.87	<0.01
Marital Status				
Single	Reference			
Married	0.69	0.46	1.03	0.07
Beneficiary category				
Non-active duty	Reference			
Active duty	0.54	0.32	0.90	0.05
Medicare eligibility				
In-eligible	Reference			
Eligible	0.98	0.38	2.53	0.97
Income (based on rank)				
Low	Reference			
High	1.50	0.41	5.43	0.54
Rank				
Officer	Reference			
Enlisted	0.94	0.28	3.11	0.92
HCC	2.88	1.38	5.98	<0.01
Procedure Type				
Open	Reference			
Minimally invasive	7.84	3.30	18.63	<0.01
Volume of center of diagnosis				
High volume	Reference			
Low volume	6.10	2.20	16.95	<0.01
MIRP availability at center of diagnosis				
Available				
Not available	1.61	0.93	2.78	0.09

Table 3 Risk-adjusted predictors of undergoing minimally invasive radical prostatectomy among TRICARE beneficiaries undergoing prostate cancer surgery in the United States

Predictors	Probability of receiving minimally invasive procedure			
	OR	95%CI		*p*-value
Age at procedure	1.01	0.99	1.03	0.64
Race				
White	Reference			
Non-white	0.93	0.67	1.30	0.68
Marital Status				
Single	Reference			
Married	1.05	0.65	1.70	0.85
Rank				
Officer				
Enlisted	0.82	0.58	1.18	0.29
HCC	0.28	0.09	0.83	0.02
Transferring Care Status				
No	Reference			
Yes	1.51	1.02	2.22	0.04
Year of procedure				
2006	Reference			
2010	33.33	20.00	50.00	<0.01

the demand for greater utilization of a particular type of care may be driven by a subset of patients who are highly motivated, and proactive in their healthcare, having strong preferences for a particular treatment option. Our findings are consistent with the findings of Tak et al.'s study, which demonstrated that patient preferences regarding participation in medical decision making was associated with greater resource utilization (i.e. longer length of stay and higher total hospitalization costs) [3].

The present study findings suggest that promoting new technology, even without clear scientific evidence showing advantages compared to standard options, may stimulate patient-induced demand thereby attracting new patients and increasing volume. Our findings are consistent with previous work done on the impact of direct-to-consumer advertising (DTCA) on healthcare utilization in the field of pharmacy [22, 23]. In an article titled, *"Just What the Patient Ordered? Direct-to-Consumer Advertising and the Demand for Pharmaceutical Products"* [22], the author demonstrates that DTCA plays a significant role in the expansion of market of a certain category of drugs. Bradford et al. evaluated the association of DTCA for osteoarthritis drugs with physicians' prescribing behavior [23]. Their work elucidates that DTCA not only increased the likelihood of the said drug being prescribed but also resulted in larger numbers of patients seen for osteoarthritis. These findings suggest that patient preferences not only impact the utilization of a certain treatment option but also increase the utilization of healthcare services as a whole. Marketing to patients therefore may also explain in part the widespread diffusion of robotic technology for MIRP in the United States, even in the absence of irrefutable scientific data showing its benefits over ORP. Our work indicates the possible magnitude of this impact and demonstrates how marketing might lead to greater utilization of a novel surgical technology.

The preference for MIRP among patients is likely borne out of a fundamental patient desire for optimal care and outcomes, although Level I evidence has shown no appreciable difference between surgical approaches [24]. In contrast, patient awareness that higher surgical volume has been consistently associated with improved outcomes following prostate cancer surgery [25] likely explains why diagnosis of prostate cancer at a military facility with a low volume of radical prostatectomies was a strong predictor of patient request for transfer of care to a civilian facility (Table 1). Additional investigation, however, is warranted to better understand our finding that non-white men and less healthy men were also more likely to transfer care from a military to a civilian facility for definitive surgical management of prostate cancer.

The percentage of patients transferring care from a military to a civilian facility increased steadily throughout the study period (Fig. 1). This finding is likely associated with the disproportionately faster and more widespread adoption of MIRP among civilian facilities compared to military facilities. These differences in adoption rates of MIRP have been attributed to differences in the financial structure of these two health care systems [10]. The military healthcare system has a salaried system of compensation for healthcare providers and funds may be allocated to preventive care. On the contrary, most civilian facilities have a fee-for-service model and healthcare delivery is reliant on generation of sufficient revenue. This is a possible incentive for adopting new technology to attract new patients and increase volume to maximize revenue [26].

Given the association between patient preferences and receipt of MIRP, some interesting questions arise. First, what is the driving force behind these patient preferences, given that the scientific literature on the benefits and risks of MIRP over ORP is mixed? [6–8, 24] Second, how can these preferences be changed to align with current evidence and cost considerations? The answer to the first question may be attributed to the increased use of internet for health-related information [27] and online information is biased towards robot-assisted radical prostatectomy [28]. Hajdenberg et al. evaluated the quality of information on robot-assisted radical prostatectomy present on the internet, and found that websites that advertise robot-assisted radical prostatectomy were more appealing than those that do not specifically advertise the procedure and instead simply provide information. Mirkin et al. in a similar effort evaluated the credibility of the information present on the internet regarding robot-assisted radical prostatectomy [29], and demonstrated that many websites claim benefits, not supported by evidence, with as many as 42% of websites failing to mention risks associated with the procedure. For the second question, the possible solutions include the need for greater regulatory control over advertisement and creation of well-balanced patient education material, so patients can make more informed decisions regarding their treatment preferences.

Limitations

This study has some limitations that need to be considered when drawing conclusion based on these results. First, we used the TRICARE database, which relied on medical claims and encounter data. Like other administrative datasets, we cannot account for some nuanced clinical characteristics that may have an impact on the association that we demonstrated, such as oncologic characteristics. However, if RP was clinically indicated, then it is generally safe to assume that all patients identified had localized prostate cancer amenable for surgical intervention, and other factors such as PSA levels, Gleason score or TNM staging may not influence results significantly [30]. Second, there exists the possibility of coding errors leading to misclassification bias. However, TRICARE has many structural similarities with Medicare, a similar database, which has been used widely for surgical outcome studies [31]. Third, we were not able to reliably account for the availability of a robot at a particular facility. Adoption of clinical innovation for the maximization of hospital revenue could be a major driver for more rapid adoption of MIRP in civilian facilities. However, it must be considered that civilian facilities are much more likely to have earlier robotic surgery capability than military facilities. The availability of specialized equipment and trained personnel are as likely (or more likely) to contribute to the more rapid and widespread adoption of MIRP in civilian facilities [10].

Conclusions

This is the first study to quantify the potential impact of patient preferences on the utilization of surgical technology using administrative data from a large population with universal insurance coverage. Low prostatectomy volume and unavailability of MIRP at the hospital of diagnosis were strong predictors of transferring care to civilian facilities despite significant financial incentives at military facilities. These findings suggest that patients' preferences induce a demand for greater utilization of MIRP. This phenomenon is particularly important in our current resource-constrained healthcare environment. Interventions aimed at cost containment, such as greater regulatory control for the advertisement of medical technology not supported by evidence, and development of balanced patient educational material, should be considered. Further work needs to focus on factors affecting patient preferences for certain healthcare technologies and treatment options, and the development of interventions to tailor these preferences according to the latest scientific evidence and cost considerations.

Appendix 1

Table 4 Demographic and clinical characteristics of TRICARE beneficiaries who were diagnosed and treated for prostate cancer at civilian facilities compared to those who transferred care from military facilities to civilian facilities after diagnosis

	Civilian facility patients	Military Facility patients Transferring Care	
Characteristic *n* (%)	779 (75.9%)	247 (24.1%)	*p*-value
Mean Age at Procedure	58.2	57.8	
Race			<0.01
White	478 (61.4%)	122 (49.4%)	
Non-white	301 (38.6%)	122 (49.4%)	
Marital Status			0.08
Married	651 (83.6%)	191 (77.3%)	
Single	80 (10.3%)	36 (14.6%)	
Unknown	48 (6.2%)	20 (8.1%)	
Sponsor rank			<0.01
Enlisted	504 (64.7%)	139 (56.3%)	
Officer	216 (27.7%)	84 (34.0%)	
Unknown	59 (7.6%)	24 (9.7%)	
Procedure Type			0.18
Open	463 (59.4%)	135 (54.7%)	
Minimally Invasive	316 (40.5%)	112 (45.3%)	
Year of Procedure			0.32
2006	144 (18.5%)	56 (22.7%)	
2007	133 (17.1%)	42 (17.0%)	
2008	177 (22.7%)	50 (20.2%)	
2009	199 (25.6%)	52 (21.0%)	
2010	126 (16.2%)	47 (19.0%)	
Median HCC	0.33	0.39	

Abbreviations

DCS: Direct Care System (Military Healthcare Facilities); DoD: Department of Defense; MDR: Military Health System Data Repository; MIRP: Minimally Invasive Radical Prostatectomy; ORP: Open Radical Prostatectomy; PCS: Purchased Care System (Civilian Healthcare Facilities)

Acknowledgements

The authors of this manuscript would like to acknowledge Dr. Stuart Lipsitz ScD, for his expertise and efforts in helping with the analytic plan of this study and Linda Kimsey, PhD, Michael W McDonald, MD and Cheryl Zogg, MSPH, MSH, for her time and efforts in reviewing the manuscript for intellectual content.

Funding

This project was funded in part by the Henry M. Jackson Foundation for the Advancement of Military Medicine. The following authors receive partial salary support from this grant: MAC, RC, WJ, PL, JSW. The Henry Jackson Foundation was not involved in the design and conduct of the study; collection, management, analysis, and interpretation of the data; preparation, review, or approval of the manuscript; and decision to submit the manuscript for publication. MAC had full access to all the data in the study and takes responsibility for the integrity of the data and the accuracy of the data analysis.

Authors' contributions

Each of the authors fulfilled authorship criteria according to the requirements set by the ICMJE, including making a substantial contribution to conception and design, or analysis and interpretation of data; drafting the article or revising it critically for important intellectual content; and giving final approval of the version to be published. MAC, JJL, MM, RC, WJ, PAL, JSW and SLC made substantial contributions to the conception or design of the work. MAC, RC, WJ, PAL, and SLC participated in the acquisition of the data. MAC, JJL, MM, PAL, JSW and SLC devised the analytical plan. MAC, RC and WJ were responsible for data analysis. MAC, JJL and RC drafted the manuscript, and MM, WJ, PAL, JSW and SLC critically revised the manuscript for intellectual content. All authors provided final approval of the version to be published and agree to be accountable for all aspects of the work in ensuring that questions related to the accuracy or integrity of any part of the work are appropriately investigated and resolved.

Competing interests

The authors declare that they have no competing interests.

Author details

[1]Center for Surgery and Public Health, Department of Surgery, Brigham and Women's Hospital, Harvard Medical School, Harvard T H Chan School of Public Health, Boston, MA, USA. [2]Division of Urology, Brigham and Women's Hospital, Harvard Medical School, Boston, MA, USA. [3]Department of Surgery, Uniformed Services University of Health Sciences, Bethesda, MD, USA.

References

1. Delamater PL, Messina JP, Grady SC, WinklerPrins V, Shortridge AM. Do more hospital beds lead to higher hospitalization rates? A spatial examination of Roemer's law. PLoS One. 2013;8(2):e54900.
2. Weeks WB, Jardin M, Dufour J-C, Paraponaris A, Ventelou B. Geographic variation in admissions for knee replacement, hip replacement, and hip fracture in France: evidence of supplier-induced demand in for-profit and not-for-profit hospitals. Med Care. 2014;52(10):909–17.
3. Tak HJ, Ruhnke GW, Meltzer DO. Association of patient preferences for participation in decision making with length of stay and costs among hospitalized patients. JAMA Intern Med. 2013;173(13):1195–205.
4. Anthony DL, Herndon MB, Gallagher PM, Barnato AE, Bynum JP, Gottlieb DJ, Fisher ES, Skinner JS. How much do patients' preferences contribute to resource use? Health Aff. 2009;28(3):864–73.
5. Alkhateeb S, Lawrentschuk N. Consumerism and its impact on robotic-assisted radical prostatectomy. BJU Int. 2011;108(11):1874–8.
6. Gandaglia G, Sammon JD, Chang SL, Choueiri TK, Hu JC, Karakiewicz PI, Kibel AS, Kim SP, Konijeti R, Montorsi F: Comparative effectiveness of robot-assisted and open radical prostatectomy in the postdissemination era. J Clin Oncol 2014:JCO. 2013.2053. 5096.
7. Trinh Q-D, Sammon J, Sun M, Ravi P, Ghani KR, Bianchi M, Jeong W, Shariat SF, Hansen J, Schmitges J. Perioperative outcomes of robot-assisted radical prostatectomy compared with open radical prostatectomy: results from the nationwide inpatient sample. Eur Urol. 2012;61(4):679–85.
8. Liu J-J, Maxwell BG, Panousis P, Chung BI. Perioperative outcomes for laparoscopic and robotic compared with open prostatectomy using the National Surgical Quality Improvement Program (NSQIP) database. Urology. 2013;82(3):579–83.
9. Leow JJ, Chang SL, Meyer CP, Wang Y, Hanske J, Sammon JD, Cole AP, Preston MA, Dasgupta P, Menon M. Robot-assisted versus open radical prostatectomy: a contemporary analysis of an all-payer discharge database. Eur Urol. 2016;70(5):837–45.
10. Leow J, Weissman J, Kimsey L, Hoburg A, Helmchen L, Jiang W, Lipsitz S, Hess D, Nguyen L, Chang S: Trends in diffusion of surgical innovation and outcomes: a comparative analysis of radical prostatectomy in military and civilian institutions. 2015.
11. Zogg CK, Jiang W, Chaudhary MA, Scott JW, Shah AA, Lipsitz SR, Weissman JS, Cooper Z, Salim A, Nitzschke SL, et al. Racial disparities in emergency general surgery: do differences in outcomes persist among universally insured military patients? J Trauma Acute Care Surg. 2016;80(5):764–75. discussion 775-767

12. Chowdhury R, Davis WA, Chaudhary MA, Jiang W, Zogg CK, Schoenfeld AJ, Jaklitsch MT, Kaneko T, Learn PA, Haider AH. Race-based differences in duration of stay among universally insured coronary artery bypass graft patients in military versus civilian hospitals. Surgery. 2017;161(4):1090–99.
13. Schoenfeld AJ, Jiang W, Harris MB, Cooper Z, Koehlmoos T, Learn PA, Weissman JS, Haider AH. Association Between Race and Postoperative Outcomes in a Universally Insured Population Versus Patients in the State of California. Ann Surg. 2016. doi:10.1097/SLA.0000000000001958.
14. Pope GC, Kautter J, Ellis RP, Ash AS, Ayanian JZ, Iezzoni LI, Ingber MJ, Levy JM, Robst J. Risk adjustment of Medicare capitation payments using the CMS-HCC model. Health Care Financ Rev. 2004;25(4):119.
15. Chang SL, Kibel AS, Brooks JD, Chung BI: The impact of robotic surgery on the surgical management of prostate cancer in the USA. BJU Int 2014.
16. Makarov DV, James BY, Desai RA, Penson DF, Gross CP. The association between diffusion of the surgical robot and radical prostatectomy rates. Med Care. 2011;49(4):333–9.
17. Aning J, Wassersug R, Goldenberg S. Patient preference and the impact of decision-making aids on prostate cancer treatment choices and post-intervention regret. Curr Oncol. 2012;19(Suppl 3):S37.
18. Hauber AB, Arellano J, Qian Y, González JM, Posner JD, Mohamed AF, Gatta F, Tombal B, Body JJ. Patient preferences for treatments to delay bone metastases. Prostate. 2014;74(15):1488–97.
19. Tol-Geerdink JJ, Willem Leer J, Weijerman PC, Oort IM, Vergunst H, Lin EN, Alfred Witjes J, Stalmeier PF. Choice between prostatectomy and radiotherapy when men are eligible for both: a randomized controlled trial of usual care vs decision aid. BJU Int. 2013;111(4):564–73.
20. Rojo MAE, Martinez-Salamanca JI, Maestro MA, Galarza IS, Rodriguez JC. Impact of cosmetic result on selection of surgical treatment in patients with localized prostate cancer. JSLS. 2014;18(4):e2014.00024.
21. Eilat-Tsanani S, Tabenkin H, Shental J, Elmalah I, Steinmetz D: Patients' perceptions of radical prostatectomy for localized prostate cancer: a qualitative study. 2013.
22. Wosinska M: Just what the patient ordered? Direct-to-consumer advertising and the demand for pharmaceutical products. Direct-to-Consumer advertising and the demand for pharmaceutical products (October 2002) HBS Marketing Research Paper 2002(02-04).
23. Bradford WD, Kleit AN, Nietert PJ, Steyer T, McIlwain T, Ornstein S. How direct-to-consumer television advertising for osteoarthritis drugs affects physicians' prescribing behavior. Health Aff. 2006;25(5):1371–7.
24. Yaxley JW, Coughlin GD, Chambers SK, Occhipinti S, Samaratunga H, Zajdlewicz L, Dunglison N, Carter R, Williams S, Payton DJ. Robot-assisted laparoscopic prostatectomy versus open radical retropubic prostatectomy: early outcomes from a randomised controlled phase 3 study. Lancet. 2016; 388(10049):1057–66.
25. Trinh Q-D, Bjartell A, Freedland SJ, Hollenbeck BK, Hu JC, Shariat SF, Sun M, Vickers AJ. A systematic review of the volume–outcome relationship for radical prostatectomy. Eur Urol. 2013;64(5):786–98.
26. Teplensky JD, Pauly MV, Kimberly JR, Hillman AL, Schwartz JS. Hospital adoption of medical technology: an empirical test of alternative models. Health Serv Res. 1995;30(3):437.
27. Tustin N. The role of patient satisfaction in online health information seeking. J Health Commun. 2010;15(1):3–17.
28. Hajdenberg J, Landau D. Patterns of robotic prostatectomy advertising on the internet: quality of the information available to US consumers through the use of Google, yahoo, Bing, and YouTube. In: ASCO Annual Meeting Proceedings, vol. 2010; 2010. p. e16538.
29. Mirkin JN, Lowrance WT, Feifer AH, Mulhall JP, Eastham JE, Elkin EB. Direct-to-consumer internet promotion of robotic prostatectomy exhibits varying quality of information. Health Aff. 2012;31(4):760–9.
30. Heidenreich A, Aus G, Bolla M, Joniau S, Matveev VB, Schmid HP, Zattoni F. EAU guidelines on prostate cancer. Eur Urol. 2008;53(1):68–80.
31. Lawthers AG, McCarthy EP, Davis RB, Peterson LE, Palmer RH, Iezzoni LI. Identification of in-hospital complications from claims data: is it valid? Med Care. 2000;38(8):785–95.

17

Sociodemographic correlates of urine culture test utilization in Calgary, Alberta

Thomas P. Griener[1,3], Christopher Naugler[1,2], Wilson W. Chan[1,3] and Deirdre L. Church[1,3,4,5*]

Abstract

Background: Many clinical practice guidelines encourage diagnosis and empiric treatment of lower urinary tract infection without laboratory investigation; however, urine culture testing remains one of the largest volume tests in the clinical microbiology laboratory. In this study, we sought to determine if there were specific patient groups to which increased testing was directed. To do so, we combined laboratory data on testing rates with Census Canada sociodemographic data.

Methods: Urine culture testing data was obtained from the Calgary Laboratory Services information system for 2011. We examined all census dissemination areas within the city of Calgary and, for each area, testing rates were determined for age and gender cohorts. We then compared these testing rates to sociodemographic factors obtained from Census Canada and used Poisson regression and generalized estimating equations to test associations between testing rates and sociodemographic variables.

Results: Per capita urine culture testing is increasing in Calgary. For 2011, 100,901 individuals (9.2% of all people) received urine cultures and were included in this analysis. The majority of cultures were received from the community (67.9%). Substantial differences in rate of testing were observed across the city. Most notably, urine culture testing was drastically lower in areas of high (≥ $100000) household income (RR = 0.07, $p < 0.0001$) and higher employment rate (RR = 0.36, $p < 0.0001$). Aboriginal – First Nations status (RR = 0.29, $p = 0.0008$) and Chinese visible minority (RR = 0.67, $p = 0.0005$) were also associated with decreased testing. Recent immigration and visible minority status of South Asian, Filipino or Black were not significant predictors of urine culture testing. Females were more likely to be tested than males (RR = 2.58, $p < 0.0001$) and individuals aged 15–39 were the most likely to be tested (RR = 1.69, $p < 0.0001$).

Conclusions: Considerable differences exist in urine culture testing across Calgary and these are associated with a number of sociodemographic factors. In particular, areas of lower socioeconomic standing had significantly increased rates of testing. These observations highlight specific groups that should be targeted to improve healthcare delivery and, in turn, enhance laboratory utilization.

Background

Lower urinary tract infection (LUTI, cystitis) can be reliably diagnosed without laboratory investigation based on a focused history of urinary symptoms (frequency, urgency and dysuria) in the absence of urethral discharge or vaginal irritation. Adult women with symptomatic, uncomplicated LUTI should receive short-course empiric antibiotic therapy and do not require urinalysis or urine culture for diagnostic confirmation of bacteriuria or pyuria. Numerous clinical practice guidelines support this and encourage the use of urine culture testing in the adult population primarily for bacterial identification and antibiotic sensitivity testing in patients not responding to therapy or with recurrent disease [1–4]. However, urine culture testing is necessary in all cases of upper urinary tract infection (pyelonephritis) and screening cultures for asymptomatic bacteriuria is also indicated in pregnancy and for those undergoing urologic procedure where bleeding is anticipated [5].

These recommendations are largely based on the following important considerations. Bacteriuria is not itself a disease state and is typically not an indication for

* Correspondence: Deirdre.church@albertahealthservices.ca
[1]Department of Pathology and Laboratory Medicine, University of Calgary, Calgary, AB, Canada
[3]Division of Microbiology, Department of Pathology and Laboratory Medicine, University of Calgary, Calgary, AB, Canada
Full list of author information is available at the end of the article

antibiotic therapy [5]. Asymptomatic bacteriuria is particularly common in the elderly population, with prevalence estimates of 3.6–19% in those aged 70 or over and living in the community [5, 6]. In nursing home residents, prevalence is estimated at up to 50%. It is not associated with increased morbidity or mortality [7]. Guidelines from the Infectious Disease Society of America (IDSA) and Choosing Wisely initiatives emphasize that even in the presence of pyuria, asymptomatic bacteriuria does not normally require treatment [5, 8]. The clinical significance of bacteriuria is therefore defined by patient signs and symptoms. Furthermore, the majority of urine specimens submitted for culture are the midstream portion of voided urine and culture results from these minimally-invasive collections have poor specificity, with a false positive rate of over 40% when compared to suprapubic needle aspiration or catheterization as gold standard [3, 9]. A positive urine culture therefore does not prove true bacteriuria, and certainly does not prove the presence of a urinary tract infection. Several strategies have been adopted by clinical microbiology laboratories to minimize reporting of contaminated specimens. The most common method is reporting of quantitative culture, for which there are established thresholds of bacterial quantity which define clinical significance [3, 5, 10]. However, in symptomatic patients, colony count thresholds likely underestimate the clinical significance of certain potential urinary pathogens while overestimating others [11]. For example, *Escherichia coli* can be associated with symptomatic disease even when isolated at quantities that are orders of magnitude below these thresholds. These combined factors minimize the value of urine culture results in both asymptomatic and symptomatic individuals.

Despite these problems, urine culture remains an important test that directs antibiotic therapy and further investigations in certain clinical settings. However, there is substantial practice variation in the use of diagnostic tests in LUTI and urine culture remains one of the highest volume tests in clinical microbiology laboratories [12]. Inappropriate testing is not without consequence as positive urine culture results likely drive unnecessary antibiotic treatment and contribute to rising rates of antibiotic resistance and other adverse events associated with antibiotic usage including *Clostridium difficile* infection [13–18]. We undertook the current ecological study to determine what variation in urine cultures testing existed across Calgary, Alberta and to determine what sociodemographic factors were associated with increased urine culture testing. Such information will allow targeted investigation into causes of potential over-utilization and more focused intervention strategies.

Methods

The study protocol was approved by the University of Calgary Conjoint Health Review Ethics Board and a waiver of consent was granted (ID#REB15–0629).

This observational study combined laboratory data with variables obtained from the 2011 Census Canada Canadian Household Survey, the most recent such survey at the time this study was completed. The study population consisted of all individuals within Calgary, Alberta who underwent urine culture testing between January 1, 2011 and December 31, 2011. All urine culture testing at Calgary Laboratory Services (CLS) is performed as part of routine patient care and samples are analyzed in a single laboratory. CLS is the only testing laboratory in Calgary, Alberta and data from the CLS laboratory information system (LIS) therefore represents a comprehensive view of urine culture testing in the entire city (2011 population 1.1 million). In addition to data for the 2011 year, the number of monthly urine cultures collected from the LIS for each month from January 2010 to December 2013 in order to measure trends in urine culture ordering.

Each patient was included only once in the analysis to avoid pseudo-replication. For each test record, the following information was extracted from the laboratory information system: urine culture result, age, sex and health care number. Health care number was used as a linking variable to determine subject postal codes from an Alberta Health database, which were then converted to their corresponding geographic coordinates and census dissemination areas (CDA). CDAs are the smallest geographic groupings used for Canadian census data and contain 300–700 individuals. The data was then permanently de-identified. We included only individuals living within the City of Calgary.

For each CDA, the following sociodemographic variables were linked from the Canadian Household Survey: median household income ≥ $CDN 100,000 (overall median household income in Calgary for 2011 was $93,410), level of education (percent with university education), percent of individuals of Aboriginal - First Nations descent (North American Indian, as defined by Statistics Canada [19]), percent of individuals immigrating to Canada within the past 5 years and percent of individuals of Chinese, South Asian (primarily Indian, Pakistani and Sri Lankan), Filipino or Black visible minority status (the four most common statuses in Calgary, as defined by Statistics Canada [20]). We then examined these data-sets for associations between these sociodemographic variables and urine culture testing rate.

For per capita testing rate (Fig. 1), the total number of urine culture tests for each year was divided by the total Calgary population as reported by the annual City of Calgary Civic census (http://www.calgary.ca). To calculate the

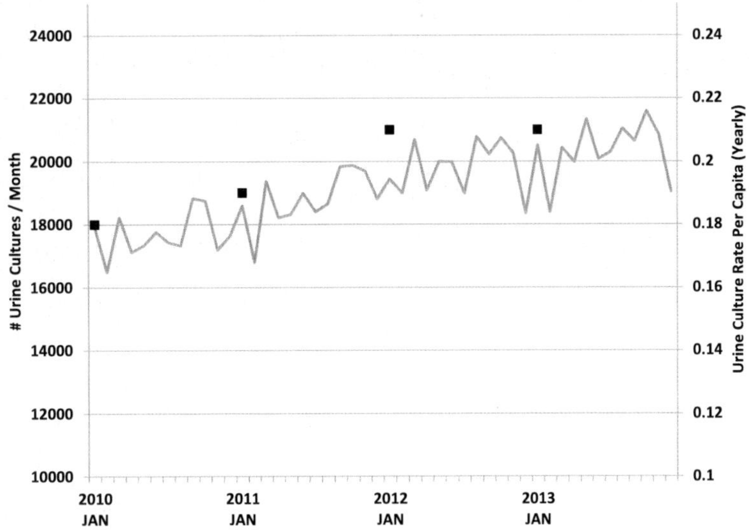

Fig. 1 Urine culture testing at CLS from January 1, 2010 to December 31, 2013 presented as the number of urine culture tests per month (grey line) and the yearly per capita urine culture test rate (black squares)

percent of testing within each age and gender group (Table 1), the total number of individuals within each group who received at least one urine culture was divided by the total population within that group in Calgary according to the 2011 Canadian census. To calculate the testing frequency for the age and gender group in each CDA, the number of individuals that received testing from that group was divided by the total number of that age group in the dissemination area. For visual representation of the data, the values were then plotted onto a dissemination area map for Calgary using the ArcGIS v9.3 geo-mapping software (Environmental System Research Institute, Redlands, California). This software tool uses Getis-Ord Gi^* statistic to produce z-scores and identify statistically significant hot (increased testing) and cold (decreased testing) spots depending on how many standard deviations the data is removed from the mean [21]. Statistical inference regarding sociodemographic variables associated with testing rate was performed using the generalized estimating equations version of Poisson regression in SAS v9.4. The reported relative risks refer to the independent contribution of each variable with the other categorical variables (age, gender, group) held constant at an arbitrary reference value. The differences in testing rates are reported as relative risk (RR) for the independent contribution of that variable to the analysis and results were considered statistically significant at a *p*-value of 0.05.

Table 1 Frequency of Urine culture testing in Calgary, Alberta for 2011

	Number of Tests	Individuals Tested	Total Population	Percent Tested
Total	219,015	100,901	1,096,830	9.2%
Male	40,294	23,009	547,475	4.2%
<15	4999	3752	100,450	3.7%
15-39	6046	4410	208,840	2.1%
40-49	4083	2653	86,935	3.1%
50-59	6130	3407	77,460	4.4%
60-69	5870	3129	41,920	7.4%
≥70	13,166	5658	31,875	17.8%
Female	132,388	77,892	549,360	14.2%
<15	10,292	7105	95,970	7.4%
15-39	53,888	34,282	205,995	16.6%
40-49	14,449	9393	84,950	11.1%
50-59	14,110	8716	75,415	11.6%
60-69	11,755	6437	43,075	15.0%
≥70	27,894	11,959	43,940	27.2%

Results

Increased testing volumes and per capita testing rates have been reported in most laboratory divisions [22]. Urine culture testing, which is the highest volume microbiology test at CLS, has seen a similar rise that exceeds Calgary's population growth (Fig. 1). Linear regression analysis of this data shows statistically significant increases in test volumes ($R^2 = 0.68$, $P < 0.001$) and year over year per capita test rates ($R^2 = 0.96$, $P = 0.002$).

Data on 225,473 urine culture results were available in our LIS for 2011, which represented 133,464 individuals who underwent urine culture testing. After excluding individuals where no postal code was available and those with postal codes outside the city of Calgary, 100,901 individuals remained and were included in our study. The majority of specimens were received from patients in the community (67.9%) and the emergency department (19.3%), with the remainder from nursing homes (2.3%), inpatients (5.3%) and various outpatient settings including pre-admission clinics and subspecialty clinics (collectively 5.2%). Overall, 9.2% of individuals in the city of Calgary were tested during the study period, including 4.2% of males and 14.2% of females (Table 1). For males and females, the highest testing rate was in individuals ≥70 years (17.8% and 27.2%, respectively), however the greatest number of specimens were received from females aged 15–39. In part, this increased testing rate is likely accounted for by screening for asymptomatic bacteriuria in pregnancy but such clinical information was not available in our study.

The ArcGIS hot spot analysis mapping illustrates significant differences in screening rates across the city (Fig. 2). Significantly increased testing is observed in the inner city and northeast quadrants of the city. The median urine culture testing rates among neighbourhoods was 9.1% with 7.5% and 10.9% as the lower and upper quartiles, respectively.

The association between sociodemographic variables and urine culture test rates are shown in Table 2 and many inequities are present. The regression model showed that females were significantly more likely to be tested than males (RR = 2.58, $p < 0.0001$). As seen in Table 2, individuals aged 15–39 were the most likely to be tested (RR = 1.69, $p < 0.0001$), followed by those ≥70 years of age (analysis control, RR = 1.0). Decreased urine culture testing was associated with higher (≥ $100000) household income (RR = 0.07, $p < 0.0001$) and higher employment rate (RR = 0.36, $p < 0.0001$). No association between university education and testing was detected. Aboriginal – First Nations individuals (RR = 0.29, $p = 0.0008$) and individuals of Chinese descent (RR = 0.672, $p = 0.0005$) were also less likely to be tested. Interestingly, recent immigration (≤ 5 years), South Asian descent, Filipino descent or Black visible minority status were not significant predictors of urine culture testing.

Discussion

Our data reveal a drastically lower rate of urine culture testing with higher household income (≥ $100000) and higher employment rate. In previous studies, we demonstrated that these factors were associated with increased 25-hydroxyvitamin D and prostate specific antigen (PSA) testing and we hypothesized that this was possibly due to greater access to health care and patient-requested testing [23, 24]. The differences in urine culture testing identified in the present study appears contrary to that hypothesis. Why such drastic differences in urine testing rates exist between higher and lower socioeconomic status groups is unclear. One possibility is that the testing differences are warranted and reflect increased rates of LUTI, complicated urinary tract infection or antibiotic resistance in lower income earners. Previous studies have demonstrated a modest association between lower household income and community-acquired urinary tract infections and asymptomatic bacteriuria [25–27]. Increased incidence of other genitourinary tract infections causing similar symptoms, such as *Neisseria gonorrhoeae* or *Chlamydia trachomatis* urethritis/vulvovaginitis, could result in greater urine culture testing as well. In support of this, an earlier study showed a similar association between lower socioeconomic indicators and prevalence of these infections in Calgary [28].

It is also possible that discrepancies in urine culture ordering are unrelated to genitourinary tract infection, but instead result from differences in the prevalence of diseases with overlapping clinical presentation. Irritative lower urinary tract symptoms (urinary urgency, incontinence and frequency) consistent with overactive bladder syndrome (OAB) and/or benign prostatic hyperplasia (BPH) increase with age and may elicit urine culture testing [29]. Previous studies have demonstrated a relationship between higher income, higher levels of education and employment status and fewer of these symptoms in both women and men [30, 31]. The authors of these studies speculated that the reduced symptoms were the result of regular health check-ups, earlier recognition of symptoms and prior treatment. This could also explain our findings as patients of lower socioeconomic status may have more persistent urinary symptoms and have more urine cultures performed while not receiving appropriate therapy for these non-infectious conditions as a result of less consistent health-care contact. Further studies are needed to determine whether this is indeed the case, as appropriate intervention would substantially improve patient care while also reducing microbiologic testing.

Concern regarding antibiotic resistant organisms could also drive increased urine culture utilization and clinical guidelines support the use of urine cultures in these instances. Resistant rates vary throughout the world; however, the Study for Monitoring Antimicrobial Resistance Trends (SMART) has established that the highest levels of antimicrobial resistance exist in the Asia-Pacific region where as many as 28.2% of LUTI pathogens possess extended spectrum β-lactamases [32]. South Asian, Chinese and Filipino people are strongly represented in Calgary's visible minority population, and increased urine culture test rates would be expected if there were concerns about antimicrobial resistance. In fact, our data reveal the opposite trend with Chinese ethnicity associated with a statistically significant decrease in testing,

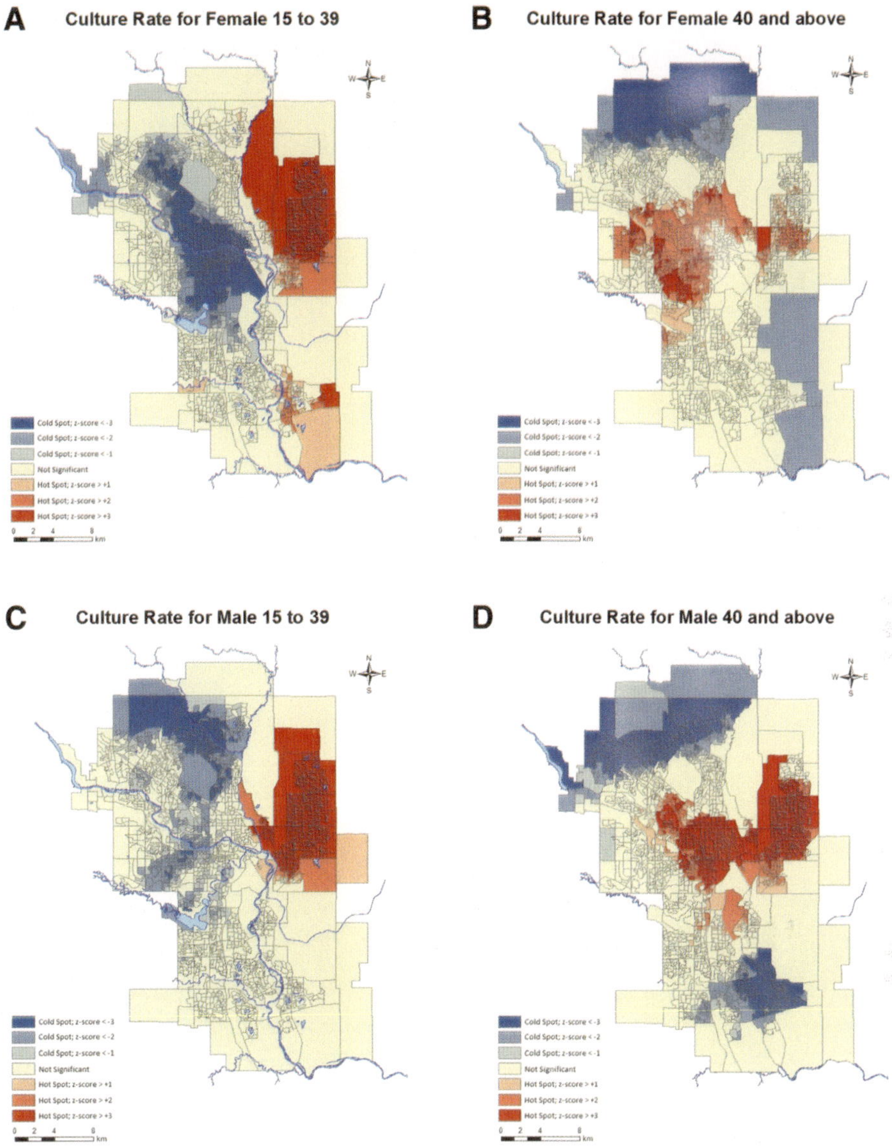

Fig. 2 Hotspot maps representing the frequency of urine culture test ordering in four age/gender groups. The testing rate (individuals tested / total individuals in dissemination area) is represented by the number of standard deviations (z-score) it is removed from the mean (yellow/beige) in the positive (red, increased testing) and negative (blue, decreased testing) direction. Culture rates are shown for Females aged 15–39 (**a**), Females aged ≥40 (**b**), Males aged 15–39 (**c**), Males aged ≥40 (**d**). Maps generated using ArcGIS v9.3 geo-mapping software

and no relationship between test rate and recent immigration, South Asian or Filipino ethnicity. The cause of this decreased testing is unclear, but could represent barriers preventing health care access. Given the risk of resistance, this is a potential cause for concern.

The main strength of this study is the large sample of patients and, because our laboratory performs testing for all of Calgary, the data presented herein represents a complete view of urine culture testing on the adult (>15) population of the city. However, the limitations of this study must be recognized when interpreting these results. Because this study was retrospective and involved a very large number of patients, we were unable to collect clinical information or assess other concurrent laboratory testing (such as urinalysis or testing for sexually transmitted infection). As a result, we cannot ascertain the clinical appropriateness of urine culture testing. However, the variability in test ordering across the city without clear explanation is highly suggestive of inappropriate utilization. Patients with underlying disease may necessitate increased urine culture testing and such patients were certainly included in this study. We attempted to minimize the impact of such patients by counting a single urine culture per individual. As well,

Table 2 Sociodemographic variables and Urine culture testing rates in Calgary, Alberta for 2011

Socio-demographic Variable	Relative Risk (RR)	RR 95% Confidence Interval		Parameter Estimate	*P*-value
Female	2.583	2.539	2.629	0.9491	<0.0001
Male[a]	1.000	Reference		Reference	Reference
Age < 15	0.586	0.548	0.627	−0.534	<0.0001
Age 15–39	1.689	1.587	1.797	0.524	<0.0001
Age 40–49	0.624	0.587	0.663	−0.472	<0.0001
Age 50–59	0.660	0.623	0.700	−0.415	<0.0001
Age 60–69	0.550	0.520	0.581	−0.599	<0.0001
Age ≥ 70[b]	1.000	Reference		Reference	Reference
Median Household Income ≥$100,000	0.074	0.038	0.147	−2.600	<0.0001
Employment Rate	0.367	0.251	0.537	−1.002	<0.0001
University Education	1.091	0.864	1.377	0.087	0.464
Recent Immigrant (≤ 5 years)	0.678	0.440	1.044	−0.389	0.077
Aboriginal – First Nations	0.289	0.140	0.596	−1.240	0.0008
Chinese	0.672	0.536	0.842	−0.398	0.0005
South Asian	0.924	0.779	1.097	−0.079	0.3656
Filipino	0.791	0.563	1.111	−0.235	0.1761
Visible Minority - Black	0.878	0.392	1.965	−0.130	0.7515

[a]Males were used as reference for females
[b]Age group ≥70 was used as a reference for the other age groups

as this is an ecological study, inferences are made based on group level variables that may not accurately represent individual level variables. Some of the differences identified may be the result of confounding variables that are not captured in this study. It is also unknown what degree of urine testing is driven by patient or physician characteristics (generalist versus specialist practice, experience, location of training, etc.) and physician variables were not controlled for in the current study. Despite these deficits, we have identified several sociodemographic groups with significantly increased rates of testing and have demonstrated substantial variation in urine culture utilization across Calgary.

Further work will be to expand these studies to investigate for mismatch between urine culture ordering practices and clinical utility. Assessment of urine culture positivity rates and antibiotic resistance rates and how they align with the test utilization rates presented in the current study will provide useful information to direct intervention strategies to improve appropriate urine culture usage.

Conclusions

Despite clinical practice guidelines recommending limited use of urine culture in diagnosing LUTI, we have shown that test rates continue to increase in Calgary and that substantial heterogeneity exists in test utilization across the city. We have also identified several patient groups with greatly increased or decreased test rates that may be indicative of inappropriate test utilization. Future investigations will now be focused on these patient groups to ascertain specific explanations for the potential over-utilization observed herein.

Abbreviations

CDA: Census dissemination area; CLS: Calgary Laboratory Services; IDSA: Infectious Disease Society of America; LIS: Laboratory Information System; LUTI: Lower urinary tract infection; RR: Relative Risk

Acknowledgments

We would like to acknowledge the crucial contributions of Jeannine Viczko, who acquired the data from the Calgary Laboratory Services laboratory information system, and Maggie Guo, who assisted with the statistical analysis and geo-mapping of the data.

Funding

This work was supported by a Canadian Institutes of Health Research foundation scheme grant to CN [RN254781-333204]. The funding agency had no input on the study.

Authors' contributions

TPG, DLC and CN conceived of the study, participated in its design. TPG analysed the data. TPC, DLC, CN and WWC all participated in interpretation of data, as well as drafting the manuscript and revising it critically. All authors have read and approve of the final manuscript.

Competing interests

The authors declare that they have no competing interests.

Author details

[1]Department of Pathology and Laboratory Medicine, University of Calgary, Calgary, AB, Canada. [2]Department of Family Medicine, University of Calgary, Calgary, AB, Canada. [3]Division of Microbiology, Department of Pathology and Laboratory Medicine, University of Calgary, Calgary, AB, Canada. [4]Department of Medicine, University of Calgary, Calgary, AB, Canada. [5]1W-410, Diagnostic and Scientific Centre, 9-3535 Research Road NW, Calgary, AB T2L 2K8, Canada.

References

1. Bonkat MG, Pickard R, Bartoletti R, Bruyère F, Geerlings SE, Wagenlehner F, Wullt W. members of the EAU Urological Infections Guidelines Panel. EAU Urological Infections Guidelines. Retrieved from: https://uroweb.org/guideline/urological-infections//. Accessed 5 Jan 2018.
2. Colgan R, Williams M. Diagnosis and treatment of acute uncomplicated cystitis. Am Fam Physician. 2011;84:771–6.
3. Scottish Intercollegiate Guidelines Network. Management of suspected bacterial urinary tract infection in adults. 2012;SIGN no 88.
4. American College of Obstetricians and Gynecologists. Treatment of Urinary Tract Infections in Nonpregnant Women, ACOG Pract. Bull. No 91, vol. 111; 2008. p. 785–94.
5. Nicolle LE, Bradley S, Colgan R, Rice JC, Schaeffer A, Hooton TM. Infectious Diseases Society of America guidelines for the diagnosis and treatment of asymptomatic bacteriuria in adults. Clin Infect Dis. 2005;40:643–54.
6. Nicolle LE. Asymptomatic bacteriuria in the Eldery. Infect Dis Clin N Am. 1997;11:647–62.
7. Nicolle LE, Bjornson J, Harding GK, MacDonell JA. Bacteriuria in elderly institutionalized men. N Engl J Med. 1983;309:1420-5.
8. Infectious Diseases Society of America. Five things physicians and patients should question. 2015. http://www.choosingwisely.org/societies/infectious-diseases-society-of-america/. Accessed 5 Jan 2018.
9. Campbell-Brown M, McFadyen IR. Bacteriuria in pregnancy treated with a single dose of cephalexin. Br J Obstet Gynaecol. 1983;90:1054–9.
10. Hooton TM, Bradley SF, Cardenas DD, Colgan R, Geerlings SE, Rice JC, et al. Diagnosis, prevention, and treatment of catheter-associated urinary tract infection in adults: 2009 international clinical practice guidelines from the Infectious Diseases Society of America. Clin Infect Dis. 2010;50:625–63.
11. Hooton TM, Roberts PL, Cox ME, Stapleton AE. Voided midstream urine culture and acute cystitis in premenopausal women. N Engl J Med. 2013;369:1883–91.
12. Llor C, Rabanaque G, López A, Cots JM. The adherence of GPs to guidelines for the diagnosis and treatment of lower urinary tract infections in women is poor. Fam Pract. 2011;28:294–9.
13. McIsaac WJ, Hunchak CL. Overestimation error and unnecessary antibiotic prescriptions for acute cystitis in adult women. Med Decis Mak. 2011;31:405–11.
14. Trautner BW. Asymptomatic bacteriuria: when the treatment is worse than the disease. Nat Rev Urol. 2011;9:85–93.
15. Phillips CD, Adepoju O, Stone N, Moudouni DKM, Nwaiwu O, Zhao H, et al. Asymptomatic bacteriuria, antibiotic use, and suspected urinary tract infections in four nursing homes. BMC Geriatr. 2012;12:73.
16. Werner NL, Hecker MT, Sethi AK, Donskey CJ. Unnecessary use of fluoroquinolone antibiotics in hospitalized patients. BMC Infect Dis. 2011;11:187.
17. Cai T, Mazzoli S, Mondaini N, Meacci F, Nesi G, D'Elia C, et al. The role of asymptomatic bacteriuria in young women with recurrent urinary tract infections: to treat or not to treat? Clin Infect Dis. 2012;55:771–7.
18. Cai T, Nesi G, Mazzoli S, Meacci F, Lanzafame P, Caciagli P, et al. Asymptomatic bacteriuria treatment is associated with a higher prevalence of antibiotic resistant strains in women with urinary tract infections. Clin Infect Dis. 2015;61:1655–61.
19. Aboriginal Group Definition. 2016; Available from: http://www12.statcan.gc.ca/nhs-enm/2011/ref/dict/pop144-eng.cfm
20. Visible Minority Definition. 2016. Available from: http://www12.statcan.gc.ca/nhs-enm/2011/ref/dict/pop127-eng.cfm
21. Mitchell A. The ESRI Guide to GIS Analysis, Volume 2: Spatial Measurements and Statistics. Redlands: 1st ed. ESRI Press; 2005.
22. Rockey M, Naugler C, Sidhu D. Laboratory utilization trends : past and future. Can Pathol. 2013;5:65–72.
23. de Koning L, Henne D, Woods P, Hemmelgarn BR, Naugler C. Sociodemographic correlates of 25-hydroxyvitamin D test utilization in Calgary, Alberta. BMC Health Serv Res. 2014;14:339.
24. Gorday W, Sadrzadeh H, de Koning L, Naugler C. Association of sociodemographic factors and prostate-specific antigen (PSA) testing. Clin Biochem. 2014;47:164–9.
25. Turck M, Goffe BS, Petersdorf RG. Bacteriuria of pregnancy. N Engl J Med. 1962;266:857–60.
26. Emiru T, Beyene G, Tsegaye W, Melaku S. Associated risk factors of urinary tract infection among pregnant women at Felege Hiwot referral hospital, Bahir Dar, north West Ethiopia. BMC Res Notes. 2013;6:292.
27. Jeon CY, Muennig P, Furuya EY, Cohen B, Nash D, Larson EL. Burden of present-on-admission infections and health care-associated infections, by race and ethnicity. Am J Infect Control. 2014;42:1296–302.
28. Bush KR, Henderson EA, Dunn J, Read RR, Singh A. Mapping the core: chlamydia and gonorrhea infections in Calgary, Alberta. Sex Transm Dis. 2008;35:291–7.
29. Wang Y, Xu K, Hu H, Zhang X, Wang X, Na Y, et al. Prevalence, risk factors, and impact on health related quality of life of overactive bladder in China. Neurourol Urodyn. 2011;30:1448–55.
30. Kim JH, Ham BK, Shim SR, Lee WJ, Kim HJ, Kwon S-S, et al. The association between the self-perception period of overactive bladder symptoms and overactive bladder symptom scores in a non-treated population and related sociodemographic and lifestyle factors. Int J Clin Pract. 2013;67:795–800.
31. Joseph MA, Harlow SD, Wei JT, Sarma AV, Dunn RL, Taylor JMG, et al. Risk factors for lower urinary tract symptoms in a population-based sample of African-American men. Am J Epidemiol. 2003;157:906–14.
32. Lu PL, Liu YC, Toh HS, Lee YL, Liu YM, Ho CM, et al. Epidemiology and antimicrobial susceptibility profiles of Gram-negative bacteria causing urinary tract infections in the Asia-Pacific region: 2009–2010 results from the Study for Monitoring Antimicrobial Resistance Trends (SMART). Int J Antimicrob Agents. 2012;40:S37–43.

18

Expression, localisation and potential significance of aquaporins in benign and malignant human prostate tissue

Johannes Bründl[1*], Sabine Wallinger[1], Johannes Breyer[1], Florian Weber[2], Matthias Evert[2], Nikolaos Theodoros Georgopoulos[3], Bernd Rosenhammer[1], Maximilian Burger[1], Wolfgang Otto[1] and Peter Rubenwolf[1,4]

Abstract

Background: To study the expression pattern, localisation and potential clinical significance of aquaporin water channels (AQP) both in prostate cancer (PC) cell lines and in benign and malignant human prostate tissue.

Methods: The AQP transcript and protein expression of HPrEC, LNCaP, DU-145 and PC3 cell lines was investigated using reverse transcriptase polymerase chain reaction (RT-PCR) and immunofluorescence (IF) microscopy labelling. Immunohistochemistry (IHC) was performed to assess AQP protein expression in surgical specimens of benign prostatic hyperplasia as well as in PC. Tissue mRNA expression of AQPs was quantified by single-step reverse transcriptase quantitative polymerase chain reaction (qPCR). Relative gene expression was determined using the 40-ΔC_T method and correlated to clinicopathological parameters.

Results: Transcripts of AQP 1, 3, 4, 7, 8, 10 and 11 were expressed in all four cell lines, while AQP 9 transcripts were not detected in malignant cell lines. IF microscopy confirmed AQP 3, 4, 5, 7 and 9 protein expression. IHC revealed highly heterogeneous AQP 3 protein expression in PC specimens, with a marked decrease in expression in tumours of increasing malignancy. Loss of AQP 9 was shown in PC specimens. mRNA expression of AQP3 was found to be negatively correlated to PSA levels ($\rho = -0.354$; $p = 0.013$), D'Amico risk stratification ($\rho = -0.336$; $p = 0.012$), ISUP grade ($\rho = -0.321$; $p = 0.017$) and Gleason score ($\rho = -0.342$; $p = 0.011$).

Conclusions: This is the first study to systematically characterize human prostate cell lines, benign prostatic hyperplasia and PC in relation to all 13 members of the AQP family. Our results indicate the differential expression of several AQPs in benign and malignant prostate tissue. A significant correlation was observed between AQP 3 expression and tumour grade, with progressive loss in more malignant tumours. Taken together, AQPs may play a role in the progression of PC and AQP expression patterns may serve as a prognostic marker.

Keywords: Aquaporins, Human prostate, Prostate cancer, Prostate cancer cell lines

Background

Water and solute movement across the epithelia lining the male reproductive tract are essential prerequisites for seminal fluid formation and homeostasis, and are of paramount significance for the modulation of the luminal environment in which sperm cells mature and reside.

The mechanism by which water crosses through epithelial borders had remained a matter of debate until the discovery and elucidation of the function of the aquaporin water channels (AQP) by the later Nobel laureate Peter Agre in the early 1990s. AQPs are a family of transmembrane pore-forming proteins that selectively allow water and other small, uncharged molecules such as urea, glycerol and pyrimidines to pass along hydrostatic and osmotic gradients. They play a fundamental role in numerous physiological processes, most notably in fluid absorption and secretion. To date, 13 different

* Correspondence: johannes.bruendl@ukr.de
[1]Department of Urology, Caritas St Josef Medical Center, University of Regensburg, Landshuter Straße 65, 93053 Regensburg, Germany
Full list of author information is available at the end of the article

mammalian AQPs have been identified at the molecular level and localised in specific tissues [1]. Analysis of several human diseases has confirmed that AQPs are functionally involved in various pathological conditions and thus may provide promising drug targets [2]. Moreover, there is strong presumptive evidence that AQPs play a role in carcinogenesis, specifically in tumour angiogenesis and cell migration [3].

To date, the presence and significance of AQPs in the human prostate remain largely uninvestigated, with reports of the individual expression of AQP 1, 3, 5 and 9 documented in previous studies [4–8]. These findings suggest that fluid reabsorption and secretion in the prostate could be modulated by AQPs. Yet, despite investigations examining expression for individual AQPs, the human prostate has not been systematically studied in relation to all 13 members of the AQP family.

The principal aim of this study was to systematically characterize the expression pattern of all 13 AQP channels in cultured normal and malignant prostate epithelial cells, as well as freshly-isolated benign and malignant human prostate tissues. This approach allowed us to systematically study expression both at the mRNA and protein level of the whole AQP family in prostate tissue, and to correlate the pattern of expression with clinicopathological parameters. The potential biological and clinical significance of our findings are discussed.

Methods

Human prostate cell lines

Cell culture

Four established human prostate cell lines, one normal human prostate epithelial cell line (HPrEC, Lifeline Cell Technology, USA), and three cancer cell lines, PC3 (Lifeline Cell Technology, USA), DU145 and LNCaP (CLS Cell Lines Service GmbH, Germany) were grown to confluency under standard culture conditions as follows: HPrEC: ProstaLife™ Basal Medium + ProstaLife™ LifeFactors Kit (37 °C; 5%CO_2); LNCaP/DU-145/PC3: DMEM + RPMI (1:1), 5% FBS (fetal bovine serum), 1% L-Glutamine (37 °C; 5%CO_2).

Ribonucleic acid isolation and transcript analysis (RT-PCR)

Confluent cultures of prostate cell lines were rinsed twice in phosphate-buffered saline (PBS) and harvested for the isolation of total RNA according to the manufacturer's recommendations. RNA was extracted using RNeasy Mini Kit (Qiagen) after incubation with Proteinase K for 10 min. RNA quantity was assessed using a Nanodrop spectrometer (Nanodrop 2000c, Thermo Scientific). RNA from cell lines was reverse transcribed to cDNA using the iScript cDNA Synthesis Kit (Biorad) in line with the manufacturer's protocol. AQP 0–12 primers were designed using the National Centre for Biotechnology Information (NCBI) database resources (primer sequences specified in Additional file 1: Table S1) with ß-actin serving as the transcript control. RT-PCR conditions were as follows: 3 min at 95 °C, followed by 30 cycles at 95 °C for 10 s, annealing for 30 s (specific annealing temperatures specified in Additional file 1: Table S1), extension at 72 °C for 30 s, and 8 min elongation at 72 °C. PCR products were analysed with 2% agarose gel electrophoresis exactly as described in [9]. Reverse transcriptase (RT)-positive and RT-negative controls were included in all PCR reactions [9, 10].

Immunofluorescence (IF) microscopy

Cells from all four human prostate cell lines were seeded at 1×10^5 cells/ml onto Multiwell glass slides. Cultures were fixed in a 1:1 (*v*/v) solution of methanol and acetone, air-dried, and incubated sequentially with the primary antibody for 16 h at 4 °C (see Additional file 2: Table S2) and the secondary antibody conjugated with Alexa 594 (Molecular Probes) for 30 min, with PBS washing between steps. Hoechst 33258 (DAPI; 0.1 mg/ml) was used to stain nuclei. Secondary antibody-only negative controls and positive control cell lines known to express the respective antigen were included as specificity controls [9, 10]. Immunolabelling was visualised by epifluorescence on a Zeiss Axio Imager Z1 microscope.

Human prostate specimens

Collection of specimens

The collection of tissues had the approval of the local research ethics committee (reference number: 17–660-101) and written patient consent was also obtained. Human prostate samples were obtained from 61 patients who underwent a suprapubic adenomectomy for benign prostatic hyperplasia (BPH, n = 15) or a robot-assisted radical prostatectomy for biopsy-proven prostate cancer (n = 46) at our department in 2014. None of these patients had undergone hormonal therapy prior to surgery.

Clinicopathological data

Clinicopathological data are summarized in Table 1. All surgical specimens were assessed histopathologically by two independent uropathologists for grading and staging based on the criteria of the 2009 UICC TNM classification and ISUP 2014 Gleason grade groups and subsequently prepared for microdissection [11].

Ribonucleic acid isolation

Paraffin wax-embedded samples were de-paraffinized in xylene and microdissected samples from five serial sections (10 μm) were pooled and collected in 50 ml of lysis buffer (Qiagen). RNA was extracted using a FFPE RNA Kit (Qiagen).

Table 1 Patient characteristics

	n (%)
Patient data	
Age (years; range)	66 (47–84)
Total number	61 (100%)
Benign prostatic hyperplasia (BPH)	15 (24.6%)
Low-risk PC (D'Amico)	16 (26.2%)
Intermediate PC (D'Amico)	16 (26.2%)
High-risk PC (D'Amico)	14 (23.0%)
PSA	
< 4 ng/ml	2 (3.3%)
4-10 ng/ml	36 (59.0%)
10-20 ng/ml	12 (19.7%)
> 20 ng/ml	5 (8.2%)
n/a	6 (9.8%)
ISUP (Gleason-Score)	
1 (6)	17 (27.9%)
2 (7a)	14 (23.0%)
3 (7b)	1 (1.6%)
4 (8)	3 (4.9%)
5 (9–10)	11 (18.0%)
No cancer	15 (24.6%)
T-stage	
pT2a	7 (11.5%)
pT2b	1 (1.6%)
pT2c	28 (45.9%)
pT3/4	10 (16.4%)
No cancer	15 (24.6%)

Real-time quantitative polymerase chain reaction (qPCR)

RNA from microdissected tissue was reverse transcribed and amplified using the iTaq Universal SYBR Green One-Step Kit (Biorad) and real-time PCR reaction was carried out on a CFX Connect Real-Time PCR Detection System (Biorad) using SYBR-Green I chemistry. Quantification was performed on MicroAmp Optical 96-Well Reaction plates. Detection of PCR products was accomplished by measuring the emitting fluorescence at the end of each reaction step. Forty amplification cycles were applied and the cycle threshold (C_T) values of AQP 3, AQP 4, AQP 7, AQP 9 were determined along with one reference gene for each AQP. The SYBR-Green assay module includes a final melting point analysis that followed the 40 cycles of quantitative PCR. Plots from the melting point analysis were manually inspected for all RNA gene assays tested to verify that primers were specific (data not shown). PBGD (porphobilinogen desaminase) was used as housekeeping gene as previously described [12]. C_T values were normalized by subtracting the C_T value of the housekeeping gene from the C_T value of the target gene (ΔC_T). RNA results were then reported as 40-ΔC_T values to ensure that the normalized gene expression obtained by the test was proportional to the corresponding mRNA expression levels [13, 14].

Immunohistochemistry

Surgical samples were fixed in 10% formalin, dehydrated, and embedded in paraffin wax. Dewaxed 4-µm tissue sections were subjected to antigen retrieval by boiling for 10 min in tris-ethylenediaminetetraacetic acid (Tris-EDTA, pH 9 for AQP 3) or citric acid (pH 6 for AQP 4, 5, 7, and 9), before labelling with pre-titrated primary antibodies (see Additional file 2: Table S2) for 16 h at 4 ° C. Secondary antibody-only controls and positive control tissues known to express the respective antigen were included as specificity controls [9, 10].

Statistical analysis

Statistical analyses were performed using SPSS version 23. The Spearman's rank correlation coefficient ρ was used as a measure of the strength and direction of the relationship between variables. Levels of mRNA-expression were stratified by quartiles.

Results

AQP expression by human prostate cell cultures in vitro

AQP gene expression was investigated by RT-PCR and immunofluorescence microscopy. In vitro, normal human prostate epithelial cells (HPrEC) as well as malignant cell lines (LNCaP, DU-145 and PC3) showed expression of AQP 1, 3, 4, 7, 8, 10 and 11 (see Fig. 1). By contrast, transcripts for AQP 0, 2, and 12 were not detected (not shown). AQP 5 mRNA transcripts were detected in the DU-145 and PC3 cancer cell lines, but not in LNCaP or HPrEC cells. Transcripts of AQP 6 were present in all cell lines except in LNCaP cells. AQP 9 transcripts were found in HPrEC, but not in malignant cell lines.

Using immunofluorescence microscopy, AQP 3, 4 and 7 were detected in normal cells as well as the three PC cell lines, whereas AQP 5 was only expressed in DU-145 and PC3 cancer cell lines, in line with the RT-PCR analysis results. Expression of AQP 9 was found in normal prostate cells (HPrEC), but was absent in all three cancer cell lines (LNCaP, DU-145, PC3), also in accordance with the transcript findings. Representative results of these experiments are shown in Fig. 2. The remaining AQPs could not be assessed for protein expression due to the lack of suitable commercially available antibodies.

AQP expression by native human prostate tissue

Having detected AQP expression at the mRNA and protein level in normal and malignant cell lines in vitro, the

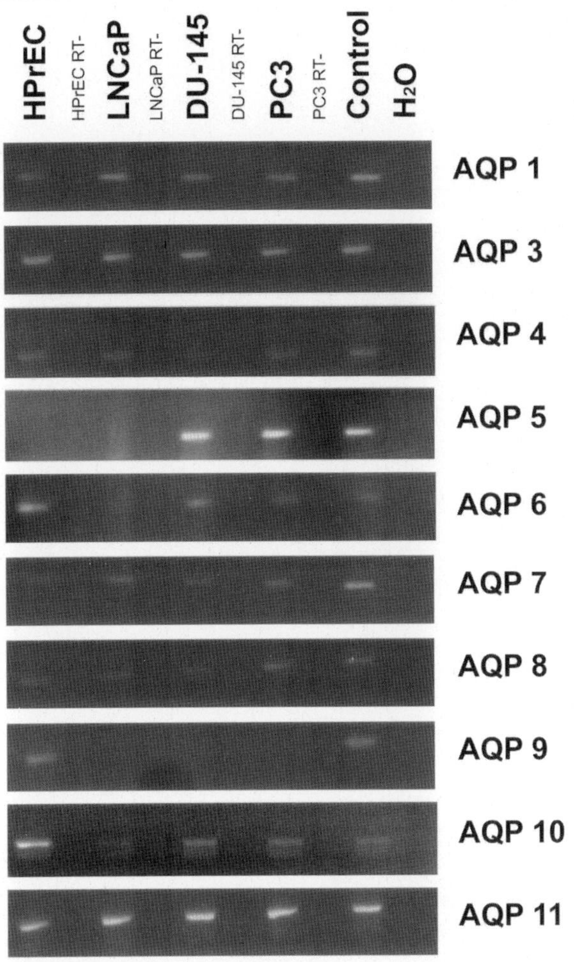

Fig. 1 AQP transcript expression: RT-PCR results of AQP 0–12 in normal prostate epithelial cells (HPrEC) and in established PC lines (LNCaP, DU-145 and PC3). AQP 1, 3, 4, 7, 8, 10 and 11 were detected in HPrEC, LNCaP, DU-145 and PC3. AQP 5 was expressed by DU-145 and PC3, but not by HPrEC and LNCaP. Transcripts of AQP 6 were present in all cell lines except in LNCaP. AQP 9 transcripts were found in HPrEC, but not in PC lines. ß-Actin, a no-template control, and positive controls were included. RT-, reverse transcriptase-negative samples

level of expression and cellular localisation of AQP protein in native, non-malignant prostate tissue was examined by immunohistochemistry. AQP 3 was strongly expressed throughout the epithelium of all specimens with benign prostatic hyperplasia (BPH). Labelling was most intense in the basal layer, less intense in the intermediate layer and weak in the luminal cells. At higher magnification, a distinct localisation pattern was apparent, with intense labelling at the intercellular borders in the basal and suprabasal compartments, as shown in Fig. 3. No immunoreactivity was seen in the submucosa, smooth muscle or endothelium. AQP 4 was not detected in any BPH specimen. AQP 5, AQP 7 and AQP 9 were found to be present in the epithelium of all benign tissues, although the expression pattern was less unequivocal compared with AQP 3 (Fig. 3).

In contrast to our observations in non-malignant (BPH) tissue, a highly heterogeneous AQP 3 protein expression was observed in prostate cancer specimens, with marked decrease in intensity and expression in tumours of increasing malignancy. Whereas intense expression with distinct labelling of the cell borders was present in the epithelium of low-risk tumours, less intense expression of AQP 3 with alternating AQP-positive and AQP-negative tumour cells was found in intermediate-risk tumours. Extensive AQP-negative compartments and abrupt transition from strongly labelled to unlabelled tumour cells were evident in tumours of high malignancy. Complete loss of expression of AQP 3 was found in one third of high-risk cancers. AQP 4 was expressed in half of the tumours tested, and expression was independent of the ISUP/Gleason grade groups. Likewise, heterogenous expression of AQP 5 and AQP 7 was found in all tumours independent of malignancy grades. Finally, AQP 9 was not detected in malignant prostatic tissue. Representative results of these studies are shown in Fig. 4.

Correlation of mRNA expression of AQP 3, AQP 4, AQP 7 and AQP 9 with clinicopathological parameters

AQP transcript expression of human prostate specimen was quantified by qPCR. The non-parametric Spearman's rank correlation indicated a negative, statistically significant correlation between mRNA expression of AQP 3 and PSA levels ($\rho = -0.354$; $p = 0.013$), D'Amico risk stratification ($\rho = -0.336$; $p = 0.012$), ISUP grade ($\rho = -0.321$; $p = 0.017$) and Gleason score ($\rho = -0.342$; $p = 0.011$). Expression of AQP 4 revealed a statistically significant positive correlation with the presence of tumour ($\rho = 0.493$; $p = 0.001$), D'Amico risk stratification ($\rho = 0.436$; $p = 0.003$), ISUP grade ($\rho = 0.434$; $p = 0.003$) and Gleason score ($\rho = 0.436$; $p = 0.003$) but not with PSA ($\rho = 0.094$; $p = 0.577$) and tumour stage ($\rho = 0.270$; $p = 0.080$). By contrast, there was no correlation between AQP 7 mRNA expression and any clinicopathological parameter investigated. Expression of AQP 9 transcripts was found to be negatively correlated with PSA ($\rho = -0.366$; $p = 0.010$). Please refer to Fig. 5.

Discussion

The expression and function of AQPs has been investigated in the majority of human tissues [9]. Previous findings have suggested that fluid reabsorption and secretion in numerous organs are modulated by AQPs. However, human prostate tissue has not yet been systematically analysed in relation to AQP channel expression. The objective of the present study was to systematically investigate the expression and localisation of AQPs not only in human prostate (normal and malignant) cell lines in vitro, but

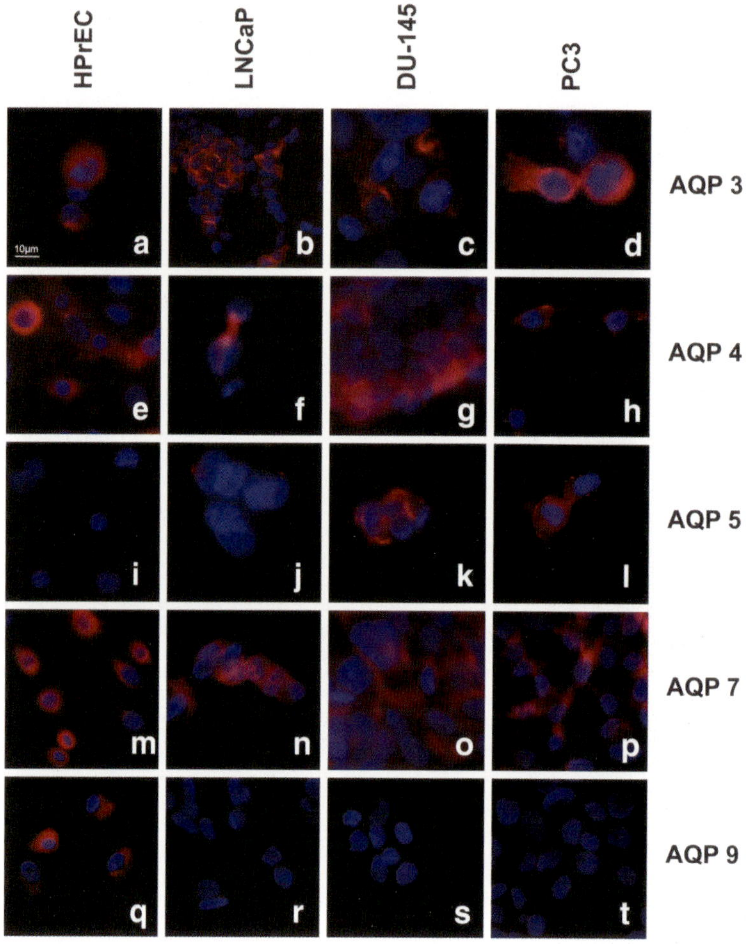

Fig. 2 Immunofluorescence labelling of HPrEC, LNCaP, DU-145 and PC3 cell lines. Intense expression of AQP 3 (**a**-**d**) AQP 4 (**e**-**h**) and AQP 7 (**m**-**p**) in all cell lines. No expression of AQP 5 was detected in HPrEC and LNCaP, but positive immunofluorescence labelling in DU-145 and PC3 (**i**-**l**). Expression of AQP 9 in HPrEC with no expression in LNCaP, DU-145 and PC3 (**q**-**t**)

also to investigate AQP expression in surgical specimens of BPH and PC of various malignancy grades.

Our study is the first to characterize human prostate tissue in relation to all 13 members of the AQP family. Transcripts for AQP 1, 3, 4, 7, 8, 10 and 11 were consistently detected in all four cell lines, while there was differential expression of AQP 5, 6 and 9. AQP 0, 2 and 12 were not detected in our study. Our mRNA transcript findings were corroborated at the protein level by immunofluorescence microscopy, where we detected AQP protein expression for those AQP family members where commercially available antibodies were able to be used. Our mRNA and protein findings in vitro are collectively in agreement with previous studies, which showed expression of AQP 1, 3, 5 in the human prostate at both the transcript and protein levels [7, 15]. Having characterized AQP expression in normal and malignant human prostate cell lines, we then investigated AQP expression in human BPH and PC specimens of various tumour grades via qPCR and immunohistochemistry.

The expression of AQPs by human prostate tissue and recent reports on their possible role in carcinogenesis in epithelial tissues raise interesting questions about the potential functional (biological) significance of AQPs in the development and progression of PC. We contend that it is particularly important to investigate whether the pattern (and localisation) of AQP expression could be of prognostic and/or of therapeutic value. Our results provide strong presumptive evidence that there is a correlation between the loss of AQP 3 expression and increased PC tumour grade. To our knowledge, this is the first report of progressive loss of AQP 3 expression in high-grade PC. Previous investigations into the significance of AQPs in non-urological tumours have almost invariably shown overexpression of AQP 3 and it has been hypothesized that AQP 3 may be a promising drug

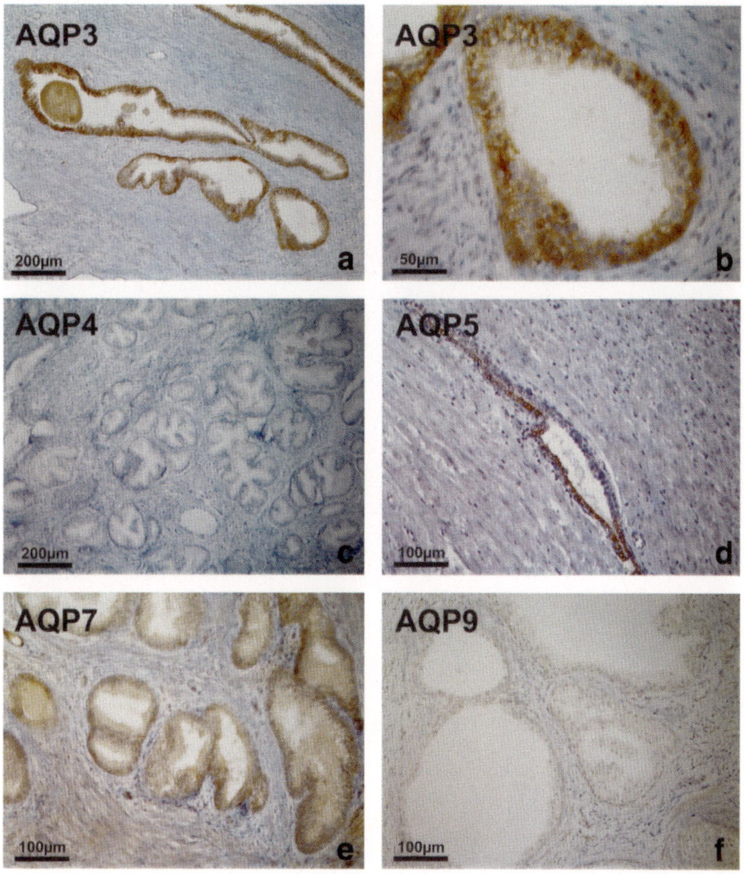

Fig. 3 AQP immunoperoxidase labelling of non-malignant prostatic tissues (BPH). Intense expression of AQP 3 throughout the epithelium from a patient with BPH. Labelling was most intense in the basal layer, less intense in the intermediate layer and weak in the luminal cells (**a**). At higher magnification, a distinct localisation pattern was apparent, with intense labelling of intercellular borders in the basal and suprabasal compartments (**b**). No immunoreactivity was seen in the submucosa, smooth muscle or endothelium. No expression of AQP 4 was detected (**c**). Heterogeneous expression of AQP 5 (**d**), diffuse expression of AQP 7 (**e**) and weak expression of AQP 9 (**f**) was observed

target in the treatment of various epithelial tumours [16–19]. The contrasting expression pattern of AQP 3 with intense labelling of AQP 3 in the case of BPH and well-differentiated PC, but non-homogeneous expression or loss of AQP 3 in the case of high-risk tumours, is noteworthy and may reflect tumour heterogeneity. Although this does not completely corroborate with cell line data, it is well known that in vitro cell lines do not necessarily reflect what happens in vivo. PC is well known for its tumour heterogeneity, which is reflected by diverse morphological manifestations and various molecular alterations associated with different tumour phenotypes [20].

With regard to clinicopathological parameters, down-regulation of AQP3 was associated with higher preoperative PSA values, higher risk according to the D'Amico classification and a higher Gleason-/ISUP-grade. Interestingly, in support of our prostate cancer findings here, we previously reported a similar observation in urothelial carcinoma, with studies suggesting that the loss of AQP 3 may play a role in bladder cancer progression. We showed a significant correlation between AQP 3 protein expression and tumour stage and grade, with AQP 3 expression being reduced or lost in urothelial carcinomas of higher grade and stage [10, 21]. Furthermore, loss of AQP 3 expression was associated with worse progression-free and cancer-specific survival in patients with muscle-invasive bladder cancer [22].

The pro-tumorigenic effect of AQP 3 loss has also been reported for non-urological tumour entities. For instance, knockdown of AQP 3 expression resulted in increased migration and proliferation in gastric adenocarcinoma cell lines [16]. By contrast, overexpression of AQP 3 has been demonstrated for most other tumour entities, such as for squamous cell carcinomas [17]. Although establishing a functional role for AQP 3 expression in BPH and PC was beyond the scope of this study, our findings suggest that progressive loss of AQP 3 expression may be associated with worse clinical PC outcomes.

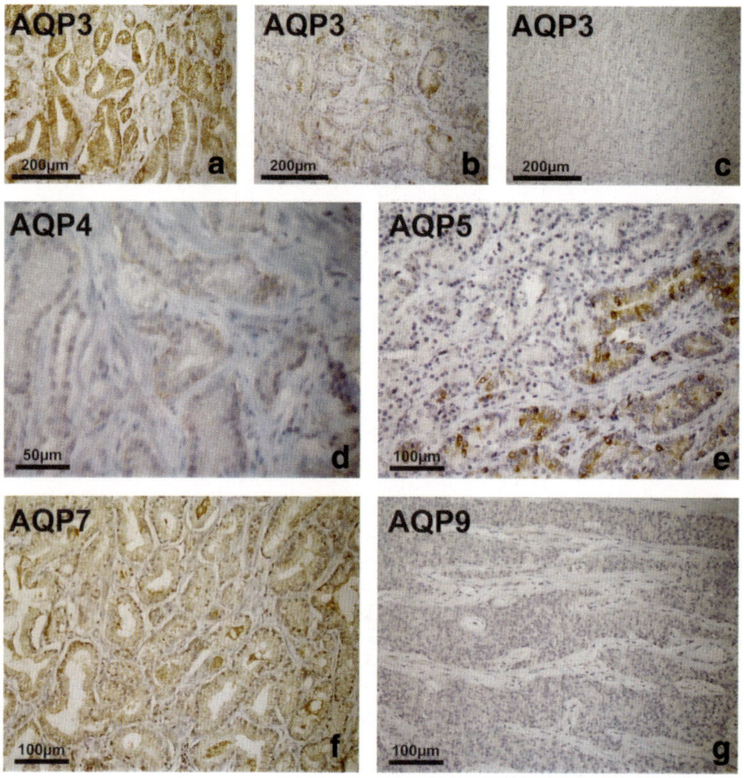

Fig. 4 AQP immunoperoxidase labelling of prostate cancer specimens. Intense expression with distinct labelling at the cell borders in a sample of a low-risk tumour (**a**), less intense expression of AQP 3 with alternating AQP-positive and AQP-negative tumour cells found in an intermediate-risk tumour (**b**). Complete loss of AQP 3 expression in a high-risk tumour (**c**). Weak expression of AQP 4 in an intermediate-risk tumour (**d**). Heterogeneous expression of AQP 5 (**e**) and expression of AQP 7 (**f**) in PC. AQP 9 was not detected (**g**)

When studying AQP 4 expression, we found expression in half of carcinomas but not in any BPH specimens in immunohistochemistry. Moreover, a significant positive correlation was observed between mRNA expression in qPCR and D'Amico risk classification, Gleason- and ISUP-grading. Differential expression of AQP 4 in benign and cancerous tissue and its potential biological and clinical roles need to be elucidated in further studies.

AQP 5 and 7 were detected both in BPH and in PC specimens of all grades. However, there was no correlation of AQP 5 and 7 mRNA expression with any clinicopathological parameter in our cohort. These findings are similar to the observations made in a recent study by Park et al. [15]. Pust et al. previously reported highly variable AQP 5 expression in PC with both negative and intense expression of AQP 5 being linked to unfavourable outcomes

Variable	Co-Variable	Spearman ρ	p-value
AQP 3	PSA	-0.354	0.013*
AQP 3	D'Amico risk stratification	-0.336	0.012*
AQP 3	ISUP grade	-0.321	0.017*
AQP 3	Gleason-Score	-0.342	0.011*
AQP 3	T-stage	-0.181	0.190
AQP 3	Presence of tumour	-0.092	0.505

Variable	Co-Variable	Spearman ρ	p-value
AQP 4	PSA	0.094	0.577
AQP 4	D'Amico risk stratification	0.436	0.003**
AQP 4	ISUP grade	0.434	0.003**
AQP 4	Gleason-Score	0.436	0.003**
AQP 4	T-stage	0.270	0.080
AQP 4	Presence of tumour	0.493	0.001**

Variable	Co-Variable	Spearman ρ	p-value
AQP 7	PSA	0.011	0.954
AQP 7	D'Amico risk stratification	-0.084	0.615
AQP 7	ISUP grade	-0.090	0.593
AQP 7	Gleason-Score	-0.084	0.615
AQP 7	T-stage	-0.140	0.402
AQP 7	Presence of tumour	-0.053	0.750

Variable	Co-Variable	Spearman ρ	p-value
AQP 9	PSA	-0.366	0,010**
AQP 9	D'Amico risk stratification	-0.191	0.162
AQP 9	ISUP grade	-0.148	0.279
AQP 9	Gleason-Score	-0.163	0.235
AQP 9	T-stage	-0.216	0.117
AQP 9	Presence of tumour	0.067	0.629

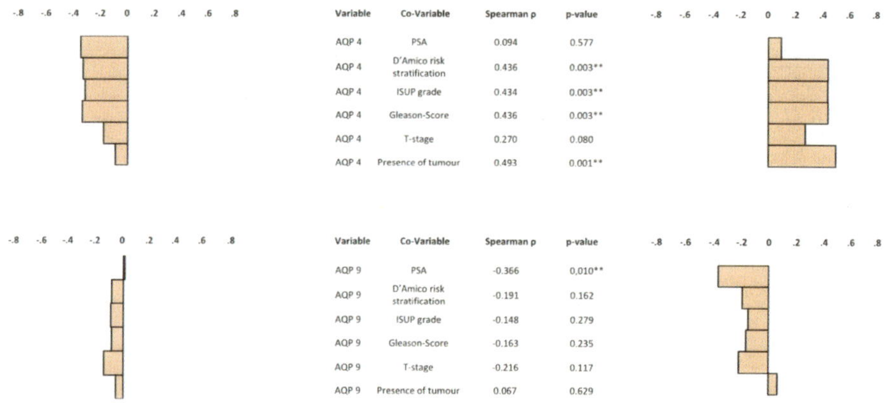

Fig. 5 Spearman correlation of mRNA expression of AQP 3, AQP 4, AQP 7 and AQP 9 with clinicopathological parameters

[23]. In contrast to our findings, Li et al. demonstrated that AQP 5 expression was upregulated and associated with advanced stage, circulating tumour cells and inferior survival rates in PC [24]. These discrepancies and a wealth of somewhat contradictory results are interesting, and indicate that further studies are required to scrutinize the significance of AQP 5 expression in PC.

AQP 9 has previously been shown to be ubiquitously expressed along the male reproductive tract [25]. In concordance with this, we found expression of AQP 9 in normal prostatic cells in vitro and in BPH in vivo, whereas loss of expression was consistently demonstrated in cancer cell lines and in PC specimens. The demonstration of an inverse correlation of AQP 9 mRNA levels in qPCR and PSA supports this. Our study is the first to report the consistent loss of AQP 9 expression in PC, the biological significance of which still remains to be established. In hepatocellular cancer, for instance, decreased expression of AQP 9 resulted in increased resistance to apoptosis [26]. In rat prostates, AQP 9 expression has been shown to be regulated by androgens [8]. Similarly, Jiang et al. and Tian et al. suggested that expression of AQP 1, 3–8, 10–12 in PC is modified by androgens, at least in rats [27, 28]. However, there are little published data on its role in the human prostate. Hence, the potential role of AQP 9 in the carcinogenesis of PC needs to be addressed in future studies.

Despite the clear differential expression of AQP demonstrated in our study (particularly AQP 3), we do accept that our observational investigation was conducted on a relatively limited number of BPH and PC specimens. As such, despite their significance, our findings would certainly be strengthened by a bigger cohort of clinical specimens. One definite weakness of our study, however, is the lack of healthy prostate tissue serving as a control. Hence, we can only speculate on the relationship between AQP expression and function in normal human prostate tissue. Nevertheless, we did observe clear differential expression of AQP and a correlation with increasing malignancy in PC. While such an approach goes beyond the scope of the present study, future studies must certainly seek to prove a functional role for AQP 3 in PC progression. This would involve mechanistic studies and silencing with the RNAi-mediated knockdown of AQP 3 to assess biological endpoints relevant to tumour progression (proliferation, migration/invasion, and/or resistance to apoptotic stimuli) in the PC cell lines studied here. In addition, pre-clinical PDX models from patients with castration resistant PC might also be helpful. This would provide mechanistic insight into how changes in AQP expression may regulate tumour biology. We are currently addressing such questions, and are carrying out further studies that include sufficient patient numbers and long-term survival data to elucidate the potential clinical significance of AQP expression and its role in PC.

Conclusions

This is the first study to demonstrate that several AQPs are expressed in human prostate cell lines, BPH and PC. Our results indicate differential expression of several AQPs in benign and malignant prostate tissue. A significant correlation was observed between AQP 3 protein expression and tumour grade, with a progressive loss of AQP 3 expression in more malignant tumours. However, it has yet to be determined whether AQPs play defined biological role(s) in the initiation and/or progression of PC and, more specifically, whether this could be of prognostic or therapeutic value.

Abbreviations

AQP: Aquaporin; BPH: Benign prostatic hyperplasia; cDNA: Complementary desoxyribonucleic acid; DMEM: Dulbecco modified Eagle's minimal essential medium; FBS: Fetal bovine serum; IF: Immunofluorescence; IHC: Immunhistochemistry; ISUP: International Society of Urological Pathology; mRNA: Messenger ribonucleic acid; PBGD: Porphobilinogen desaminase; PBS: Phosphate-buffered saline; PC: Prostate cancer; PDX: Patient derived xenograft; qPCR: Quantitative polymerase chain reaction; RNA: Ribonucleic acid; RPMI: Roswell Park Memorial Institute medium; RT-PCR: Reverse-transcriptase polymerase chain reaction; TNM: TNM Classification of Malignant Tumours; Tris-EDTA: Tris-ethylenediaminetetraacetic acid; UICC: Union internationale contre le cancer

Acknowledgments

The authors would like to thank Stefanie Götz and Nina Mierswa for excellent technical and Ralph Wirtz for statistical support.

Authors' contributions

All authors have read and approved the manuscript. Study concept and design: JB1 (Johannes Bründl), SW, ME, MB, WO, PR. Acquisition of data: JB1, JB2 (Johannes Breyer), BR. Analysis and interpretation of data: SW, FW, PR. Drafting of the manuscript: JB1, SW, NG, PR. Critical revision of the manuscript for important intellectual content: JB2, ME, NG, BR, MB, WO, PR. Statistical analysis: JB1, JB2. Administrative, technical, or material support: SW, WO. Supervision: MB, ME, PR.

Competing interests

All authors have declared that they have no competing interests.

Author details

[1]Department of Urology, Caritas St Josef Medical Center, University of Regensburg, Landshuter Straße 65, 93053 Regensburg, Germany. [2]Institute of Pathology, University of Regensburg, Regensburg, Germany. [3]Department of Biological Sciences, School of Applied Sciences, University of Huddersfield, Huddersfield, UK. [4]Department of Urology, Frankfurt University Medical Center, Frankfurt, Germany.

References

1. Magni F, Sarto C, Ticozzi D, Soldi M, Bosso N, Mocarelli P, Kienle MG. Proteomic knowledge of human aquaporins. Proteomics. 2006;6(20):5637.
2. Jeyaseelan K, Sepramaniam S, Armugam A, Wintour EM. Aquaporins: a promising target for drug development. Expert Opin Ther Targets. 2006; 10(6):889.
3. Saadoun S, Papadopoulos MC, Hara-Chikuma M, Verkman AS. Impairment of angiogenesis and cell migration by targeted aquaporin-1 gene disruption. Nature. 2005;434(7034):786.

4. Hwang I, Jung SI, Hwang EC, Song SH, Lee HS, Kim SO, Kang TW, Kwon D, Park K. Expression and localization of aquaporins in benign prostate hyperplasia and prostate cancer. Chonnam medical journal. 2012;48(3):174.
5. Mobasheri A, Airley R, Hewitt SM, Marples D. Heterogeneous expression of the aquaporin 1 (AQP1) water channel in tumors of the prostate, breast, ovary, colon and lung: a study using high density multiple human tumor tissue microarrays. Int J Oncol. 2005;26(5):1149.
6. Mobasheri A, Marples D, Young IS, Floyd RV, Moskaluk CA, Frigeri A. Distribution of the AQP4 water channel in normal human tissues: protein and tissue microarrays reveal expression in several new anatomical locations, including the prostate gland and seminal vesicles. Channels. 2007;1(1):29.
7. Wang J, Tanji N, Kikugawa T, Shudou M, Song X, Yokoyama M. Expression of aquaporin 3 in the human prostate. Int J Urol. 2007;14(12):1088.
8. Wang J, Tanji N, Sasaki T, Kikugawa T, Song X, Yokoyama M. Androgens upregulate aquaporin 9 expression in the prostate. Int J Urol. 2008; 15(10):936.
9. Rubenwolf PC, Georgopoulos NT, Clements LA, Feather S, Holland P, Thomas DF, Southgate J. Expression and localisation of aquaporin water channels in human urothelium in situ and in vitro. Eur Urol. 2009;56(6):1013.
10. Rubenwolf PC, Otto W, Denzinger S, Hofstadter F, Wieland W, Georgopoulos NT. Expression of aquaporin water channels in human urothelial carcinoma: correlation of AQP3 expression with tumour grade and stage. World J Urol. 2014;32(4):991.
11. Mottet N, Bellmunt J, Bolla M, Briers E, Cumberbatch MG, De Santis M, Fossati N, Gross T, Henry AM, Joniau S, et al. EAU-ESTRO-SIOG guidelines on prostate Cancer. Part 1: screening, diagnosis, and local treatment with curative intent. Eur Urol. 2017;71(4):618.
12. Boormans JL, Hermans KG, Made AC, van Leenders GJ, Wildhagen MF, Collette L, Schroder FH, Trapman J, Verhagen PC. Expression of the androgen-regulated fusion gene TMPRSS2-ERG does not predict response to endocrine treatment in hormone-naive, node-positive prostate cancer. Eur Urol. 2010;57(5):830.
13. Breyer J, Wirtz RM, Otto W, Erben P, Worst TS, Stoehr R, Eckstein M, Denzinger S, Burger M, Hartmann A. High PDL1 mRNA expression predicts better survival of stage pT1 non-muscle-invasive bladder cancer (NMIBC) patients. Cancer Immunol Immunother. 2018;67(3):403.
14. Breyer J, Wirtz RM, Otto W, Laible M, Schlombs K, Erben P, Kriegmair MC, Stoehr R, Eidt S, Denzinger S, et al. Predictive value of molecular subtyping in NMIBC by RT-qPCR of ERBB2, ESR1, PGR and MKI67 from formalin fixed TUR biopsies. Oncotarget. 2017;8(40):67684.
15. Park JY, Yoon G. Overexpression of Aquaporin-1 is a prognostic factor for biochemical recurrence in prostate adenocarcinoma. Pathol Oncol Res. 2017;23(1):189.
16. Huang Y, Zhu Z, Sun M, Wang J, Guo R, Shen L, Wu W. Critical role of aquaporin-3 in the human epidermal growth factor-induced migration and proliferation in the human gastric adenocarcinoma cells. Cancer Biol Ther. 2010;9(12):1000.
17. Kusayama M, Wada K, Nagata M, Ishimoto S, Takahashi H, Yoneda M, Nakajima A, Okura M, Kogo M, Kamisaki Y. Critical role of aquaporin 3 on growth of human esophageal and oral squamous cell carcinoma. Cancer Sci. 2011;102(6):1128.
18. Niu D, Kondo T, Nakazawa T, Yamane T, Mochizuki K, Kawasaki T, Matsuzaki T, Takata K, Katoh R. Expression of aquaporin3 in human neoplastic tissues. Histopathology. 2012;61(4):543.
19. Verkman AS, Hara-Chikuma M, Papadopoulos MC. Aquaporins--new players in cancer biology. J Mol Med (Berl). 2008;86(5):523.
20. Tolkach Y, Kristiansen G. The heterogeneity of prostate Cancer: a practical approach. Pathobiology. 2018;85(1–2):108.
21. Rubenwolf PC, Denzinger S, Otto W. Aquaporin 3 protein expression in transitional cell carcinoma: a potential marker with regard to tumour progression and prognosis? Eur Urol. 2012;61(3):627.
22. Rubenwolf P, Thomas C, Denzinger S, Hartmann A, Burger M, Georgopoulos NT, Otto W. Loss of AQP3 protein expression is associated with worse progression-free and cancer-specific survival in patients with muscle-invasive bladder cancer. World J Urol. 2015;33(12):1959.
23. Pust A, Kylies D, Hube-Magg C, Kluth M, Minner S, Koop C, Grob T, Graefen M, Salomon G, Tsourlakis MC, et al. Aquaporin 5 expression is frequent in prostate cancer and shows a dichotomous correlation with tumor phenotype and PSA recurrence. Hum Pathol. 2016; https://doi.org/10.1016/j.humpath.2015.09.026.
24. Li J, Wang Z, Chong T, Chen H, Li H, Li G, Zhai X, Li Y. Over-expression of a poor prognostic marker in prostate cancer: AQP5 promotes cells growth and local invasion. World J Surg Oncol. 2014; https://doi.org/10.1186/1477-7819-12-284.
25. Pastor-Soler N, Bagnis C, Sabolic I, Tyszkowski R, McKee M, Van Hoek A, Breton S, Brown D. Aquaporin 9 expression along the male reproductive tract. Biol Reprod. 2001;65(2):384.
26. Jablonski EM, Mattocks MA, Sokolov E, Koniaris LG, Hughes FM Jr, Fausto N, Pierce RH, McKillop IH. Decreased aquaporin expression leads to increased resistance to apoptosis in hepatocellular carcinoma. Cancer Lett. 2007; 250(1):36.
27. Jiang J, Tian JC, Xia JY, Zhu YS, Jiang R. Expressions of aquaporins decrease in the prostate and seminal vesicles of castrated rats. Zhonghua Nan Ke Xue. 2015;21(4):300.
28. Tian JC, Xia JY, Jiang J, Jiang R, He YZ, Lin H. Effect of androgen deprivation on the expression of aquaporins in rat prostate and seminal vesicles. Andrologia. 2016;48(3):268.

19

Reflex erection in the rat: reciprocal interplay between hemodynamic and somatic events

Alexander Andreev-Andrievskiy[1,2,3*], Evgeniia Lagereva[2,3] and Anfisa Popova[1,2,3]

Abstract

Background: Penile erection is a complex reflex under spinal control and modulated by the brain. The hemodynamic events under autonomic control and the perineal muscles somatic activity are interconnected during the reflex erection at the spinal level, however if the afferent feedback on the corpus cavernosum pressure during an erection affects the somatic activity (perineal muscles contractions) and vice versa is not known. This study was aimed to test this hypothesis using a rat model.

Methods: Intracavernous pressure (ICP) and bulbocavernosus (BC) muscle EMG were recorded during reflex erections elicited with dorsal penile nerve (DNP) electrical stimulation in anaesthetized acutely spinalized SD rats with surgically (bilateral cavernous nerve section, CnX, $n = 8$) and pharmacologically (trimetaphan infusion, TMPh, $n = 8$) abolished pressor response, or with surgically (bilateral section of the motor branch of the pudendal nerve, PnX, $n = 7$) and pharmacologically (1 mg/kg d-tubocurarine, $n = 8$) blocked perineal muscles contractions, or with interrupted afferent input from the penis (bilateral crush of the dorsal penile nerve, DPnX, $n = 7$). Control rats ($n = 8$) received no intervention.

Results: Moderate positive correlations were found between net parameters of pressor and somatic activity during DNP-stimulation induced reflex erection in spinal rats, particularly the speed of pressor response development was positively correlated to EMG parameters. No changes of EMG activity were found in CnX rats, while the decrease of BC EMG in TMPh-treated males can be attributed to direct inhibitory action of TMPh on neuromuscular transmission. Pressor response latency was increased and ICP front slope decreased in dTK and PnX rats, indicating that perineal muscles contraction augment pressor response. DPN crush had little effect on ICP and EMG.

Conclusion: Afferent input on the level of intracavernous pressure and the perineal muscles activity has minimal impact on, correspondingly, the somatic and the autonomic components of the reflex erection in spinal males, once the reflex has been initiated.

Keywords: Reflex erection, Dorsal penile nerve, Intracavernous pressure, Bulbocavernosus muscle, Correlation

Background

Penile erection is a complex reflex under spinal control and modulated by the brain [1, 2]. The sensory information from the penis is conveyed by the dorsal penile nerve, as the sensory branch of the pudendal nerve [3], to the spinal centers, displaying pattern generator and integrative properties [4–6]. The efferents include the autonomic proerectile parasympathetic neurons, the sympathetic neurons and the somatic afferents innervating the perineal muscles.

Reflex erection can be triggered by the descending input from the supraspinal sites [7] and the afferentation from the genitalia: tactile stimulation of the penis or electrical stimulation of the dorsal penile nerve. In rodents, when reflex erections are scored visually, the response includes penile tumescence, phasic penile glans engorgements and dorsoventral movements of the penis

* Correspondence: aandrievsky@gmail.com
[1]Lomonosov Moscow State University, Biology faculty, 1-12 Leninskie gory, Moscow 119234, Russia
[2]Institute for biomedical problems RAS, 76A Khoroshevskoe shosse, Moscow 123007, Russia
Full list of author information is available at the end of the article

[8, 9]. Instrumental recordings during reflex erection in the rat [10] or mouse [11] reveal tonic pressure increase mediated by the parasympathetic neurons [12], superimposed with suprasistolic pressure peaks in the corpora cavernosum [10, 13] and spongiosum [14, 15]. The phasic pressure peaks arise concurrently with the perineal muscles EMG bursts and contractions [16], and denervation of the muscles abolishes these phasic events [17]. Apart from the crucial role the perineal muscles play in penile movements during copulation and glans erection, changes of reflex erection in paralyzed rats imply some auxiliary role of these muscles in initiation and/or maintaining the tonic pressure increase during the erection [12].

Persistence of reflex erections after thoracic spinal transection clearly illustrates self-sufficiency of the spinal level of erection control [8]. Tracing studies revealed profuse collaterals of the spinal preganglionic neurons within the spinal cord [5, 18–21], as well as ascending to supraspinal structures [3, 18, 22]. Numerous interneurons in the lumbar and sacral segments receive the afferent input from the penis [23, 24]. Glutamate [25, 26], acetylcholine [27], noradrenalin [28], serotonin [29–31], dopamine [32], GABA [33, 34], oxytocin [20, 35] and prostaglandins [36] are involved in erection control and provide ample neurochemical basis for complex regulation of the autonomic and somatic processes constituting an erection.

The hemodynamic and the somatic events during reflex erection are obviously time matched. The integration of these two components can be realized "directly" within the spinal cord, and there is also a possibility of "indirect" reciprocal influence of the afferent feedback on the level of somatic and autonomic activity, i.e. the afferent input on the level of intracavernous pressure could affect somatic activity and, vise versa, the perineal muscles proprioceptor feedback could modulate the parasympathetic or sympathetic neurons. It can be speculated, that this afferent interplay, if present, underlies the efficiency of physiotherapeutic treatments for erectile dysfunction based on stimulation/training of perineal muscles [37]. This study was aimed to investigate if the reciprocal afferent interplay between the autonomic and the somatic components of the reflex erectile response actually occurs. To this end we recorded intracavernous pressure and bulbocavernosus muscle EMG during reflex erection induced with DNP electrical stimulation in anaesthetized spinal rats with surgically or pharmacologically blocked hemodynamic or somatic component of the reflex response.

Methods

Animals and housing

Mature male SD rats weighing 500–600 g and 7–8 months of age were used in the study. Rats were purchased from the Institute of cytology and genetics SB RAS Animal resource center and were specific pathogen free. Males were housed in groups of 2–3 in semi-transparent cages (floor area 1500 cm^2, Tecniplast, Italy) at 20–26 °C, 30–70% RH and 12-h light-dark cycle (lights on at 09:00). Standard rat chow (Assortiment agro, Russia) and reverse osmotic water were provided ad libitum. Wood chips were used for bedding; paper tissues and wooden sticks were offered to enrich the environment.

The study was approved by the Bioethics commission of MSU Institute for Mitoengeneering and performed in compliance with the European Convention for the Protection of Vertebrate Animals used for Experimental and Other Scientific Purposes.

Experimental deign

Males were randomly divided into 6 experimental groups: 1) CnX animals ($n = 8$) that underwent bilateral ablation of the cavernous nerve, 2) TMPh (n = 8) group that received ganglionic blocker trimetophan; 3) PnX ($n = 7$) rats that were subject to bilateral sectioning of the pudendal nerve motor branch, 4) dTK ($n = 8$) rats that were paralyzed with d-tubocurarine, 5) DPnX ($n = 8$) rats had the dorsal penile nerve crush and 6) control rats ($n = 8$) that received no intervention. An on-line tool (https://www.graphpad.com/quickcalcs/randomize1/) was used for randomization. The sample size was calculated using G*Power (version 3.2) basing on the in-lab data on the parameters variability. After surgical preparation, two reflex erections were elicited in each animal before (baseline) and two more – after the experimental interventions were applied. The whole procedure was performed in urethane-anaesthetized animals. Intracavernous pressure and perineal muscles EMG were the primary outputs, with blood pressure and heart rate continuously monitored as indication of the animal's general condition. Correction for baseline values collected in the same animal was used in order to minimize the inter-individual variability.

Preparation

Experiments were performed with urethane-anesthetized rats (1.0–1.2 g/kg) using a procedure modified from Pescatori et al. [10]. Firstly, thoracic vertebral column was reached and cleared of the surrounding muscles. T9 vertebra was identified [38] and after laminectomy the spinal cord was transected at T8-T9 level. After the hemostasis was reached, the muscles and the skin were sutured in layers. Secondly, the right carotid and the left jugular vein were cannulated with PE50 tubing for direct blood pressure recording and fluid delivery correspondingly. The trachea was intubated to secure normal breezing or artificial ventilation if needed. Next, the penis was excised form the prepuce, cleared of the connective tissue and the left (chosen by convention) corpus cavernosum was cannulated with G23 injection needle on the ventro-lateral surface ≈5 mm distal to the crus for intracavernous pressure recording. The dorsal nerve of the penis was isolated bilaterally and placed on stainless steel electrodes. The bipolar G30 stainless steel electrodes spaced 3 mm apart (isolated for the whole length except for the bevel) were inserted into the left bulbocavernosus for EMG recording. All exposed tissues were covered with saline-soaked tissues to prevent dehydration and a small piece of cotton wool soaked in mineral oil was used to cover the DNP.

In addition to this general procedure, further preparation of the CnX, PnX and DPnX was performed. In CnX animals, access to the prostate was reached by bluntly separating the abdominal wall muscles, and the cavernous nerve was isolated bilaterally at the site of emergence from the major pelvic ganglion. The ligature was placed under both nerves and passed through a length of PE 100 tubing; after the baseline responses recording the ligature was pulled through the tubing so that the loop severed the nerve. In PnX rats, the motor branch of the pudendal nerve was accessed by gently separating the perineal muscles. Similarly to CnX rats, the ligature and a piece of tubing were used to form makeshift loop scissors around the nerve bilaterally. In DPnX rats the loose ligature knot was placed over the dorsal nerve of the penis distally to the stimulating electrodes and was tightened to crush the nerve after the baseline responses registration.

Experimental protocol

Four reflex erections were elicited with DNP electrical stimulation with 4 V square pulses of 1 ms duration delivered at 5 Hz for 20 s; the intervals between the stimulations were 5–7 min. Analog BP, ICP and EMG signals were amplified, recorded at 5 kHz sampling rate and analyzed using PowerLab 8/30 and LabChart Pro. After the first two "baseline" responses the experimental interventions were applied. In CnX and PnX rats the cavernous nerves and the motor branches of the pudendal nerve correspondingly were severed; in DPnX animals the dorsal penile nerve was crushed. TMPh rats received 60 mg/kg trimetaphan as a bolus through the jugular catheter, followed by continuous infusion at 20 mg/kg/h. To maintain normal blood pressure in TMPh rats, angiotensin II was infused constantly at 15–75 mkg/kg/h rate (to the effect [39]). dTK rats were injected with 1 mg/kg d-tubocurarine into the lateral tail veins and immediately provided with artificial ventilation at 80 breaths per minute and 9–12 mmHg end tidal pressure (KTR-5 animal ventilator, Hugo Sachs Elektronik, Germany). After the treatments were applied, two more DPN stimulations were performed. The animals were euthanized prior to recovery from anesthesia via decapitation.

Data handling and analysis

No a priori inclusion or exclusion criteria has been developed or used. Thus, all the collected data were included into the analysis.

The pressor response in the cavernous bodies was quantified on the basis of ICP/MAP ratio; to minimize the contribution of phasic pressure peaks, ICP traces were low-pass filtered (cut-off frequency 0.1 Hz) before division by MAP. Response amplitude (ICP A), area under the curve (ICP AUC), front slope (ICP IR, increase rate), latency (LP) and time to maximum (T_{MAX}) were calculated. For EMG, cyclic analysis was performed to determine mean amplitude (EMG A), duration and frequency of each burst, AUC was calculated as a product of amplitude and duration. EMG activity was present mainly after the end of DNP electric stimulation; usually moderate to negligible EMG during the stimulation was distorted with stimulus artifacts and discarded from the analysis. The values for the two first responses were averaged to estimate the "baseline", and averaging of the next two responses produced "treatment" values. The person preforming the original recordings analysis was blinded to the treatments.

Spearman's correlations were calculated to estimate the relations between the ICP and EMG parameters for the pooled sample of "baseline" responses that were first averaged within the animal. For the "treatment" data, statistical analysis was performed using two-way ANOVA (factors "Group" and "Time") on the values corrected for the group baseline means, followed with Sidak's post-test. The correlations and differences were considered significant at $p < 0.05$. The data are presented as mean ± standard error of the mean.

Results

Reflex erectile response

For the "baseline" reflex responses, before the "treatments" were applied, the onset of the pressor component occurred on average 4.2 ± 0.3 s after the DNP stimulation start, ICP/MAP increased with an average slope of 2.06 ± 0.13 a.u./min and reached maximum amplitude of 0.651 ± 0.016 a.u. 29.7 ± 0.6 s after the response start. The first tonic pressure wave was often followed by a second one, and less frequently three waves were observed. The incidence of 1, 2 and 3-wave responses was 38.9, 55.6 and 5.6% correspondingly. The response lasted 83.7 ± 2.1 s and the AUC, as an integral characteristic of the erection intensity, was 28.51 ± 1.37 a.u. × s (Fig. 1a).

Bulbocavernosus EMG activity started simultaneously with the pressor response, but could be reliably quantified after the end of DNP stimulation only (Fig. 1a). EMG bursts, on average 9.4 ± 0.4 per response, were differentiated into three types. The most frequent (94.4 ± 1.4% of all bursts) "single" bursts (Fig. 1b) of varying shape and

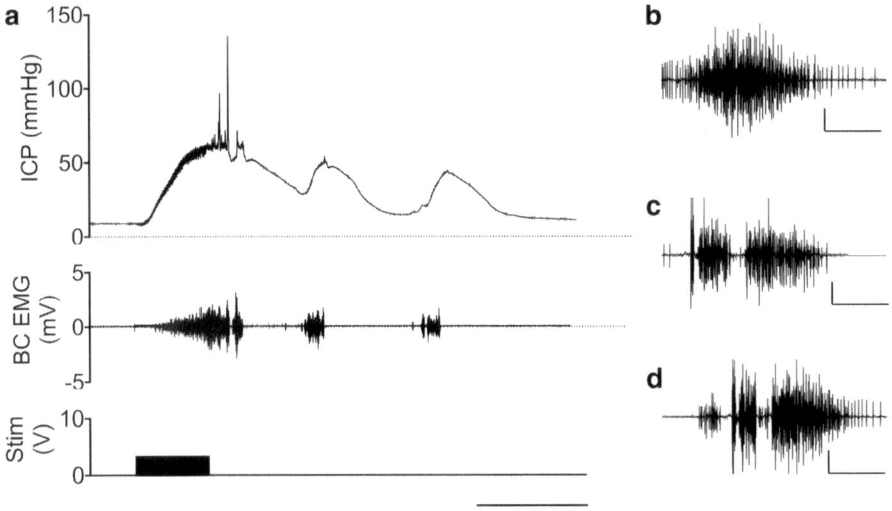

Fig. 1 A representative reflex erection recording (**a**). Electrical stimulation of the dorsal penile nerve induced one to three (as in this recording) waves of tonic intracavernous pressure increase and bursts of bulbocavernosus muscle electromyogram. Concurrent with the perineal muscles contractions phasic peaks of intracavernous pressure occurred. Scale bar - 30 s. A "single" (**b**), "double" (**c**) and "serial" (**d**) bulbocavernosus EMG bursts. Scale bars - 2 mV/500 ms

usually moderate amplitude, "double" bursts separated with 50–100 ms pause (Fig. 1c) and resembling "intromission" bursts [16] (5.0 ± 0.9%), and the most rare serial bursts (Fig. 1d), separated with 50–100 ms pauses in EMG activity (0.5 ± 0.5% of total number of EMG bursts per response). The amplitude of the dual and the serial bursts was approximately twice the single bursts amplitude. EMG bursts were associated with the front and the plateau of tonic pressure waves, at that, the dual and the serial bursts were always associated with the ICP plateau and produced phasic pressure peaks.

The response pattern, i.e. the number of tonic pressure waves and the pattern of EMG activity, was relatively stable within one animal, so that the correlation coefficients between the quantitative parameters of the first and the second "baseline" responses ranged ≈0.90–0.95.

Correlations of hemodynamic and perineal muscles activity parameters

Parameters of the intracavernous pressor response and the bulbocavernosus muscle EMG were correlated during the reflexive erection (Table 1). Particularly, positive correlations were found between AUCs under the ICP/MAP and EMG curves, rate of ICP/MAP increase and EMG amplitude and EMG AUC, between ICP/MAP amplitude and EMG frequency, while latency of the ICP rise after the start of dorsal penile nerve stimulation was negatively correlated with the bulbocavernosus muscle electrical activity.

Changes of hemodynamic and somatic activity after surgical and pharmacological interventions

Blood pressure was unaffected by either of the treatments ($F(5, 40) = 1.57$, $p = 0.1905$) or time ($F(1, 40) = 1.73$, $p = 0.1955$). HR did not vary with the treatment ($F(5, 40) = 0.65$, $p = 0.6618$), but increased over the duration of the experiment ($F(1, 40) = 38.47$, $p < 0.0001$), particularly "after the treatment" HR was greater than the "baseline" in the control, trimetaphan and d-tubokurarine treated rats ($p < 0.05$, Sidak's post test), but not in CnX, PnX and DPnX animals. No differences in BP or HR were found between any of the groups and the control rats either before or after the treatments (Additional file 1: Table S1).

In control rats, virtually no difference was found between baseline and "post-treatment" values of ICP/MAP or EMG parameters.

Bilateral ablation of the cavernous nerve or ganglionic blockade with trimetaphan prevented ICP rise after dorsal penile nerve electrical stimulation (Fig. 2a-g, Additional file 1: Table S1). Trimetaphan administration

Table 1 Spearman's correlations between ICP and EMG parameters

Spearman r(n = 46)		ICP				
		AUC(a.u. × s)	*A(a.u.)*	*IR(a.u./s)*	*LP(s)*	*Tmax(s)*
EMG	*AUC (mV×s)*	**0.354**	0.180	**0.370**	**−0.314**	−0.148
	A (mV)	0.121	0.181	**0.321**	−0.122	−0.201
	F (Hz)	−0.106	**0.303**	0.157	−0.119	0.010

Correlations significant at $p < 0.05$ are highlighted with **bold** text

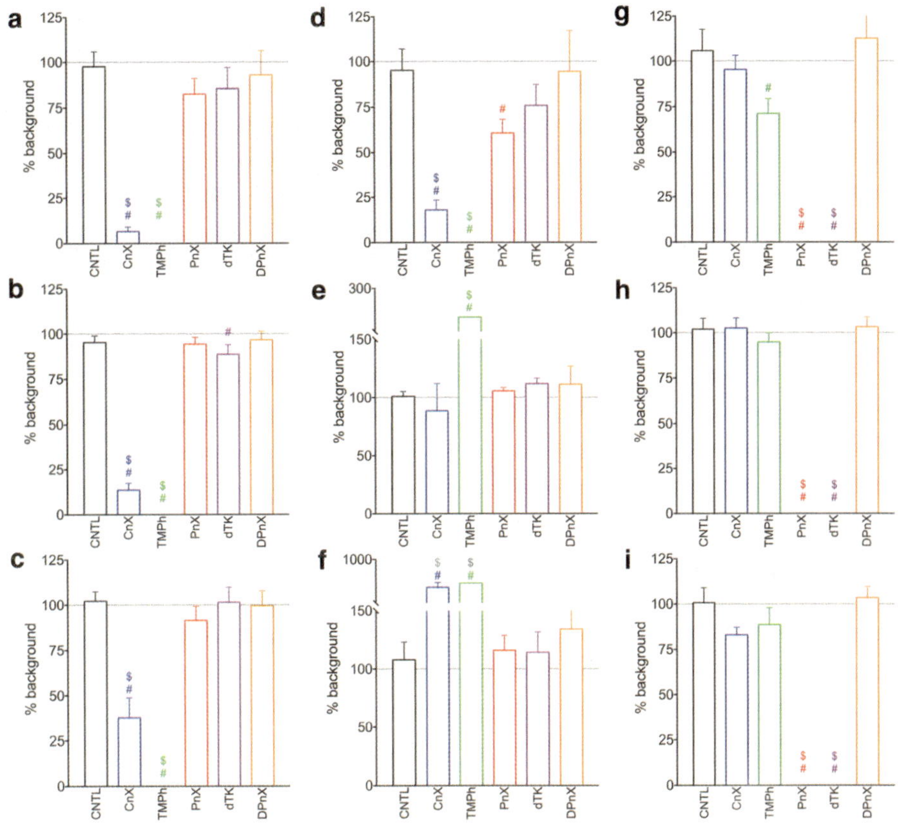

Fig. 2 Erectile response (ICP/MAP) AUC (**a**), amplitude (**b**), duration (**c**), front slope (**d**), latency (**e**) and time to maximum (**f**), bulbocavernosus muscle EMG AUC (**g**), frequency (**h**) and duration (**i**) in control rats (CNTL, $n = 8$), animals with surgically (cavernous nerve crush, CnX, $n = 8$) or pharmacologically (trimetaphan administration, TMPh, $n = 7$) abolished erectile response, rats with surgically (motor branch of the pudendal nerve crush, PnX, $n = 8$) or pharmacologically (d-tubokurarine administration, dTK, $n = 8$) abolished perineal muscles activity, or after sensory dorsal penile nerve crush (DPnX, $n = 7$). The data are presented as percent of baseline (before the treatment) values. $ - $p < 0.05$ vs. control, # - $p < 0.05$ vs. baseline, Sidak's post-test

was more effective, whereas some erectile response persisted in CnX animals due to incomplete sectioning of the diffuse cavernous nerve. No change of total bulbocavernosus muscle electrical activity was observed in CnX rats, while a 29 ± 8% decrease in EMG AUC followed TMPh administration, which was governed by reduced EMG average amplitude (− 15 ± 10%) and total EMG duration (− 11 ± 9%). Interestingly, EMG average amplitude was actually increased in CnX rats (11 ± 8%), and it was counterbalanced by shorter EMG total duration (− 17 ± 4%), resulting in EMG AUC little different from AUC before the nerve section (− 5 ± 8%). All EMG changes in CnX rats, however, did not reach statistical significance level ($p > 0.05$, Sidak's post test).

Bilateral section of the pudendal nerve motor branch or d-tubokurarine administration resulted in complete loss of the bulbocavernosus muscle electrical activity and contractions after the DNP stimulation (Fig. 2g-i, Additional file 1: Table S1). Area under the ICP/MAP curve was somewhat lower in PnX (− 18 ± 8%) and dTK (− 15 ± 11%) animals (Fig. 2a), peak amplitude was decreased in dTK (− 11 ± 5%), but not PnX (− 6 ± 4%) rats (Fig. 2b), while pressor response duration was unaffected. ICP/MAP increase rate was diminished in PnX animals by 40 ± 8% ($p < 0.05$), and a comparable decrease (− 24 ± 11%) in curarized animals was not significant. Latency to ICP/MAP rise was longer in both PnX and dTK rats by ≈15% ($p > 0.05$, Sidak's post-test), but the Tmax, measured from the response start, was unchanged.

In rats with dorsal penile nerve crush (located distally to the stimulating electrodes) no significant changes of either ICP/MAP or EMG parameters were found, however somewhat higher EMG AUC (+ 12 ± 16%) and longer latency of ICP/MAP rise (+ 13 ± 12%) should be noted.

Discussion

Here we report existence of positive correlations between quantitative parameters of the reflex erection hemodynamic and somatic components in the spinal rat. Surgical or pharmacological blockade of the muscle activity resulted in a slower intracavernous pressure increase and in a generally smaller response, while electrical activity of the perineal muscles was not affected in rats with abolished pressor response. Interruption of the sensory input from the penis had little impact on the reflex erectile response in spinal rats.

Reflex erectile response

Intracavernous pressor response in the DNP-stimulation induced reflex erection model we report here can be described as a tonic pressure wave(s) superimposed with phasic pressure peaks. It is reminiscent of the events during penile reflex tests in intact males [40], the apomorphine-induced erections [41], noncontact erections and, to a lesser extent, copulation [13] and can be mimicked with simultaneous stimulation of the cavernous nerve and the motor branch of the pudendal nerve [42]. Consistently with previous findings [10], the duration of ICP tonic increase was much longer in our experiments compared to penile reflexes tests with intact males, presumably due to disinhibition of the spinal centers and the intensive nerve stimulation used. In this regard it should be noted, that despite presumably the same neural pathways are activated during DPN electrical stimulation and tactile stimulation of the penile skin, they are not equivalent. At the very least, a mixed nature of dorsal penile nerve, that contains a portion of NO-ergic axons, that could directly induce intracavernous pressure increase upon electrical stimulation, should be mentioned [43].

In contrast to slower pressure events, the phasic pressure peaks are difficult to reliably measure, due to interference the cavernous tissue trabeculae create by mechanically obstructing the orifice of the cannula and the limitations of the catheter technique, when the long and relatively narrow fluid filled tubing can act as a low-pass filter. However, in case the peaks were registered (Fig. 1a), they did resemble those described previously in other erection models [13]. A similar pattern of pressor response is also found in the rat corpus spongiosum during reflex erections [14, 15]. The BS electrical activity in our study was also similar to the recordings made previously during reflex erections and mating [10, 16, 44]. Of particular interest, distinct EMG patterns that were recorded during intromissions [16], can be also observed in spinal males after DNP stimulation (Fig. 1b-d). Thus the responses we observed are in good accord with the existing data.

Correlations of hemodynamic and perineal muscles activity parameters

Analysis of the quantitative parameters of ICP and BC EMG elicited with DNP stimulation revealed weak (≈ 0.3) but significant correlations between ICP and EMG responses, particularly, parameters that characterize the erection onset (latency and ICP increase rate) and EMG activity. Basing on the correlations found, several assumptions could be made: a) that the perineal muscles activity facilitates cavernous pressure increase, b) that the perineal muscles activity promotes greater erection intensity, or, alternatively, c) that the higher the intracavernous pressure and the faster it grows during the erection onset, the greater the muscle activity. The results of the transection and pharmacological experiments in this study indicate that the first two assumptions are true, while the latter is not.

Pressor response inhibition has minimal impact on perineal muscles activity

After the pressor response was abolished via the cavernous nerve sectioning no changes of bulbocavernosus EMG were found, except for reduction of total EMG duration (insignificant), while in trimetaphan treated rats the EMG AUC was markedly reduced. The discrepancy between the denervation and ganglionic blockade results are explained by direct inhibitory action of trimetaphan on the neuromuscular transmission [45, 46], though not interfering with acetylcholine action directly [47]. Use of trimetaphan, rather than a more specific ganclionic blocker [48], could be considered a limitation of our study, however the differences in results obtained with TMPh and CnX rats underscore that abolished pressor response, and consequently, lack of the corresponding afferent input from the penis do not affect the perineal muscles motoneurons.

Ganglionic blockade leads to a marked drop in blood pressure, and ICP is directly dependent on the blood pressure level. To overcome the possible impact of low blood pressure on the outcomes of the study, we continuously infused angiotensin II to maintain arterial pressure within the normal range. It could be speculated that angiotensin itself could affect the pressor or somatic responses after DNP stimulation. However, unlike other systemic vasoconstrictors, particularly, adrenergic agonists, angiotensin displays pro-erectile properties [39], and low angiotensin concentrations have been shown to facilitate muscle contractions [49] through increased quantal content [50]. Thus, EMG inhibition found in trimetaphan treated rats can be attributed to direct effects of this ganglionic blocker on neuromuscular transmission and could not be governed by angiotensin.

The hemodynamic component of the reflex erection could affect the perineal muscles activity either "directly" through collaterals of the autonomic preganglionic neurons within the spinal cord or interneurons [5, 21, 23], or reflexively, as a result of afferent activity on the intracavernous pressure or penis distension. Our experiments were aimed to test the "reflex hypothesis". Saline infusion into the penis can increase firing rate in the cavernous nerve, however, this activity persists after distal cavernous nerve crush [51], implying that the afferent feedback is conveyed by other routes, possibly, the dorsal penile nerve. The penile skin contains different types of sensory nerve endings, and electrophysiological studies reveal at least two types of slowly adapting neurons in the rat that could provide the afferent signal about penis engorgement. Interestingly, the reported adaptation period of tens of seconds in these slowly adapting units corresponds well with the erection duration [52]. The penile afferents innervate diverse regions in the spinal cord [19, 23, 53], and reach as far as the major pelvic ganglion [25] and could affect the motoneurons innervating the perineal muscles through pudendo-pudendal reflex [54] or other possible mechanisms. However, in our experiments rats with abolished pressor response had mostly unchanged perineal muscles EMG, thus the afferent feedback on the level of pressure increase does not seriously affect the bulbocavernosus motoneurons.

Pressor response is decreased in absence of perineal muscles activity

After denervation of the perineal muscles or curarization the ICP rise was slower, the time to ICP/MAP maximum was somewhat longer, while the pressor response amplitude, and AUC, as an integral characteristic of the response intensity, were reduced. The pressor response changes in absence of the perineal muscles activity were relatively small, with the exception of the response onset latency that was increased by 40% in PnX and 25% in dTK rats. The longer pressor response latency we report here is in accord with findings of Giuliano at all made in a similar model with gallamine-paralyzed animals [12]. It should be mentioned, that the DPN stimulation was much longer in this study, while in our experiments a relatively brief electrostimulation was used to trigger the reflex response. Thus, our experiments provide more clear-cut data on the impact of perineal muscles contractions on the reflex erection pressor component. In intact males, denervation of the perineal muscles prevents glans erections in the penile reflexes tests [17] and impairs the ability of the male to reach an intromission during copulation [55].

The slower reflex pressor response in rats with blocked perineal muscles contractions can be explained by several possible mechanisms. One of them is a "mechanistic" explanation, namely that the muscles contractions facilitate penile veins occlusion or pump additional blood from penile crus and/or bulb and thus promote faster pressure increase. Alternatively, the action could be realized through diffusion of the motoneuron activity in the spinal cord or influence of the perineal muscle afferents. Little is known about the proprioreceptor feedback from the perineal muscles, however, in humans, spindles have been identified in the bulbocavernosus muscle [56] and stimulation of the perineal nerve elicits a reflex efferent activity [57]. Moreover, physiotherapeutic electrostimulation of the ischiocavernous muscle improves penile rigidity [37]. In the rat, contractions of the perineal muscles induce afferent firing in the cavernous nerve, that are abolished after neuromuscular blockade [51]. Thus, our results support the idea that the perineal muscles play an auxiliary role in initiating/maintaining erection, possibly by promoting compression of the penile veins and thus limiting the venous drainage, however, they do not rule out the other, "neurophysiological", explanation.

In the reflex erection model used in our study, DPN crush, and thus interruption of the afferent feedback from the penis, had little impact on either pressor or somatic component of the reflex response. This result is in accord with previous report by Giuliano et al. in a similar model [42], where sectioning the dorsal penile nerve had little impact on the intracavernous pressure rise induced with DNP stimulation. Quite on the contrary, experiments with penile skin desensitization or sectioning of the pudendal nerve during copulation indicate that the sensation from the penile skin is critical to induce adequate somatic activity, for males with desensitized penises reached fewer intromissions than intact animals [55, 58]. Interestingly, male thrusting rate during a mount approximates ≈20 Hz in the rat [58], thus leaving ≈50 ms to initiate somatic events corresponding to an intromission, which is in good accord with the latencies of spinal components of pudendal and micturitions reflexes [51, 59]. In our experiments phasic tactile stimulation, like the one occurring during copulation, was presumably absent or minimal, but it can be speculated that slow adapting afferents were activated during the tonic intracavernous pressure waves. Thus, results of DPN crush experiments further support our conclusion that the feedback on the degree of penile tumescence does not affect the somatic perineal activity.

Conclusion

In summary, our results indicate that once the reflex erection is initiated, there is little interplay between the pressor and the somatic components of the response, at least in the acutely spinalized rats. The somatic perineal muscles activity, however, augments the pressor response by mechanically accelerating the pressure increase.

Acknowledgements
The authors thank Innokentiy Skulachev, head of MSU Institute for Mitoengeneering, LLC for support of this study.

Funding
The study was financed by MSU Institute for Mitoengeneering, LLC.

Authors' contributions
AAA designed the study analyzed the data and drafted the manuscript. AP took part in animal experiments, data analysis and contributed to the manuscript draft. EL took part in animal experiments, data analysis and contributed to the manuscript draft. All authors read and approved the final manuscript.

Competing interests
The authors declare that they have no competing interests.

Author details
[1]Lomonosov Moscow State University, Biology faculty, 1-12 Leninskie gory, Moscow 119234, Russia. [2]Institute for biomedical problems RAS, 76A Khoroshevskoe shosse, Moscow 123007, Russia. [3]MSU Institute for mitoengeneering, LLC, 1-73A Leninskie gory, Moscow 119234, Russia.

References
1. Steers WD. Neural pathways and central sites involved in penile erection: neuroanatomy and clinical implications. Neurosci Biobehav Rev. 2000;24: 507–16.
2. Giuliano F, Rampin O. Neural control of erection. Physiol Behav. 2004;83: 189–201.
3. Tajkarimi K, Burnett AL. The role of genital nerve afferents in the physiology of the sexual response and pelvic floor function. J Sex Med. 2011;8:1299–312.
4. Sachs BD, Garinello LD. Hypothetical spinal pacemaker regulating penile reflexes in rats: evidence from transection of spinal cord and dorsal penile nerves. J Compar Physiol Psychol. 1980;94:530–5.
5. Morgan CW, de Groat WC, Felkins LA, Zhang SJ. Axon collaterals indicate broad intraspinal role for sacral preganglionic neurons. Proc Natl Acad Sci U S A. 1991;88:6888–92.
6. Lu Y, Inokuchi H, McLachlan EM, Li JS, Higashi H. Correlation between electrophysiology and morphology of three groups of neuron in the dorsal commissural nucleus of lumbosacral spinal cord of mature rats studied in vitro. J Comp Neurol. 2001;437:156–69.
7. Giuliano F, Bernabé J, Brown K, Droupy S, Benoit G, Rampin O. Erectile response to hypothalamic stimulation in rats: role of peripheral nerves. Am J Physiol Regul Integr Comp Physiol. 1997;273:R1990–7.
8. Sachs BD, Garinello LD. Spinal pacemaker controlling sexual reflexes in male rats. Brain Res. 1979;171:152–6.
9. Hart BL, Melese-D'Hospital PY. Penile mechanisms and the role of the striated penile muscles in penile reflexes. Physiol Behav. 1983;31:807–13.
10. Pescatori ES, Calabro A, Artibani W, Pagano F, Triban C, Italiano G. Electrical stimulation of the dorsal nerve of the penis evokes reflex tonic erections of the penile body and reflex ejaculatory responses in the spinal rat. J Urol. 1993;149:627–32.
11. Allard J, Edmunds NJ. Reflex penile erection in anesthetized mice: an exploratory study. Neuroscience. 2008;155:283–90.
12. Rampin O, Giuliano F, Dompeyre P, Rousseau JP. Physiological evidence of neural pathways involved in reflexogenic penile erection in the rat. Neurosci Lett. 1994;180:138–42.
13. Bernabé J, Rampin O, Sachs BD, Giuliano F. Intracavernous pressure during erection in rats: an integrative approach based on telemetric recording. Am J Phys. 1999;276:R441–9.
14. Schmidt MH, Valatx JL, Sakai K, Debilly G, Jouvet M. Corpus spongiosum penis pressure and perineal muscle activity during reflexive erections in the rat. Am J Phys. 1995;269:R904–13.
15. Nout YS, Schmidt MH, Tovar CA, Culp E, Beattie MS, Bresnahan JC. Telemetric monitoring of corpus spongiosum penis pressure in conscious rats for assessment of micturition and sexual function following spinal cord contusion injury. J Neurotrauma. 2005;22:429–41.
16. Holmes GM, Chapple WD, Leipheimer RE, Sachs BD. Electromyographic analysis of male rat perineal muscles during copulation and reflexive erections. Physiol Behav. 1991;49:1235 46.
17. Monaghan EP, Breedlove SM. The role of the bulbocavernosus in penile reflex behavior in rats. Brain Res. 1992;587:178–80.
18. Johnson RD, Chadha HK, Dugan VP, Gupta DS, Ferrero SL, Hubscher CH. Bilateral Bulbospinal projections to pudendal Motoneuron circuitry after chronic spinal cord Hemisection injury as revealed by Transsynaptic tracing with pseudorabies virus. J Neurotrauma. 2011;28:595–605.
19. Rose RD, Collins WF. Crossing dendrites may be a substrate for synchronized activation of penile motoneurons. Brain Res. 1985;337:373–7.
20. Tang Y, Rampin O, Calas A, Facchinetti P, Giuliano F. Oxytocinergic and serotonergic innervation of identified lumbosacral nuclei controlling penile erection in the male rat. Neuroscience. 1997;82:241–54.
21. Marson L, Platt KB, McKenna KE. Central nervous system innervation of the penis as revealed by the transneuronal transport of pseudorabies virus. Neuroscience. 1993;55:263–80.
22. Hubscher CH, Reed WR, Kaddumi EG, Armstrong JE, Johnson RD. Select spinal lesions reveal multiple ascending pathways in the rat conveying input from the male genitalia. J Physiol. 2010;588:1073–83.
23. Tang Y, Rampin O, Giuliano F, Ugolini G. Spinal and brain circuits to motoneurons of the bulbospongiosus muscle: retrograde transneuronal tracing with rabies virus. J Comp Neurol. 1999;414:167–92.
24. Staudt MD, Truitt WA, McKenna KE, de Oliveira CVR, Lehman MN, Coolen LM. A pivotal role of lumbar spinothalamic cells in the regulation of ejaculation via Intraspinal connections. J Sex Med. 2012;9:2256–65.
25. Aïoun J, Rampin O. Anatomical evidence for glutamatergic transmission in primary sensory neurons and onto postganglionic neurons controlling penile erection in rats: an ultrastructural study with neuronal tracing and immunocytochemistry. Cell Tissue Res. 2005;323:359–75.
26. Rampin O. Spinal control of erection by glutamate in rats. Am J Physiol Regul Integr Comp Physiol. 2004;286:710R–718.
27. Vargas VM, Torres D, Corona F, Vergara M, Gómez LE, Delgado-Lezama R, et al. Cholinergic facilitation of erection and ejaculation in spinal cord-transected rats. Int J Impot Res. 2004;16:86–90.
28. Yaici ED, Rampin O, Calas A, Jestin A, McKenna KE, Leclerc P, et al. α2a and α2c adrenoceptors on spinal neurons controlling penile erection. Neuroscience. 2002;114:945–60.
29. Holmes GM, Bresnahan JC, Beattie MS. Inhibition of pudendal reflexes in spinal rats. Reassessing the role of serotonin. Physiol Behav. 2001;74:57–64.
30. Xu C, Giuliano F, Sun XQ, Brisorgueil M-J, Leclerc P, Vergé D, et al. Serotonin 5-HT2A and 5-HT5A receptors are expressed by different motoneuron populations in rat Onuf's nucleus. J Comp Neurol. 2007;502:620–34.
31. Rubio-Casillas A, Rodríguez-Quintero CM, Rodríguez-Manzo G, Fernández-Guasti A. Unraveling the modulatory actions of serotonin on male rat sexual responses. Neurosci Biobehav Rev. 2015;55:234–46.
32. Hsieh GC. Central mechanisms regulating penile erection in conscious rats: the dopaminergic systems related to the Proerectile effect of Apomorphine. J Pharmacol Exp Ther. 2003;308:330–8.
33. Paredes RG, Holmes GM, Sachs BD, Agmo A. Electromyographic activity of rat ischiocavernosus muscles during copulation after treatment with a GABA-transaminase inhibitor. Behav Neural Biol. 1993;60:118–22.
34. Dorfman VB, Vega MC, Coirini H. Age-related changes of the GABA-B receptor in the lumbar spinal cord of male rats and penile erection. Life Sci. 2006;78:1529–34.
35. Giuliano F, Bernabé J, McKenna K, Longueville F, Rampin O. Spinal proerectile effect of oxytocin in anesthetized rats. Am J Physiol Regul Integr Comp Physiol. 2001;280:R1870–7.
36. Miura A, Kawatani M, Maruyama T, de Groat WC. Effect of prostaglandins on parasympathetic neurons in the rat lumbosacral spinal cord. Neuroreport. 2002;13:1557.

37. Derouet H, Nolden W, Jost WH, Osterhage J, Eckert RE, Ziegler M. Treatment of erectile dysfunction by an external ischiocavernous muscle stimulator. Eur Urol. 1998;34:355–9.
38. de Medinaceli L. An anatomical landmark for procedures on rat thoracic spinal cord. Exp Neurol. 1986;91:404–8.
39. MacKenzie LD, Heaton JPW, Adams MA. Impact of systemically active Neurohumoral factors on the erectile response of the rat. J Sex Med. 2011;8:2461–71.
40. Bernabé J, Rampin O, Giuliano F, Benoit G. Intracavernous pressure changes during reflexive penile erections in the rat. Physiol Behav. 1995;57:837–41.
41. Ishizuka O, Gu B-J, Nishizawa O, Mizusawa H, Anderson KNE. Effect of apomorphine on intracavernous pressure and blood pressure in conscious, spinalized rats. Int J Impot Res. 2002;14:128–32.
42. Giuliano F, Rampin O, Bernabé J, Rousseau JP. Neural control of penile erection in the rat. J Auton Nerv Syst. 1995;55:36–44.
43. Baba K, Yajima M, Carrier S, Akkus E, Reman J, Nunes L, et al. Effect of testosterone on the number of NADPH diaphorase-stained nerve fibers in the rat corpus cavernosum and dorsal nerve. Urology. 2000;56:533–8.
44. Holmes GM, Sachs BD. Erectile function and bulbospongiosus EMG activity in estrogen-maintained castrated rats vary with behavioral context. Horm Behav. 1992;26:406–19.
45. Ardc D, Tdw D. The influence of certain ganglionic blocking agents on neuromuscular transmission. Br J Anaesth. 1958;30:217–25.
46. Gergis SD, Sokoll MD, Rubbo JT. Effect of sodium nitroprusside and trimetaphan on neuromuscular transmission in the frog. Can Anaesth Soc J. 1977;24:220–7.
47. Nakamura K, Hatano Y, Mori K. The site of action of trimethaphan-induced neuromuscular blockade in isolated rat and frog muscle. Acta Anaesthesiol Scand. 1988;32:125–30.
48. Santajuliana D, Hornfeldt BJ, Osborn JW. Use of ganglionic blockers to assess neurogenic pressor activity in conscious rats. J Pharmacol Toxicol Methods. 1996;35:45–54.
49. Wali FA. Effect of angiotensin II on mechanical and electrical responses of frog, chick and rat skeletal muscle. Arch Int Pharmacodyn Ther. 1986;282:314–27.
50. Augusto Oliveira F, Silveira PE, Lopes MJ, Kushmerick C, Naves LA. Angiotensin II increases evoked release at the frog neuromuscular junction through a receptor sensitive to A779. Brain Res. 2007;1175:48–53.
51. Steers WD, Mallory B, de Groat WC. Electrophysiological study of neural activity in penile nerve of the rat. Am J Phys. 1988;254:R989–1000.
52. Kitchell RL, Gilanpour H, Johnson RD. Electrophysiologic studies of penile mechanoreceptors in the rat. Exp Neurol. 1982;75:229–244.
53. Dobberfuhl AD, Oti T, Sakamoto H, Marson L. Identification of CNS neurons innervating the Levator Ani and Ventral Bulbospongiosus muscles in male rats. J Sex Med. 2014;11:664–77.
54. McKenna KE, Nadelhaft I. The pudendo-pudendal reflex in male and female rats. J Auton Nerv Syst. 1989;27:67–77.
55. Sachs BD, Liu YC. Copulatory behavior and reflexive penile erection in rats after section of the pudendal and genitofemoral nerves. Physiol Behav. 1992;51:673–80.
56. Peikert K, May CA. Muscle spindles in the human bulbospongiosus and ischiocavernosus muscles. Muscle Nerve. 2015;52:55–62.
57. Yang CC, Bradley WE. Reflex innervation of the bulbocavernosus muscle. BJU Int. 2001;85:857–63.
58. Contreras JL, Agmo A. Sensory control of the male rat's copulatory thrusting patterns. Behav Neural Biol. 1993;60:234–40.
59. Mallory B, Steers WD, de Groat WC. Electrophysiological study of micturition reflexes in rats. Am J Phys. 1989;257:R410–21.

Does anchoring vaginal mesh increase the potential for correcting stress incontinence?

Zoltán Fekete[1,2*], Szilvia Kőrösi[2], László Pajor[1], Zoltán Bajory[1], Gábor Németh[2] and Zoltan Kozinszky[3]

Abstract

Background: This study aims to explore the feasibility of anchoring a four-arm transvaginal mesh (TVM) to the mid-*urethra* to correct an anterior compartment POP–Quantification stage II–III (Q II–III) and concomitant genuine SUI.

Methods: We analysed clinical data from 248 patients with stage II–III anterior prolapse and concomitant SUI who had undergone surgery at a tertiary referral centre in Hungary between January 2008 and June 2010. One hundred and twenty-four women treated with anterior *colporrhaphy* and 62 patients implanted with a conventional permanent TVM were selected as historical matched controls. Sixty-two patients received a modified permanent TVM, where the mesh was fixed to the mid-*urethra* with two stitches for the purpose of potentially correcting SUI. Surgical complications were classified using the Clavien–Dindo (CD) classification system.

Results: The anti-SUI efficacy was minimally higher in the mTVM group than in the original TVM group ($p = 0.44$, 96.8% vs 91.9%, respectively), while prosthesis surgery was more effective than anterior *colporrhaphy* in improving the anterior compartment POP–Q status (96.8, 90.3% vs 64.5%, respectively). Anchoring the mesh did not increase the extrusion rate ($p = 0.11$). The de novo urge symptoms were not more prevalent among those who had received additional periurethral stitches ($p = 1.00$, 11.3% vs 12.9%). The incidence of reoperation observed in the mTVM group was non-significantly lower than that in the TVM group ($p = 0.15$, 6.5% vs 16.1%); however, the difference did not reach the level of significance. The early postoperative complication profile was more favourable among the mTVM patients (classified as CD I: 8.1%; CD II: 1.6%; and CD IIIb: 1.6%) as compared to the TVM group ($p = 0.013$).

Conclusions: The new, modified mesh surgery represents an effective procedure for prolapse and concomitant SUI with a decreased risk of short- and long-term complications.

Keywords: Modified transvaginal mesh, Transobturator tape, Anterior colporrhaphy, Complications, SUI with POP–Q II, Clavien–Dindo classification

Background

Coexisting stress urinary incontinence (SUI) and pelvic organ prolapse (POP) are highly prevalent (63–80%) [1], and the cumulative risk of surgery for POP or SUI by the age of 80 years has been estimated at 11.1% [2, 3]. Despite the availability of a wide variety of prolapse surgery, there is no consensus on the optimal treatment. Vaginal prosthetic surgery has been proposed for anterior compartment POP–Quantification (Q) stage II–III (International Continence Society/International Urogynecological Association) [4] in view of the low recurrence rate (6.7–24%) [5–8] relative to that after classical anterior *colporrhaphy* (30–40%) [6, 8, 9]. A recent Cochrane review confirms the superiority of repairing prolapse of the mid-anterior vaginal wall with permanent mesh over native tissue repair [8]. However, a worldwide spread of a range of vaginal mesh operations has resulted in a huge number of complications (e.g. infection, extrusion and de novo urge symptoms). As a consequence, the US Food and Drug Administration has published warnings with the aim of restricting the utilization of vaginal prosthesis to centres with specially trained surgeons after patients have been thoroughly informed [10]. Furthermore, it is assumed that a combination of a synthetic mesh with the sling operation [11–13] will substantially increase the cure rate of concomitant SUI. In contrast, the combined

* Correspondence: fekete.zoltan@med.u-szeged.hu
[1]Department of Urology, University of Szeged, Hungary, Semmelweis u. 1, Szeged H-6725, Hungary
[2]Department of Obstetrics and Gynaecology, University of Szeged, Hungary, Semmelweis u. 1, Szeged H-6725, Hungary
Full list of author information is available at the end of the article

techniques represent an increased complication rate and elevated financial burden.

It is well known that the supporting position of the prosthesis differs slightly with the transvaginal mesh (TVM) and transobturator tape (TVT-O). The TVT-O sling is located under the mid-*urethra*, whereas the TVM elevates the whole anterior and middle compartment [14]. TVM produces a significantly weaker anti-SUI effect compared to that of the TVT-O since TVM elevates the urinary bladder neck [7]. Furthermore, we hypothesise that the original TVM operation can be followed by residual SUI as the strengthening of the back arms may result in a backward sliding of the entire mesh, leading to a lack of suspension of the *urethra*.

We propose a modification of the four-arm TVM procedure in an attempt to achieve a better SUI correction, without any decrease in prolapse repair efficacy. We have developed a new method where the mesh is sutured to the mid-*urethra* in order to prevent the backward sliding, and, in this way, the anterior arms mainly elevate the middle part of the urethra, potentially leading to effective anti-incontinence. In other words, the anchored mesh takes over the function of the *pubourethral ligament*, which should normally stabilize the *urethra*, but is loose in SUI.

We demonstrate an alternative operative method for POP–Q II–III repair and anti-incontinence with the TVM fixed to the mid-*urethra*. The efficacy and short- and long-term complication profiles of this new surgical technique were compared with those of historical controls involving original TVM and anterior *colporrhaphy* operations at our departments.

Methods

The prospective longitudinal cohort study comprised 62 women who presented for the correction of SUI in conjunction with symptomatic anterior compartment POP–Q II–III at the Departments of Urology and Obstetrics and Gynaecology, University of Szeged, Hungary, between January 2010 and June 2010. The trial was conducted in accordance with the IDEAL consensus. After the idea (IDEAL stage 1) of concomitant surgery for SUI and POP was developed, ten operations were performed with a high cure rate of both symptoms in all cases after four weeks (IDEAL stage 2). Based on these data, TVM or *anterior colporrhaphy* and delayed TVT-O for SUI and coexisting POP repair have been replaced by the new surgery in our departments (IDEAL stage 3) [15]. The patients were monitored during monthly outpatient appointments in the first six months; thereafter, check-ups occurred every half year. The Institutional Review Board regularly reviewed the clinical data on the patients.

Our work was carried out in accordance with the Code of Ethics of the World Medical Association (Declaration of Helsinki) for experiments involving humans and was approved by the Ethics Committee, Faculty of Medicine, University of Szeged (Protocol No. 194/2010). The Institutional Review Board supervised patient monitoring. Written informed consent was obtained from all participants after the advantages and possible complications of the modified surgery were explained in detail.

All the patients who exhibited coexisting symptoms (both SUI and POP–Q II–III) were recruited prospectively into the study. The symptomatic POP–Q stage II–III anterior prolapse is defined as the maximum extent of the prolapsed anterior vaginal wall being within 1 cm above and 6 cm below the hymen [4, 16]. According to the international POP guidelines (the EBU and NICE guidelines) [17, 18], if the condition disrupts the patient's life and nonsurgical treatment options have not helped, it should be treated surgically. POP repair was considered effective if a significant (> 1 cm) improvement was measured at points Aa, Ba and C and in total vaginal length (TVL) during the follow-up in accordance with the POP–Q system (International Continence Society) [4, 16]. Anti-incontinence efficacy was determined if no further SUI was diagnosed by urodynamic examination.

In all cases, urodynamic examinations comprising uroflowmetry, cystometrography and abdominal leak point pressure tests were performed before surgery to objectively determine the coexisting symptomatic SUI based on the international guidelines (the EBU and NICE guidelines) [15, 16]. The abdominal leak point pressure test was used as a standardised examination method for the evaluation of SUI with urine leakage as a sign. If the intraabdominal pressure recorded at the point of urine leakage was less than 40 cmH_2O, the origin of the SUI was set as intrinsic *sphincter* deficiency (ISD) [19]. In the case of ISD, preoperative pelvic floor muscle training (PFMT) was recommended. If the patient was unwilling to do PFMT or the training was unsuccessful, a modified TVM operation was recommended. This was also recommended in the case of suspected urethral hypermobility – i.e. if the intraabdominal pressure at the point of urine leakage was higher than 60 cmH_2O. Preoperative irritating voiding symptoms were not an exclusion criterion before the study.

All the data were collected prospectively. Further inclusion criteria in the study were negative urinary culturing and ineffective non-surgical treatment or patient's unwillingness to receive conservative treatment. The exclusion criteria were as follows: occult SUI, a history of mesh use or anti-incontinence pelvic procedures, antidepressant therapy, pregnancy, whether the patient was in the puerperal period and up to six months post-partum, and cancer of the pelvic organs.

There are no clear international recommendations on surgical anterior compartment POP–Q II repair, but an increasing body of evidence suggests that TVM is a better treatment option for anterior wall prolapse ≥ stage II than traditional anterior *colporrhaphy* [7, 20, 21]. We have modified the transobturator TVM operation reported by Sergent et al. [7] by inserting two additional stabilizing sutures which fix the anterior edge of the mesh to the paraurethral tissues at the level of the mid-*urethra.* All operations were carried out with 100% polypropylene monofilament permanent meshes produced by Aspide® SURGIMESH® PROLAPSE (Aspide Médical, La Talaudière, France). The implanted vaginal prosthesis has pores which are 1.6 × 1.7 mm in size and is approved for anterior vaginal repair.

Surgery was performed under general anaesthesia with the patient in the lithotomy position with an indwelling urinary catheter. The anterior vaginal wall was incised longitudinally throughout its thickness from the cervix to 1 cm below the urethral meatus, under the mid-*urethra.* The thickness of the dissection, the location of the vaginal incision, the placement of the mesh and the closure of the incision varied only minimally, and the length of the incision varied only between 6 and 7 cm. Before insertion, all sterile meshes were soaked in iodic fluid (Betadine®). The Surgimesh® device was introduced beneath the dissection. Its four arms were then passed through the obturator membrane. The posterior part of the mesh was anchored to the anterior side of the cervix using two Prolene® 2–0 sutures (Ethicon, Issy-les-Moulineaux, France).

The mesh was then spread by securing its anterior parts beneath the mid-*urethra* using two Vicryl 2–0® absorbable sutures (Ethicon, Issy-les-Moulineaux, France) and promoting the proper elevation and closure of the *urethra* (Fig. 1). The mesh was then adjusted in a tension-free manner beneath the distal part of the urethra and bladder, and the anterior vaginal wall was closed using Monocryl® 3–0 absorbable sutures (Ethicon, Issy-les-Moulineaux, France) with a slight colpectomy. All the operations were performed by the same two experienced senior surgeons, and there were no differences in the operative processes.

Prophylactic preoperative antibiotics (cefazolin 1 g, amoxicillin and clavulanic acid 1.2 g or gentamycin 160 mg) were administered intravenously. A urinary catheter was removed on the morning of the postoperative day. A vaginal gauze pack (gauze soaked in Betadine iodine) was placed for 12 h. The post-voided residual urine was measured by ultrasonography before each patient was discharged. All the patients participated in topical intravaginal oestrogen cream treatment for at least twelve months following the operation (Ovestin® 1 mg/gram daily), but none of the patients took part in preoperative oral hormone replacement therapy. The follow-up period after the modified TVM operation was 36 months.

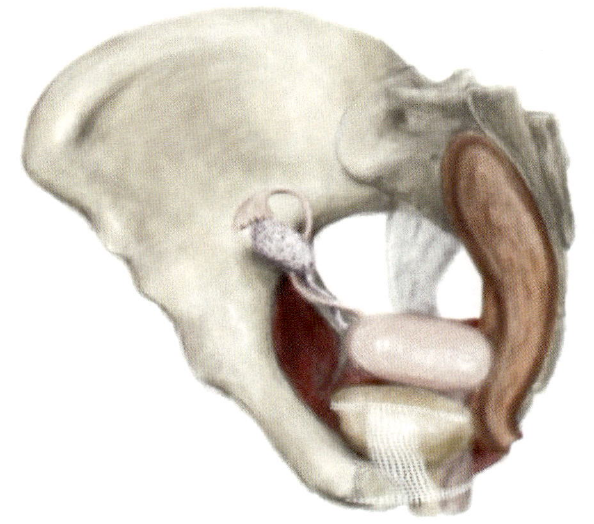

Fig. 1 Anchoring stitches stabilize the mesh position under the mid-urethra

The historical controls comprised 62 patients with genuine SUI verified by urodynamic examination with grades of POP II–III who had originally undergone a TVM operation (control group I). A further 124 patients with anterior compartment symptomatic POP–Q II and any SUI corrected by anterior *colporrhaphy* operations (control group II) were also operated on by the same two senior surgeons at the departments. The data on the historical controls were retrieved retrospectively from the medical database between January 2008 and December 2009. Eligibility for the operation and consistent collection of outcome measurements (operative characteristics and post-operative findings) were tied to a follow-up schedule which was routinely established in the historical groups. This schedule was followed for the mTVM group as well. The follow-up period in the control groups was also three years. Baseline and follow-up evaluations after six weeks to three years were performed by an experienced urogynaecologist. All the patients were given an appointment for the subsequent medical consultation according to a follow-up arrangement (Table 1). When a patient missed an appointment, a urogynaecologist reminded her by telephone, and, hence, there was no registered loss due to lack of follow-up in our samples. For each case, we matched controls in each control arm (groups I and II) who were as similar as possible in age, systemic diseases, and previous parity and vaginal operations.

The factors studied were the demographic and patient data, the intraoperative findings and postoperative factors. Furthermore, the incidence of systemic chronic diseases that might have a detrimental effect on the healing process (i.e. in *diabetes mellitus* and autoimmune diseases) was also recorded, and displacement of the implant due to chronic coughing in airway

Table 1 Schedule of assessments/data collection for both

Assessment	Recruitment before intervention phase	Intervention (Surgery)	Follow-up				
			6 weeks	6 months	1 years	2 years	3 years
Written informed consent[a]	x						
Gynaecological examination: incontinence symptoms	x	x	X	x	x	x	X
Gynaecological examination: prolapse	x	x	X	x	x	x	X
Urodynamic examination	x				x		X
Adverse events		x	X	x	x	x	X
Urine culture	x			x	x	x	X

[a]available in the modified transvaginal mesh operated women

diseases was also considered. As concerns the long-term postoperative complications of the sling and mesh procedures, we determined the rejection rate, the presence of de novo urge symptoms (DNUS) or urinary tract infection (UTI), and the need for reoperation. The diagnosis of DNUS was set if detrusor pressure changes were detected in cystometrographic pressures after the surgeries. The postoperative complications that led to reoperation were infection, recurrent descent or incontinence, implant extrusion, chronic pelvic pain and total retention. Prosthetic extrusion was diagnosed by the presence of exposed graft material in the vagina. Post-void residual urine is a measurement of the urine that remains in the bladder less than 20 min following voiding which identifies urinary retention. Bladder volumes that suggest urinary retention are commonly defined as greater than 500 to 600 ml [22, 23]. DNUS was classified as a sudden involuntary contraction of the muscular wall of the bladder causing urinary urgency, an immediate unstoppable urge to urinate with a postoperative onset.

Operative and perioperative complications (six weeks after the procedures) described after mTVM and historical operations were collated, overall frequency within all cases were calculated, and severity was graded using the Clavien–Dindo classification comprising all the follow-up periods. More specifically, additional medication due to deviation from the normal postoperative course (pain, fever, wound infection and minimal bleeding) was categorized as Grade I, UTIs requiring antibiotic treatment and SUI/POP without any postoperative correction, DNUS or blood transfusion were grouped as Grade II, and reoperation performed in general anaesthesia was graded as IIIb [22].

Statistical analysis

The SPSS 17.0 program package was used to analyse the data. The non-parametric design of the continuous variables was verified with the Shapiro–Wilk test. The categorical and continuous variables were compared with the χ^2 test and Kruskal–Wallis test, respectively. Univariate logistic regression was employed to determine the odds for continuous variables. Multiple logistic regression was used to adjust the comparisons of the groups in terms of age, previous parity, postmenopausal stage, previous vaginal operations, chronic systemic diseases, POP–Q stage and urge symptoms due to inequalities between cases and controls. A two-tailed p-value of < 0.05 was judged as significant. The power of the statistical tests ranged between 74 and 99% in the study.

Results

Table 2 presents the baseline characteristics of the participants in the study groups. Maternal age and BMI were significantly higher among the mesh-operated patients ($p < 0.001$ and $p = 0.004$, respectively). The vast majority was postmenopausal in all groups; however, the highest rate was noticed disproportionally among those who had undergone mTVM (97%).

There was a trend of patients with modified mesh having vaginal deliveries and vaginal operations at the highest rate; however, the differences between the groups were not significant. No significant differences were observed between groups in any type of chronic systemic diseases.

Table 3 lists the operative characteristics and complications, while Table 4 provides the odds and adjusted odds of the differences in baseline and surgical characteristics in the three study groups. The operation took a similar amount of time in the mTVM group as compared with the anterior *colporrhaphy* (Adjusted odds rate (AOR): 1.03) or TVM (AOR: 0.97) control group. The estimated blood loss during the operation was significantly lower in the mTVM group than in control group I (AOR: 0.96, $p < 0.001$) and control group II (AOR: 0.96, $p < 0.001$). The occurrence of bladder injury and the need for immediate postoperative blood transfusion were negligible in all the study groups.

The reoperation rate was significantly the lowest in the mTVM group at 6.5% as compared to that in the anterior *colporrhaphy* group (32.1%) (AOR: 0.07, $p < 0.001$) and that of 16.1% in the TVM group (AOR: 0.22, $p = 0.15$). The rate of implant removal was lower among those mesh-operated patients who had undergone the modified

Table 2 Baseline characteristics of patients who presented for operation for POP–Q II–III and genuine SUI between January 2006 and December 2012

	Modified TVM group ($N = 62$)	Control group I (historical controls: TVM) (N = 62)	Control group II (historical controls: anterior colporrhaphy) ($N = 124$)	*p* value
Age (y) (mean ± S.D.)	62.9 ± 7.7	59.7 ± 10.1	55.9 ± 11.1	< 0.001
BMI (kg/m^2) (mean ± S.D.)	29.4 ± 2.9	28.4 ± 3.0	27.8 ± 3.8	0.004
Previous vaginal deliveries (mean ± S.D.)	2.3 ± 1.2	2.1 ± 0.6	2.1 ± 0.8	0.71
Postmenopausal women, n (%)	60 (96.8)	47(75.8)	92 (74.2)	0.001
Previous vaginal operations, n (%)	24 (38.7)	14 (22.6)	36 (29.0)	0.14
Chronic systemic diseases, n (%)	17 (27.4)	16 (25.8)	18 (14.5)	0.06
Diabetes mellitus, n (%)	10 (16.1)	10 (16.1)	9 (7.3)	0.09
Autoimmune diseases, n (%)	4 (6.5)	3 (4.8)	5 (4.0)	0.77
Airway diseases, n (%)	5 (8.1)	3 (4.8)	6 (4.8)	0.64

All recruited patients presented for anterior compartment POP–Q II–III (pelvic organ prolapse) and genuine SUI (stress urinary incontinence). The modified transvaginal mesh (mTVM) group comprised patients who received a four-arm mesh that was fixed to the mid-urethra. Control groups I and II include historical controls who had participated in TVM and anterior colporrhaphy without any Kelly–Stoeckel suture, respectively
Chronic systemic diseases include diabetes mellitus, airway diseases and autoimmune diseases

technique than those with the original TVM (AOR: 0.13, 1.6% vs 9.7%, respectively); however, the difference did not reach a significant level. One reoperation occurred in the mTVM group due to apical compartment POP (1.6%), another (1.6%) was performed due to anterior compartment descent after the removal of the extruded mesh, a third (1.6%) for SUI and a fourth (1.6%) for postoperative pain. In addition, reoperation due to postoperative POP had a frequency of 8.1%, and one patient (1.6%) required reoperation due to SUI in the original TVM group. The *colporrhaphy* patients needed more reoperations (32.1%), and the difference was robust (AOR: 0.007). All the cases involving POP recurrence (3.2 and 9.7%, AOR: 2.94) following the two mesh operations were found in the untreated compartment, posteriorly behind the mesh-supported area. The recurrence of anterior compartment POP (35.5%, $p < 0.001$) and SUI (38.7%, $p < 0.001$) or reoperation due to recurrence of SUI (8.9%, AOR: 0.11, $p = 0.06$) and POP (25.0%, AOR: 0.05, $p < 0.001$) during the follow-up period was typical of the anterior *colporrhaphy* patients. As expected, slightly more cases of SUI were cured in the mTVM group than in the TVM group (96.8% vs 91.9%), although the differences were not significant (AOR: 2.98). Prolapse repair was achieved in a significantly higher proportion of the patients who underwent mTVM compared to their anterior *colporrhaphy* counterparts (96.8% vs 64.5%, AOR: 14.16 $p < 0.001$). Modification of the TVM displayed a moderate effect on POP recurrence compared to the original operation (9.7%) (AOR: 2.94, $p = 0.27$). Urinary tract infection was not more prevalent after the prosthesis operations than after anterior *colporrhaphy*. The rate of extrusion was nearly four times higher in the TVM group than in the mTVM group (AOR: 0.13, $p = 0.11$), with extrusion appearing earlier in the group that underwent a non-modified operation. All implants were removed because of the extrusion of the vaginal wall. No rectal or bladder *fistula*, pelvic abscess or *haematoma* was observed in any of the groups.

Modifying the TVM technique led to a signicantly higher elevation of point Aa compared to the traditional TVM (AOR: 4.83) with a significantly reduced shortening of the vagina (AOR: 0.41). The mTVM significantly improved the prolapse status (POP–Q of Aa, AOR: 142.9; Ba, AOR: 5.95; and C, AOR: 25.0) compared to that of anterior colporrhaphy, whereas the total vaginal length was significantly shortened ($p < 0.001$) (Table 5).

Table 6 demonstrates the postoperative complications within six weeks according to the Clavien–Dindo classification. A total complication rate of 11.3% in the mTVM group, 35.5% in the TVM group and 22.6% in the *colporrhaphy* group was noted with significant differences ($p = 0.013$). Subanalyses were performed indicating that the complications occurred with a non-significantly lower prevalence among the mTVM participants compared to the anterior *colporrhaphy* group (AOR: 0.56, $p = 0.3$), whereas the difference was significantly lower in the mTVM group than among the TVM participants (AOR: 0.29, $p = 0.02$) (data are not shown). CD I complications predominantly occurred in the two groups of women operated on with prostheses, whereas the historical anterior *colporrhaphy* operations were followed mostly by CD II.

Discussion

The most striking result of this study is that the transvaginal implantation of the four-arm mesh sutured to the mid-*urethra*, a new modification of the TVM procedure [7], is highly effective in the repair of an *anterior* prolapse (POP–Q II–III) and in genuine stress urinary incontinence (SUI). Success rates of 96.8 and 96.8% were

Table 3 Operative characteristics and postoperative complications of patients who presented for operation for POP–Q II–III and genuine SUI between January 2006 and December 2012

	Modified TVM group (N = 62)	Control group I (historical controls: TVM) (*N* = 62)	Control group II (historical controls: anterior colporrhaphy) (N = 124)	*p* value
POP grading				
grade II	50 (80.6)	59 (95.2)	124 (100)	< 0.001
grade III	12 (19.4)	3 (4.8)	0 (0)	
Urge symptoms	8 (12.9)	2 (3.2)	7 (5.6)	0.08
Duration of operation (min) (mean ± S.D.)	37.8 ± 7.4	38.8 ± 6.0	34.9 ± 7.9	< 0.001
Estimated blood loss (ml) (mean ± S.D.)	48.7 ± 21.8	83.8 ± 41.2	74.0 ± 33.4	< 0.001
Intraoperative bladder injury, n (%)	1 (1.6)	0 (0)	0 (0)	0.22
Blood transfusion, n (%)	0 (0)	0 (0)	1 (0.8)	0.61
Reoperation, n (%)	4 (6.5)	10 (16.1)	40 (32.3)	< 0.001
POP–Q, n (%)	2 (3.2)	5 (8.1)	31 (25.0)	< 0.001
SUI, n (%)	1 (1.6)	1 (1.6)	11 (8.9)	0.04
Vaginal wall extrusion, n (%)	1 (1.6)	6 (9.7)	0 (0)	0.11
Postoperative bleeding, n (%)	0 (0)	3 (4.8)	1 (0.8)	0.06
Postoperative pain, n (%)	1 (1.6)	0 (0)	0 (0)	0.22
Total retention, n (%)	0 (0)	1 (1.6)	1 (0.8)	0.61
Successful treatment of POP–Q, n (%)	60 (96.8)	56 (90.3)	80 (64.5)	< 0.001
Successful treatment of SUI, n (%)	60 (96.8)	47 (75.8)	76 (61.3)	< 0.001
Urinary tract infection, n (%)	11 (17.7)	14 (22.6)	23 (18.5)	0.75
De novo urge incontinence, n (%)	7 (11.3)	8 (12.9)	0 (0)	< 0.001
Average time to observed extrusion (months) (mean ± S.D.)	1 ± 0	13.7 ± 8.3	n.m.[a]	0.13

All recruited patients presented for anterior compartment POP–Q II–III (pelvic organ prolapse) and genuine SUI (stress urinary incontinence). The modified transvaginal mesh (mTVM) group comprised patients who received a four-arm mesh that was fixed to the mid-urethra. Control groups I and II include historical controls who participated in TVM and anterior colporrhaphy without any Kelly–Stoeckel suture, respectively. n.m.[a], not measurable

demonstrated for genuine SUI and prolapse, respectively. This surgical procedure for prosthetic placement provided a minimally better SUI reconstructive effect than that of the TVM procedure in our historical control group (91.9%) or that reported in the literature (69–90.3%) [24–26]. With regard to the POP repair, mTVM (96.8%) proved significantly more effective than historical anterior colporrhaphy (64.5%), but only minimally higher than that of the non-modified, transobturator mesh technique in our database (90.3%) and that demonstrated in the literature (with a rate of 82.3–100%) [5, 20, 21, 26–29]. Fixing the *anterior* arm of the mesh to the *periurethral* tissue elevates point Aa significantly more effectively than the original TVM with less vaginal shortening.

TVM supports the whole of the anterior and middle compartments, but does not elevate the middle of the *urethra* and, hence, theoretically allows for urethral dorsal rotation, which may lead to residual SUI, especially if the mesh is able to migrate a bit more posteriorly toward the cervix. It is also possible that mesh movements could be responsible for DNUS with the traditional TVM method. Using stabilizing sutures to fix the mesh to the paraurethral tissues at the level of the mid-*urethra*, where the *pubourethral* ligament originally held it, helps to elevate the middle region, this being considered the treatment of SUI that is at least as effective as the TVT-O technique (91.2% in our non-published data and 92% in the literature) [30]. In other words, anchoring the anterior part of the mesh to the mid-*urethra* imitates the mechanism of action of the mid-*urethral* sling as an additional procedure for SUI correction. The original TVM has a limited anti-SUI mechanism.

Furthermore, our results suggest a better anatomical success rate after the mesh is fixed to the mid-*urethra*, which may be explained by the lack of shrinkage and less folding of the mesh. By contrast, our results might allow for the speculation that prosthesis stabilization with sutures to prevent any backward movement could lead to prolapse recurrence in the untreated middle compartment, i.e. in the area not supported by the mesh.

We attribute our lower anatomical recurrence of mTVM to a wider suspension area of the insertion of a smooth, non-folded mesh. To check on this, we have launched a further study at our department, in which the posterior arms of the TVM are anchored towards the pericervical ring to provide apical support.

Table 4 Crude odds ratios (OR) and adjusted OR (AOR) for confounders in various comparisons of patients who presented for operation for POP–Q II–III and genuine SUI between January 2006 and December 2012

	Modified TVM group vs Control group I (historical controls: TVM)			Modified TVM group vs Control group II (historical controls: anterior colporrhaphy)		
	p value	Unadjusted OR (95% CI)	Adjusted OR[a] (95% CI)	*p* value	Unadjusted OR (95% CI)	Adjusted OR[a] (95% CI)
Age	0.05	1.04 (1.00–1.08)	1.02 (0.97–1.08)	< 0.001	1.07 (1.04–1.11)	1.05 (1.01–1.10)
BMI	0.05	1.13 (1.00–1.29)	1.12 (0.96–1.30)	0.001	1.14 (1.04–1.25)	1.13 (1.01–1.26)
Previous vaginal deliveries	0.26	1.28 (0.83–1.98)	1.57 (0.90–2.76)	0.45	1.15 (0.84–1.58)	1.18 (0.79–1.76)
Postmenopausal women	0.001	9.6 (2.09–4.35)	11.58 (1.78–75.1)	< 0.001	10.44 (2.41–45.2)	8.09 (0.98–67.05)
Previous vaginal operations	0.08	2.16 (0.99–4.74)	2.16 (0.86–5.44)	0.19	1.54 (0.81–2.93)	1.29 (0.59–2.80)
Chronic systemic diseases	1.00	1.09 (0.49–1.41)	0.95 (0.37–2.41)	0.045	2.23 (1.05–4.71)	1.84 (0.77–4.41)
Diabetes mellitus	1.00	1.00 (0.38–2.60)	0.77 (0.16–4.46)	0.07	2.46 (0.94–6.11)	0.86 (0.19–3.88)
Autoimmune diseases	1.00	1.36 (0.29–6.33)	3.23 (0.41–25.67)	0.48	1.64 (0.43–0.34)	1.99 (0.34–11.59)
Airway disorders	0.72	1.72 (0.40–2.58)	0.90 (0.15–5.54)	0.51	1.73 (0.51–5.89)	0.4 (0.08–2.14)
POP–Q III vs II	0.02	4.71 (1.26–17.5)	6.32 (1.07–37.52)	< 0.001	1.24 (1.10–4.40)	1.36 (1.08–4.10)
Urge symptoms	0.09	4.44 (0.90–21.74)	4.85 (0.91–25.94)	0.10	2.48 (0.85–7.18)	3.02 (0.84–10.90)
Duration of operation	0.41	0.98 (0.93–1.03)	0.97 (0.91–1.03)	0.22	1.05 (1.01–1.09)	1.03 (0.98–1.09)
Estimated average blood loss	< 0.001	0.96 (0.95–0.98)	0.96 (0.94–0.98)	< 0.001	0.96 (0.94–0.97)	0.96 (0.94–0.98)
Intraoperative bladder injury[b]	1.00	1.02 (0.98–1.05)	n.m.[b]	0.33	1.02 (0.99–1.05)	n.m.[b]
Blood transfusion	n.m[b]	n.m[b]	n.m.[b]	1.00	0.99 (0.98–1.01)	n.m.[b]
Reoperation[b]	0.15	0.36 (0.11–1.21)	0.22 (0.04–1.10)	< 0.001	0.15 (005–0.43)	0.07 (0.02–0.32)
POP	0.44	0.38 (0.07–2.04)	0.26 (0.04–1.96)	< 0.001	0.10 (0.02–0.43)	0.05 (0.006–0.41)
SUI	1.00	1.00 (0.06–16.39)	0.19 (0.01–5.7)	0.06	0.17 (0.02–1.34)	0.11 (0.06–0.89)
Vaginal wall extrusion	0.11	0.15 (0.02–1.31)	0.13 (0.009–1.71)	n.m	n.m.[b]	n.m.[b]
Bleeding	0.24	0.95 (0.90–1.01)	n.m.[b]	1.00	0.99 (0.98–1.01)	0.89 (0.68–1.12)
Postoperative pain	1.00	1.02 (0.98–1.05)	n.m.[b]	0.33	1.02 (0.99–1.05)	n.m.[b]
Total retention	1.00	0.98 (0.95–1.02)	n.m.[b]	1.00	0.99 (0.98–1.01)	n.m.[b]
Successful treatment of POP–Q	0.27	3.22 (0.62–16.67)	2.94 (0.47–18.6)	< 0001	16.5 (3.85–70.77)	14.16 (3.09–65.00)
Successful treatment of SUI	0.004	9.58 (2.09–43.9)	72.2 (8.56–606.65)	< 0.001	18.95 (4.43–81.13)	96.2 (7.40–1250.0)
Urinary tract infection	0.66	0.74 (0.31–1.79)	0.70 (0.26–1.87)	1.00	1.95 (0.43–2.19)	0.92 (0.34–2.45)
De novo urge symptoms	1.00	0.86 (0.29–2.53)	0.89 (0.25–3.22)	< 0.001	1.13 (1.03–1.23)	1.10 (1.06–1.19)
Average time to extrusion observed	0.99	n.m.[b]	n.m.[b]	n.m.[b]	n.m.[b]	n.m.[b]

All recruited patients presented for anterior compartment POP–Q II–III (pelvic organ prolapse) and genuine SUI (stress urinary incontinence). The modified transvaginal mesh (mTVM) group comprised patients who received a four–arm mesh that was fixed to the mid-urethra. Control groups I and II include historical controls who participated in TVM and anterior colporrhaphy without any Kelly–Stoeckel suture, respectively

OR, Odds ratio; 95% CI, 95% confidence interval,

Adjusted OR[a], All variables were adjusted for age, previous parity, postmenopausal stage, previous vaginal operations and chronic systemic diseases, POP–Q stage and urge symptoms. n.m.[b], not measurable

TVM corrects SUI subjectively in only 83.3% of cases [7]. Furthermore, subvesical mesh towards the obturator spaces in a total of 74 patients with a stage ≥2 anterior prolapse was associated with a symptomatic SUI repair in 72% of the cases, and cystocele was corrected in 97% [27]. The current trend is to resolve the concomitant SUI and POP in a single hospitalization session so as to reduce medical costs and improve the patient's satisfaction, but the optimum use of anti-incontinence procedures during pelvic reconstructive surgery remains a matter of debate [31]. A combination of mesh with a mid-*urethral* sling in one session has been scarcely studied [12, 32]. When TVM was combined with a TVT-O operation [12, 32], the success rate for SUI was 87.8–93.2% and that for anterior wall repositioning was 94.4–96%, i.e. a similar anti-incontinence and anatomical reconstruction rate than those in our study, though that follow-up was for up to 60 months. More studies are needed to evaluate whether the additional insertion of a TVT-O sling into a mesh provides any additional improvement in the SUI and POP cure rate as compared with a single TVM or modified TVM.

Table 5 Patients' preoperative and postoperative POP-Q status

	Control group I (historical controls: TVM) (N = 62)			*p* value	Unadjasted OR (95% CI)	Adjusted OR[a] (95% CI)	Modified TVM group (*N* = 62)			*p* value	Unadjasted OR (95% CI)	Adjusted OR[a] (95% CI)	Control group II (historical controls: anterior colporrhaphy) (*N* = 124)		
	Pre-operative	Post-operative	Mean difference				Pre-operative	Post-operative	Mean difference				Pre-operative	Post-operative	Mean difference
Aa	−0.97 ± 0.6	−1.37 ± 0.55	−0.40 ± 0.61	< 0.001	4.55 (2.38–9.09)	4.83 (2.26–10.31)0.6	− 0.55 ± 0.69	− 1.68 ± 0.74	− 1.13 ± 0.80	< 0.001	43.5 (1.61–125)	142.9 (28.57–500.0)	−0.97 ± 0.36	− 0.76 ± 0.69	0.21 ± 0.60
Ba	−0.42 ± 0.64	− 1.74 ± 1.0	−2.16 ± 1.04	0.50	1.12 (0.8–1.56)	1.17(0.71–1.52)	−0.53 ± 1.08	−1.76 ± 0.94	−2.3 ± 1.08	< 0.001	6.49 (3.65–11.63)	5.95 (3.27–10.87)	− 0.49 ± 0.75	− 0.94 ± 1.48	− 0.45 ± 1.17
C	−6.55 ± 1.16	−6.82 ± 0.85	−0.27 ± 0.6	0.70	0.90 (0.54–1.52)	1.20(0.66–2.16)	− 6.53 ± 0.82	− 6.76 ± 0.67	− 0.23 ± 0.58	< 0.001	23.81 (3.34–166.67)	25.0 (3.70–166.7)	− 6.74 ± 0.61	− 6.45 ± 0.83	0.29 ± 0.62
TVL	8.25 ± 0.67	7.9 ± 0.62	−0.35 ± 0.48	0.018	0.37 (0.16–0.86)	0.41(0.16–0.99)	7.82 ± 0.42	7.66 ± 0.60	−0.16 ± 0.41	< 0.001	n.m.[b]	n.m.[b]	7.91 ± 0.29	7.91 ± 0.29	0.0 ± 0.0

All recruited patients presented for anterior compartment POP-Q II–III (pelvic organ prolapse) and genuine SUI (stress urinary incontinence). The modified transvaginal mesh (mTVM) group comprised patients who received a four-arm mesh that was fixed to the mid-urethra. Control groups I and II include historical controls who participated in TVM and anterior colporrhaphy without any Kelly-Stoeckel suture, respectively

OR, Odds ratio; 95% CI, 95% confidence interval,

Adjusted OR[a], All variables were adjusted for age, previous parity, postmenopausal stage, previous vaginal operations and chronic systemic diseases, POP-Q stage and urge symptoms. n.m.[b], not measurable

Table 6 Clavien–Dindo classification for postoperative surgical complications among patients who presented for operation for POP–Q II–III and genuine SUI between January 2006 and December 2012

Clavien–Dindo grade[a]	Complications	Modified TVM group (*N* = 62)	Control group I (historical controls: TVM) (*N* = 62)	Control group II (historical controls: anterior colporrhaphy) (*N* = 124)	*p* value
I	Non–pharmacologically treated postoperative bleeding, fever, wound infection	5 (8.1)	12 (19.4)	11 (8.9)	0.013
II	Urinary tract infection, post–void residual volume, blood transfusion, treatment for de novo urge symptoms	1 (1.6)	7 (11.3)	16 (12.9)	
IIIb	Reoperation for vaginal wall extrusion	1 (1.6)	3 (4.8)	1 (0.8)	
Total complications		7 (11.3)	22 (35.5%)	28 (22.6)	0.015

CD, Clavien–Dindo. [a]No grade IIIa, IVa, IVb or V complication occurred. [b]Data are expressed as n (%)

Surprisingly, the double-sling extrusion rate was extremely low (0–10%) [12, 32]. The corresponding figures were 1.6% in our mTVM group and 9.7% among our TVM participants, which is in agreement with the mean value of 11.6% (ranging from 3.9 to 16%) reported in the literature [4, 20, 24, 27, 33, 34]. The extrusion rate generally correlates well with the prosthesis breadth; however, we observed a remarkably higher extrusion rate for mesh compared to that for modified mesh. One can speculate that the lack of stabilizing sutures led to a "folding/wrinkling" of the edge of the mesh, resulting in a lifting up and compressing of the mucosa and deranged periprosthetic vasculature. The reported incidence of prosthesis exposure for double-sling operations is not clear-cut. A wider and double prosthesis involves a greater chance of bacterial colonization, and the enhanced preparation may additionally impair blood supply to the vaginal wall.

Anterior *colporrhaphy* is inferior to mesh procedures with regard to the effectiveness of POP repair and anti-incontinence both in our database and as reported by others (37–85 and 54%, respectively) [20, 33, 35, 36]. The mTVM greatly improved the POP–Q status in all examined compartments in the vagina compared to that of colporrhaphy. However, the perioperative complication rate is diminished after non-mesh surgery (22.6%) compared to that after implant surgery (35.5%). This is supported by the literature data [20, 28, 35]; however, our modified mesh procedure produced the lowest complication rate in our dataset (11.3%). The robustly lower complication rate after the mTVM can be partly explained by the fact that the surgeons in the study received more training at the time. It is of note that there are no studies which illustrate the perioperative, short-term complications of these genitourinary surgeries.

In a single TVM series with the Perigee technique, the average blood loss was found to be 180 ml [33], which was much higher than in our mTVM data series (48.7 ml), and the mean procedure duration was also shorter in the mTVM group (37.8 min vs. 60.9 min) [36].

One of the most frequent long-term complications we observed with synthetic mesh materials in our series was DNUS (11.3% and 12.9), which is an important indicator of the level of patient satisfaction. Post-operative urodynamic examinations showed detrusor muscle action in all the cases suffering from DNUS. The average detrusor muscle pressure was 7.75 cmH_2O postoperatively, whereas no sign of detrusor or intravesical pressure elevation was detected preoperatively. We believe that one possible reason for this is the fact that the mesh cannot slide backwards and cannot press the *urethra* to the bladder neck after the TVM is modified. The average reported prevalence of de novo dyspareunia following vaginal placement of a polypropylene mesh is 14% [37], i.e. significantly higher than in our study (1.6%) (the data are not presented in a table). Mesh+sling operations impair the pelvic blood circulation and induce de novo urge symptoms and pelvic pain; however, the reported extrusion rate was 10% [32].

Our study had some limitations. The baseline characteristics of the patients were not equally distributed in the groups, and, hence, statistical adjustments were used in multivariate analyses. A further limitation of the study is its non-randomized manner. The surgeons became better trained in the operative techniques, a fact which may somehow bias the results. Moreover, it was not an aim of the study to determine the subjective curative rate of SUI or POP; however, the prospectively collected objective curative frequency was noted. Furthermore, different types of complications occur after anterior *colporrhaphy* compared to mesh operations (i.e. extrusion does not occur after *colporrhaphy*), and the total complication rate should be interpreted with caution.

Conclusions

In summary, use of a modified transvaginal mesh resulted in a higher rate of treatment success than the traditional mesh operation or non-mesh reconstructive surgery (*colporrhaphy)* for repair of anterior vaginal-wall prolapse and stress incontinence. By seeking a balance between the highly effective anti-incontinence and POP repair of the prosthesis operations and the less harmful non-mesh repairs, the mTVM could be a reasonable choice with a high SUI and coexisting POP reconstructive effect, thus ensuring lower rates of intra- and postoperative adverse events. Further randomized studies are therefore necessary to compare the efficacy of this novel intervention with that of double-sling procedures.

Abbreviations:

CD: Clavien–Dindo classification system; DNUS: De novo urge symptoms; ISD: Intrinsic sphincter deficiency; mTVM: Modified transvaginal mesh operation; PFMT: Pelvic floor muscle training; POP: Pelvic organ prolapse; POP–Q II: Pelvic organ prolapse quantification system stage II; SUI: Stress urinary incontinence; TVL: Lotal vaginal length; TVM: Transvaginal mesh operation; TVT-O: Transobturator tape operation; UTI: Urinary tract infection

Authors' contributions

Z F.: Study design, Data collection, Manuscript writing. SK Data collection. L P. Manuscript writing, Z B Data analysis, Study design, G N Study design. Z K Study design, Data analysis, Manuscript writing. All authors read and approved the final version of the manuscript.

Competing interests

The authors declare that they have no competing interests.

Author details

[1]Department of Urology, University of Szeged, Hungary, Semmelweis u. 1, Szeged H-6725, Hungary. [2]Department of Obstetrics and Gynaecology, University of Szeged, Hungary, Semmelweis u. 1, Szeged H-6725, Hungary. [3]Department of Obstetrics and Gynaecology, Blekinge Hospital, Karlskrona, Sweden.

References

1. Molander U, Milsom I, Ekelund P, Mellström D. An epidemiological study of urinary incontinence and related urogenital symptoms in elderly women. Maturitas. 1990;12(1):51–60.
2. Olsen A, Smith V, Bergstrom J, Colling J, Clark A. Epidemiology of surgically managed pelvic organ prolapse and urinary incontinence. Obstet Gynecol. 1997;89(4):501–6.
3. Rodríguez-Miasa NL, Martínez-Franco E, Aguado J, Sánchez E, Amat-Tardiu L. Pelvic organ prolapse and stress urinary incontinence, do they share the same risk factors? Eur J Obstet Gynecol Reprod Biol. 2015;190:52–7.
4. Persu C, Chapple CR, Cauni V, Gutue S, Geavlete P. Pelvic organ prolapse quantification system (POP–Q) – a new era in pelvic prolapse staging. J Med Life. 2011;4(1):75–81.
5. Letouzey V, Deffieux X, Gervaise A, Mercier G, Fernandez H, de Tayrac R. Transvaginal cystocele repair using a tension-free polypropylene mesh: more than 5 years of follow-up. Eur J Obstet Gynecol Reprod Biol. 2010;151(1):101–5.
6. Hiltunen R, Nieminen K, Takala T, Heiskanen E, Merikari M, Niemi K, Heinonen PK. Low-weight polypropylene mesh for anterior vaginal wall prolapse: a randomized controlled trial. Obstet Gynecol. 2007;110(2):455–62.
7. Sergent F, Resch B, Diguet A, Verspyck E, Marpeau L. Vaginal prolapse and stress urinary incontinence: combined treatment by a single prosthesis. Prog Urol. 2006;16(5):361–7.
8. Maher C, Feiner B, Baessler K, Christmann-Schmid C, Haya N, Marjoribanks J. Transvaginalmesh or grafts compared with native tissue repair for vaginal prolapse. Cochrane Database Syst Rev. 2016;(Issue 2) Art. No.: CD012079. DOI: 10.1002/14651858.CD012079
9. Hannestad YS, Rortveit G, Sandvik H, Hunskaar S. A community-based epidemiological survey of female urinary incontinence: the Norwegian EPINCONT. J Clin Epid. 2000;53(11):1150–7.
10. US Food and Drug Administration. UPDATE on Serious Complications Associated with Transvaginal Placement of Surgical Mesh for Pelvic Organ Prolapse: FDA Safety Communication. 2011. http://wayback.archive-it.org/7993/20170722150848/https://www.fda.gov/MedicalDevices/Safety/AlertsandNotices/ucm262435.htm
11. Abbott S, Unger CA, Evans JM, Jallad K, Mishra K, Karram MM, Iglesia CB, Rardin CR, Barber MD. Evaluation and management of complications from synthetic mesh after pelvic reconstructive surgery: a multicenter study. Am J Obstet Gynecol. 2014;210(2):163. e1–8
12. Yonguc T, Bozkurt IH, Sen V, Aydogdu O, Yonguc GN, Gunlusoy B. Double-sling procedure for the surgical management of stress urinary incontinence with concomitant anterior vaginal wall prolapse. Int Urol Nephrol. 2015;47(10):1611–7.
13. van der Ploeg JM, Oude Rengerink K, van der Steen A, van Leeuwen JH, Stekelenburg J, Bongers MY, Weemhoff M, Mol BW, van der Vaart CH, Roovers JP. Transvaginal prolapse repair with or without the addition of a midurethral sling in women with genital prolapse and stress urinary incontinence: a randomised trial. BJOG. 2015;122(7):1022–30.
14. Rane A, Kannan K, Barry C, Balakrishnan S, Lim Y, Corstlaans A. Prospective study of the perigee system for the management of cystocoeles – medium-term follow up. Aust NZ J Obstet Gynaecol. 2008;48(4):427–32.
15. McCulloch P, Altman DG, Campbell WB. No surgical innovation without evaluation: the IDEAL recommendations. Lancet. 2009;374(9695):1105–12.
16. Reid F. Assessment of pelvic organ prolapse: a practical guide to the pelvic organ prolapse quantification. Obstet Gynaecol Reprod Med. 2014;24(6):170–6.
17. Urinary incontinence in women: management 2015 NICE guidelines [CG171] https://www.nice.org.uk/guidance/cg171 Urinary Incontinence EBU Guideline 2016 https://uroweb.org/guideline/urinary-incontinence
18. Urinary Incontinence EBU Guideline 2016 November. https://uroweb.org/guideline/urinary-incontinence
19. Majoros A, Hamvas A, Keszthelyi A, Romics I. Value of testing the abdominal leak point pressure in the differential diagnosis of urinary stress incontinence. Orv. Hetilap. 2003;144(47):2321–5. [Article in Hungarian]
20. Altman D, Väyrynen T, Engh ME, Axelsen S, Falconer C. Nordic transvaginal mesh group. Anterior colporrhaphy versus transvaginal mesh for pelvic-organ prolapse. N Engl J Med. 2011;364(19):1826–36.
21. Cervigni M, Natale F, La Penna C, Panei M, Mako A. Transvaginal cystocele repair with polypropylene mesh using a tension-free technique. Int Urogynecol J Pelvic Floor Dysfunct. 2008;19(4):489–96.
22. Tubach F, Brouwer T, Dahmani S, Mantz J, Desmonts JM. Predictive factors of early postoperative urinary retention in the postanesthesia care unit. Anesth Analg. 2005;101(2):592–6.
23. Lamonerie L, Marret E, Deleuze A, Lembert N, Dupont M, Bonnet F. Prevalence of postoperative bladder distension and urinary retention detected by ultrasound measurement. Br J Anaesth. 2004;92(4):544–6.
24. Dindo D, Demartines N, Clavien PA. Classification of surgical complications: a new proposal with evaluation in a cohort of 6336 patients and results of a survey. Ann Surg. 2004;240(2):205–13.
25. Serati M, Sorice P, Bogani G, Braga A, Cantaluppi S, Uccella S, Caccia G, Salvatore S, Ghezzi F. TVT for the treatment of urodynamic stress incontinence: efficacy and adverse effects at 13-year follow-up. Neurourol Urodyn. 2017;36(1):192–7.
26. Nauth MA, Fünfgeld C. Correction of cystocele and stress incontinence with anterior trans obturator mesh. Eur J Obstet Gynecol Reprod Biol. 2007; 136(2):249–53.
27. Sergent F, Sentilhes L, Resch B, Verspyck E, Medeiros R, Descamps P, Marpeau L. Treatment of concomitant prolapse and stress urinary incontinence via a transobturator subvesical mesh without independent suburethral tape. Acta Obstet Gynecol Scand. 2010;89(2):223–9.

28. Maher C. Anterior vaginal compartment surgery. Int Urogynecol J. 2013; 24:1791–802.
29. Dwyer PL, O'Reilly BA. Transvaginal repair of anterior and posterior compartment prolapse with atrium polypropylene mesh. BJOG. 2004;111(8):831–6.
30. Giberti C, Gallo F, Cortese P, Schenone M. Transobturator tape for treatment of female stress urinary incontinence: objective and subjective results after a mean follow-up of two years. Urology. 2007;69(4):703–7.
31. Goldman HB. SUI surgery at the time of vaginal POP repair: is a surgical algorithm possible or desirable? Neurourol Urodyn. 2011;30(5):758–61.
32. Wu CJ, Chuang FC, Chu LC, Kung FT, Huang KH, Wu MP. Concomitant trocar-guided transvaginal mesh surgery with a midurethral sling in treating advanced pelvic organ prolapse associated with stress or occult stress urinary incontinence. Taiwan J Obstet Gynecol. 2013;52(4):516–22.
33. Maher C, Feiner B, Baessler K, Schmid C. Surgical management of pelvic organ prolapse in women. Cochrane Database Syst Rev. 2013;4:CD004014.
34. Barski D, Otto T, Gerullis H. Systematic review and classification of complications after anterior, posterior, apical, and total vaginal mesh implantation for prolapse repair. Surg Technol Int. 2014;24:217–24.
35. Nguyen JN, Burchette RJ. Outcome after anterior vaginal prolapse repair: a randomized controlled trial. Obstet Gynecol. 2008;111(4):891–8.
36. Kapur K, Dalal V. Mesh repair of vaginal wall prolapse. Med J Armed Forces India. 2014;70(2):105–110.
37. Deffieux X, Letouzey V, Savary D, Sentilhes L, Agostini A, Mares P, Pierre F. Prevention of complications related to the use of prosthetic meshes in prolapse surgery: guidelines for clinical practice. Eur J Obstet Gynecol Reprod Biol. 2012;165(2):170–80.

Assessment of the use of contrast enhanced ultrasound in guiding microdissection testicular sperm extraction in nonobstructive azoospermia

Shijun Zhang[1], Jing Du[1], Ruhui Tian[2], Shaowei Xie[1], Fenghua Li[1*] and Zheng Li[2]

Abstract

Background: The aim of this study is to assess the value of contrast-enhanced ultrasound (CEUS) as a new non-invasive approach to locate the testicular area in which spermatogenesis is most likely to be found in non-obstructive azoospermic testes and to evaluate the accuracy of CEUS as a predictor of successful sperm retrieval.

Methods: CEUS was performed in 120 nonobstructive azoospermia (NOA) patients. Microdissection testicular sperm extraction (M-TESE) was performed on the best and poorest perfusion areas selected by CEUS and on conventional areas.

Results: In the 187 testicles that underwent M-TESE, the sperm retrieval rates (SRRs) in the best perfusion area and poorest perfusion area over the maximal longitudinal section and conventional area were 63.1, 34.7 and 47.1%. According to receiver operating characteristic (ROC) analysis, the arrival times (AT) ≤27 s, time-to-peak intensity (TTP) ≤45 s, and peak intensity (PI) ≥11 dB were the best predictors of positive sperm retrieval. The location of the best perfusion area was able to guide M-TESE to improve the success rates.

Conclusions: Testicle CEUS is suggested to be performed in all patients with NOA. If AT≤27 s, TTP ≤ 45 s or PI≥11 dB are found in the best perfusion area, M-TESE is strongly recommended.

Keywords: Contrast-enhanced ultrasound, Microdissection testicular sperm extraction, Non-obstructive azoospermia, The sperm retrieval rate, Johnson score

Background

Microdissection testicular sperm extraction (M-TESE) combined with intracytoplasmic sperm injection (ICSI) has become a successful treatment strategy for patients with non-obstructive azoospermia (NOA). However, under certain conditions, sperm retrieval may be challenging. The sperm retrieval success rate for patients with NOA ranges from 42 to 62% and seems to be related to the method of retrieval, patient selection or histological patterns [1–3]. NOA is caused by testicular failure, which can be attributed to genetic disorders (such as sexual chromosomal abnormalities, translocation and microdeletions of the Y chromosome), cryptorchidism, testicular torsion, radiation and toxins [4, 5]. It is well established that isolated regions of spermatogenic tissue may exist in the testes of men with NOA [6, 7]. Some studies have suggested a correlation between testicular perfusion and focal spermatogenesis [8, 9]. Testicular sperm extraction has been improved by the guidance of Doppler ultrasound in several studies, but Doppler ultrasound could not precisely localize seminiferous tubules containing sperm [2, 8, 10–13] because it was not able to show the testicle microvasculature. In this study, the microvasculature within the testicle was depicted by contrast enhanced ultrasound (CEUS), and spermatozoa residuals were most likely to be found in hyperperfused

* Correspondence: fenghuali61@163.com
[1]Department of ultrasound, Renji Hospital, School of Medicine, Shanghai Jiaotong University, 160 Pujian RD, Shanghai 200127, China
Full list of author information is available at the end of the article

regions of non-obstructive azoospermic testes. Therefore, our study aimed to assess the accuracy of CEUS as a non-invasive approach to guide sperm retrieval and to evaluate whether it could be used as a predictor of successful sperm retrieval.

Methods

This prospective study was approved by the institutional review board, and written informed consent was obtained from all patients.

All the patients were collected in Renji hospital between 2015 and 2016. In the CEUS group, CEUS bilateral testis was performed in 120 consecutive patients with NOA. The control group was collected from the NOA patients, retrospectively, in 2015, and they did not receive CEUS. The diagnosis of NOA was based on the complete medical history and a physical examination, and at least three different semen specimens were analysed to confirm azoospermia according to the guidelines of WHO [14]. A relevant clinical history and examination were recorded, including age, testis volume, FSH value, and karyotype analysis. No patient had prior biopsies.

The testicle volume was calculated by the Lambert formula, length × height × width ×0.71 [15]. CEUS was performed with a PHILIPS IU22 scanner equipped with a 9 MHz L9–3 transducer, which was capable of simultaneously displaying the low mechanical index (MI) mode and a grey-scale image on a split screen. The testicles were held with a hand during CEUS to keep them from moving in the scrotum, and the epididymis was kept to the backside of the testicles. Under these conditions, the testicle was in a fixed position, which was essential to locate the best perfusion area for M-TESE. The maximal longitudinal section of the testicle was selected for CEUS, and the MI for CEUS was 0.06; then, a dose of 2.4 ml of sulfur hexafluoride microbubbles (SonoVue, Bracco, Milan, Italy) was injected into a cubital vein in a bolus via a 20-gauge needle, followed by a flush with 5 mL of 0.9% normal saline. CEUS clips until 150 s after the injection were recorded continuously for further quantitative analysis. CEUS was performed on the contralateral testicle in the same manner.

All images were analysed independently by two investigators (SJZ who has 11 years of experience in testes US, and SWX who has 10 years' experience in testes US). For every testicle, the best and poorest perfusion areas over the maximal longitudinal section were chosen, and the main vessels were not included in these areas. The distance between the best/poorest perfusion area and upper pole/anterior of the testicle was measured to locate potential spermatogenesis during M-TESE (Fig. 1). Time-intensity curves (TICs) were derived from the imaging sequences, and the regions of interest (ROIs) were manually placed on the best and poorest perfusion areas on CEUS. In quantitative analysis of CEUS, the following parameters were considered:

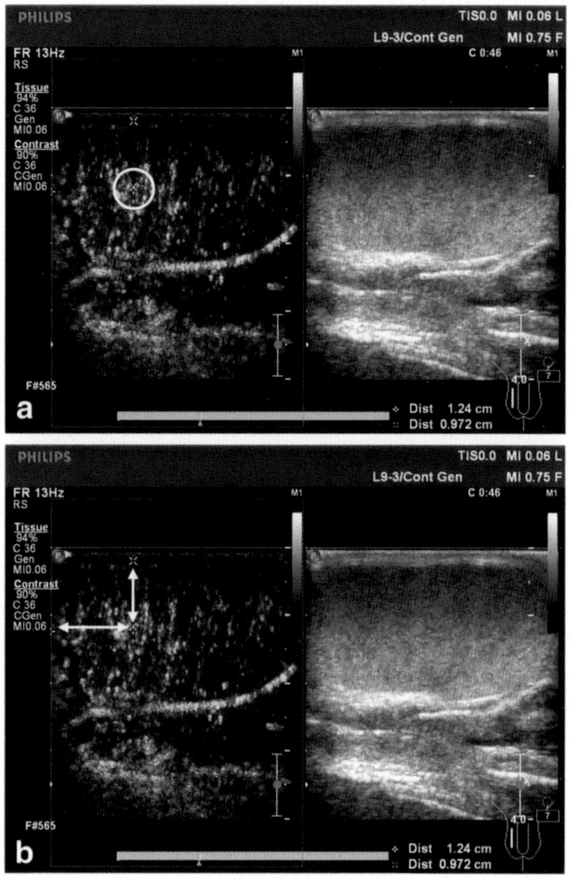

Fig. 1 The best perfusion area analysis and location. **a**: The best perfusion area (white circle) was selected. **b**: The distance between the best perfusion area and upper pole/anterior of the testicle was measured

Arrival time (AT) - the time from the injection of the agent to the point when the first contrast bubbles appeared in the testicle;

Time-to-peak intensity (TTP) - the time it took for the image intensity to reach the maximum from the injection of the agent;

Peak intensity (PI): the maximal intensity of the TIC;

Area under the curve (AUC): the area under the TIC.

The PI of the whole testicle (PIT) and AUC of the whole testicle (AUCT) were also analysed.

AT and TTP indicated the microbubble flow velocity in blood vessels. The TTP also indicated the testicle capillaries. PI indicated the maximum number of microbubbles in the capillaries, so it represented the number of capillaries. PIT indicated the number of capillaries in the entire testicle, and AUCT indicated the microbubble distribution in the entire testicle [16].

All patients underwent sperm retrieval one week after CEUS. In the CEUS group, the testicle was held in the same position as in CEUS. An incision in the equatorial plane along the mid portion at the anterior of testicle was made while the epididymis was fixed at the backside of the testicle. The mid-portion of the tunica albuginea was widely and equatorially opened in an avascular region, and with the use of an operating microscope, and seminiferous tubules that appeared larger, opaquer, and whiter were selected for seeking sperm [17]. Then, the seminiferous tubules in the best and poorest perfusion areas on CEUS were obtained separately using M-TESE. All specimens were examined by an embryologist for the surgical procedures. Any viable sperm present was cryopreserved for future ICSI. Specimens taken from the best perfusion area were sent for pathological analysis, and a Johnson score was determined for each specimen. If there was no sperm found in the testicle, the contralateral testicle underwent M-TESE in the same manner. The control group patients underwent M-TESE in the same manner without CEUS guidance. The testicle tunica albuginea was opened randomly at the upper, mid, and lower portions for seeking sperm.

Student's t-test and the chi-square test were used to compare the SRR and CEUS parameters. The correlation between the CEUS parameters and Johnson score were analysed by correlation analysis. All statistical analyses were performed using SPSS 16.0 (SPSS Inc., Chicago, USA), with $p < 0.05$ considered to be statistically significant.

Results

In the CEUS group, the mean age of 120 patients was 28.3 (21–38) years, and the mean testis volume was 7.3 ml (1.8–11.6 ml). The FSH value range was 4.25 IU/L-46.43 IU/L, and the mean value was 13.49 IU/L. There were 187 testes from 120 patients who received M-TESE. Sixty-seven patients received bilateral and 53 patients received unilateral M-TESE. Sperm was retrieved from 79 testes, and the overall sperm retrieval rate was 65.8% (79/120). In the control group, sperm was retrieved from 19 patients, and the SRR was 47.5% (19/40). The SRR of the control group was lower than CEUS-guided M-TESE ($P < 0.05$). In the 187 CEUS-guided procedures, the sperm retrieval rates (SRRs) in the best perfusion area, poorest perfusion area (over the maximal longitudinal section) and conventional area were 63.1, 34.7 and 47.1%, respectively($p < 0.05$). The correlation between the Johnson score and CEUS parameters obtained in the best perfusion area are shown in Table 1. PI and PIT had a positive correlation with the Johnson score ($P < 0.006$; $P < 0.031$). However, AT and TTP had a higher negative correlation ($P < 0.001$). AUC and AUCT had no correlation ($P > 0.05$). According to ROC analysis, AT≤27 s, TTP ≤ 45 s, and PI≥11 dB were the best cut-off point for predicting positive sperm retrieval (Fig. 2).

Table 1 Correlation of the CEUS parameters obtained in the best perfusion area with the Johnson score and area under ROC

	PI	AUC	PIT	AUCT	TTP	AT
Correlation coefficient(r)	0.488	0.314	0.394	0.212	−0.651	− 0.597
P	0.006	0.09	0.031	0.261	< 0.001	< 0.001
Area under ROC	0.746	0.617	0.632	0.569	0.796	0.768

Discussion

It was established that isolated regions of spermatogenic tissue may exist in the testes of men with NOA. M-TESE provides an optimal technique for sperm extraction with the guidance of an operating microscope to observe larger and opaquer seminiferous tubules. These seminiferous tubules are most likely to have ongoing spermatogenesis. In addition, M-TESE could prevent the main testicular blood supply from being damaged. Nevertheless, SRR is unsuccessful in many patients with NOA. Spermatogenesis is not distributed equally throughout the testis. Studies of patients with NOA showed that sperm quality was highest in areas with high tissue perfusion [11]. Therefore, locating areas with high perfusion would be helpful for sperm retrieval. Colour Doppler ultrasound, power Doppler ultrasound, laser flowmetry, and magnetic resonance spectroscopy have been used to locate the foci of spermatogenesis in previous studies [18]. However, these methods could only detect the main arteries in the testes, and the microvasculature was not able to be imaged. However, the high-density microvasculature greatly contributed to the high blood testicular perfusion, which was correlated with focal spermatogenesis [8, 9].

The microbubble agent used in this method (SonoVue™) is an intravascular agent and therefore does not "leak" into surrounding tissue, which provides a true representation of the microvascular supply to the testicle area. With the CEUS method, we were able to locate the high perfusion area where a rich amount of microvasculature exists before M-TESE. In our results, the SRR of the best perfusion area over the maximal longitudinal section was higher than those the poorest perfusion area and equatorial area. The best perfusion area had the densest microvasculature in the whole testicle, so the blood supply was rich in this area. It has been demonstrated that the foci of spermatogenesis might be found in regions with improved blood supply. Therefore, M-TESE performed in the best perfusion area had the best chance of detecting normal sperm. In our study, the SRR in the best perfusion area over the maximal longitudinal section was the highest, 63.1%. The CEUS group had a higher SRR than the control group. Herwig et al.

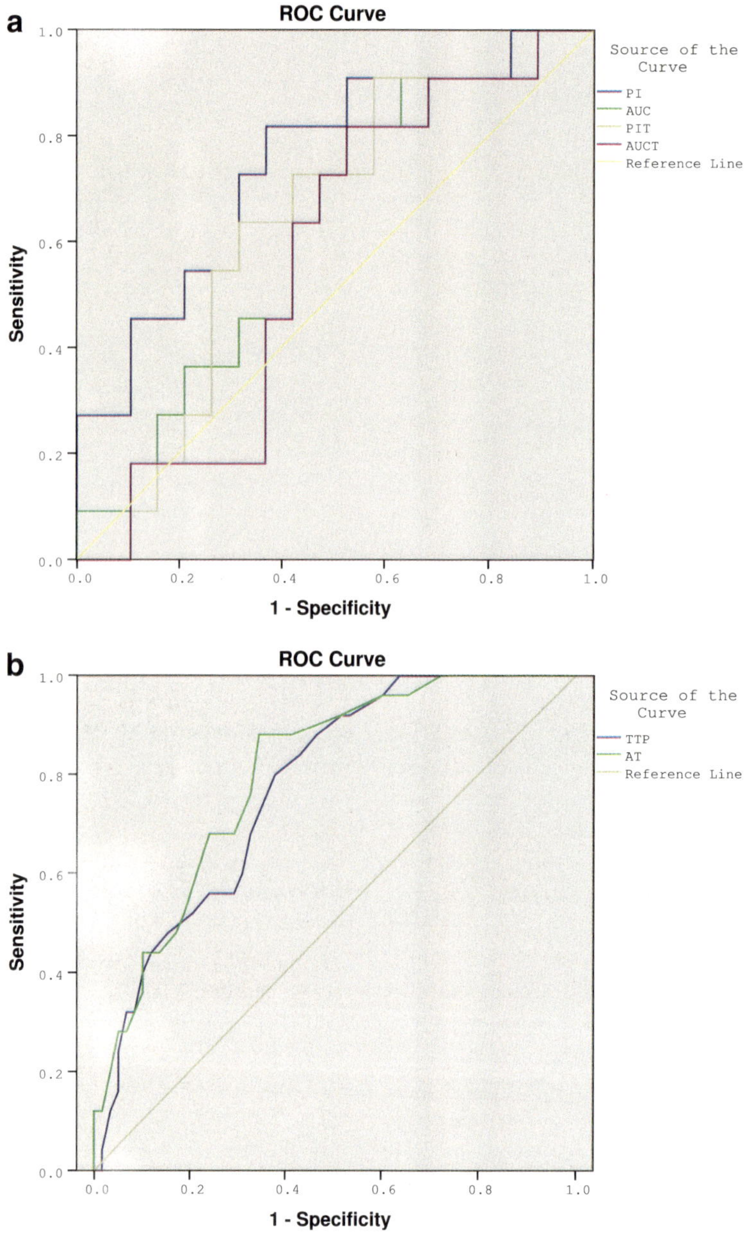

Fig. 2 ROC curve. PI, TTP and AT were the best predictors of positive sperm retrieval. The two images respectively showed the ROC curves of PI, AUC, PIT, AUCT (a) and TTP, AT (b) in predicting positive sperm retrieval

[11] used a laser Doppler flowmeter and colour Doppler ultrasound to measure testicle tissue perfusion before TESE, and they found that sperm quality and quantity were highest in areas of high tissue perfusion. This conclusion was similar to ours. However, in Ullrich's study, no significant accumulation of sperm-positive samples could be found in the main testicular vessels [18]. This conclusion did not conflict with ours, and the high perfusion area was not mostly near the main vessels, but instead occurred at positions with rich microvasculature. During M-TESE, an operating microscope cannot be used to identify the microvasculature, but CEUS could provide a new approach to image the testicle microvasculature.

In the best perfusion area from the maximal longitudinal section on CEUS of 187 testicles, we obtained pathological Johnson scores. Although sperm quality was high in areas of high tissue perfusion [11], not all of the CEUS parameters had a significant correlation with the Johnson score. In our results, PI, AT and TTP showed a relatively high correlation with the Johnson score. Pinggera et al. [10] investigated the value of the resistive index (RI) of intratesticular arteries as an indicator for normal sperm retrieval, and they found that a low RI might suggest a normal sperm count in andrological patients. When blood flows through a vessel, a lower resistance could increase blood flow. A large microvasculature and low RI may cause a high PI and low AT and TTP. According to the ROC curve, we obtained the cut-off values of the quantitative parameters to make them better predictors of successful sperm retrieval. Simultaneously, we also knew the suggested location of positive spermatogenesis. Testicles during CEUS were kept at the same position as during M-TESE. According to the measurements of the best perfusion area location over the maximal longitudinal section, the M-TESE operator could accurately find this area. With this approach, the SRR could be increased.

However, there are some limitations to our study. The best perfusion area was selected from images of the maximal longitudinal section for the testicle, so this area provided the best perfusion in one image, if not in the whole testicle. We hope additional studies will be able to use 3-Dimensional CEUS to study the whole testicle. Another limitation is the heterogenous patient population. The next research steps will include controls for age, testicular volume, and other pre-op values, such as AZFc mutations, among other factors.

Conclusions

CEUS is able to show the microvascular distribution in testicles. The location of the best perfusion area over the maximal longitudinal section is able to guide M-TESE to improve the success rate. By using CEUS guided M-TESE, the SRR can be significantly increased. From our results, we propose that all patients with NOA receive testicle CEUS. If AT≤27 s, TTP ≤ 45 s or PI≥11 dB are found in the best perfusion area, M-TESE in this area is strongly recommended.

Abbreviations

AT: The arrival time; AUC: Area under the curve; AUCT: The AUC of the whole testicle; CEUS: Contrast-enhanced ultrasound; ICSI: Intracytoplasmic sperm injection; M-TESE: Microdissection testicular sperm extraction; NOA: Non-obstructive azoospermia; PI: The peak intensity; PIT: The PI of the whole testicle; ROIs: The regions of interest; SRR: Sperm retrieval rate; TICs: The time-intensity curves; TTP: The time-to-peak intensity

Acknowledgements

We thank Dr. Qiang Liu, Department of Pathology, Renji Hospital, School of Medicine, Shanghai Jiao Tong University, Shanghai, China, for reviewing all testicle biopsies. We thank Dr. Caixia Zhu, Xiaoling Wang, and Dr. Xuesong Liu, Department of Ultrasound, Renji Hospital, School of Medicine, Shanghai Jiao Tong University, Shanghai, China, for their assistance in this study.

Funding

Sources of Funding: The study was funded by the Science and Technology Commission of Shanghai Municipality (Project 15411966300) in the design of the study and collection of data, in writing the manuscript, by the Shanghai ability construction project of the Clinical Assistant Department (Project SHDC22015003) in the analysis of data, and by the fund for cultivating scientific research seed plan of Renji Hospital (Project RJZZ14-012) in interpretation of data.

Authors' contributions

SJZ and SWX performed the ultrasound examinations and CEUS. RHT and ZL performed M-TESE after ultrasound examinations. SJZ and FHL developed the study concept, participated in its design and wrote the manuscript. JD and FHL analysed the data and corrected the draft. All of the authors read and approved the final manuscript.

Competing interests

The authors declare that they have no competing interests.

Author details

[1]Department of ultrasound, Renji Hospital, School of Medicine, Shanghai Jiaotong University, 160 Pujian RD, Shanghai 200127, China. [2]Department of Andrology, Shanghai General Hospital, Shanghai Jiaotong University, 100 Haining RD, Shanghai 200080, China.

References

1. Dabaja AA, Schlegel PN. Microdissection testicular sperm extraction: an update. Asian J Androl. 2013;15:35–9.
2. Tunc L, Alkibay T, Kupeli B, Tokgoz H, Bozkirli I, Yucel C. Power Doppler ultrasound mapping in nonobstructive azoospermic patients prior to testicular sperm extraction. Arch Androl. 2005;51:277–83.
3. Donoso P, Tournaye H, Devroey P. Which is the best sperm retrieval technique for nonobstructive azoospermia? A systematic review. HumReprod Update. 2007;13:539–49.
4. Ezeh UI. Beyond the clinical classification of azoospermia: opinion. Hum Reprod. 2000;15:2356–9.
5. Raman JD, Schlegel PN. Testicular sperm extraction with intracytoplasmic sperm injection is successful for the treatment of nonobstructive azoospermia associated with cryptorchidism. J Urol. 2003;170:1287–90.
6. Hauser R, Temple-Smith PD, Southwick GJ, de Kretser D. Fertility in cases of hypergonadotropic azoospermia. Fertil Steril. 1994;63:631–6.
7. Foresta C, Garolla A, Bettella A, Ferlin A, Rossato M, Candiani F. Doppler ultrasound of the testicular testis in azoospermic subjects as a parameter of testicular function. Hum Reprod. 1998;13:3090–3.
8. Har-Toov J, Eytan O, Hauser R, Yavetz H, Elad D, Jaffa AJ. A new power Doppler ultrasound guiding technique for improved testicular sperm extraction. Fertil Steril. 2004;81:430–4.
9. Herwig R, Tosun K, Pinggera GM, Soelder E, Moeller KT, Pallwein L, et al. Tissue perfusion essential for spermatogenesis and outcome of testicular sperm extraction (TESE) for assisted reproduction. J Assist Reprod Genet. 2004;21:175–80.
10. Pinggera GM, Mitterberger M, Bartsch G, Strasser H, Gradl J, Aigner F, et al. Assessment of the intratesticular resistive index by colour Doppler ultrasonography measurements as a predictor of spermatogenesis. BJU Int. 2008;101:722–6.
11. Herwig R, Tosun K, Schuster A, Rehder P, Glodny B, Wildt L, et al. Tissue perfusion-controlled guided biopsies are essential for the outcome of testicular sperm extraction. Fertil Steril. 2007;87:1071–6.
12. Souza CA, Cunha-Filho JS, Fagundes P, Freitas FM, Passos EP. Sperm recovery prediction in azoospermic patients using Doppler ultrasonography. Int Urol Nephrol. 2005;37:535–40.
13. Eytan O, Har-Toov J, Fait G, Yavetz H, Hauser R, Yogev L, et al. Vascularity index distribution within the testis: a technique for guiding testicular sperm extraction. Ultrasound in Med. 2001;27:1171–6.
14. World Health Organization. WHO Laboratory Manual for the Examination and Processing of Human Semen[M]. Geneva: World Health Organization; 2010.
15. Sakamoto H, Saito K, Oohta M, Inoue K, Ogawa Y, Yoshida H. Testicular volume measurement: comparison of ultrasonography, orchidometry, and water displacement. Urology. 2007;69:152–7.
16. Yang C, Lee DH, Mangraviti A, Su L, Zhang K, Zhang Y, et al. Quantitative correlational study of microbubble-enhanced ultrasound imaging and magnetic resonance imaging of glioma and early response to radiotherapy in a rat model. Med Phys. 2015;42(8):4762–72.

22

Role of lymph node dissection in the management of upper tract urothelial carcinomas

Runqi Guo[†], Yuze Zhu[†], Gengyan Xiong, Xuesong Li, Kai Zhang[*] and Liqun Zhou[*]

Abstract

Background: Lymph node dissection (LND) is not routinely performed during radical nephroureterectomy (RNU) in upper tract urothelial carcinomas (UTUC) and the role of LND has been controversial. We aim to investigate whether patients with LND had improved survival in UTUC patients.

Methods: We performed a systematic literature search of PubMed, Embase, and Cochrane library for citations published prior to January 2016, describing LND performed among UTUC patients and conducted a standard meta-analysis of survival outcomes.

Results: Eleven eligible studies containing 7516 patients satisfied the inclusion criteria. Pooled HRs for cancer-specific survival (CSS) and recurrence-free survival (RFS) were 1.17 ($P = 0.18$) and 1.33 ($P = 0.19$) respectively. However, the patients in the LND group had more advanced tumour stages and grades ($P < 0.001$). Further subgroup analysis showed that among muscle-invasive UTUC patients, the pooled HR for CSS and RFS were 1.10 ($P = 0.42$) and 0.92 ($P = 0.72$) respectively. Besides, no difference was found in CSS and RFS between pN0 and pNx individuals in overall populations and in patients with muscle-invasive UTUC, while pN+ patients had significantly worse prognosis when compared to pN0 patients.

Conclusions: LND during RNU allows more accurate staging and prediction of survival, but it remains uncertain whether LND independently improves survival in patients with UTUC. However, standard use of LND should be further investigated in a multi-center, prospective evaluation to obtain a definitive statement regarding this matter.

Keywords: Lymph node dissection, Recurrence, Survival, Upper urinary tract, Urothelial carcinoma

Background

Urothelial carcinomas are the fourth most common tumors [1]. However, upper tract urothelial carcinomas (UTUC) are comparatively uncommon compared to bladder cancer and occupy only 5–10% of urothelial carcinomas [2, 3]. Approximately 30% of patients suffered from muscle-invasive UTUC at presentation and the incidence of lymph node metastasis ranges from 30% to 40% at surgery [4, 5].

Radical nephroureterectomy (RNU) with bladder cuff resection and regional lymph node dissection (LND) is the backbone of management [3, 6, 7]. Generalizing results from previous bladder cancer researches [8–13], it seems reasonable to believe that LND in conjunction with RNU may provide not only utile staging and prognostic information but also a therapeutic benefit in selected patients with UTUC. Nevertheless, the therapeutic benefit of LND in improving survival remains controversial [14–16].

For these reasons, we systematically reviewed the published studies and performed a meta-analysis of studies in which data were reported for the treatment of LND to assess whether patients who achieved LND had improved cancer-specific survival (CSS) or recurrence-free survival (RFS) compared with patients who did not achieve LND, as a means for providing data for standardizing the indication of LND and assisting in creating a better management strategy for UTUC.

* Correspondence: kaizhangpku@163.com; zhoulqmail@sina.com
[†]Equal contributors
Department of Urology, Peking University First Hospital and Institute of Urology, National Research Center for Genitourinary Oncology, Beijing 100034, China

Methods

Search strategy

We systematically reviewed PubMed, Embase, and Cochrane library for citations published prior to January 2016, describing LND performed among patients with UTUC. The search strategy included the terms: lymphadenectomy or lymph node excision or lymphatic metastases, and upper tract urothelial neoplasms or upper tract urothelial cancer or transitional cell carcinoma of the upper urinary tract. Two authors independently reviewed article titles and abstracts for eligibility, and divergences were settled by consensus.

Inclusion and exclusion criteria of trials

Studies were included if they met all the following criteria: (1) prospective randomized studies or well-designed non-randomized controlled experiments; (2) studies analyzing the relationship between LND and UTUC prognosis; (3) clearly described outcome assessment by representing it in CSS or RFS; (4) sufficient survival information with hazard ratios (HR) and corresponding 95% confidence interval (CI), or Kaplan–Meier curves comparing survival among pathologic subgroups that were stratified according to LN status (pN0, negative node; pNx, skipping LND; pN+, positive node) or between LND and NLND; and (5) demographics and pathologic characteristics of patients were stratified according to LN status or according to the presence or absence of LND. Studies were excluded if they met one of the following criteria: (1) the article was a review or meta-analysis; (2) No available data could be able to extracted from the previously published studies; (3) the article deal with recurrent UTUC, metastatic carcinoma, previous or concurrent invasive bladder tumors or neoadjuvant chemotherapy; and (4) (potentially) overlapping study populations were reported for the same outcome.

Data extraction

All studies identified were independently reviewed by two reviewers. Titles and abstracts were screened for initial inclusion and final agreement on study inclusion was made by discussion and consensus with other authors. Two reviewers extracted data from all the included studies independently. Divergences were settled through consensus.

Quality assessment

The quality of the cohort studies was evaluated using the modified Newcastle-Ottawa Scale, which met the demands of this study [17]. This scale assesses risk in three domains: patient selection, comparability of LND and NLND groups and assessment of outcome (Table 1). To compare the two cohorts, we concentrated on the following variables that had been identified as independent predictors in previous multivariate studies: age, gender, tumor grade and tumor stage [18–21]. Each study was assessed by two reviewers independently. Any divergences were settled by discussion or through arbitrament by a third reviewer if no agreement could be reached.

Table 1 Newcastle-Ottawa quality assessment scale

Check list
Selection
•How representative was the control group (lymph node dissection) in comparison with the general elderly population for transitional cell carcinoma of the upper urinary tract? (if yes, one point; no point, if the patients were selected or selection of group was not described)
•How representative was the research group (non-lymph node dissection) in comparison with the elderly population for transitional cell carcinoma of the upper urinary tract? (if data from the same community as the control group, one point; no point, if drawn from a different source or selection of group was not described)
•Assignment for treatment: any detail report? (if yes, one point)
Comparability
•Group comparable for the grade of tumor, clinical TNM staging system (if yes, two points; one point was assigned, if one of these two characteristics had differences; no star was assigned, if the two groups differed)
•Group comparable for age, gender (if yes, two points; one star was assigned, if one of these two characteristics had differences; no point was assigned, if the two groups differed)
Outcome assessment
•Comprehensively evaluated the outcome? (yes, one point for information ascertained by record or International Classification of Diseases; no point, if this information was not reported)
•Adequacy of follow-up (one star, if follow-up > 90%)

Data analysis and synthesis

We use log HR and the variance as the summary outcome measure from all trials in the meta-analysis. For each trial, HR with the 95% CI of the survival rate was derived and calculated using either the fixed-effects model or the random-effects model [22]. Chi-square test was used to assess the heterogeneity between studies. For P values less than 0.1, the assumption of homogeneity was deemed invalid. Therefor, we calculated pooled estimates using random effects modeling, which provides more conservative estimates than fixed effects modeling when heterogeneity was present.

Publication bias is considered as a concern for meta-analyses. In our study, publication bias was assessed by funnel plots and Egger's regression [23]. Review manager version 5.3 (Cochrane Collaboration, Oxford, UK) was used for data analysis. A P value of less than 0.05 was considered statistically significant.

Results

Study identification and quality assessment

A total of 658 studies were identified. After excluding duplicates, 144 articles remained, 127 of which were excluded: 106 were apparent irrelevant studies, 4 were case, series/case reports, and 17 were letters/reviews/comments. 17 were reviewed in depth, and a full examination of the text was performed. Five studies were excluded because of insufficient outcome and one was excluded due to potentially overlapping study populations. At last, 11 studies involving 7516 UTUC patients were included into this meta-analysis [14, 15, 16, 24–30, 31] (Fig. 1) (Table 2).

The quality assessment of included cohort studies was performed using the modified Newcastle-Ottawa Scale. Studies that scored > 7 were considered as having low risk of bias, scores of 5–7 indicated moderate risk of bias, and scores of < 5 indicated high risk of bias, and the total scores are shown in Table 3. Most studies were deemed to be of moderate risk of bias and we only scored 3 of 11 studies as having low risk of bias. Commonly identified concern was the comparability of LND and NLND groups, especially regarding tumor grade and TNM staging.

Meta-analysis results

Cancer-specific survival

Of the 10 studies that referred to CSS, there was significant heterogeneity among them ($I^2 = 80\%$, $Chi^2 = 45.96$, $P < 0.00001$). Thus, a random-effects model was used to calculate the pooled HR and corresponding 95% CI. No statistically significance was found between the LND group and the NLND group (HR = 1.17, 95% CI: 0.93–1.48, $P = 0.18$) (Fig. 2 A1). Besides, patients with pN0 did not have better CSS compared with those with pNx (HR = 0.99, 95% CI: 0.81–1.22, $P = 0.95$) with significant heterogeneity ($I^2 = 94\%$, $Chi^2 = 35.97$, $P < 0.00001$) (Fig. 2 A2), while patients with pN+ showed poor CSS compared with those with pN0 (HR = 3.38, 95% CI: 1.94–5.89, $P < 0.0001$) with significant heterogeneity ($I^2 = 93\%$, $Chi^2 = 71.90$, $P < 0.00001$) (Fig. 2 A3).

To explore the source of apparent heterogeneity, we compared the differences in tumor stage and tumor grade between the groups, thereby demonstrating the features between the groups using Chi-square tests and Fisher's exact tests for categorical variables (Table 4). The results showed that there was remarkable significant difference in tumor stage and tumor grade between the LND group and NLND group ($P < 0.001$), which might have significant association with the heterogeneity.

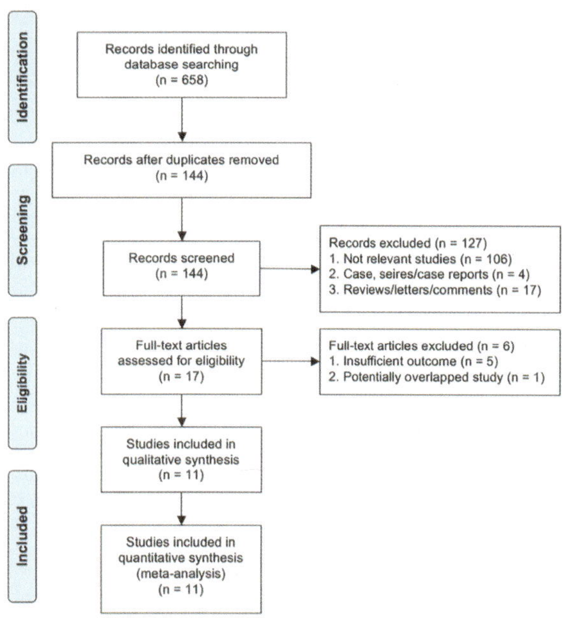

Fig. 1 Flowchart of study selection

Recurrence-free survival

Significant heterogeneity was observed in the four studies that focused on RFS ($I^2 = 89\%$, $Chi^2 = 26.57$, $P < 0.00001$), hence we utilzed the random-effects model. The pooled HR for RFS was 1.33 (95% CI: 0.87–2.06, $P = 0.19$), which indicate that LND was not associated was better RFS in patients with UTUC (Fig. 2 B1). Meanwhile, in consideration of pN0/pNx, no significant difference in RFS between pN0 and pNx was found (HR = 0.98, 95% CI: 0.62–1.55, $P = 0.93$) and there was significant heterogeneity among them ($I^2 = 85\%$, $Chi^2 = 19.82$, $P = 0.0002$) (Fig. 2 B2). In contrast, pN+ showed poor RFS compared with those pN0 (HR = 3.46, 95% CI: 2.00–5.97, $P < 0.0001$) with significant heterogeneity ($I^2 = 78\%$, $Chi^2 = 13.95$, $P < 0.003$) (Fig. 2 B3).

Subgroup analysis

We performed subgroup analysis according to pT statuses, among patients with muscle-invasive UTUC. Data for CSS in patients with muscle-invasive UTUC were reported in four studies, and there was heterogeneity among those studies ($I^2 = 63\%$, $Chi^2 = 8.04$, $P = 0.05$); hence, we utilzed the random-effects model. However, no statistically significance was found between the two groups (HR = 1.10, 95% CI: 0.88–1.37, $P = 0.42$) (Fig. 2 C1).

Additionally, the results of the subsequent analyses showed no difference in RFS between the LND group and the NLND group among muscle-invasive UTUC individuals (HR = 0.92, 95% CI: 0.58–1.46, $P = 0.72$) and there was relatively high heterogeneity in this subgroup ($I^2 = 88\%$, $Chi^2 = 16.48$, $P = 0.0003$) (Fig. 2 C2).

Furthermore, among the patients with muscle-invasive UTUC, no significant difference between pN0

Table 2 Characteristics of included studies in meta-analysis

Study	Type of study	Gender	Patients (n)	Follow-up median (month)	Median age (year)	Node status (overall)/ LND or NLND	Extent of LND	Tumor location	Pathologic tumor stage	Tumor grade	Outcome
Kondo T et al 2014 [31]	Prospective	Male 112 Female 54	166	23.7	72.4	pN0 69 pNx 86 pN+ 11	Renal pelvis tumor: LN from the renal hilar to the inferior mesenteric artery. Tumor of upper 2/3 ureter: LN from the renal hilar to the aortic bifurcation. Tumor of lower 1/3 ureter: the ipsilateral pelvic LN	Renal pelvis 90 Ureter 76	≤pT1 62 pT2 27 pT3 72 pT4 5	Low 71 High 95	CSS
Ouzzane A et al 2013 [16]	Retrospective	Male 484 Female 228	714	27.0	70.0	pN0 204 pNx 460 pN+ 50	NA	Renal pelvis 388 Pelvis+ureter 90 Multifocal 236	pTa/Tis 209 pT1 168 pT2 74 pT3 224 pT4 39	G1 71 G2 244 G3 399	CSS, RFS
Mason RJ et al. 2012 [15]	Retrospective	Male 654 Female 375	1029	19.8	68.6	pN0 199 pNx 753 pN+ 77	NA	Renal pelvis 538 Pelvis+ureter 213 Ureter 250	pTa/Tis 108 pT1 463 pT2 160 pT3 244 pT4 54	Low 340 High 689	CSS, RFS
Burger M et al 2011 [30]	Retrospective	Male 542 Female 243	785	34.0	68.0	pN0 136 pNx 595 pN+ 54	Hilar & regional LN adjacent to ipsilateral great vessel	NA	pTa 165 pTis 10 pT1 196 pT2 148 pT3 222 pT4 44	G1 100 G2 226 G3 459	CSS, RFS
Abe T et al 2010 [29]	Retrospective	Male 195 Female 98	293	NA	69.2	pN0 130 pNx 141 pN+ 22	Tumor of renal pelvis tumor & upper 2/3 ureter: Hilar & regional LN adjacent to ipsilateral great vessel Lower ureteral tumor: ipsilateral pelvic LN	Renal pelvis 157 Pelvis+ureter 24 Ureter 112	pTa/Tis 53 pT1 66 pT2 56 pT3 101 pT4 17	Low 185 High 108	RFS
Lughezzani et al 2010 [14]	Retrospective	Male 1666 Female 1158	2824	43.0	72.0	pN0 1835 pNx 747 pN+ 242	NA	Renal pelvis 1913 Ureter 911	pT1 867 pT2 500 pT3 584 pT4 873	G1 156 G2 935 G3 1234 G4 499	CSS
Roscigno M et al 2009 [28]	Retrospective	NA	1130	45.0	69.1	pN0 412 pNx 578 pN+ 140	Renal pelvis and proximally ureteral tumor: LN from the renal hilar to the inferior mesenteric artery Mid and lower ureteral tumors: LN from the renal hilar to the bifurcation of the common iliac artery and ipsilateral pelvic LN	NA	pT1 317 pT2 269 pT3–4544	Low 291 High 839	CSS
Kondo T et al. 2007 [27]	Retrospective	Male 113 Female 56	169	37.3	67.5	LND 81 NLND 88	Renal pelvis tumor: LN from the renal hilar to the inferior mesenteric artery Tumor of upper 2/3 ureter: LN from the renal hilar to the aortic bifurcation	Renal pelvis 100 Upper ureter 9	≤pT1 45 pT2 34 pT3 79 pT4 9	NA	CSS

Table 2 Characteristics of included studies in meta-analysis *(Continued)*

Study	Type of study	Gender	Patients (n)	Follow-up median (month)	Median age (year)	Node status (overall)/ LND or NLND	Extent of LND	Tumor location	Pathologic tumor stage	Tumor grade	Outcome
							Tumor of lower 1/3 ureter: ipsilateral pelvic LN	Midureter 20 Lower ureter 40			
Secin FP et al. 2007 [26]	Retrospective	Male 166 Female 86	252	37.2	69.0	pN0 105 pNx 119 pN+ 28	NA	NA	pTa 71 pTis 12 pT1 46 pT2 35 pT3 72 pT4 8	G1 64 G2 38 G3 143	CSS
Brausi MA et al 2007 [25]	Retrospective	Male 59 Female 23	82	64.7	LND 67.8 NLND 67.1	LND 40 NLND 42	Renal pelvis and upper ureteral tumor: LN from the renal hilar to the inferior mesenteric artery Mid ureteral tumors: LN from the renal hilar to the bifurcation of the common iliac artery Lower ureteral tumor: ipsilateral pelvic LN	Renal pelvis 47 Pelvis+ureter 7 Ureter 28	pT2 38 pT3 36 pT4 8	G2 44 G3 38	CSS
Miyake H et al.. 1998 [24]	Retrospective	Male 53 Female 19	72	49	LND 64 NLND 67	LND 35 NLND 38	Renal pelvis and upper ureteral tumor: LN from the renal hilar to the inferior mesenteric artery Mid ureteral tumor: LN from the renal hilar to the bifurcation of the common iliac artery Lower ureteral tumor: ipsilateral pelvic LN	Renal pelvis 40 Pelvis+ureter 3 Ureter 29	pTa 11 pT1 25 pT2 18 pT3 14 pT4 4	G1 12 G2 33 G3 37	CSS

LND Lymph node dissection, *NLND* Non-LND, *NA* Not available, *pN+* Positive lymph node, *pN0* Negative lymph node, *pNx* Not undergo lymph node dissection, *CSS* cancer-specific survival, *RFS* recurrence-free survival

Table 3 Assessment for quality of included studies

Study	Selection			Comparability		Outcome assessment		Score
	1	2	3	1	2	1	2	
Kondo T et al 2014 [31]	1	1	1	2	0	1	1	7
Ouzzane A et al 2013 [16]	1	1	1	0	2	1	1	7
Mason RJ et al 2012 [15]	1	1	1	0	1	1	1	6
Burger M et al 2011 [30]	1	1	1	0	1	1	1	6
Abe T et al 2010 [29]	1	1	1	0	2	1	1	7
Lughezzani et al 2010 [14]	1	1	1	0	2	1	1	7
Roscigno M et al 2009 [28]	1	1	1	0	1	1	1	6
Kondo T et al 2007 [27]	1	1	1	1	2	1	1	8
Secin FP et al 2007 [26]	1	1	1	1	1	1	1	7
Brausi MA et al 2007 [25]	0	1	1	2	2	1	1	8
Miyake H et al 1998 [24]	1	1	1	2	1	1	1	8

and pNx was found in CSS and RFS (HR = 0.97, 95% CI: 0.64–1.47, $P = 0.87$; and HR = 0.97, 95% CI: 0.64–1.47, $P = 0.87$, respectively) and there was significant heterogeneity ($I^2 = 94\%$, $Chi^2 = 35.97$, $P < 0.00001$; and $I^2 = 89\%$, $Chi^2 = 18.80$, $P < 0.00001$, respectively) (Fig. 2 C3 & 2C4). However, patients with pN+ showed poor CSS and RFS in comparison with those with pN0 (HR = 3.27, 95% CI: 2.83–3.78, $P < 0.00001$; and HR = 2.10, 95% CI: 1.05–4.20, $P = 0.0002$, respectively) (Fig. 2 C5and C6).

Publication bias

The publication bias was detected using a funnel plot of the meta-analysis result. The basic symmetry of the funnel plots suggested that there was no obvious publication bias (Fig. 3). The Egger's test for CSS and RFS did not show any evidence of publication bias.

Discussion

Radical cystectomy with pelvic LND for muscle-invasive bladder cancer is relatively standardized because it improves tumor staging and survival of patients [32, 33]. However, potential benefit of LND during RNU on survival for UTUC is still controversial [15, 30]. On the basis of the latest European guidelines on UTUC, LND should be performed in conjunction with RNU not only for better tumor staging but also for prognosis improvement [3]. Nevertheless, this recommendation is only Level III evidence. Thus, we reviewed the published studies and conducted a meta-analysis to clarify the prognostic value of LND in patients with UTUC.

In the present research, 11 studies were eligible and the HRs of cumulative survival rates were summarized quantitatively. Our analysis revealed that pN+ patients had significantly worse prognosis when compared to pN0 patients. The same results were observed when restricting the analyses to patients with muscle-invasive carcinomas, who should, anyway, be systematically considered for staging LND in light of this growing body of data.

However, no difference was found in survival or disease recurrence when comparing pN0/pNx individuals and the LND/NLND groups. The sample size of the included studies could explain these results. Most of the early years studies include small numbers of patients (less than 200), while larger series (more than 1000) with more events only emerged recently. Besides, the decision to perform LND was left to the discretion of the surgeon, it is possible that those NLND patients had less aggressive disease than LND patients, and that a true benefit to LND does exist. An increased risk of cancer-related death is usually related to higher tumor stage and grade. In this comparison, there was no significant difference in CSS and RFS between the LND group and the NLND group, which may reversely suggest the possible therapeutic value of LND for patients with more aggressive tumors. Nevertheless, the results remained no significant difference when controlling for tumor stage. Conversely, in a review by Kondo and Tanabe [34], it was highlighted that when the regional nodes were completely dissected, the patients with the advanced stage had significantly higher survival compared with those without LND.

Interestingly, pNx was not associated with poor CSS and RFS in patients with muscle-invasive carcinomas and in overall population. Several explanations may account for our results. First, pNx individuals were most likely identified by their surgeons as low risk for nodal metastases. It is also possible that pNx individuals may harbor micrometastatic lymph node deposits, which could be either destroyed or removed during the surgery, without being identified as pN1 by the pathologist. Furthermore, the lack of standardized anatomical limits

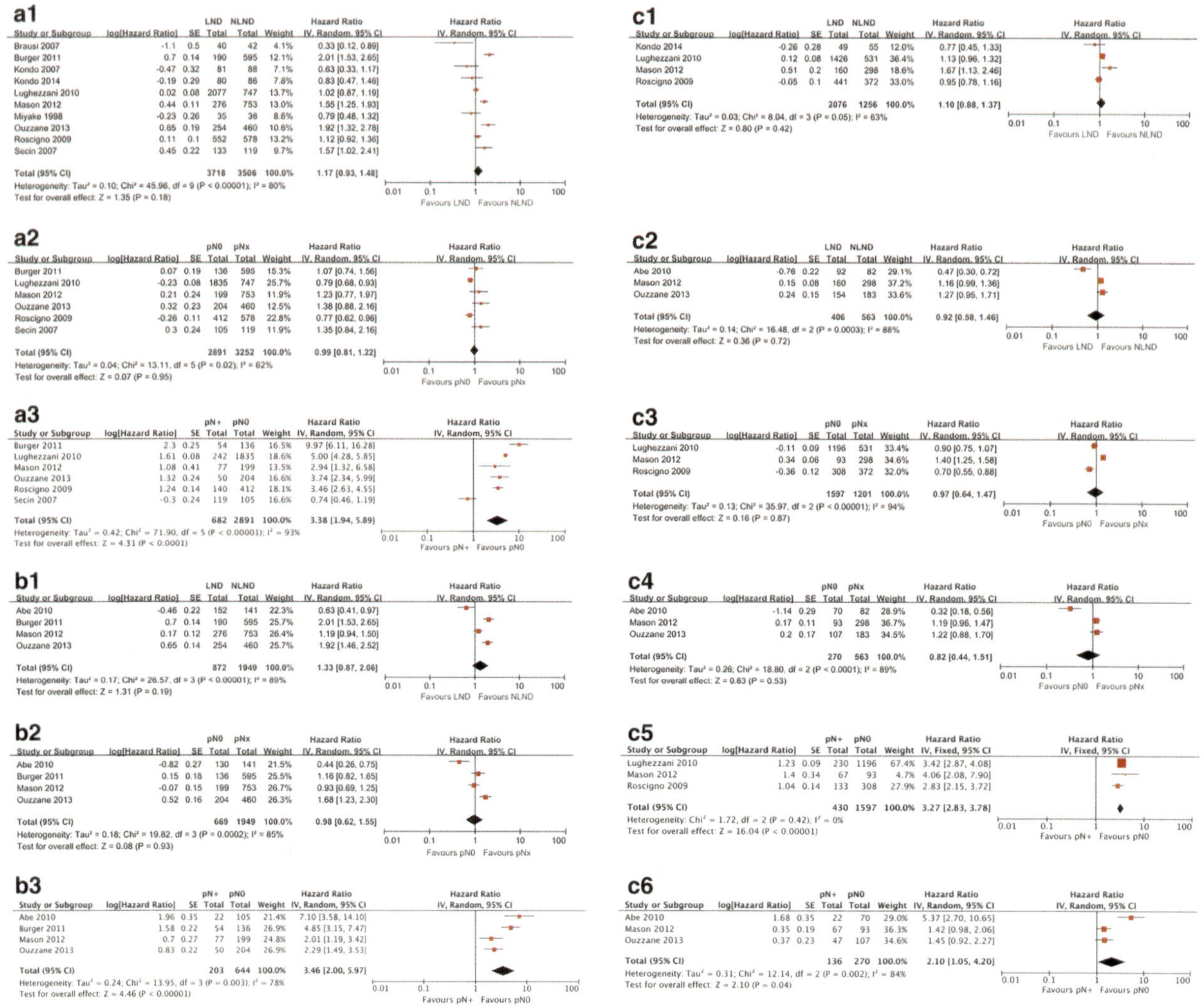

Fig. 2 Forest plot comparing survival and subgroup analysis of different pT statuses. (**A1**) CSS in patients receiving LND versus NLND; (**A2**) CSS in patients considered pN0/pNx; (**A3**) CSS in patients considered pN+/pN0; (**B1**) RFS in patients receiving LND versus NLND; (**B2**) RFS in patients considered pN0/pNx; (**B3**) RFS in patients considered pN+/pN0; (**C1**) CSS in muscle-invasive UTUC patients receiving LND versus NLND; (**C2**) RFS in muscle-invasive UTUC patients receiving LND versus NLND; (**C3**) CSS in patients of muscle-invasive UTUC considered pN0/pNx; (**C4**) RFS survival in patients of muscle-invasive UTUC considered pN0/pNx; (**C5**) CSS in patients of muscle-invasive UTUC considered pN+/pN0; (**C6**) RFS survival in patients of muscle-invasive UTUC considered pN+/pN0. CSS, cancer-specific surviva; LND: lymph node dissection; NLND: non-lymph node dissection; pN0: Negative lymph node; pNx: Not undergo lymph node dissection; RFS, recurrence-free survival; UTUC: upper tract urothelial carcinoma.

Table 4 Chi-square tests for two groups

Variable	LND (n, %)	NLND (n, %)	*P* value
Tumor stage			< 0.001
≤T1	1210 (31.3)	1684 (46.2)	
T2	722 (18.7)	637 (17.5)	
T3	1204 (31.2)	990 (27.2)	
T4	726 (18.8)	335 (9.2)	
Tumor grade			< 0.001
Low grade or ≤ G2	1610 (35.4)	1281 (43.2)	
High grade or > G2	2936 (64.6)	1682 (56.8)	

LND lymph node dissection, *NLND* non LND

and indication for the LND could account for our results: some patients certainly had very limited dissection and unsuitable for tumor location, leading to a wrong histological report of pN0 stage even though they had nodal metastasis not including in the LND.

It is noteworthy that 49.0% RNU patients were staged as pNx in our studies. In 2009, Roscigno et al. pointed out that patients with pN0 disease had a better prognosis than pNx disease in patients with muscle-invasive carcinomas [28]. It is conceivable that, despite a higher pNx rate at tertiary care centers, the extent of LND in those in whom it was performed was substantially greater than the LND extent in the community. Under this premise, a more important stage migration towards

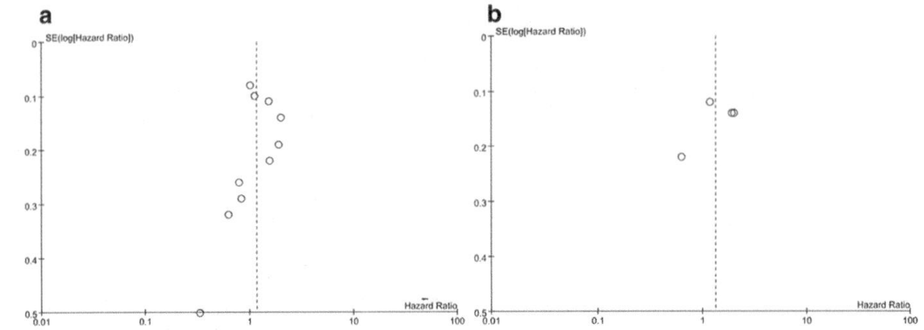

Fig. 3 Funnel plot for the evaluation of potential publication bias. (**a**) cancer-specific survival; (**b**) recurrence-free survival

true pN0 status may have occurred at tertiary care centers than in the current population-based series [14]. Taken together, our findings suggest that pNx individuals have no better prognosis than pN0 individuals.

Without standardized criteria for who should receive LND and how extensive LND should be, comparisons between series proved to be challenging. It was reported that the patients with incomplete LND in showed lower survival than those with complete LND, which reached statistical significance. Five-year CSS in the patients with pT2 or higher and pT3 or higher was 77.9% and 73.2% in the patients with complete LND, but just 54.0% and 43.7% in those with incomplete LND and 59.0% and 47.3% in those with NLND [34].

The most important finding of our study is that LND patients had no worse prognosis than NLND patients, especially in those with muscle-invasive carcinomas. According to a recent review, carrying out LND for UTUC is unlikely to be time-consuming and to increase the risk of major complications [34]. Although the current quality of evidence is generally not high, which may lead to biased and uncertain results, it might still suggest that the role of LND in UTUC is of importance, as UTUC is likely to simulate the biological behavior of bladder cancer because of the same histology among the two diseases.

Limitation should also be considered. First, the sources of the publications were limited, thus potentially introducing inevitable publication bias. Second, although 11 eligible studies involving 7516 patients were included in this meta-analysis, most of them were retrospective studies and the sample sizes of some selected studies are small, which might render the results less reliable. Third, marked heterogeneity of studies was seen in pooled-analysis of CSS and RFS. Furthermore, 7 of the 11 included studies provided the extent of LND, but the indication and extent of LND were not standardized. Last but not the least, as the included studies spanned a 10-year interval, the year in which the surgery occurred could be associated with different survival rates due to better imaging, earlier diagnosis and improved perioperative strategies of care. In the future, the role of LND should be further examined by validating templates of regional lymph nodes, and by prospective studies with larger numbers of patients. Then, we will discuss whether LND can be a standard treatment for UTUC.

Conclusions

LND during RNU allows more accurate staging and prediction of survival, but it remains uncertain whether LND independently improves survival in patients with UTUC. However, standard use of LND should be further investigated in a multi-center, prospective evaluation to obtain a definitive statement regarding this matter.

Abbreviations

CI: Confidence interval; CSS: Cancer-specific survival; HR: Hazard ratios; LND: Lymph node dissection; RFS: Recurrence-free survival; RNU: Radical nephroureterectomy; UTUC: Upper tract urothelial carcinomas

Acknowledgements

This work was supported by grants from the Collaborative Research Foundation of Peking University Health Science Center and National Taiwan University, College of Medicine (BMU20120318), Natural Science Foundation of Beijing (7152146) and the Clinical Features Research of Capital (No.Z151100004015173).

Funding

Not applicable.

Authors' contributions

GRQ participated in data collection and management, data analysis and manuscript writing. ZYZ participated in data analysis and manuscript writing. XGY participated in data collection and manuscript writing. LXS participated in project development, critical revision and manuscript editing. ZK participated in project development, critical revision and supervision. ZLQ participated in project development, critical revision and supervision. All the authors approved the final manuscript.

Competing interest

The authors declare that they have no competing interests.

References

1. Oxford Centre for Evidence-based Medicine Levels of Evidence (May 2009). Produced by bob Phillips, Chris ball, Dave Sackett, Doug Badenoch, Sharon Straus, Brian Haynes, Martin Dawes since November 1998. Updated by Jeremy Howick March 2009.
2. Siegel RL, Miller KD, Jemal A. Cancer statistics, 2015. CA Cancer J Clin. 2015; 65:5–29.
3. Rouprêt M, Babjuk M, Compérat E, Zigeuner R, Sylvester RJ, Burger M, et al. European Association of Urology guidelines on upper urinary tract urothelial cell carcinoma: 2015 update. Eur Urol. 2015;68:868–79.
4. Corrado F, Ferri C, Mannini D, Corrado G, Bertoni F, Bacchini P, et al. Transitional cell carcinoma of the upper urinary tract: evaluation of prognostic factors by histopathology and flow cytometric analysis. J Urol. 1991;145:1159–63.
5. Schatteman P, Chatzopoulos C, Assenmacher C, De Visscher L, Jorion JL, Blaze V, et al. Laparoscopic nephroureterectomy for upper urinary tract transitional cell carcinoma: results of a Belgian retrospective multicentre survey. Eur Urol. 2007;51:1633–8.
6. NCCN Clinical practice guidelines in oncology: bladder cancer. Including upper tract tumors and urothelial carcinoma of the prostate. Version 2.2015. National Comprehensive Cancer Network Web site http://www.nccn.org/professionals/physician_gls/pdf/bladder.pdf. Accessed May 2015.
7. Cornu JN, Rouprêt M, Carpentier X, Geavlete B, de Medina SG, Cussenot O, et al. Oncologic control obtained after exclusive fexible ureteroscopic management of upper urinary tract urothelial cell carcinoma. World J Urol. 2010;28:151–6.
8. Koppie TM, Vickers AJ, Vora K, Dalbagni G, Bochner BH. Standardization of pelvic lymphadenectomy performed at radical cystectomy: can we establish a minimum number of lymph nodes that should be removed? Cancer. 2006;107:2368–74.
9. Leissner J, Hohenfellner R, Thüroff JW, Wolf HK. Lymphadenectomy in patients with transitional cell carcinoma of the urinary bladder: significance for staging and prognosis. BJU Int. 2000;85:817–23.
10. Herr HW, Bochner BH, Dalbagni G, Donat SM, Reuter VE, Bajorin DF. Impact of the number of lymph nodes retrieved on outcome in patients with muscle invasive bladder cancer. J Urol. 2002;167:1295–8.
11. Konety BR, Joslyn SA, O'Donnell MA. Extent of pelvic lymphadenectomy and its impact on outcome in patients diagnosed with bladder cancer: analysis of data from the surveillance, epidemiology and end results program data base. J Urol. 2003;169:946–50.
12. Abdel-Latif M, Abol-Enein H, El-Baz M, Ghoneim MA. Nodal involvement in bladder cancer cases treated with radical cystectomy: incidence and prognosis. J Urol. 2004;172:85–9.
13. Liedberg F, Mansson W. Lymph node metastasis in bladder cancer. Eur Urol. 2006;49:13–21.
14. Lughezzani G, Jeldres C, Isbarn H, Shariat SF, Sun M, Pharand D, et al. A critical appraisal of the values of lymph node dissection at nephroureterectomy for upper tract urothelial carcinoma. Urology. 2010;75:118–24.
15. Mason RJ, Kassouf W, Bell DG, Lacombe L, Kapoor A, Jacobsen N, et al. The contemporary role of lymph node dissection during nephroureterectomy in the management of upper urinary tract urothelial carcinoma: the Canadian experience. Urology. 2012;79:840–5.
16. Ouzzane A, Colin P, Ghoneim TP, Zerbib M, De La Taille A, Audenet F, et al. The impact of lymph node status and features on oncological outcomes in urothelial carcinoma of the upper urinary tract (UTUC) treated by nephroureterectomy. World J Urol. 2013;31:189–97.
17. Taggart DP, D'Amico R, Altman DG. Effect of arterial revascularisation on survival: a systematic review of studies comparing bilateral and single internal mammary arteries. Lancet. 2001;358:870–5.
18. Clements T, Messer JC, Terrell JD, Herman MP, Ng CK, Scherr DS, et al. High-grade ureteroscopic biopsy is associated with advanced pathology of upper-tract urothelial carcinoma tumors at definitive surgical resection. J Endourol. 2012;26:398–402.
19. Li CC, Chang TH, Wu WJ, Ke HL, Huang SP, Tsai PC, et al. Significant predictive factors for prognosis of primary upper urinary tract cancer after radical nephroureterectomy in Taiwanese patients. Eur Urol. 2008;54:1127–34.
20. Lughezzani G, Burger M, Margulis V, Matin SF, Novara G, Roupret M, et al. Prognostic factors in upper urinary tract urothelial carcinomas: a comprehensive review of the current literature. Eur Urol. 2012;62:100–14.
21. Shariat SF, Godoy G, Lotan Y, Droller M, Karakiewicz PI, Raman JD, et al. Advanced patient age is associated with inferior cancer-specific survival after radical nephroureterectomy. BJU Int. 2010;105:1672–7.
22. DerSimonian R, Laird N. Meta-analysis in clinical trials. Control Clin Trials. 1986;7:177–88.
23. Green S. Cochrane handbook for systematic reviews of interventions version 5.1.0 [updated march 2011]. The Cochrane collaboration. Chichester: Wiley; 2011.
24. Miyake H, Hara I, Gohji K, Arakawa S, Kamidono S. The significance of lymphadenectomy in transitional cell carcinoma of the upper urinary tract. Br J Urol. 1998;82:494–8.
25. Brausi MA, Gavioli M, De Luca G, Verrini G, Peracchia G, Simonini G, et al. Retroperitoneal lymph node dissection (RPLD) in conjunction with nephroureterectomy in the treatment of infiltrative transitional cell carcinoma (TCC) of the upper urinary tract: impact on survival. Eur Urol. 2007;52:1414–8.
26. Secin FP, Koppie TM, Salamanca JI, Bokhari S, Raj GV, Olgac S, et al. Evaluation of regional lymph node dissection in patients with upper urinary tract urothelial cancer. Int J Urol. 2007;14:26–32.
27. Kondo T, Nakazawa H, Ito F, Hashimoto Y, Toma H, Tanabe K. Impact of the extent of regional lymphadenectomy on the survival of patients with urothelial carcinoma of the upper urinary tract. J Urol. 2007;178:1212–7.
28. Roscigno M, Shariat SF, Margulis V, Karakiewicz P, Remzi M, Kikuchi E, et al. Impact of lymph node dissection on cancer specific survival in patients with upper tract urothelial carcinoma treated with radical nephroureterectomy. J Urol. 2009;181:2482–9.
29. Abe T, Shinohara N, Muranaka M, Sazawa A, Maruyama S, Osawa T, et al. Role of lymph node dissection in the treatment of urothelial carcinoma of the upper urinary tract: multi-institutional relapse analysis and immunohistochemical re-evaluation of negative lymph nodes. Eur J Surg Oncol. 2010;36:1085–91.
30. Burger M, Shariat SF, Fritsche HM, Martinez-Salamanca JI, Matsumoto K, Chromecki TF, et al. No overt influence of lymphadenectomy on cancer-specific survival in organ-confined versus locally advanced upper urinary tract urothelial carcinoma undergoing radical nephroureterectomy: a retrospective international, multi-institutional study. World J Urol. 2011;29:465–72.
31 Kondo T, Hara I, Takagi T, Kodama Y, Hashimoto Y, Kobayashi H, et al. Template-based lymphadenectomy in urothelial carcinoma of the renal pelvis: a prospective study. Int J Urol. 2014;21:453–9.
32 Dhar NB, Klein EA, Reuther AM, Thalmann GN, Madersbacher S, Studer UE. Outcome after radical cystectomy with limited or extended pelvic lymph node dissection. J Urol. 2008;179:873–8.
33 Holmer M, Bendahl PO, Davidsson T, Gudjonsson S, Månsson W, Liedberg F. Extended lymph node dissection in patients with urothelial cell carcinoma of the bladder: can it make a difference? World J Urol. 2009;27:521–6.
34 Kondo T, Tanabe K. Role of lymphadenectomy in the management of urothelial carcinoma of the bladder and the upper urinary tract. Int J Urol. 2012;19:710–21.

Decreased expression of BRAF-activated long non-coding RNA is associated with the proliferation of clear cell renal cell carcinoma

Sheng Xue[1†], Sheng-Qun Jiang[2†], Qing-wen Li[1], Sheng Wang[1], Jian Li[1], Shuai Yang[1], Hai-Min Zhang[3], Yun-Fei Xu[3], Long-Sheng Wang[3] and Jun-Hua Zheng[4*]

Abstract

Background: BRAF-activated long non-coding RNA (BANCR) has been associated with various types of cancer. Nevertheless, the role of BANCR in clear cell renal cell carcinoma (ccRCC) is still not fully understood. This study aims to investigate the relationship between ccRCC and BANCR.

Methods: Expression of BANCR in TCGA renal cancer data sets was analyzed. The expression pattern of BANCR in Immortalized normal human proximal tubule epithelial cell line HK-2 and ccRCC cell lines (ACHN, CAKI-1, A498 and 786-O) was detected by real-time quantitative RT-PCR (qRT-PCR). ccRCC tissues with adjacent normal renal tissues diagnosed by pathological methods from 62 patients were used to detect the expression of BANCR, and its correlation with prognosis of ccRCC patients was assessed by Kaplan-Meier method. The LV-BANCR vector was used to examine the influence of BANCR on the proliferation, migration, invasion, apoptosis and cell cycle distribution of ccRCC cells in vitro.

Results: BANCR was downregulated in renal cancer according to TCGA data sets. Compared with adjacent normal renal tissues and normal human proximal tubule epithelial cell line HK-2, BANCR expression was significantly decreased in ccRCC tissues and ccRCC cell lines, and its low expression was associated with poor prognosis. Moreover, in the condition of BANCR overexpression by LV-BANCR vector, the proliferation, migration, invasion capacity of ccRCC cells was inhibited, while the apoptosis was increased and the G1 cell cycle arrest was induced in vitro.

Conclusions: BANCR is downregulated in ccRCC tissues and cell lines, and is associated with ccRCC progression. Thus, BANCR may represent a novel prognostic biomarker and a potential therapeutic target for ccRCC patients.

Keywords: Clear cell renal cell carcinoma, Long non-coding RNAs, BANCR

Background

Renal cell carcinoma (RCC) is one of the most commonly diagnosed urological cancers in the world [1]. In 2016 in the United States, there were approximately 62,700 cases of renal cancer and renal pelvis cancer that resulted in 14,240 deaths [2]. Among all subtypes of RCC, clear cell renal cell carcinoma (ccRCC) accounts for about 70% of RCC cases [3]. For localized RCC, it has been estimated that more than 25% patients encounter metastases at first visit, while another 25% experience local advancement [4]. Moreover, RCC has shown strong resistance to radiotherapy and chemotherapy [5, 6]. Over the last decade, great progress has been made in genetic and epigenetic variations concerning RCC; Yet, the precise mechanism of RCC pathogenesis still remains unclear. Thus, elucidating the pathogenesis of RCC and identifying available biomarker is of utmost importance.

LncRNAs are no-coding RNAs that are longer than 200 nucleotides, and are characterized by not translated

* Correspondence: zhengjunhua2016@163.com
[†]Sheng Xue and Sheng-Qun Jiang contributed equally to this work.
[4]Department of Urology, Shanghai General Hospital, Shanghai Jiao Tong University School of Medicine, Shanghai 200072, China
Full list of author information is available at the end of the article

into proteins [7, 8]. Multitudinous long noncoding RNAs (lncRNA) have shown to be involved in various types of tumorigenesis [9–11]. During the last decade, accumulated evidence has demonstrated that lncRNAs have an important role in tumorigenesis, invasion and metastasis of human cancers [12–14]. BRAF- activated non-coding RNA (BANCR) has been originally identified in melanoma cells [15]. BANCR has abnormal expression in various cancers, such as bladder cancer [16], colorectal cancer [17], melanoma [18], endometrial cancer [19], gastric cancer [20], and hepatocellular carcinoma [21]. For example, Wang et al. have reported that BANCR promotes endometrial cancer cell invasion and proliferation by modulating ERK/MAPK signaling pathway [19].

In this current study, we aimed to explore the expression and clinical significance of lncRNA BANCR in ccRCC cell lines and 62 clinical ccRCC samples, and investigate the biological functions of BANCR in ccRCC cells.

Methods

Patients and specimens

A total of 62 pathologically diagnosed ccRCC tissues and matched adjacent normal tissue specimens were collected from the Department of Urology, Shanghai Tenth People's Hospital of Tongji University between 2007 and 2010. The fresh ccRCC tissues and paired adjacent normal tissues were collected from patients underwent radical nephrectomy and were frozen in liquid nitrogen to protect the protein or RNA away from degradation. All diagnosis was pathologically confirmed of clear cell renal cell carcinoma, other pathological patterns of renal cancer were not included in the present study. Patients who have received chemotherapy or radiotherapy before surgery were excluded. The median follow-up time was 34 months until December 2011 and the follow-up was carried out mainly through telephone and outpatient service. The study was submitted and approved by the Ethics Committees of Shanghai Tenth People's Hospital. Each patient included in the study provided written consent after receiving oral and written information regarding the course and purpose of the study; and all the consents were saved by the ethics committee.

Cell lines and plasmid transfection

Immortalized normal human proximal tubule epithelial cell line HK-2 was obtained from the American Type Culture Collection (ATCC, USA). Human renal cancer cell lines A498 and 786-O were purchased from the Cell Bank of Type Culture Collection of Chinese Academy of Sciences (CCCAS, China). HK-2 cells were incubated in KSFM medium (Gibco), while RCC cell lines A498 and 786-O were cultured in RPMI-1640 medium (HyClone). Both cell medium were supplemented with 10% fetal bovine serum (Gibco), and all cells were cultured in a humidified atmosphere containing 5% CO^2 at 37 °C.

Recombinant lentiviruses carrying BANCR sequences (LV-BANCR) and a negative control sequence (LV-NC) were constructed (Hanyin, Shanghai, China). The LV-BANCR or LV-NC was infected into A498 and 786-O cells according to the manufacturer's protocols. qRT-PCR was performed to detected the expression of BANCR.

RNA extraction and qRT-PCR

Total RNA from tissues or cells were extracted by using Trizol reagent (Invitrogen, CA, USA) according to the manufacturer's protocols. For qPCR assay, qualified total RNA was reverse-transcribed to cDNA by SuperScript Frist-Strand cDNA System (Invitrogen CA, USA). The expression of BANCR was measured by real-time PCR using SYBR EX TAQ (Takara). GAPDH was used as an internal control. The prime sequences were as follows: GAPDH, 5'-GTAAGACCCCTGGACCACCA-3′ (forward), 5'-CAAGGGGTCTACATGGCA ACT-3′ (reverse); BANCR, 5'-ACAGGACTCCATGGCAAACG-3′ (forward), 5'-ATGAAGAAAGCCTGGTGCAGT-3′.

Cell proliferation and colony formation assay

Cell Counting Kit-8 (CCK8) assay was performed to evaluate the proliferation capacity of ccRCC cells. Briefly, A498 and 786-O cells were transfected with LV-BANCR or LV-NC for 48 h, and then seeded into 96-well plates at a density of 5×10^3 per well. After incubation for different time (0 h, 24 h. 48 h, 72 h, and 96 h), 10 ul CCK-8 reagent was added to each well and further incubated for 4 h. At the end, cell proliferation ability was examined by measuring the absorbance at 450 nm, using an enzyme-labeled analyzer.

For colony formation assays, cells infected with LV-BANCR or LV-NC were plated in 6-well plates. 10 days later, methanol-fixed and then stained with 0.1% crystal violet.

Protein extraction and western blot assay

Total protein was extracted using RIPA lysis buffer added by protease inhibitors and phosphatase inhibitors. After measuring concentration using Bio-Rad assay system, protein was separated by SDS-PAGE minigel and transferred onto Nitrocellulose (NC) membrane (Bio-Rad). The blots were probed with primary antibodies (abcam) overnight and then incubated with secondary antibodies at room temperature for 1 h, signals were detected.

Flow cytometry

For cell cycle distribution analysis, cells were harvested and fixed in 70% of pre-cooling ethanol overnight. Cells were then centrifuged and resuspended in PBS containing propidium iodide (PI; BD Biosciences) and RNase (100 μg/ml) as well as Triton X-100 (0.2%) for 30 min. Finally, flow cytometry (FACS, BD Biosciences) was used to analyzed cell cycle distribution.

Cell apoptosis were examined using Annexin V-FITC detection kit (BD Biosciences) in accordance with the manufacture' s protocol. Cells were harvested, washed with PBS and then resuspended with Annexin V-FITC and propidium iodide (PI) stained at room temperature in the dark for 15 min. Flow cytometry was performed to analyzed cell apoptosis rate.

Wound-healing assay

To determine cell migration, A498 and 786O cells were transfected with negative control or LV-BANCR were seeded into 6-well plates. After the cell reached about 90% confluence, three separate wounds were scratched by a sterile 100 μl pipet tip through the cells. Floating cells were removed by PBS. 24 h later, images of the scratches were got by an inverted microscope (Olympus).

Matrigel invasion assay

Matrigel-coated invasion chambers with a pore size of 8 μm (Costar, NY, USA) were used according to manufacturer's direction. After being starved for 24 h, transfected cells were collected. Equal numbers of the indicated cells (5×10^4) were seeded into the upper chambers in 200 μl serum-free medium, while a 600ul medium containing 10% fetal bovine serum was added to the bottom chamber. At 24 h post- incubation, cells remaining on the surface of the upper membrane were scraped off using a cotton swab, and the invasive cells were stained using 0.1% crystal violet for 30 min, and then photographed using a light microscope.

Statistical analysis

SPSS version 23.0 software (IBM) was used for statistical analysis of the present study. Date from three independent experiments are shown as mean ± SD. The differences between each group were analyzed by a Wilcoxon signed-rank test, a Student's t test, or a chi-square test. Kaplan-Meier method and univariate analysis was used to estimate the overall survival. $P < 0.05$ was considered statistically significant.

Results

BANCR is down-regulated in ccRCC tissues and cell lines

We analyzed the expression of BANCR in TCGA renal cancer data sets. The results indicated that BANCR expression was markedly down-regulated in renal cancer

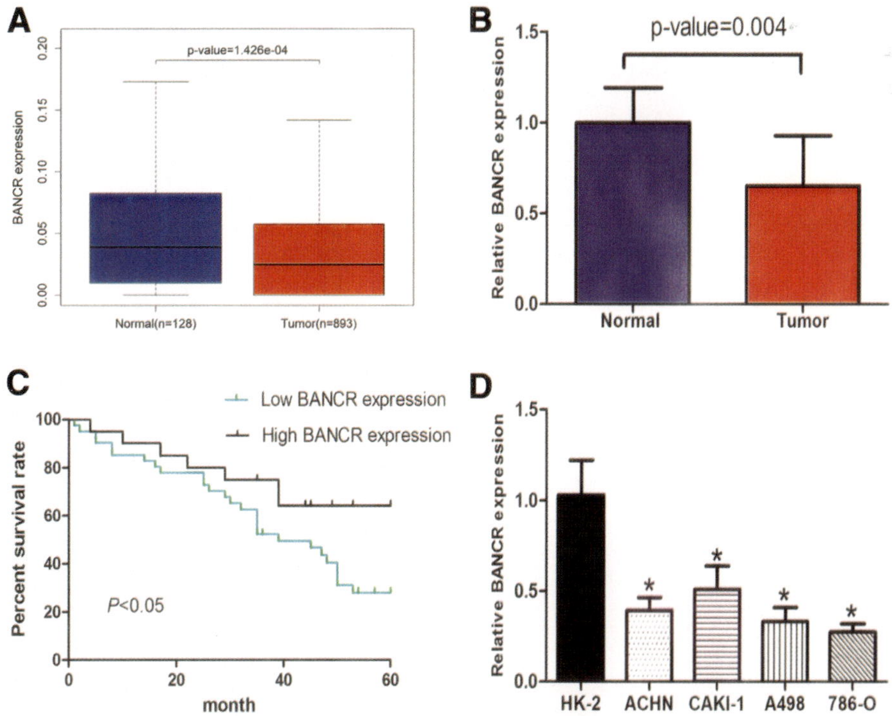

Fig. 1 Expression of BANCR in TCGA, ccRCC tissues and cell lines. **a** BANCR expression was lower in renal cancer tissues compared to normal renal tissues from TCGA dataset (*$p < 0.05$). **b** BANCR expression was lower in clear cell renal cancer tissues compared with adjacent normal renal tissues (*$p < 0.05$). **c** BANCR expression was associated with overall survival of ccRCC patients (*$p < 0.05$). **d** High expression of BANCR was found in HK2 cell (*$p < 0.05$)

tissues compared to normal renal tissues ($p < 0.01$) (Fig. 1a). Furthermore, we examined the expression of BANCR in 62 ccRCC tissues and matched normal renal tissues by qRT-PCR. Briefly, the expression of BANCR was obviously down-regulated in 67.7% (42 of 62) cancer tissues compared with adjacent normal renal tissues of ccRCC patients (Fig. 1b, $p < 0.01$).

To evaluate its clinical significance, we further performed the Kaplan-Meier analysis to evaluate the prognostic significance of BANCR. Our results indicated that patients with higher expression of BANCR had a significant better overall survival compared with patients with lower BANCR expression (log-rank test, $p < 0.05$) (Fig. 1c).

Moreover, we investigated the expression of BANCR in different ccRCC cell lines in vitro. The BANCR expression was significantly decreased in 786-O, A498, ACHN, CAKI-1 cells compared to HK2 cells (Fig. 1d). To sum up, these results revealed that BANCR may suppress ccRCC progression, thus might be a good diagnostic biomarker for ccRCC.

Overexpression of BANCR inhibited ccRCC cell proliferation in vitro

To explore the possible biological significances of BANCR on ccRCC cells in vitro, we constructed LV-BANCR (cells overexpressing BANCR) and a negative control (LV-NC) cells (Fig. 2a and b). Furthermore, the cell proliferation capacity of A498 and 786-O were detected by CCK-8 assay as well as cell clone assay. Briefly, cell proliferation of 786-O and A498 cells was significantly inhibited by LV-BANCR compared to negative control ($p < 0.05$, Fig. 2c and d). The above results indicated that BANCR may inhibit ccRCC cells proliferation.

Overexpression of BANCR induced apoptosis and cell cycle arrest in ccRCC cell lines

We further investigated whether LV-BANCR promoted cell apoptosis and/or induced cell cycle distribution. After transfection with LV-BANCR or negative control for 48 h, cells were analyzed by flow cytometry. As

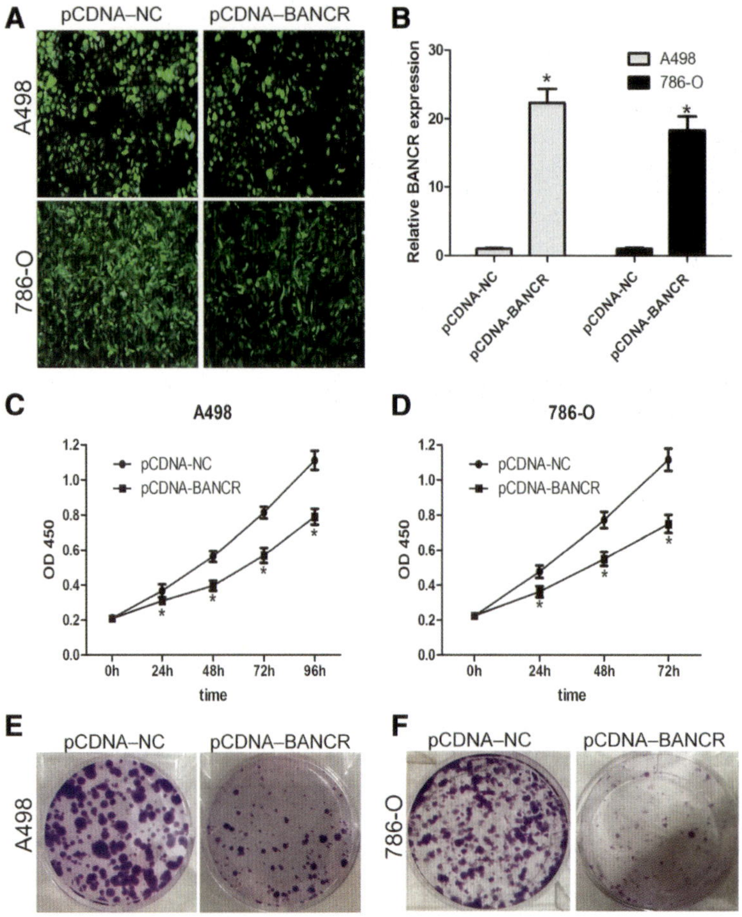

Fig. 2 Overexpression of BANCR inhibited ccRCC cell proliferation in vitro. **a** LV-BANCR was effectively transfected into A498 and 786-O cells. **b** The expression of BANCR was examined by q-PCR. CCK-8 assay **(c, d)** and cell clone formation assay **(e, f)** were performed to detect cell proliferation ability of A498 and 786-O cells. Data are represented as mean ± SD. $^*P < 0.05$

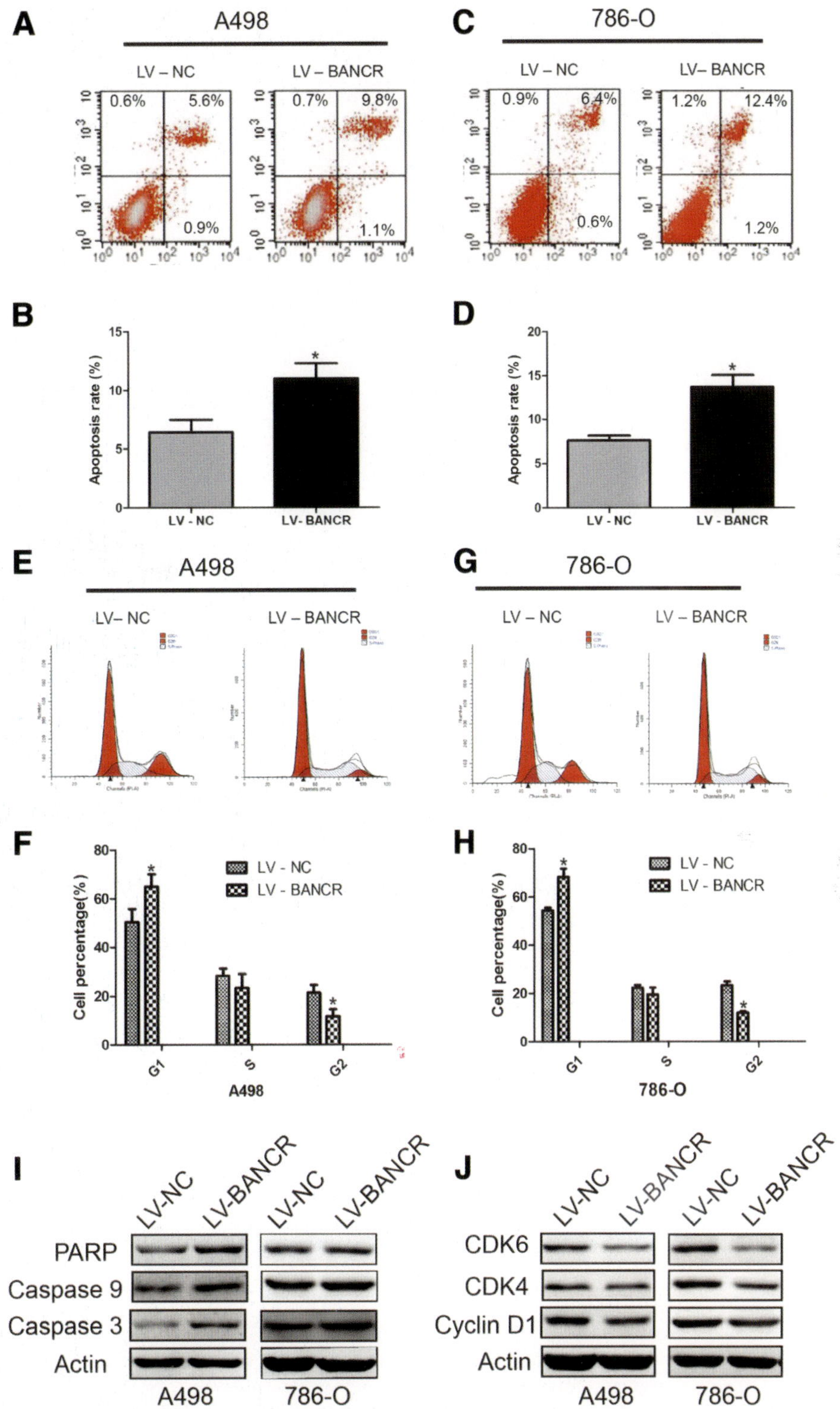

Fig. 3 BANCR overexpression induce apoptosis and cell cycle arrest in A498 and 786-O cells. Cell apoptosis of A498 (**a** and **b**) and 786-O (**c** and **d**) after BANCR overexpression was detected by flow cytometry. Cell cycle distribution of A498 (**e** and **f**) and 786-O (**g** and **h**) following BANCR overexpression was determined by flow cytometry. **i** The expression of PARP, caspase 3 and caspase 9 were examined by Western bloting assay in the two cells after BANCR overexpression. **j** The expression of Cycling D1, CDK4 and CDK6 were detected by Western bloting both in A498 and 786-O cells after BANCR overexpression. Data are shown as mean ± SD. *$p < 0.05$

shown in Fig. 3a-d, higher apoptotic rate was observed in A498 and 786-O cells transfected with LV-BANCR compared with the LV-NC group. It is well known that members of caspases, including caspase 3 and caspase 9, have a vital role in the process of apoptosis. The cleavage of PARP (nuclear DNA repair enzyme poly (ADP-ribose) polymerase) acts as a biomarker for cell apoptosis, and it is a target of caspase 3. In this study, the expressions of these three proteins were examined in LV-BANCR or LV-NC cells. Briefly, we found that the expression of caspase-3, caspase-9 and PARP were obviously upregulated by LV-BANCR group in both A498 and 786-O cells (Fig. 3i).

Moreover, G0/G1 phase cell cycle arrest was induced in LV-BANCR group in both two cell lines (Fig. 3e-h). Cyclin D1 was closely involved in cell cycle distribution. Meanwhile, CDK4 and CDK6 have shown to play vital role in cell cycle G1 phase [22], thus we further examined their expression in fLV-BANCR or LV-NC cells. It was found that the expression of cyclin D1, CDK4, as well as CDK6 were all downregulate after BANCR overexpression (Fig. 3j).

To conclude, these results suggest that BANCR overexpression causes cell proliferation inhibition by increasing cell apoptosis rate and inducing cell cycle arrest.

BANCR overexpression inhibited ccRCC cell migration and invasion

We explored the effect of lncRNA BANCR on ccRCC cells migration and invasion ability. As for wound healing assay, the migration viability of both A498 and 786-O cells was obviously decreased after LV-BANCR transfection compared with negative control ($p < 0.05$; Fig. 4a-b). Furthermore, BANCR overexpression reduced cell invasion in both A498 and 786-O cells (Fig. 4c). The results indicated that the overexpression of BANCR significantly suppresses ccRCC cells migration and invasion.

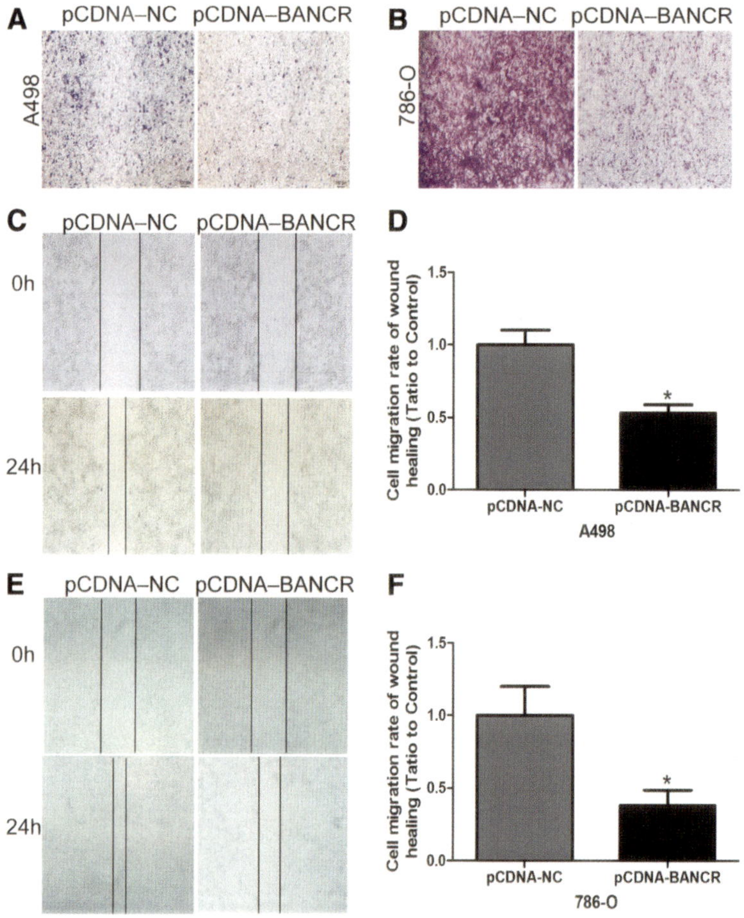

Fig. 4 BANCR overexpression inhibited ccRCC cell migration and invasion. The migration ability of A498 (**a** and **b**) and 786-O (**c** and **d**) cell examined using the Wound-healing assay. The invasion ability of A498 (**e**) and 786-O (**f**) cell examined using the Matrigel invasion assay. Data are shown as mean ± SD. *$p < 0.05$

Discussion

Over the last decade, lncRNAs have gained increasing attention as a class of non-coding genes. It has been reported that lncRNAs are essential in tumorigenesis and tumor progression [23, 24]. For example, it has been reported that a higher lncRNA UCA1 expression was found in esophageal squamous cell carcinoma tissues compared with normal tissues, while down-regulation of UCA1 decreases esophageal squamous cell ability of migration and proliferation [25].

As reported, morbidity of RCC is increasing annually [26]. Consequently, early diagnosis based on full understanding of molecular pathways is of great importance for RCC patients. Over the past few years, much attention has been given to the role of lncRNAs in RCC. For example, lncRNA CADM1-AS1 has been reported to be decreased in tumor tissues of ccRCC patients, while a worse survival in ccRCC patients was correlated with relative lower CADM1-AS1 expression [27].

lncRNA BANCR has been reported in various cancers, however, its biological functions as well as prognosis value in different cancer patients were contradictory [28–31]. As a tumor suppressor, BANCR was reported in lung cancer [32, 33]. On the contrary, BANCR was reported to promote tumor growth in various cancers [15, 18, 21, 34]. In contrast, BANCR was shown to be decreased in bladder cancer and colorectal cancer [16].

This is the first study to determine expression of BANCR and its biological function in ccRCC. Present study results revealed that that BANCR was obviously down-regulated in ccRCC tissues and cell lines. Moreover, the OS (overall survival) was worse in ccRCC patients with low BANCR expression. We further studied the effects of BANCR on the proliferation, migration, invasion, apoptosis and cell cycle distribution of ccRCC cells in vitro.

As the weakness of this study, molecular mechanism through which BANCR was decreased in ccRCC and the molecular mechanism involved in BANCR overexpression induced proliferation inhibition in ccRCC cell lines should be further investigated.

Conclusions

In conclusion, all the above reported evidences suggest that lncRNA BANCR may be a suppressor gene and a novel target gene for the prognosis as well as therapy of ccRCC.

Abbreviations

ATCC: American Type Culture Collection; BANCR: BRAF-activated long non-coding RNA; CCK8: Cell Counting Kit-8; ccRCC: clear cell renal cell carcinoma; NC: Nitrocellulose; PI: Propidium iodide

Funding

This study was supported by National Science Foundation of China (31570775 and 81602216). The funding body didn't play role in the design of the study and collection, analysis, and interpretation of data and in writing the manuscript.

Authors' contributions

ZJH and XS conceived and designed the experiments; XS and JSQ performed the experiments; LQW, JSQ, WLS and WS analyzed the data; LJ, ZHM, XYF and YS contributed reagents/materials/analysis tools; ZHM, XYF and WLS wrote the paper. All authors read and approved the final manuscript.

Competing interests

The authors declare that they have no competing interests.

Author details

[1]Department of Urology, The First Affliated Hospital of Bengbu Medical College Bengbu, Bengbu, Anhui, China. [2]Department of Ophthalmology, The First Affliated Hospital of Bengbu Medical College Bengbu, Bengbu, Anhui, China. [3]Department of Urology, Shanghai Tenth People's Hospital, Tongji University, Shanghai, China. [4]Department of Urology, Shanghai General Hospital, Shanghai Jiao Tong University School of Medicine, Shanghai 200072, China.

References

1. Siegel RL, Miller KD, Jemal A. Cancer statistics, 2017. CA Cancer J Clin. 2017; 67(1):7–30.
2. Siegel RL, Miller KD, Jemal A. Cancer statistics, 2016. CA Cancer J Clin. 2016; 66(1):7–30.
3. Znaor A, Lortet-Tieulent J, Laversanne M, Jemal A, Bray F. International variations and trends in renal cell carcinoma incidence and mortality. Eur Urol. 2015;67(3):519–30.
4. Cindolo L, Patard JJ, Chiodini P, Schips L, Ficarra V, Tostain J, de La Taille A, Altieri V, Lobel B, Zigeuner RE, et al. Comparison of predictive accuracy of four prognostic models for nonmetastatic renal cell carcinoma after nephrectomy: a multicenter European study. Cancer. 2005;104(7):1362–71.
5. Wang Q, Wang S, Sun SQ, Cheng ZH, Zhang Y, Chen G, Gu M, Yao HJ, Wang Z, Zhou J, et al. The effects of RNA interference mediated VEGF gene silencing on biological behavior of renal cell carcinoma and transplanted renal tumor in nude mice. Cancer Biomark. 2016;16(1):1–9.
6. Sternberg CN, Davis ID, Mardiak J, Szczylik C, Lee E, Wagstaff J, Barrios CH, Salman P, Gladkov OA, Kavina A, et al. Pazopanib in locally advanced or metastatic renal cell carcinoma: results of a randomized phase III trial. J Clin Oncol. 2010;28(6):1061–8.
7. Esteller M. Non-coding RNAs in human disease. Nat Rev Genet. 2011;12(12): 861–74.
8. Harries LW. Long non-coding RNAs and human disease. Biochem Soc Trans. 2012;40(4):902–6.
9. Ponting CP, Oliver PL, Reik W. Evolution and functions of long noncoding RNAs. Cell. 2009;136(4):629–41.
10. Cheetham SW, Gruhl F, Mattick JS, Dinger ME. Long noncoding RNAs and the genetics of cancer. Br J Cancer. 2013;108(12):2419–25.
11. Yang L, Xue Y, Liu J, Zhuang J, Shen L, Shen B, Yan J, Guo H. Long noncoding RNA ASAP1-IT1 promotes cancer stemness and predicts a poor prognosis in patients with bladder cancer. Neoplasma. 2017;64(6):847–55.
12. Huarte M, Rinn JL. Large non-coding RNAs: missing links in cancer? Hum Mol Genet. 2010;19(R2):R152–61.
13. Tsai MC, Spitale RC, Chang HY. Long intergenic noncoding RNAs: new links in cancer progression. Cancer Res. 2011;71(1):3–7.
14. Wang C, Mao ZP, Wang L, Wu GH, Zhang FH, Wang DY, Shi JL. Long non-coding RNA MALAT1 promotes cholangiocarcinoma cell proliferation and invasion by activating PI3K/Akt pathway. Neoplasma. 2017;64(5):725–31.
15. Flockhart RJ, Webster DE, Qu K, Mascarenhas N, Kovalski J, Kretz M, Khavari PA. BRAFV600E remodels the melanocyte transcriptome and induces BANCR to regulate melanoma cell migration. Genome Res. 2012;22(6):1006–14.
16. He A, Liu Y, Chen Z, Li J, Chen M, Liu L, Liao X, Lv Z, Zhan Y, Zhuang C, et al. Over-expression of long noncoding RNA BANCR inhibits malignant phenotypes of human bladder cancer. J Exp Clin Cancer Res. 2016;35(1):125.

17. Shi Y, Liu Y, Wang J, Jie D, Yun T, Li W, Yan L, Wang K, Feng J. Downregulated long noncoding RNA BANCR promotes the proliferation of colorectal Cancer cells via Downregualtion of p21 expression. PLoS One. 2015;10(4):e0122679.
18. Li R, Zhang L, Jia L, Duan Y, Li Y, Bao L, Sha N. Long non-coding RNA BANCR promotes proliferation in malignant melanoma by regulating MAPK pathway activation. PLoS One. 2014;9(6):e100893.
19. Wang D, Wang D, Wang N, Long Z, Ren X. Long non-coding RNA BANCR promotes endometrial Cancer cell proliferation and invasion by regulating MMP2 and MMP1 via ERK/MAPK signaling pathway. Cell Physiol Biochem. 2016;40(3–4):644–56.
20. Zhang ZX, Liu ZQ, Jiang B, Lu XY, Ning XF, Yuan CT, Wang AL. BRAF activated non-coding RNA (BANCR) promoting gastric cancer cells proliferation via regulation of NF-kappaB1. Biochem Biophys Res Commun. 2015;465(2):225–31.
21. Zhou T, Gao Y. Increased expression of LncRNA BANCR and its prognostic significance in human hepatocellular carcinoma. World J Surg Oncol. 2016;14(1):8.
22. Wang LS, Chen SJ, Zhang JF, Liu MN, Zheng JH, Yao XD. Anti-proliferative potential of glucosamine in renal cancer cells via inducing cell cycle arrest at G0/G1 phase. BMC Urol. 2017;17(1):38.
23. Wu J, Zhang J, Shen B, Yin K, Xu J, Gao W, Zhang L. Long noncoding RNA lncTCF7, induced by IL-6/STAT3 transactivation, promotes hepatocellular carcinoma aggressiveness through epithelial-mesenchymal transition. J Exp Clin Cancer Res. 2015;34:116.
24. Taheri M, Omrani MD, Ghafouri-Fard S. Long non-coding RNA expression in bladder cancer. Biophys Rev. 2017;8:1–9.
25. Li JY, Ma X, Zhang CB. Overexpression of long non-coding RNA UCA1 predicts a poor prognosis in patients with esophageal squamous cell carcinoma. Int J Clin Exp Pathol. 2014;7(11):7938–44.
26. Petejova N, Martinek A. Renal cell carcinoma: review of etiology, pathophysiology and risk factors. Biomed Pap Med Fac Univ Palacky, Olomouc, Czechoslovakia. 2016;160(2):183–94.
27. Yao J, Chen Y, Wang Y, Liu S, Yuan X, Pan F, Geng P. Decreased expression of a novel lncRNA CADM1-AS1 is associated with poor prognosis in patients with clear cell renal cell carcinomas. Int J Clin Exp Pathol. 2014;7(6):2758–67.
28. Fan YH, Ye MH, Wu L, Wu MJ, Lu SG, Zhu XG. BRAF-activated lncRNA predicts gastrointestinal cancer patient prognosis: a meta-analysis. Oncotarget. 2017;8(4):6295–303.
29. Liu XF, Hao JL, Xie T, Pant OP, Lu CB, Lu CW, Zhou DD. The BRAF activated non-coding RNA: a pivotal long non-coding RNA in human malignancies. Cell Prolif. 2018;27:e12449.
30. Yu X, Zheng H, Chan MT, Wu WKK. BANCR: a cancer-related long non-coding RNA. Am J Cancer Res. 2017;7(9):1779–87.
31. He A, Feng S, Chen Z, Liu Y, Mei H. Long non-coding RNA BRAF activated non-coding RNA as a potential novel molecular biomarker for metastasis and prognosis in various cancers. Minerva Med. 2017;108(3):293–8.
32. Sun M, Liu XH, Wang KM, Nie FQ, Kong R, Yang JS, Xia R, Xu TP, Jin FY, Liu ZJ, et al. Downregulation of BRAF activated non-coding RNA is associated with poor prognosis for non-small cell lung cancer and promotes metastasis by affecting epithelial-mesenchymal transition. Mol Cancer. 2014;13:68.
33. Jiang W, Zhang D, Xu B, Wu Z, Liu S, Zhang L, Tian Y, Han X, Tian D. Long non-coding RNA BANCR promotes proliferation and migration of lung carcinoma via MAPK pathways. Biomed Pharmacother. 2015;69:90–5.
34. Guo Q, Zhao Y, Chen J, Hu J, Wang S, Zhang D, Sun Y. BRAF-activated long non-coding RNA contributes to colorectal cancer migration by inducing epithelial-mesenchymal transition. Oncol Lett. 2014;8(2):869–75.

Posterior urethral valves: 10 years audit of epidemiologic, diagnostic and therapeutic aspects in Yaoundé gynaeco-obstetric and paediatric hospital

Faustin Felicien Mouafo Tambo[6,7], Paul Nkemtendong Tolefac[1*], Marcelin Ngowe Ngowe[2], Jacqueline Ze Minkande[3,4], Landry Mbouche[7], Georgette Guemkam[5], Neville Alemnju Telelen[2], Fru Fobuzshi Angwafo III[6,7] and Aurelien Maurice Sosso[6]

Abstract

Background: The incidence of posterior urethral valve (PUV) is estimated at 1:5000–1:8000 males. It is the most common paediatric urologic urgency and the most common cause of male obstructive uropathy and chronic renal failure in children. The study aimed to describe the experience of Yaoundé gynaeco-obstetrics and paediatric hospital in the management of PUV.

Methods: Retrospectively, medical records were retrieved over a ten year period and all data recorded and analyzed for study objectives. Patients were called and evaluated for outcomes regarding morbidity and mortality.

Results: A total of 18 patients all males were managed over the ten year period, given prevalence of 13 cases/100,000 admissions and an admission rate of 2 per annum. The median age at presentation was 22 months and 13 (72.2%) participants presented late. Voiding urethrocystogram was done in all the participants where it showed dilated and elongated posterior urethral valves in 16 (88.9%) of the cases. Endoscopic valve ablation resulted in the relief of obstruction in all but 3 (16.7%) participants that had residual valves and 2 (11.2%) participants that had urethral stenosis. Type I valves were most common in 14 (78.0%) participants. The mean duration of follow up was 34.56 ± 21.47 months. Complications at final follow up were: 10 (55.6%) chronic renal failure, 2 (11.2%) end-stage renal failure. The case fatality rate was 5.6%.

Conclusion: Many patients present late in our setting with already established complications. There is the need to counsel parents/guardians on the importance of long-term follow up after relief of obstruction.

Keywords: Posterior urethral valves, Epidemiologic, Diagnostic, Yaoundé, Late presentation

Background

Posterior urethral valve (PUV) is the most common lower urinary tract congenital anomaly in boys with an incidence of 1: 5000–1:8000 males [1–5]. It is the leading cause of bladder outlet obstruction and renal insufficiency in male children [6–8]. The incidence is unknown in our sub-region. In Nigeria, Uba et al. [3] in Jos, reported 3–8 cases per annum and Jaja et al. [9] in Port Harcourt observed that it accounted for 1 in 2447 children seen in their hospital.

This disease was first described by Morgagni in 1717 and later by Langenbeck in 1802 [10, 11]. The exact embryology and aetiology of this condition are not known.

PUV has detrimental and wide-ranging effects on the global development of the kidney, bladder and the entire urinary system. This result from persistent and unrelieved pressure on the bladder leading to bladder diverticular, hydronephrosis and chronic to end-stage renal diseases (ESRD). The anomaly is associated with high mortality and morbidity including urosepsis, overflow urinary incontinence, chronic kidney diseases (CKD),

* Correspondence: ptolefac15@gmail.com
[1]Specialized Internship Program, Faculty of Medicine and Biomedical Sciences, University of Yaoundé 1, Yaoundé, Cameroon
Full list of author information is available at the end of the article

hypertension, chronic anaemia, failure to thrive, poor quality of life and even death [5, 12].

Early diagnosis can be made prenatally by regular and routine prenatal ultrasounds. The routine use of this modality has significantly increased early diagnosis and management of this pathology in most developed countries. As prenatal hydronephrosis usually prompts an early and complete work up at birth with a voiding cysto-urethrogram (VCUG) leading to early postnatal diagnosis [4]. Prenatal ultrasound uptakes are still at low levels in our environment.

Initial continuous catheter drainage and or vesicostomy and eventual management by endoscopic valve resection, usually ameliorate the obstructive uropathy. However, it has been noted that even after surgical treatment of valves and relief of obstruction, about 70% of older children and adolescents continue to have persistent bladder dysfunction, poor quality of life, and worsening CKD and ESRD [4, 11]. Long-term management of PUV constitutes a challenge in the practice of pediatric urology in our environment due to lack of specialized centers as well as the paucity of trained pediatric urologists and nephrologists to evaluate and monitor these children [3]. In the few highly specialized centers where valve ablation is done, most patients fail to turn up for follow-up visits due to an erroneous belief that it has been cured following the initial relief of the obstruction.

This study aimed to describe the epidemiologic, diagnostic and therapeutic aspects of PUV in Yaoundé Gynaeco-Obstetric and Paediatric Hospital (YGOPH), Cameroon. YGOPH is a tertiary care hospital located in the city of Yaoundé with a modern theatre that operates among other cases patients with PUV. These patients with PUV are usually operated in this center by a group of surgeons from China and Cameroon owing to the Cameroon-China cooperation.

Methods

Study design and setting

This was a retrospective descriptive cross-sectional study carried out over a period of 10 years (April 2005–March 2016) in the pediatric surgical unit of Yaoundé gynaeco-obstetric and pediatric hospital (YGOPH). YGOPH is a tertiary hospital located in the city of Yaoundé. Among other units in the hospital is the pediatric surgical unit that manages cases of pediatric surgery. It receives cases from Yaoundé and its environs. Cases of posterior urethral valves are usually received in the service all year round. The pediatric surgery unit is fully equipped material resources including a hospitalization section (12 beds), outpatient surgical consultations, minor theatre and the major theatre as well as human resources such as two pediatric surgeons, two urologists, one orthopedic surgeon and several nurses. Over the past years, corporation between this hospital and China has allowed these children to benefit from endoscopic resection of the valve by electrocautery. At hospitalization and after fluid and electrolyte stabilization, vesicostomy is usually done to relieve obstruction after which an interval endoscopic valve resection is programmed. Endoscopic valve resection is usually done by a team of Cameroonian and Chinese surgeons owing to the Cameroon-China cooperation in this hospital.

Data collection

We included all cases of posterior urethral valves that had a confirmed endoscopic diagnosis, and we excluded all those whose medical files could not be seen as well as those with files not containing relevant information such as endoscopic findings and valve types. Those with alternative endoscopic intraoperative diagnosis were also excluded. The study was divided into two phases: Phase I was a was a retrospective analysis of children aged 15 years and below managed for PUV at the paediatric surgical unit of YGOPH for 10 years between April 2005 to March 2016. Phase II was a cross-sectional evaluation of the clinical and kidney functions of all the patients operated between the said period. Information on the age at presentation, clinical features, and anthropometric measures, results of investigations: hemoglobin level, serum electrolytes, white cell count, urea and creatinine, urine culture as well as information on prenatal ultrasound, postnatal abdominal ultrasound, voiding cysto-urethrogram (VCUG) were obtained. At each follow-up, weight, height, blood pressure, serum creatinine, and full blood count and urine culture, complications developed were noted. After stabilizing the patients by controlling infection, correction of fluid, electrolyte balance, catheter drainage and or vesicostomy was done while awaiting definitive valve ablation which was programmed by a group of surgeons. After valve ablation, a urethral catheter was left in situ for 3–5 days to allow the oedema to subside and to enable measurement of urinary output. Intravenous fluids were given and adjusted to meet the need of patients while serum electrolytes were monitored. Patients were then subsequently discharged on antibiotic prophylaxis and followed up in an outpatient clinic at pediatric nephrology consultation at the mother and child center, Chantal Biya Foundation with voiding history, abdominopelvic ultrasonography, and serial serum creatinine estimation.

Statistical analysis

Data collected with the aid of case report forms were entered into WHO epi info version 3.5.4 and analyzed using WHO epi info version 3.5.4 and statistical package for social scientists (SPSS) software version 20. The results were presented as tables and charts. Mean and standard deviation were determined for continuous variables and frequency and percentage for categorical variables. Continuous variables were compared with t-test, and categorical variables with Chi-Square test or the McNemar test were appropriate. Level of significance was set at a p-value 0f < 0.05.

Ethical considerations

Ethical clearance was obtained from the ethical committee of YGOPH and the institutional review board of the University of Douala.

Definition of terms

Late presentation is defined in this study as a patient presenting after 30 days of life.

Results

Sociodemographic and clinical characteristics of posterior urethral valves

There were 140,444 admissions of ages 0 days to 15 years patients in the pediatric surgery unit of YGOPH between April 2005 and March 2016, out of which 25 were treated for posterior urethral valves (PUV). According to hospital records 25 patients were hospitalized for PUV during the study period, 7 participants were excluded, in five of them the medical files were missing, and in the remaining two the files were incomplete with missing vital information such as endoscopic findings, types of valves and VCUG findings (Table 1).

As shown in Table 2, the most common clinical features were voiding dysfunction (characterized by dribbling, poor stream, and straining) in all 18 (100%) participants, supra-pubic distension from palpable bladder in 9 (50.0%) participants. Others included recurrent UTI in 11 (61.1%) participants, anaemia in 10 (55.6%) participants, urine retention with suprapubic bladder in 9 (50.0%) participants, fever with core temperature > 38 ° C in 7 (38.9%) participants, failure to thrive in 5 (27.8%) participants, ascites in 4 (22.4%) participants; associated congenital malformations noted were umbilical hernia in 4 (22.2%) participants, cryptorchidism in 2 (11.1) participants, vaginal hydrocele in 1 (5.6%) participants and inguinal hernia 1 (5.6%) participants, 15 (83.3%) did urine culture at presentation, 6 (40.0%) of the urine culture were sterile. The most frequently isolated bacteria were *Escherichia coli* in 4 (26.7%) and *Klebsiella sp.* in 3 (20.0%). The bar chart in Fig. 1 that follows is a distribution of the bacteria isolated.

Table 1 Age distribution at presentation

Age group / months	Frequency (n)	Percentage (%)
≤1 month	5	27.8
2-12 months	3	16.7
13-48 months	4	22.2
49-84 months	4	22.2
85-120 months	2	11.1
Total	18	100

Their age at presentation ranges from 1st day of life to 108 months (9 years) with a median age of 22 months. The diagnosis was made in 13 (72.2%) participants after 1 month and in 10 (55.6%) after 1 year as shown in Table 1. This gives a prevalence of 13 cases of PUV/100, 000 admissions in our pediatric surgery unit and an annual admission rate of 2 cases of PUV per annum

Table 2 Clinical features at presentation

Clinical Feature	Frequency (n)	Percentage (%)
Voiding dysfunctions	18	100
Fever	7	38.9
Convulsion	2	11.1
Gastroenteritis	2	11.1
Respiratory Distress	2	11.1
Sepsis	2	11.1
CKD	2	11.1
Recurrent UTI	11	61.1
Failure to thrive	5	27.8
History Neonatal infection	4	22.2
Jaundice	2	11.1
Lower limb oedema	1	5.6
Abdominal Distension/Ascites	4	22.2
Urine retention	9	50.0
Umbilical hernia	4	22.2
Inguinal hernia	1	5.6
Vaginal hydrocele	1	5.6
Cryptorchidism	2	11.1
Anaemia	10	55.6

Diagnosis of posterior urethral valves

VCUG was diagnostic in 16 (88.9%) patients, showing dilated and elongated posterior urethra. Figure 2 is a VCUG of a 2.3 year-old toddler showing dilated and elongated PUV (white arrow). There was associated vesico-ureteric reflux in 10 (55.6%) patients; bladder diverticular in 3 (16.7%) and multiple trabeculated bladder in 8 (44.4%). Abdominal Ultrasound was diagnostic in 7 (38.9%) showing dilated and elongated posterior urethral valves. In 16 (88.9%) participants there was suspicion of PUV by the presence of bilateral hydronephrosis (BHN). Out of the participants with BHN, 6 (37.5%) had stage I BHN, 6 (37.5%) had stage II BHN, 2 (12.5%) had stage III BHN and 2 (12.5%) had stage IV BHN. Other ultrasound findings included vesico-ureteric reflux 9 (50.0%), trabeculated bladder 11 (61.1%). 10 (55.6%) participants did a prenatal ultrasound between 18th to 28th weeks of

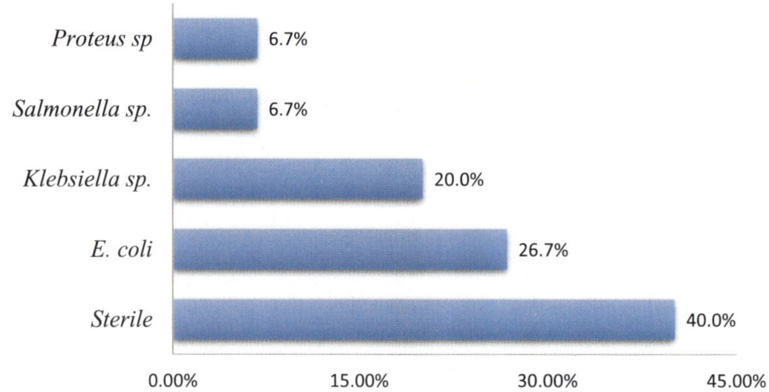

Fig. 1 Bacteria isolated in the urine of patients

pregnancy. 2 (20%) of the prenatal ultrasounds were suggestive of PUV by showing bilateral hydronephrosis.

Management of posterior urethral valves

All participants benefited from primary endoscopic valve resection by electrocautery. In 6 (33.3%) participants vesicostomy for urinary drainage was done before definitive endoscopic valve resection. Valve resection resulted in improvement of urinary symptoms in all but (3) 16.7% of participants that had residual valves that necessitated a second endoscopic resection and in 2 (11.2%) participants it was complicated by urethral stenosis that necessitated urethral dilatation. The delay between diagnosis and primary endoscopic valve resection ranges between 0 and 46 months (median = 1 month) whereas the mean delay between vesicostomy and urethrocystoscopy ranges between 0 and 12 months. The most frequent valves were type I in 14 (77.8%) participants. Type II and type III valves had an equal prevalence of 11.2% each.

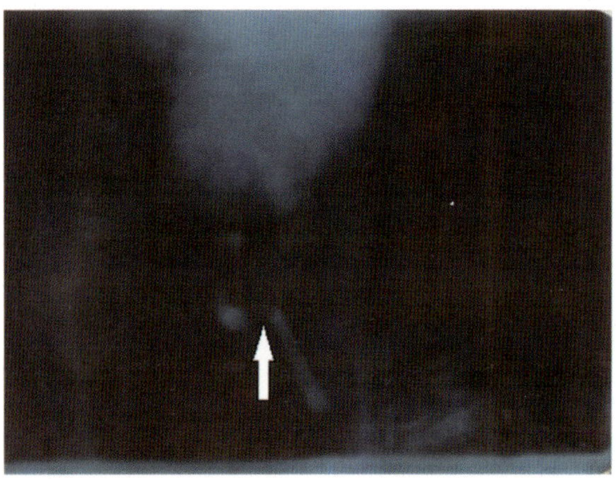

Fig. 2 VCUG showing dilated and elongated PUV (White arrow) in a 2 year 3 months old toddler

Complications of posterior urethral valves

At presentation, 6 (33.3%) patients were in renal insufficiency with serum creatinine greater than 132.6 μmol/l. However, determination of glomerular filtration rate (GFR) using Swartz formula showed a mean GFR of 51.0 ± 43.83 ml/min/1.73m^2 with a range of 11.40–148.5 ml/min/1.73m^2 and most of the participants having a GFR between 15 and 29 ml/min/1.73m^2. Half of the participants were in chronic renal failure (GFR < 60) and16.70% in ESRD (GFR < 15) requiring dialysis. GFR could not be gotten for three participants with serum creatinine because their heights were not taking on admission. For the nine participants followed up (prospective phase), at diagnosis of posterior urethral valves, 4 (44.4%) patients were in chronic renal failure (GFR < 60) and 1 (11.1%) patients in ESRD (GFR < 15). At the final follow up, 5 (55.6%) participants were in CRF (GFR < 60) with 1 (11.1%) participants in ESRD (GFR < 15). The change in the percentage of patients with CRF before surgery and at follow up was not statistically significant using the McNemar test with the level of significance set at p-value of 0.05 (p-value =1). In general, as shown on the curve below (Fig. 3), there is a modest improvement of GFR and hence renal functions following relief of the obstruction.

The mean duration of follow up was 34.6 ± 21.5 months with a range of 6–73. 9 (50%) participants were lost to follow up. One death was recorded in 2013 with the cause of death being ESRF and urosepsis. This gives a mortality/case fatality rate (CFR) of 5.6%.

Discussion

The indexed study described the experience in the management of posterior urethral valves in a tertiary care center in Cameroon. The prevalence of PUV and admission rate in the surgical unit of this institution was estimated at 13 cases / 100,000 admissions and 2 cases per annum respectively. An earlier review of childhood obstructive uropathy in Nigeria by Jaja et al. [9] in 2012 suggested that the condition is certainly not as rare as

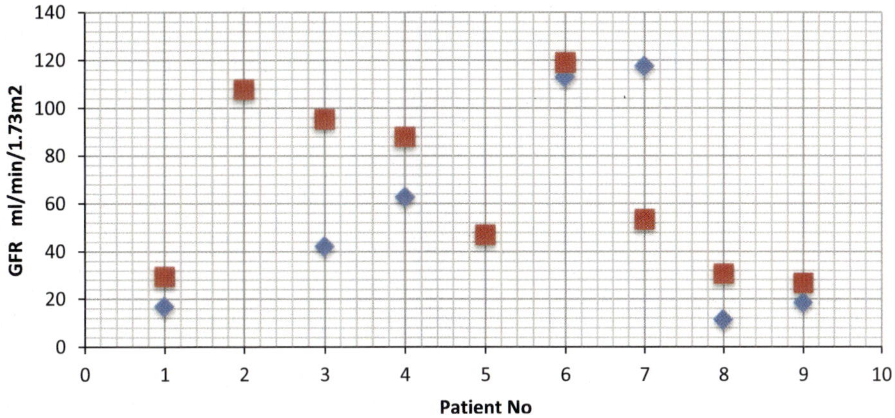

Fig. 3 Variations of GFR before surgery (blue) and at final follow up (red) for 9 patients

the paucity of reports on the prevalence in English literature may suggest [3]. In the present study, the rate of two children with PUV diagnosed yearly is comparable to earlier studies conducted in Cameroon by Angwafo et al. [13] and Chiabi et al. [14] where the rate ranges between 3 and 4 cases per annum. From this, we can conclude that this disease has a constant rate of presentation in our hospitals. This was equally similar to studies conducted elsewhere in Africa by Talabi et al. [2] where they got 3 per annum and Uba et al. [3] of 3–8 per annum. The low prevalence in our environment may be related to early death in the perinatal and neonatal periods as a result of severe obstruction, superimposed infection, acute renal failure and pulmonary hypoplasia, who never get to the hospital and were therefore never diagnosed [3, 15].

While the diagnosis of posterior urethral valves can be made prenatally [16, 17], only 10 (55.6%) patients did a prenatal ultrasound. In 2 (11.2%) of the ultrasounds, there was suspicion of PUV. This is consistent with reports by Okafor et al. [18] and Talabi et al. [2] of 6.5 and 8.1% respectively. A study conducted in Nigeria in 2010 by Ohagwu et al. [19] showed that negative attitude, long distances to service providers, considerably heavy financial cost, long waiting periods, and unsatisfactory previous scan experience are major barriers to prenatal ultrasound in Nigeria, and these barriers have indirectly made prenatal diagnosis of PUV difficult in our setting. Low level of detection of PUV by prenatal ultrasounds can also be explained by the lack of experts in prenatal imaging hence missed diagnosis.

The median age of diagnosis in the study of 22 months suggested that patients with this condition presented late in our environment. 72.7% presented after the age of 1 month and 55.5% presented after the age of 1 year. This is similar to studies done earlier in Cameroon by Chiabi et al. [14] where 50% of patients presented after 1 year. It is also similar to studies conducted in Nigeria by Orumah et al. [6], Odetunde et al. [1] and Ikuerowo et al. [20] where they found out that 56.8, 52 and 57.1% of patients respectively presented after the age of 1 year. Factors that might have contributed to late presentation noted include a suboptimal prenatal ultrasound utilization, [19] poverty, ignorance on the part of parents, the paucity of specialist care, late referral by primary care providers.

All the participants presented with voiding dysfunction ranging from dribbling 11 (61.1%), dysuria 8 (44.4%) and **pollakiuria** 6 (33.3%). This is similar to the study conducted earlier in Cameroon by Chiabi et al. [14] where the most common urinary symptoms were dribbling (61.7%) and dysuria (54%) and in another study by India by Bhaumik et al. [21] where 79% presented with dribbling. Again, the similarity was noted in studies conducted in Nigeria by Odetunde et al. [1] and Orumuah et al. [6] where 100 and 92% respectively presented with voiding anomaly. It is therefore important to have a high index of suspicion of PUV in neonates and infants presenting with urinary symptoms. We also found out that at hospitalization, nine (50.0%) of the participants had a palpable bladder/urine retention, which is comparable to a study conducted in a Nigerian tertiary hospital in 2015 by Orumuah et al. [6] where about a third of participants had a palpable bladder.

In our setting, participants were not routinely subjected to screening tests to detect other congenital anomalies due to financial constraints and the limited availability of screening facilities. However, associated congenital anomalies noted included 4 umbilical hernias (22.2%), one inguinal hernia (5.6%), one hydrocele (5.6%), and two cryptorchidism (11.2%). Similar congenital malformations were described in studies by Chiabi et al. [14] and Orumuah et al. [6]. Previous studies have also noted congenital defects in the cardiovascular, urogenital, gastrointestinal, and central nervous systems of males with PUV [6, 22, 23].

The gold standard for the diagnosis of PUV is VCUG [21]. This was done in all cases and demonstrated dilatation and elongation of the posterior urethral in (16) 88.9%, and can be compared to earlier studies in 2015 by Talabi et al. [2] where it showed dilated and elongated posterior urethral valves in 83.8% of the cases.

Biological investigations conducted at presentation revealed complications such as renal insufficiency, urinary tract infections, and anemia and electrolyte imbalances. (10) 55.6% patients had altered renal functions with glomerular filtration rate < 60 ml/min/1.73m^2 at presentation which is comparable with 40.5% reported by Talabi et al. [2]. 71.4% reported by Odetunde et al. [1] in Nigeria, but in conflict with 15.4% reported by Dahab et al. [24]. Elevated serum creatinine level has been documented to be associated with poor prognosis in PUV patients, and this may not be reversed even with the relief of the obstruction. 60% of those who did urine cultures had a positive culture with the most commonly cultured germs being *Escherichia coli*. This was different from Talabi et al. [2] where the most common cultured bacteria was *Klebsiella sp*. These complications were similar to those observed in Nigeria [1, 6] and in Yaoundé [14].

Various operative techniques have been described for PUV resection. In this study, all the patients benefited from endoscopic valve resection. Type I valves were most common in 14 (78.0%) participants, which is comparable to what was found in a study in Nigeria [6]. Valve resection resulted in the relief of obstruction in all but three (16.7%) patients that had residual valves and thus needed repeat valve ablation to attain satisfactory passage of urine. This was similar to a study conducted by Mirshermirani et al. [12] and Sudarsanan et al. [25] where 15.3 and 13% respectively had residual valves. Endoscopic valve resection resulted to urethral stricture in two (11.2%) patients. This is comparable to 7.1, 5 and 8.2% obtained by Mirshermirani et al. [12], Shittu et al. [26] and Sudersanan et al. [25] respectively. Hence, the rate of complication in our low-resource setting remains relatively low and is comparable to that in the developed world which generally have greater resources and medical expertise. This comparison could be explained by the fact that the surgeries done in our setting are conducted by a team of both Cameroonian and Chinese surgeons thanks to the long-standing Cameroon-China cooperation.

The mortality rate of 5.6% recorded in our study is comparable to 4.9% reported in Nigeria [3], 5.1% in Iran [12] and 3.8% in Canada [27], but higher mortality rates were observed in Cameroon (21%) [14] in earlier studies conducted in Nigeria (9–13.5%) [2, 6, 18]. Studies have been reported with zero mortality rate [25] and other studies reported with mortality as high as 69% [1]. The reinforcement of our local team with surgeons from China, may explain the relatively low mortality in our series which is similar to that in the developed world.

The majority of the patients were lost to follow-up. Unfortunately, the reason for this is not known. However, it may be due to the reluctance of parents to continue hospital visits in the presence of satisfactory urine stream after relief of the obstruction. This, combined with the long distances required to travel to the hospital and poverty may also contribute to losses a follow-up. Educating parents and guardians about the importance of long-term follow-up and issues such as ongoing renal deterioration even after relief of obstruction should, therefore, be incorporated into the management of this disease.

Limitations

Though our study has described very important clinico-biological characteristics of PUV in a major pediatric surgery unit in Cameroon, the applicability may be limited by:

- Cross-sectional nature and inability to establish spatial relationships
- A relatively small sample size of 18 participants
- Being solely hospital-based since many patients with PUV die during the neonatal period and infancy without an established diagnosis.
- Incomplete and absent information on many parameters as a result of its retrospective nature.

However, the study provides a documented perspectives of PUV over 10 years, providing much-needed evidence in a setting where the availability of data is a challenge. We, therefore, recommend a large multicentre case-control or cohort study to assess the relationship of most of the variables associated with PUV. In spite of these limitations, our study may serve as a pilot study for future studies on PUV and may provide data on clinical decision making in our local context.

Conclusion

The rarity of posterior urethral valves with a rate of two cases per year, routine prenatal ultrasound and investigations of neonates presenting with urinary symptoms will lead to earlier detection. With early presentation, diagnosis, and, therefore, treatment, the outcome is expected to improve as valve ablation leads to satisfactory urinary stream in most of the patients in the series. The rate of complications and mortality remains relatively low. However, there is a need to further educate parents on the symptoms of the disease and the benefits of long-term follow–up of patients.

Abbreviations

BHN: Bilateral hydronephrosis; CKD: Chronic kidney disease; CRF: Chronic renal failure; ESRD: End stage renal disease; GFR: Glomerular filtration rate; PUV: Posterior urethral valves; VCUG: Voiding cysto-urethrogram; YGOPH: Yaoundé Gynaeco – Obstetric and Paediatric Hospital

Acknowledgements
We express our sincere gratitude to all doctors, nurses and medical students who took part in the management of the patient. Special thanks also goes to Papa Federick who contributed immensely in data analysis.

Authors' contributions
Conception and design of the original manuscript (FFMT, PNT, MNN, LM, NAT, & GG), Drafting of the manuscript (FFMT, NAT, PNT), Critical revision of the manuscript for important intellectual content (MNN, JZM, FFA, GG, AMS & LM), Correction of final manuscript (all authors), supervision (PNT, MNN, FFMT, AMS). All authors read and approved the final manuscript.

Competing interests
The authors declare that they have no competing interests.

Author details
[1]Specialized Internship Program, Faculty of Medicine and Biomedical Sciences, University of Yaoundé 1, Yaoundé, Cameroon. [2]Department of Surgery, Faculty of Health Sciences, University of Buea, Buea, Cameroon. [3]Department of Anaesthesia and Intensive Care, Faculty of Medicine and Biomedical Sciences, University of Yaoundé 1, Yaoundé, Cameroon. [4]Department of Anaesthesia and Intensive Care, Yaoundé Gynaeco-Obstetric and Paediatric Hospital, Yaoundé, Cameroon. [5]Paediatric Nephrology Unit, Mother and Child Centre, Chantal Biya Foundation, Yaoundé, Cameroon. [6]Departmennt of Surgery and Subspecialties, Faculty of Medicine and Biomedical Sciences, University of Yaoundé 1, Yaoundé, Cameroon. [7]Paediatric Surgery Unit, Yaoundé Gynaeco-Obstetric and Paediatric Hospital, Yaoundé, Cameroon.

References
1. Odetunde OI, Odetunde OA, Ademuyiwa AO, Okafor HU, Ekwochi U, Azubuike JC, et al. Outcome of late presentation of posterior urethral valves in a resource-limited economy: challenges in management. Int J Nephrol. 2012;2012:e345298.
2. Talabi AO, Sowande OA, Etonyeaku AC, Salako AA, Adejuyigbe O. Posterior urethral valves in children: pattern of presentation and outcome of initial treatment in Ile-Ife, Nigeria. Niger J Surg Off Publ Niger Surg Res Soc. 2015; 21(2):151–6.
3. Uba AF, Chirdan LB, Ihezue CH, Ramyil VL, Dakum NK. Posterior urethral valves in children: pattern of presentation and outcome of initial treatment in Ile-Ife, Nigeria. Afr J Urol. 2007;13:124–31.
4. Thomas J. Etiopathogenesis and management of bladder dysfunction in patients with posterior urethral valves. Indian J Urol IJU J Urol Soc India. 2010;26(4):480–9.
5. Desai D. A review of urodynamic evaluation in children and its role in the management of boys with posterior urethral valves. Indian J Urol. 2007; 23(4):435.
6. Orumuah AJ, Oduagbon OE. Presentation, management, and outcome of posterior urethral valves in a Nigerian tertiary hospital. Afr J Paediatr Surg. 2015;12(1):18.
7. Hodges SJ, Patel B, McLorie G, Atala A. Posterior urethral valves. ScientificWorldJournal. 2009;9:1119–26.
8. Uthup S, Binitha R, Geetha S, Hema R, Kailas L. A follow-up study of children with posterior urethral valve. Indian J Nephrol. 2010;20(2):72–5.
9. Jaja T, Anochie IC, Eke FU. Posterior urethral valve in childhood in Port Harcourt, Nigeria. Port Harcourt Med J. 2012;6(1):10–6.
10. Morgagni G, Alexander B. The seats and causes of diseases investigated by anatomy; in five books, containing a great variety of dissections, with remarks. To which are added ... copious indexes. London: A. Millar; and T. Cadell, his successor [etc.]; 1769. p. 796. [cited 2016 Jan 20]. Available from: http://archive.org/details/seatscausesofdis02morg
11. Nasir AA, Ameh EA, Abdur-Rahman LO, Adeniran JO, Abraham MK. Posterior urethral valve. World J Pediatr. 2011;7(3):205–16.
12. Mirshemirani A, Khaleghnejad A, Rouzrokh M, Sadeghi A, Mohajerzadeh L, Sharifian M. Posterior urethral valves; a single center experience. Iran J Pediatr. 2013;23(5):531–5.
13. Angwafo F, Andze G, Biouele JM, Sosso MA, Edzoa T, Niat G. Les valves de l'urètre postérieur chez l'enfant : à propos de 22 cas. J Urol (Paris). 1995; 101(3):132–7.
14. Chiabi A, Angwafo F, Obama MT, Takou V, Zoung JK. Posterior urethral valves in children: a review of 28 cases in Yaounde, Cameroon. Clin Mother Child Heal. 2006;1(2) [cited 2016 Jan 18]. Available from: http://www.ajol.info/index.php/cmch/article/view/35799
15. Tolefac PN, Tamambang RF, Yeika E, Mbwagbaw LT, Egbe TO. Ten years analysis of stillbirth in a tertiary hospital in sub-Sahara Africa: a case control study. BMC Res Notes. 2017;10(1):447.
16. Ka H, Df T, Rj A, Hc I, Se S. Prenatally detected posterior urethral valves: is gestational age at detection a predictor of outcome? J Urol. 1994;152(2 Pt 2):698–701.
17. ACOG Practice Bulletin No. 101: Ultrasonography in pregnancy. - PubMed - NCBI [Internet]. [cited 2016 Apr 11]. Available from: http://www.ncbi.nlm.nih.gov/pubmed/19155920
18. Okafor HU, Ekenze SO, Uwaezuoke SN. Posterior urethral valves: determinants of outcome in a developing country: posterior urethral valve outcome. J Paediatr Child Health. 2013;49(2):115–9.
19. Ohagwu CC, Abu PO, Odo MC, Chiegwu HU. Maternal perception of barriers to utilization of prenatal ultrasound in prenatal care in the northern part of Nigeria. Clin Mother Child Heal. 2010;7(1) [cited 2016 Apr 10] Available from: http://www.ajol.info/index.php/cmch/article/view/60569
20. Ikuerowo SO, Balogun BO, Akintomide TE, Ikuerowo AOA, Akinola RA, Gbelee HO, et al. Clinical and radiological characteristics of Nigerian boys with posterior urethral valves. Pediatr Surg Int. 2008;24(7):825–9.
21. Bhaumik K, Chatterjee I, Basu KS, Samanta N, Das S. Posterior urethral valve : its clinical, biochemical and imaging patterns. J Indian Assoc Pediatr Surg. 2003;8(3):153.
22. Heikkila J. Posterior urethral valves are often associated with cryptorchidism and inguinal hernias. J Urol. 2008;180(2):715–7.
23. Mondal K, Maheshwari A, Aneja S, Seth A. A case of Down syndrome with a posterior urethral valve. Indian J Nephrol. 2012;22(5):403–5.
24. Dahab H, Khalafallah AH, Mosaab. Posterior urethral valve presentation, management and outcome. Glob J Med Res. 2013;13(5) [cited 2016 Apr 18] Available from: http://medicalresearchjournal.org/index.php/GJMR/article/view/406.
25. Sudarsanan B, Nasir AA, Puzhankara R, Kedari PM, Unnithan GR, Damisetti KRP. Posterior urethral valves: a single center experience over 7 years. Pediatr Surg Int. 2009;25(3):283–7.
26. Shittu OB, Asinobi AO. Long-term outcome of posterior urethral valves ablation using the Mohan's urethral valvotome. West Afr J Med. 2004; 23(1):35–7.
27. Warren J, Pike J, Leonard M. Posterior urethral valves in Eastern Ontario - a 30 year perspective. Can J Urol. 2004;11(2):2210–5.

Detection of micro-metastases by flow cytometry in lymph nodes from patients with penile cancer

Lu Zhang[1], Jin Hu[1], A. Ali Zirakzadeh[1,4], Jesper Rosvall[2], Mats Hedlund[2], Ping Sheng Hu[3], Robert P.A. Wallin[1], Amir Sherif[4†] and Ola Winqvist[1*†]

Abstract

Background: The tumor draining lymph node concept was first described in penile cancer for staging. Immunohistochemistry and histopathology evaluations are routinely used in clinical practice to examine lymph nodes for metastasis. However, these methods are time-consuming with low diagnostic accuracy and micro-metastases might be missed. In this study, we aim to evaluate detection of metastatic cells in draining lymph nodes by flow cytometry.

Methods: To assess the sensitivity of micro-metastasis detection by FACS (Fluorescence-activated cell sorting), HeLa cells were titrated into Peripheral blood mononuclear cells (PBMCs) and expression of pan-cytokeratin AE1/AE3 was analyzed. Single cell suspensions were separately prepared from 10 regional lymph nodes obtained from 5 patients with invasive penile cancer undergoing radical surgery and lymph node dissection. Lymph node dereived cells were examined for cell surface expression of EpCAM, E-cadherin and intracellular expression of pan-cytokeratin AE1/AE3 by FACS.

Results: Ten lymph nodes from 5 penile cancer patients were investigated in a head-to-head comparison between FACS and pathology examination of sections. All metastatic lymph nodes verified by pathology examination were also identified by FACS. Two additional lymph nodes with micro-metastases were diagnosed by FACS only.

Conclusions: FACS analyses of pan-cytokeratin AE1/AE3 stained single cells from tumor draining lymph nodes can be used to detect micro-metastases in patients with penile cancer patients.

Keywords: Penile cancer, Tumor draining lymph nodes, Flow cytometry, Micro-metastasis detection, Pan-cytokeratin AE1/AE3

Background

The concept of sentinel lymph nodes as the tumor draining lymph nodes was introduced by Cabanas in 1977 investigating patients with penile cancer [1]. It is widely accepted that the histological status of the regional lymph nodes in patients with solid tumors, including penile cancer, is an important predictor for patient survival [2–4]. Routine histopathology exam of penile cancer is performed by visual examination of hematoxylin and eosin (H&E)-stained slices under microscope by pathologists. However, this method is generally considered to be time-consuming and most importantly metastasis may be missed in this examination. For instance, one study in colon cancer found that 19.4% of lymph nodes, which contained micro-metastasis by immunohistochemistry (IHC), were not revealed by H&E examination [5]. Although IHC is not routinely used in penile cancer, it has been suggested that metastasis may also be missed in IHC, as evidenced by that examination of multiple IHC sections with automated computer-assisted image analysis detect additional metastasis [6], suggesting that examination of additional sections from every node increase the sensitivity [7]. However, both methods are extensive workloads for application in routine clinical practice. In addition, a 5 μm-thick section from a lymph node, which is normally examined in routine examinations, represents less than 0.1% of the node. Therefore, micro-metastasis may be missed in clinical pathology examination.

* Correspondence: ola.winqvist@sll.se
†Amir Sherif and Ola Winqvist contributed equally to this work.
[1]Department of Medicine, Immunology and Allergy Unit, Karolinska University Hospital, SE-171 76 Stockholm, Sweden
Full list of author information is available at the end of the article

Our previous studies have demonstrated that flow cytometry can be used to detect micro-metastasis in lymph nodes from patients with colon, renal and head and neck cancer using cytokeratin antibodies [8–10]. In colon cancer the standard for IHC is to detect the presence of aberrant cytokeratin 20 staining in lymph nodes, while in renal cancer cytokeratin 18 is used to demonstrate metastasis. Moreover, it has been found that penile cancer cells are mainly keratinizing squamous cells [11], which express several cytokeratins including 1, 4, 5/6, 8, 13, 18, 19 and 20 [12]. Therefore, a Pan-cytokeratin reagent [13, 14], which is a cocktail of cytokeratin detecting antibodies, can be used to detect the presence of squamous cells in patients with penile cancer. Keratinizing squamous cells are found primarily in HPV negative penile cancer patients but to a less content in HPV positive patients [15]. Moreover, ectopic presence of epithelial cells in lymph nodes is considered as a result of metastasis [16]. These cells can be detected using EpCAM antibody which recognizes an adhesion molecule expressed on the cell surface of most epithelial cells [8]. In addition, the expression of E-cadherin, a type I cell adhesion molecule, has been associated with metastasis [17, 18].

In this paper, we evaluated the use of EpCAM, E-cadherin, and cytokeratins for detection of metastasis in tumor draining lymph nodes from penile cancer patients by flow cytometry.

Methods

Patients

Five patients with invasive penile cancer, 70–80 years old, from Södersjukhuset, Stockholm and Norrlands Universitetssjukhus, Umeå, Sweden, (2014–2015), were included (Table 1), with a preoperative staging; cT1-2 N0-1 M0. The study was approved by the regional ethical committee and written informed consent was obtained from all participants (EPN-Stockholm, dnr: 2013/835–32).

Preparation of specimens

At surgery one piece of primary tumor was removed for the extraction of tumor cells as positive control. Lymph nodes (LNs) were identified and one half of LNs respectively underwent routine histopathology and immunological evaluation by flow cytometry. Venous blood was drawn and peripheral blood mononuclear cells (PBMC) were purified by ficoll-hypaque (Pharmacia, Amersham). Single cell suspensions from tissue specimens (if available to get) were obtained by gentle pressure using a loose-fit glass-homogenizer. Cells were washed twice and resuspended in AIM V® (Life technologies).

Cell culture

The HeLa cell line CCL2 (ATCC) (HPV18 positive) was cultured in RPMI 1640 medium (Sigma) supplemented with 10% fetal bovine serum (FBS), 1% penicillin/streptomycin (Hyclone), and 1% L-glutamine (Hyclone). For flow cytometry detection, cells were detached with Trypsin-EDTA solution (Sigma).

Identification of cancer cells in mixed cultures by flow cytometry

HeLa cells were added to PBMC, diluted in steps of three (3%, 1%, 0.33%, 0.11%, respectively), and kept in FACS-buffer (PBS containing 2% FCS and 0.05% NaN_3). PBMCs alone were used as a negative control.

For surface staining, cells were washed and resuspended in FACS-buffer. Then cells were either directly labeled with an EpCAM antibody conjugated with PE (eBioscience) for 30 min at 4 °C, or incubated with an E-cadherin antibody (Dako) for 30 min at 4 °C, followed by incubation with goat-anti-mouse IgG conjugated with allphycocyanine (APC) (Jackson Immunoresearch) for 30 min in the dark.

For intracellular staining, cells were permeabilized with cytofix/cytoperm buffer (Becton Dickinson) for 30 min at 4 °C, washed and resuspended with 0.3% saponin (Sigma) in FACS-buffer. Direct labeling was performed by incubation of cells with anti-human pancytokeratin AE1/AE3 antibody conjugated with Alexa Fluor® 488 (eBiosience) for 30 min at 4 °C; indirect labeling was performed by incubation of cells with E-cadherin antibody or CK5/CK6 antibody

Table 1 Patient characteristics and lymph node detection

Patient	Age	Clinical tumor staging	pT- stages	Total no. of excised lymph nodes	Total no. of metastatic lymph nodes	Treatment after radical surgery	*Survival (months from the first surgery)
1	80	T2N0M0	pT2	7	0	Total amputation of penis 1.5 months later	Alive
2	77	T1N0M0	pT1	4	0	No	Alive
3	78	T2N1M0	pT2	8	1	No	Alive
4	78	T1N0M0	pT1a	4	2	Repeat Surgery 2 months later to remove bilateral lymph nodes inguinal and iliacal (yield 11/14 metastatic nodes)	4 months
5	70	T2N0M0	pT2	4	0	No	Alive

*Clinically determined during surgery. Alive, still alive at the latest follow-up in 6 August 2016

(Dako), followed by incubation with goat-anti-mouse IgG conjugated APC for 30 min in the dark. An aliquot of the cells was stained with irrelevant conjugated antibodies as isotype controls.

Single-cell suspension from tumor draining lymph nodes was isolated by loose-fit glass homogenizer. Tumor cells were collected from tumor tissue using GentleMACS Dissociator (Miltenyi Biotec) in 10 ml RPMI 1640 medium (Sigma), containing 1% collagenase/Hyaluronidase solution (StemCell Technologies). Direct labeling with pancytokeratin AE1/AE3 antibody conjugated with Alexa Fluor® 488 was performed as above.

Cells were investigated using the LSR-FORTESSA (Becton Dickinson). Collected data were analyzed using FACS DIVA software (Becton Dickinson).

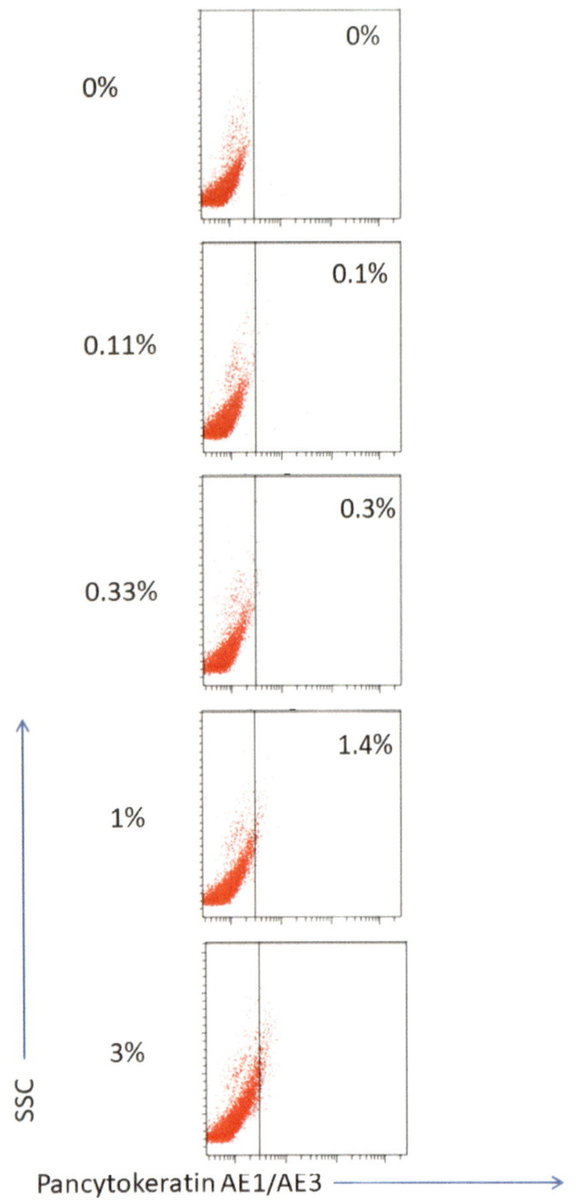

Fig. 1 Detection of HeLa cells mixed with PBMCs. Hela cells were added to PBMCs and diluted in steps of three (3%, 1%, 0.33%, 0.11%, respectively), then stained with Pancytokeratin AE1/AE3 and detected by flow cytometry

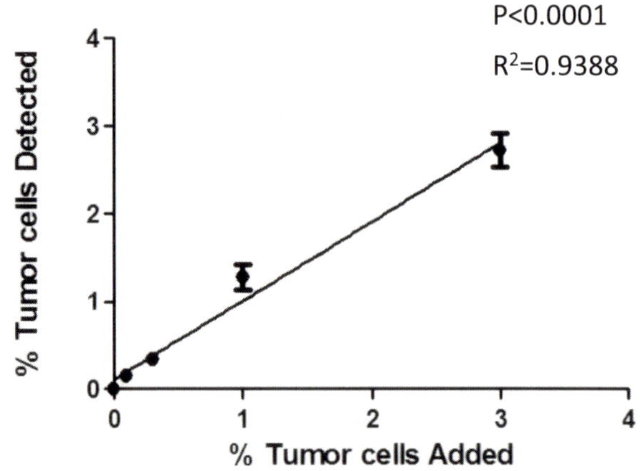

Fig. 2 Sensitivity of flow cytometry detection assay. Y axis displayed the percentage of tumor cell added in the mixed cells. X axis demonstrate the percentage of tumor cells detected by flow cytometry. The linage regression analysis demonstrated a significant correlation between added and detected cells ($p < 0.0001$, $r^2 = 0.9388$)

Statistical evaluation

Comparisons between added and detected cells were evaluated by linear regression using the software GraphPad Prism. *P* value less than 0.05 was regarded as significant.

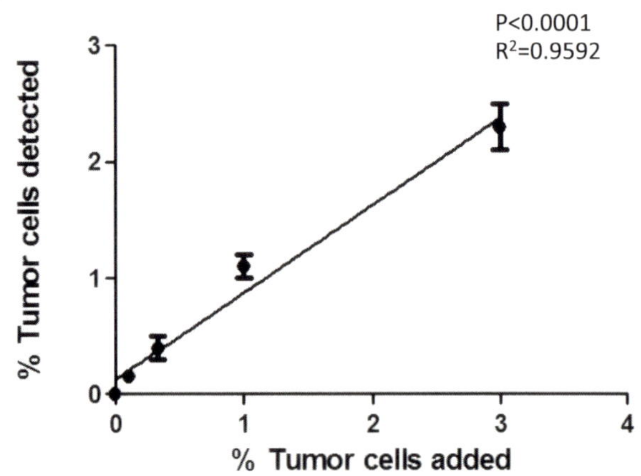

Fig. 3 Stability of flow cytometry detection assay. To test for repeat measurement and stability over time, the same samples were run again after ~ 12 h. Y axis displayed the percentage of tumor cell added in the mixed cells. X axis demonstrate the percentage of tumor cells detected by flow cytometry. The comparison between added and detected cells demonstrated a significant correlation ($p < 0.0001$, $r^2 = 0.9592$)

Results

Identification of tumor cells in mixed cultures using flow cytometry

To the best of our knowledge there are no penile cancer cell lines available. Since there is a resemblance between HPV positive penile cancer cells and cervical cancer cells [19] we decided to use HeLa cells for initial set up of the flow cytometry protocol. First, we tested HeLa cells for their cell surface expression of the epithelial marker EpCAM and E-cadherin, but no positive signal was found (data not shown). Next, we performed intracellular staining using E-cadherin and CK5/CK6 antibody. However again we failed to demonstrate any positive signal (data not shown). Therefore, we decided to use the pan-cytokeratin AE1/AE3 antibody mix which recognize subfamily A and B cytokeratins, and now we were able to detect a positive signal in HeLa cells compared to isotype control (data not shown). The HeLa cells in our cultures only expressed low amounts of cytokeratin allowing a stringent evaluation of the flow cytometry detection of tumor cells in a mixed leukocyte environment. Thus, in order to imitate the presence of metastatic cells in a lymph node we added decreasing number of HeLa cells into PBMCs from 3 to 0.11% in a serial dilution. When 3% HeLa cells were added, we detected 3.2% pan-cytokeratin AE1/AE3 positive cells (Fig. 1). HeLa cells were further titrated and when the lowest number of cells were

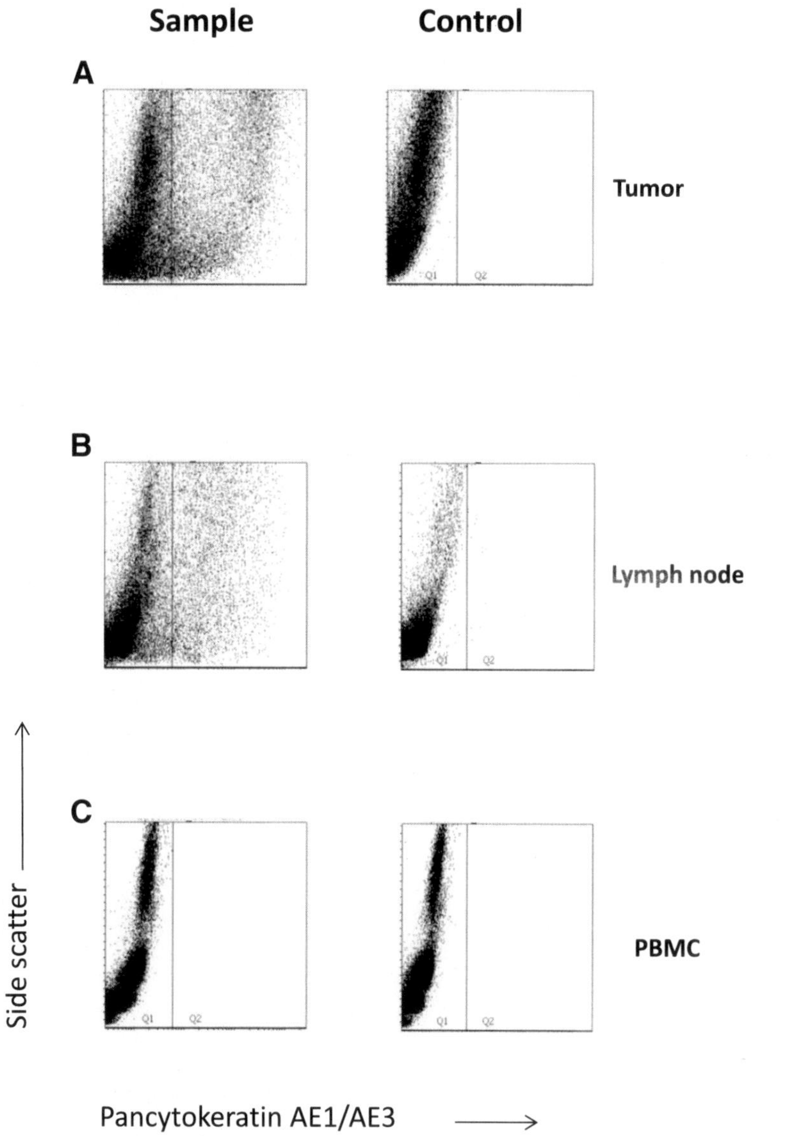

Fig. 4 Detection of tumor cells using flow cytometry. Cell suspensions from the tumor (**a**), Lymph node (**b**) and peripheral blood mononuclear cells (PBMC) (**c**), from patient 9, were intracellularly stained with antibodies against Pancytokeratin AE1/AE3. Right panels were stained with isotype control

added (0.11%) we detected 0.1% pan-cytokeratin AE1/AE3 positive cells in the mixed culture, demonstrating that the method can detect a small number of metastatic cells with precision and accuracy (Fig. 1).

Stability of the method

For evaluating the stability of the method we used PBMCs from 5 different donors, adding decreasing number of HeLa cells from 3 to 0.11%, and compared the number of added vs. detected pan-cytokeratin positive cells at five different occasions (Fig. 2). The linear regression analysis demonstrated a significant correlation between added and detected cells ($p < 0.0001$, $r^2 = 0.9388$) (Fig. 2). The result indicates a linear and reliable detection of pan-cytokeratin positive cells from 0.11 to 3% of tumor cells in PBMCs. The detection of pan-cytokeratin positive cells demonstrated a good inter assay variability even when samples from different donors were used. To test for repeat measurement and stability over time, the same samples were run again after ~ 12 h. The comparison between added and detected cells demonstrated a significant correlation ($p < 0.0001$, $r^2 = 0.9592$) (Fig. 3), indicating that the method is stable over time.

Identification of Pan-cytokeratin positive cells from patients with penile cancer

Next, we started to investigate the expression of pan-cytokeratin in single cells from penile tumors as a positive control (Fig. 4a). A large proportion of penile tumor derived cells were positive with a strong intracellular pan-cytokeratin staining when investigated by FACS (Fig. 4a). The pan-cytokeratin staining of penile cancer cells was in the order of 1–2 log stronger than seen in HeLa cells (Fig. 1).

A total of 10 lymph nodes were harvested from 5 patients with penile cancer (Table. 2). Lymph nodes were divided and sent for routine pathology and investigations with flow cytometry and intracellular pan-cytokeratin staining for a head to head comparison. We received one LN from patient 1 and we found 16.7% pan-cytokeratin-positive cells (Fig. 4b, left panel), demonstrating the presence of metastatic cells. When testing PBMCs from peripheral blood from the patients with penile cancer we were unable to detect any pan-cytokeratin positive cells, suggesting that no circulating metastatic cells were present, at least not above detection limit of 0.11% (Fig. 4c). Compared with the cells suspension from the tumor tissue, we found 47.6% pan cytokeratin positive cells (Fig. 4a). Two lymph nodes from patient 3 were investigated and we found 8.6% and 9.7% pan cytokeratin positive cells respectively (Table. 2) while we found one lymph node from patient 4 containing 2.1% pan cytokeratin positive cells (Table 2). Those lymph nodes were considered as metastatic lymph nodes.

Table 2 Investigation of PBMCs, Lymph nodes and cell suspensions extract from tumor tissues from patients with penile cancer

Patient No.	PBMC (%)	Lymph Node (%)	Cells suspension extract from tumor tissue (%)
1	0.4	0.2	ND
2	0.1	16.7	47.6
3	0.6	8.6	ND
3		9.7	
4	0.1	2.1	33.4
4		0.4	
4		1.1	
5	1.1	0.5	ND
5		0.1	
5		0.2	

In this study, we found Pan-cytokeratin-positive cells in a total of 4 LNs (4/10) (40%) from 3 of the 5 investigated penile cancer patients using flow cytometry (Table 3). In contrast routine pathology demonstrated metastatic cells in 3 LNs (3/17) from 2 out of 5 patients. Thus, the flow cytometry investigation using pan cytokeratin detection resulted in an upstaging of two patients, patients nos. 1 and 3. One LN from patient no.1 displayed Pan-cytokeratin-positive cells by FACS, whereas the pathology report was negative (pN0) in seven investigated LNs from the same patient. Thus, patient no. 1 was upgraded from pN0 to pN1. In addition, patient no. 3 was upgraded from pN1 to pN2 with FACS analysis. In patient no. 4 routine pathology identified 2 metastatic LN (2/4) whereas flow cytometry identified pan-cytokeratin positive cells only in 1 LN (1/3). Finally, in agreement with the pathology investigation patients 2 and 5 were staged as pN0 with both routine histopathology and flow cytometry (Table 3).

Discussion

In this study, we investigated markers expressed by penile cancer cells using flow cytometry for identifying metastatic cells in the lymph nodes. We demonstrate that penile cancer cells could be detected in very small amounts. This detection method is sensitive and reliable. In our earlier studies, antibodies against CK20, EpCAM and CA19–9 were used to detect metastatic colon cancer cells and antibodies against CK18, CA9, and Cadherin 6 were used to detect renal cancer cells in lymph nodes [8, 9]. Here we add Pancytokeratin AE1/AE3 staining for detection of metastatic penile cancer cells to the list of solid tumors that may be evaluated for lymphatic dissemination by flow cytometry. Thus, tumors with specific markers, not present in lymph nodes, are likely candidates for flow cytometry based detection of metastatic cells.

Table 3 Comparison of Pathology results and Pancytokeratin AE1/3 FACS results

Patient	Pathology results		pN staging (by standard pathology)	FACS results		pN staging (FACS)
	Total no. of [a]LNs received	Total no. of metastatic LNs		Total no. of LNs tested	Total no. of metastatic LNs	
1	7	0	pN0	1	1	**pN1**
2	1	0	pN0	1	0	pN0
3	2	1	pN1	2	2	pN2
4[b]	4	2	pN2	3	1	pN1
5	3	0	pN0	3	0	pN0

[a]LNs stand for lymph nodes
[b]The second metastatic LN identified by pathology was never subjected to flow cytometry analysis

The gold standard to evaluate lymph node metastasis is by pathology examination with or without out immunohistochemistry. However pathology examination is time consuming and costly since it involves technicians for preparation of sections and a skilled pathologist for ocular evaluation of the specimens. When using flow cytometry to detect metastasis in lymph nodes, the total time for preparation, staining of cells and evaluation is approximately 2-h were all the steps can be conducted by a technician. In addition, multiple samples can be prepared and analyzed at the same time. If compared with gold standard methodology, the flow cytometry assay is time saving and cost effective while maintaining sensitivity. There are many studies trying to improve the sensitivity in micro-metastasis detection. Some studies suggest detecting tumor antigen mRNA expression using the polymerase chain reaction (PCR) technique [20, 21]. These methods indeed improve the sensitivity of detection; however, they are time consuming and not easy to apply in clinical routine.

Since there are no penile cancer cell lines available, we used HeLa cells, a cervical cancer cell line which is HPV infected. Since studies on penile cancer found HPV negative tumors with keratinized cells expressing pancytokeratin AE1/AE3, there is a need to evaluate the method in HPV positive cases. Spiking Hela cells into PBMCs was used to estimate the accuracy of the metastasis detection in lymph nodes from patients with penile cancer. When we investigated the surface marker EpCAM and the cell adhesion marker E-cadherin, they both failed to detect tumor cells. From our cell spiking results, flow cytometry could detect as low as 0.11% of pancytokeratin AE1/AE3 stained tumor cells in the mixed leukocyte environment, demonstrating the method to be sensitive in detecting metastatic cells.

When applying our method to samples from penile cancer patients, FACS-results were in good agreement with routine pathology. However, two LNs were reclassified as metastatic due to presence of pan-cytokeratin positive cells identified by FACS. The results agree with our hypothesis: Since one section from a lymph node represents less than ~ 0.1% of the node [9] we assume that running single cell suspension through flow cytometry could obtain more information. In this small proof of concept study, we demonstrated that Pancytokeratin AE1/AE3 antibodies were useful for detecting metastatic penile cancer cells in lymph nodes. The technique to identify metastatic cells in lymph nodes from patients with penile cancer by staining for specific tumor markers and detection by flow cytometry needs to be systematically evaluated for sensitivity and specificity in a larger study where serial sectioning and pathology evaluation should be carried out head to head with flow cytometry based tumor specific marker identification.

Conclusion

Intracellular pan-cytokeratin AE1/AE3 staining with flow cytometry can be used to detect micro-metastasis in tumor draining lymph nodes. Large scale head to head comparisons between FACS and routine pathology assessment are warranted.

Abbreviations

FACS: Fluorescence-activated cell sorting; H&E: Hematoxylin and eosin; IHC: Immunohistochemistry; LNs: Lymph nodes; PBMC: Peripheral blood mononuclear cells; PCR: Polymerase chain reaction

Acknowledgements

This work was supported by the Swedish Cancer Foundation, the Wallenberg Foundation, the Swedish Medical Research Council, the Karolinska Research Network Program in Immune Modulatory Therapies for Autoimmunity and Cancer and the Swedish Research Council funding for clinical research in medicine (ALF) in Västerbotten, VLL, Sweden. This investigation was also supported by a grant from the Cancer Research Foundation in Northern Sweden. We also acknowledge doctor research nurses Britt-Inger Dahlin and Kerstin Almroth (Department of Surgical and Perioperative Sciences, Urology and Andrology, Umeå University) for the great assistance in the work.

Funding

This work was supported by the Swedish Cancer Foundation, the Wallenberg Foundation, the Swedish Medical Research Council, the Karolinska Research Network Program in Immune Modulatory Therapies for Autoimmunity and Cancer and the Swedish Research Council funding for clinical research in medicine (ALF) in Västerbotten, VLL, Sweden. This investigation was also supported by a grant from the Cancer Research Foundation in Northern Sweden.

Authors' contributions

LZ was a major contributor in all the experiments and writing the manuscript. JH collected samples from patients and participated in flow cytometry analysis. A.AZ collected samples from patients and participated in flow cytometry analysis. AS made substantial contributions to conception and design, acquisition of data, analysis and interpretation of data. He is also the national & official PI of the study and has written the research programme together with author OW and also written the complete application to the ethical committee and further, has partly funded the study; has been involved in drafting the manuscript or revising it critically for important intellectual content. JR has made substantial contributions to acquisition of data, analysis and interpretation of data and has been the junior local instigator at one of the urological centers; has been involved in drafting the manuscript or revising it critically for important intellectual content. MH has made substantial contributions to acquisition of data, or analysis and interpretation of data and has been the senior local instigator at one of the urological centers; has been involved in drafting the manuscript or revising it critically for important intellectual content. PSH, RW, and OW had contributions to conception and design the experiments. AS and OW also involved in revising the manuscript critically for important intellectual content. All authors have given final approval of the version to be published; and finally have agreed to be accountable for all aspects of the work.

Competing interests

The authors declare that they have no competing interests.

Author details

[1]Department of Medicine, Immunology and Allergy Unit, Karolinska University Hospital, SE-171 76 Stockholm, Sweden. [2]Department of Urology, South General Hospital, Karolinska Institutet, Stockholm, Stockholm, Sweden. [3]Cancer Biotherapy Center, Affiliated Hospital of Guizhou Medical University, Guiyang, China. [4]Department of Surgical and Perioperative Sciences, Urology and Andrology, Umeå University, Umeå, Sweden.

References

1. Cabanas RM. An approach for the treatment of penile carcinoma. Cancer. 1977;39(2):456–66.
2. Balch CM, Soong SJ, Gershenwald JE, Thompson JF, Reintgen DS, Cascinelli N, Urist M, McMasters KM, Ross MI, Kirkwood JM, et al. Prognostic factors analysis of 17,600 melanoma patients: validation of the American joint committee on Cancer melanoma staging system. Journal of clinical oncology : official journal of the American Society of Clinical Oncology. 2001;19(16):3622–34.
3. Ravi R. Correlation between the extent of nodal involvement and survival following groin dissection for carcinoma of the penis. Br J Urol. 1993;72(5 Pt 2):817–9.
4. Pandey D, Mahajan V, Kannan RR. Prognostic factors in node-positive carcinoma of the penis. J Surg Oncol. 2006;93(2):133–8.
5. Tschmelitsch J, Klimstra DS, Cohen AM. Lymph node micrometastases do not predict relapse in stage II colon cancer. Ann Surg Oncol. 2000; 7(8):601–8.
6. Weaver DL, Krag DN, Manna EA, Ashikaga T, Harlow SP, Bauer KD. Comparison of pathologist-detected and automated computer-assisted image analysis detected sentinel lymph node micrometastases in breast cancer. Modern pathology : an official journal of the United States and Canadian Academy of Pathology, Inc. 2003;16(11):1159–63.
7. Lim J, Govindarajulu S, Sahu A, Ibrahim N, Magdub S, Cawthorn S. Multiple step-section frozen section sentinel lymph node biopsy--a review of 717 patients. Breast. 2013;22(5):639–42.
8. Karlsson M, Nilsson O, Thorn M, Winqvist O. Detection of metastatic colon cancer cells in sentinel nodes by flow cytometry. J Immunol Methods. 2008; 334(1–2):122–33.
9. Hartana CA, Kinn J, Rosenblatt R, Anania S, Alamdari F, Glise H, Sherif A, Winqvist O. Detection of micrometastases by flow cytometry in sentinel lymph nodes from patients with renal tumours. Br J Cancer. 2016;115(8): 957–66.
10. Hayry V, Kagedal A, Hjalmarsson E, Neves da Silva PF, Drakskog C, Margolin G, Georen SK, Munck-Wikland E, Winqvist O, Cardell LO. Rapid nodal staging of head and neck cancer surgical specimens with flow cytometric analysis. Br J Cancer. 2018;118(3):421–7.
11. Bleeker MC, Heideman DA, Snijders PJ, Horenblas S, Dillner J, Meijer CJ. Penile cancer: epidemiology, pathogenesis and prevention. World J Urol. 2009;27(2):141–50.
12. Suo Z, Holm R, Nesland JM. Squamous cell carcinomas. An immunohistochemical study of cytokeratins and involucrin in primary and metastatic tumours. Histopathology. 1993;23(1):45–54.
13. Thompson LD, Wieneke JA, Miettinen M, Heffner DK. Spindle cell (sarcomatoid) carcinomas of the larynx: a clinicopathologic study of 187 cases. Am J Surg Pathol. 2002;26(2):153–70.
14. Zarbo RJ, Crissman JD, Venkat H, Weiss MA. Spindle-cell carcinoma of the upper aerodigestive tract mucosa. An immunohistologic and ultrastructural study of 18 biphasic tumors and comparison with seven monophasic spindle-cell tumors. Am J Surg Pathol. 1986;10(11):741–53.
15. Cubilla AL, Lloveras B, Alejo M, Clavero O, Chaux A, Kasamatsu E, Velazquez EF, Lezcano C, Monfulleda N, Tous S, et al. The basaloid cell is the best tissue marker for human papillomavirus in invasive penile squamous cell carcinoma: a study of 202 cases from Paraguay. Am J Surg Pathol. 2010; 34(1):104–14.
16. Iken S, Schmidt M, Braun C, Valentino A, Lehr HA, Schaefer SC. Absence of ectopic epithelial inclusions in 3,904 axillary lymph nodes examined in sentinel technique. Breast Cancer Res Treat. 2012;132(2):621–4.
17. Beavon IR: The E-cadherin-catenin complex in tumour metastasis: structure, function and regulation. Eur J Cancer 2000, 36(13 Spec No):1607–1620.
18. van Roy F, Berx G. The cell-cell adhesion molecule E-cadherin. Cellular and molecular life sciences : CMLS. 2008;65(23):3756–88.
19. Gregoire L, Cubilla AL, Reuter VE, Haas GP, Lancaster WD. Preferential association of human papillomavirus with high-grade histologic variants of penile-invasive squamous cell carcinoma. J Natl Cancer Inst. 1995; 87(22):1705–9.
20. Luo J, Yang K, Wen YG: Nested polymerase chain reaction technique for the detection of Gpc3 and Afp mRNA in liver cancer micrometastases. Genet Mol Res : GMR 2017, 16(1).
21. Kim YJ, Chung WC, Choi S, Jung YD, Lee J, Chae SY, Jun KH, Chin HM. The detection of messenger RNA for carcinoembryonic antigen and cytokeratin 20 in peritoneal washing fluid in patients with advanced gastric Cancer. The Korean journal of gastroenterology = Taehan Sohwagi Hakhoe chi. 2017; 69(4):220–5.

Impact of early changes in serum biomarkers following androgen deprivation therapy on clinical outcomes in metastatic hormone-sensitive prostate cancer

Hiromi Sato[1], Shintaro Narita[1*], Norihiko Tsuchiya[2], Atsushi Koizumi[1], Taketoshi Nara[1], Sohei Kanda[1], Kazuyuki Numakura[1], Hiroshi Tsuruta[1], Atsushi Maeno[1], Mitsuru Saito[1], Takamitsu Inoue[1], Shigeru Satoh[3], Kyoko Nomura[4] and Tomonori Habuchi[1]

Abstract

Background: Less evidence is known about the role of early changes in serum biomarker after androgen deprivation therapy (ADT) in patients with metastatic hormone-sensitive prostate cancer (mHSPC). Here we evaluated the impact of pre-treatment prognostic factors and early changes in serum biomarkers on prostate specific antigen (PSA) progression-free and overall survival rates in mHSPC.

Methods: We retrospectively reviewed the medical records of 60 mHSPC patients (median age 72 years) treated with ADT whose laboratory data at baseline and following 12 weeks were available.

Results: Forty-four patients (73%) had PSA progression and 27 patients (45.0%) died during a median follow-up of 34 months. The multivariable Cox hazard model demonstrated that a log-transformed baseline PSA level ($p = 0.003$) and an extent of bone disease (EOD) score of ≥3 ($p = 0.004$) were statistically associated with an increased risk for PSA progression whereas one unit increase in a log-transformed PSA change (baseline-12 weeks) was associated with a decreased risk for PSA progression ($p = 0.004$). For overall survival, a high level of alkaline phosphatase (ALP) at 12 weeks was associated with increased risk ($p = 0.030$) whereas a one-unit increase in the log-transformed PSA change was associated with decreased risk ($p = 0.001$).

Conclusions: An increased level of PSA at baseline, or an EOD score of ≥3 may be a good predictor of PSA progression, and a high level of ALP at 12 weeks may be a risk predictor of death. A larger decline in PSA at 12 weeks from the baseline was associated with both PSA progression-free and overall survival time. Early changes in serum biomarkers may be useful in predicting poor outcomes in patients with mHSPC who are initially treated with ADT.

Background

Prostate cancer is the second leading cause of cancer death among men worldwide [1]. Although androgen deprivation therapy (ADT) has been a standard treatment for metastatic prostate cancer, its response and duration vary. Recent studies have shown that an early chemohormonal therapy with docetaxel results in improved overall survival (OS) than ADT alone in patients with metastatic hormone-sensitive prostate cancer (mHSPC) [2, 3]. Sweeney et al. reported that the benefit of early chemotherapy for mHSPC was more apparent in the subgroup with a high-volume disease [2]. In addition, some prostate cancer patients who received chemotherapy experienced severe toxicities, particularly in Asian patients [4, 5]. Therefore, it is important to predict a poor response to ADT in order to screen appropriate candidates for the administration of early chemotherapy combined with ADT.

Several candidate biomarkers have been found to have prognostic value in predicting poor outcomes in patients

* Correspondence: nari6202@gipc.akita-u.ac.jp; naritashintaro@gmail.com
[1]Department of Urology, Akita University School of Medicine, 1-1-1 Hondo, Akita 010-8543, Japan
Full list of author information is available at the end of the article

with mHSPC treated with ADT [6], and risk stratification models in mHSPC using these risk factors have been proposed [6, 7]. Furthermore, recent studies showed that dynamic changes in serum biomarkers at the cancer's early stage, including prostate specific antigen (PSA) or alkaline phosphatase (ALP) changes, had a higher impact on clinical outcome in patients with mHSPC and/or castration-resistant prostate cancer than that of pretreatment variables [8, 9]. However, there is less evidence about the impact of early changes in serum biomarker after ADT in patients with mHSPC, and the comparison to pretreatment prognostic factors, including the categorized definition of high-tumor burden in recent trials, still needs to be investigated.

In order to predict PSA progression and poor survival in patients with mHSPC, initially treated with ADT, we assess the impact of the early changes in serum biomarkers at 12 weeks along with pretreatment prognostic factors such as a high-volume disease in the CHAARTED trial on PSA progression-free survival and OS.

Methods

Study population

We retrospectively reviewed the medical records of 80 consecutive primary metastatic prostate cancer patients treated with ADT at the Akita University Hospital in Japan between 2000 and 2015. Sixty patients whose laboratory data at 12 weeks post ADT were available and included in this study. Our institutional review board approved this study.

Treatment and evaluation

All patients were treated with a maximal androgen blockage (MAB) as an initial therapy. MAB therapy consisted of a chemical or surgical castration in combination with bicalutamide. Sequential treatments after first-line ADT were administered at physician's discretion. PSA examination was routinely performed at least every three months. Radiographic examination was routinely performed before ADT, and thereafter at physician's discretion. PSA progression was defined according the Prostate Cancer Clinical Trials Working Group 2 (PCWG2) criteria [10]. OS was calculated as the time from ADT initiation to the date of death.

Statistical analyses

All pretreatment variables were evaluated when prostate cancer was diagnosed. The extent of bone disease (EOD) scores for each patient was classified by bone scintigraphy according to the definition reported by Soloway et al. at initial diagnosis [11]. Eastern cooperative oncology group performance-status score (ECOG-PS) and the presence of bone pain were evaluated by inquiry and physical examination. A high-volume disease in the CHAARTED trial was defined as the presence of visceral metastases or ≥ 4 bone metastatic lesions with ≥ 1 beyond the vertebral bodies and pelvis, and a low-volume disease was defined as other than the definition of a high-volume disease [2].

There were missing values for the levels of Hb, ALP, and LDH at baseline ($n = 4$) and following 12 weeks ($n = 5$), and for the EOD scores ($n = 5$), and CHAARTED criteria ($n = 5$). We replaced the missing data with the mean or the median according to the distribution of the corresponding variable. Missing values for the EOD scores and CHAATED criteria were not imputed for ethical reasons. Because similar results were obtained before and after imputation, we present only the results with imputation.

PSA progression-free survival and OS curves were estimated using the Kaplan-Meier method, and the comparison of survival curves was statistically tested using a log-rank test. The subjects were split into three groups according to their disease status and PSA change and compared. The three groups were a group with a high-volume disease in the CHAARTED trial, a group with a low-volume disease in the CHAARTED trial and larger PSA change larger than or equal to the median, and a group with a low-volume disease in the CHAARTED trial and PSA change smaller than the median.

To identify independent prognostic factors for PSA progression-free survival and death, Cox proportional hazard model was applied to calculate the hazard ratio (HR) along with the 95% confidence interval (95%CI) adjusting for the following variables: patient age; biopsy Gleason score; EOD score; ECOG-PS; the presence of bone pain; the presence of visceral metastases; high- or low-volume disease in the CHAARTED trial; log-transformed baseline PSA level and log-transformed PSA change (baseline-12 weeks after ADT); low ($\leq$ mean g/dl) or high (>mean, g/dl) Hemoglobin (Hb) level (baseline and 12 weeks after ADT); low ($\leq$median, IU/L) or high (>median, < IU/L) ALP levels (baseline and 12 weeks after ADT); and low ($\leq$median, IU/L) or high (>median, IU/L) LDH levels (baseline and 12 weeks after ADT). The selected cut-off points were 1 for ECOG-PS, 8 for the biopsy Gleason score, and 3 for the EOD score. The final multivariable Cox proportional hazards models were determined using PROC PHREG in statistical analysis system (SAS) and SCORE option and were based on a subset of model selection methods (i.e., stepwise, forward, and backward) using a $p < 0.05$ as entry criterion, and a $p \geq 0.05$ as removal criterion. The best model (Model I) was determined with the highest chi-square statistic and lowest score for Akaike information criterion (AIC). Because of high correlation between a log-transformed baseline PSA level and a log-transformed PSA change (Pearson coefficient 0.979, $p < 0.0001$), Model II was built where a log-transformed baseline PSA level was removed from Model I.

All statistical analyses were performed using SPSS software version 19.0 and SAS (version 9.4, NC, USA). All reported p-values were two-sided, and considered statistically significant at $p < 0.05$.

Results

The baseline patient characteristics in this study are shown in Table 1. The median age was 72 years (range, 56–93 year). Forty-four patients (73%) had PSA progression and 27 patients (45.0%) died of cancer progression (except one patient who died of other disease) during a median follow-up of 34 months. The median PSA level at pre-treatment and 12 weeks after the initiation of MAB therapy were 195 ng/ml and 2.6 ng/ml, respectively. The median percentage change in the PSA level at 12 weeks was 98.5% {Interquartile range (IQR), 94.4–99.6%}. A negative change in PSA levels from baseline to 12 weeks was observed in only two patients.

Table 1 Patient characteristics

Variables		n = 60
Age, y, median (IQR)		72.0 (56–93)
ECOG-PS, No. (%)	0	55 (91.7)
	1	5 (8.3)
Baseline PSA level, ng/ml, median (IQR)		195.0 (53.0–610.9)
Baseline Hb level, g/dl, median (IQR)		13.2 (12.0–14.5)
Baseline ALP level, IU, median (IQR)		320.0 (232.0–620.5)
Baseline LDH level, IU, median (IQR)		203.0 (174.0–251.0)
Biopsy Gleason Score, No. (%)	≤8	18 (30.0)
	≥9	42 (70.0)
Site of metstasis, No. (%)	Bone	100 (100)
	Lymphnode	26 (43.3)
	Visceral	2 (3.3)
Presence of bone pain, No. (%)		25 (41.7)
EOD score, No. (%)	1	28 (46.7)
	2	7 (11.7)
	3	11 (18.3)
	4	9 (15.0)
CHAARTED criteria, No. (%)	unknown	5 (8.3)
	low	25 (41.7)
	high	30 (50.0)
	unknown	5 (8.3)
PSA level at 12 weeks, ng/ml, median (IQR)		2.6 (0.5–9.3)
Hb level at 12 weeks, g/dl, median (IQR)		12.5 (11.3–13.3)
ALP level at 12 weeks, IU, median (IQR)		284.0 (233.5–536.0)
LDH levelat 12 weeks, IU, median (IQR)		198.0 (177.0–247.5)
PSA change (baseline-12wks), ng/ml, median (IQR)		159.5 (34.4–546.9)
PSA change at 12 weeks,%, median (IQR)		98.5 (94.4–99.6)

IQR Interquartile range, *ECOG* Eastern Cooperative Oncology Group, *PSA* prostate specific antigen, *Hb* hemoglobin, *ALP* alkaline phosphatase, *LDH* lactate dehydrogenase, *EOD* extent of bone disease

Using the Kaplan-Meier method to investigate PSA progression-free survival, the data showed that the 1- and 2-year PSA progression-free survival rates of the group of PSA change at 12 weeks of ≥98.5% were markedly higher than those of the group with PSA change at 12 weeks of < 98.5% (85.8% and 58.5 vs 29.3% and 7.3, respectively, $P < 0.001$; Fig. 1a). Using the Kaplan-Meier method to investigate OS (Fig. 1b), the data showed that the 2- and 5-year OS rates of the group with PSA change at 12 weeks of ≥98.5% were markedly higher than the group with PSA change at 12 weeks of < 98.5% (96 and 80% vs 50 and 18%, respectively, $p < 0.001$). Median OS was 103 months for patients with a PSA change at 12 weeks of ≥98.5%, while 38 months for a PSA change at 12 weeks of < 98.5%. When we analyzed the difference in OS based on a percentage reduction in the PSA level for the two subgroup in the CHAARTED trial, OS in patients in the low-volume disease in the CHAARTED trial with a PSA change at 12 weeks of < 98.5% was comparable with that in the high-volume disease ($p = 0.954$; Fig. 2). In addition, patients in the low-volume disease in CHAARTED with a PSA change at 12 weeks of < 98.5% tended to have a poor survival compared with those in the low-volume disease in CHAARTED with a PSA change of ≥98.5% at 12 weeks ($p = 0.051$). The results suggested that the low-volume disease included patients with a poor survival, and that the early change of serum biomarkers might help predict prognosis more precisely.

Results of univariable and multivariable survival analyses using the Cox regression model for PSA progression-free survival are shown in Table 2. The univariable analyses show that the factors significantly associated with PSA progression are a low Hb level at baseline ($p = 0.001$) and at 12 weeks ($p = 0.043$), visceral metastases ($p = 0.001$), an EOD score of ≥3 ($p < 0.001$), a high-volume group in the CHAARTED trial ($p = 0.007$), and a high ALP level at 12 weeks ($p = 0.001$). The best model is shown in Model I selected based on a subset of model selection methods, AIC (i.e., 229.7), and chi-square statistic (i.e., 45.5) which had three variables: a log-transformed baseline PSA level, a log-transformed PSA change, and an EOD score. In the final multivariable model, a log-transformed baseline PSA level (HR 3.

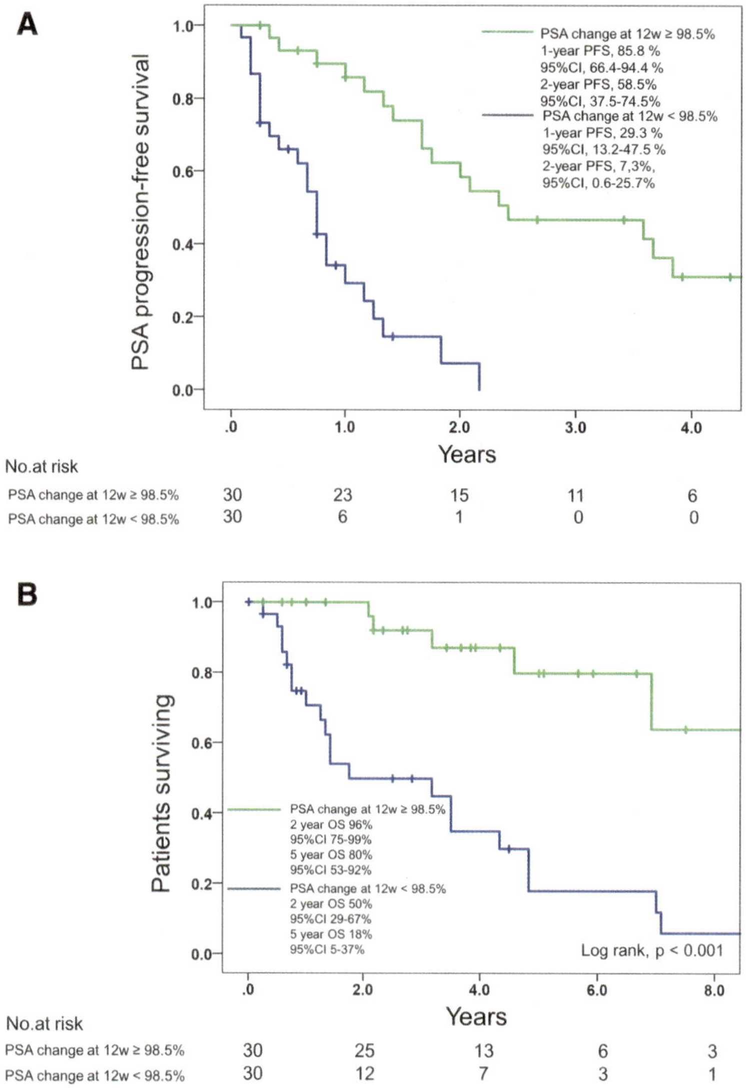

Fig. 1 a Time to PSA progression-free survival according to the percentage change in the PSA level at 12 weeks. **b** Overall survival according to the percentage change in the PSA level at 12 weeks

62, 95% CI 1.57–8.36) and an EOD score of ≥3 (HR 3. 14, 95% CI 1.45–6.82) was statistically associated with increased risk for PSA progression, whereas a one-unit increase in a log-transformed PSA change (baseline-12 weeks) was associated with a decreased risk of PSA progression (HR 0.30, 95%CI 0.13–0.68). To avoid collinearity between a log-transformed baseline PSA level and a log-transformed PSA change, Model II was built where a log-transformed baseline PSA level was removed from Model I that indicated that an EOD score of ≥3 (HR 3.47, 95% CI 1.65–7.33) was an only significant factor associated with increased risk of PSA progression. However, AIC of Model II was higher than Model I and chi-square statistic of Model II was lower than Model I, suggesting that Model I has a better goodness of fit compared to Model II.

Results of the univariable and multivariable survival analyses using Cox regression model for OS are shown in Table 3. Univariable analyses show that the factors significantly associated with a decreased risk for death was a one-unit increase in a log-transformed baseline PSA level ($p = 0.035$) and a log-transformed PSA change (baseline-12 weeks; $p = 0.014$), whereas factors associated with an increased risk for death are bone pain ($p = 0.049$), visceral metastases ($p = 0.029$), an EOD score of ≥3 ($p = 0.004$), a low level group of Hb levels at 12 weeks ($p = 0.025$), and a high level group of ALP levels at 12 weeks ($p = 0.002$). The best model is shown to be Model I, which was selected based on a subset of model selection methods, AIC (i.e.,122.9), and score chi-square value (i.e., 26.5) with five variables of log-transformed PSA- at baseline and PSA change, EOD

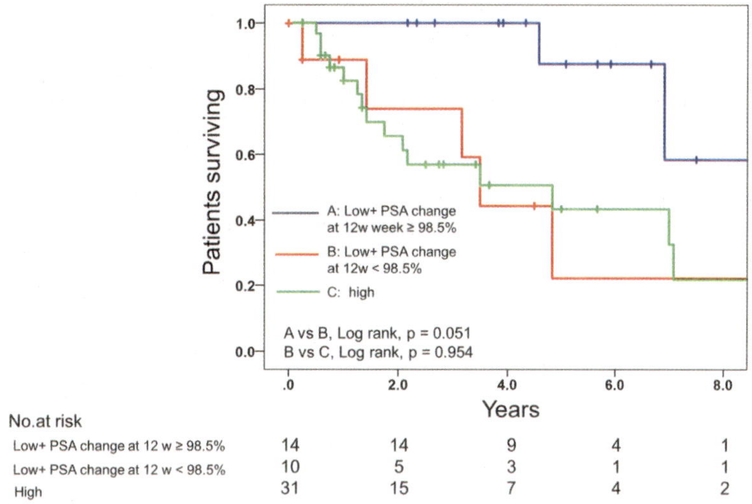

Fig. 2 Comparison of overall survival in patients with dichotomized according to subgroups in the CHAARTED trial and percentage change in the PSA level at 12 weeks. The low-volume disease in the CHAARTED trial was dichotomized according to the percentage change in the PSA level at 12 weeks

score, Hb and ALP levels at 12 weeks. In Model I, a high level group of ALP at 12 weeks (HR 3.37, 95% CI 1.01–11.23) was statistically associated with shortened OS time, but no other factors became significant. To avoid the collinearity effect on the OS, Model II was built where a log-transformed baseline PSAlevel was removed from Model I that demonstrated that the *p*-values for a log-transformed PSA change, Hb level at 12 weeks, and ALP level at 12 weeks became closer to significance levels (Hb level was almost significant, but did not reach the significance level). A one-unit increase in a log-transformed PSA change was associated with a decreased risk for OS (HR 0.68, 95% CI 0.54–0.85) whereas a high ALP level at 12 weeks was positively associated with an increased risk for death (HR 3.57,

Table 2 Univariable and multivariable analysis for PSA progression-free survival in patients with mHSPC treated with ADT

					Multivariable					
		Univariable			Model I (Base line PSA adjusted) (*n* = 52; chi-square 45.5; AIC 229.7)			Model II (*n* = 52; chi-square 13.2; AIC 234.7)		
Factors	Group	HR	95% CI	*p* value	HR	95% CI	*p* value	HR	95% CI	*p* value
Age	Continuous	0.99	0.95–1.03	0.642						
ECOG-PS	1 vs 0	1.13	0.40–3.17	0.820						
Log-transformed baseline PSA level (ng/dL)	Continuous	1.14	0.95–1.36	0.156	3.62	1.57–8.36	0.003			
Baseline Hb level (g/dl)	Low vs normal	3.31	1.68–6.51	0.001						
Baseline ALP level (IU/l)	High vs normal	1.58	0.84–2.972	0.157						
Baseline LDH level (IU/l)	High vs normal	1.23	0.66–2.29	0.510						
Presence of bone pain	Yes vs No	1.52	0.81–2.84	0.191						
Biopsy Gleason score	≥8 vs ≤7	2.60	0.62–10.82	0.190						
Visceral metastasis	Yes vs No	28.62	4.03–203.21	0.001						
EOD score	≥3 vs ≤2	3.89	1.91–7.92	<0.001	3.14	1.45–6.82	0.004	3.47	1.65–7.33	0.001
Sub-group in the CHAARTED trial	high vs low	2.44	1.28–4.65	0.007						
Log-transformed PSA change (baseline-12wks)	Continuous	1.10	0.92–1.32	0.281	0.30	0.13–0.68	0.004	1.04	0.87–1.25	0.66
Hb level at 12 weeks	Low vs normal	1.94	1.02–3.67	0.043						
ALP level at 12 weeks	High vs normal	3.19	1.67–6.11	0.001						
LDH level at 12 weeks	High vs normal	1.17	0.59–2.31	0.652						

mHSPC metastatic hormone-sensitive prostate cancer, *ADT* androgen deprivation therapy, *ECOG* Eastern Cooperative Oncology Group, *PSA* prostate specific antigen, *Hb* hemoglobin, *ALP* Alkaline phosphatase, *LDH* Lactate dehydrogenase, *EOD* extend of bone metastasis, *HR* hazard ratio, *CI* confidence interbal

Table 3 Univariable and multivariable analysis for overall survival in patients with mHSPC treated with ADT

					Multivariable					
		Univariable			Model I (Base line PSA adjusted) (*n* = 52; chi-square 26.5; AIC 122.9)			Model II (*n* = 52; chi-square 22.8; AIC 121.1)		
Factors	Group	HR	95% CI	*p* value	HR	95% CI	*p* value	HR	95% CI	*p* value
Age	Continuous	1.01	0.96–1.07	0.702						
ECOG-PS	1 vs 0	1.10	0.26–4.76	0.895						
Log-transformed baseline PSA level (ng/dL)	Continuous	0.81	0.67–0.99	0.035	1.25	0.58–2.71	0.572			
Baseline Hb level(g/dl)	Low vs normal	1.90	0.85–4.27	0.120						
Baseline ALP level (IU/l)	High vs normal	1.34	0.60–3.02	0.480						
Baseline LDH level (IU/l)	High vs normal	1.08	0.48–2.43	0.846						
Presence of bone pain	Yes vs No	2.23	1.00–4.98	0.049						
Biopsy Gleason score	≥8 vs ≤7	0.55	0.16–1.89	0.345						
Visceral metastasis	Yes vs No	5.37	1.18–24.32	0.029						
EOD score	≥3 vs ≤2	3.85	1.55–9.59	0.004	1.97	0.61–6.39	0.256	2.05	0.65–6.46	0.222
Sub-group in the CHAARTED trial	high vs low	2.03	0.86–4.82	0.109						
Log-transformed PSA change (baseline-12wks)	Continuous	0.78	0.64–0.95	0.014	0.55	0.26–1.18	0.123	0.68	0.54–0.85	0.001
Hb level at 12 weeks	Low vs normal	2.44	1.12–5.31	0.025	2.54	0.92–7.00	0.071	2.58	0.95–7.04	0.060
ALP level at 12 weeks	High vs normal	3.47	1.59–7.58	0.002	3.37	1.01–11.23	0.048	3.57	1.11–11.53	0.030
LDH level at 12 weeks	High vs normal	1.74	0.75–4.00	0.197						

mHSPC metastatic hormone-sensitive prostate cancer, *ADT* androgen deprivation therapy, *ECOG* Eastern Cooperative Oncology Group, *PSA* prostate specific antigen, *Hb* hemoglobin, *ALP* Alkaline phosphatase, *LDH* Lactate dehydrogenase, *EOD* extend of bone metastasis, *HR* hazard ratio, *CI* confidence interba

95%CI 1.11–11.53). The goodness of the model fitness was indistinguishable between Model I (chi-square 26. 5; AIC 122.9) and Model II (chi-square 22.8; AIC 121.1).

Discussion

In this study, we assessed the prognostic markers for PSA progression-free survival and OS in patients with mHSPC based on early changes in serum biomarkers post-ADT along with the pretreatment risk factors. We found that the level of PSA at baseline as well as PSA change from baseline to 12 weeks were strong prognostic factors of PSA progression. In addition, an EOD score of ≥3 was significantly associated with poor PSA progression free survival. For the risk of death, a large decline in PSA change was associated with a decreased risk, whereas a higher ALP level at 12 weeks was associated with an increased risk. Although the high-volume disease, as defined in the CHAARTED trial, was statistically associated with the PSA progression-free survival, it was not selected in the multivariable model, and was not associated with OS. These findings suggest that the early changes in serum biomarkers have the potential to better predict progression and/or poor prognosis in mHSPC initially treated with ADT compared with the application of only pretreatment variables as predictors.

PSA-related variables, including initial PSA levels and PSA kinetics, have been the most frequently assessed biomarkers in mHSPC [6]. In PSA kinetic variables, PSA nadir and time to PSA nadir are promising biomarkers for mHSPC [12, 13]. However, previous studies reported that the median time to PSA nadir was six to 10 months [12, 13], which means that the prognosis was predictable more than half a year later following the initiation of ADT. In previous phase III trials, ADT had commenced within 120 days before randomization. Therefore, it might be reasonable to predict patients with poor prognosis using early changes (up to three months) in serum biomarkers post-ADT. Park et al. reported that the shorter PSA half-time calculated as log 2 divided by the slope of the linear regression of log PSA vs time using pre- and post-treatment PSA levels assayed every three months were independent risk factors for poor cancer specific survival in patients with mHSPC [8]. A recent study has shown that a velocity of PSA decline > 11 ng/mL per month was significantly associated with an increased risk of progression to castration-resistant prostate cancer after initial ADT [14]. PSA velocity, which is calculated as the slope of log PSA vs. time based on the least squares method using at least two post baseline PSA measurements [15], may achieve a more accurate prediction of outcomes. Although further studies are needed to identify what is the best marker among PSA-related variables to predict the outcome among mHSPC patients, PSA change at 12 weeks is a simple and convenient biomarker for the prediction of clinical outcomes.

Previous studies revealed several cut-off points of the serum PSA level after the administration of ADT to predict the prognosis of mHSPC patients [2, 16]. Hussain et al. investigated prognostic factors based on the absolute PSA level after ADT treatment in 1134 newly-diagnosed cases of mHSPC in the SWOG trial. Their study showed that a PSA of ≤4 ng/mL after 7 months of ADT was a strong predictor of survival [16]. In the phase III trial assessing the impact of concomitant treatment with ADT plus docetaxel in mHSPC reported by Sweeney et al., a complete serological response was defined as a PSA level of ≤0.2 ng/mL [2]. Further studies with a larger number of patients are required because the small number of patients in the dichotomized subgroup is a limitation of our study, although the current study demonstrated that a median percentage of PSA level (98.5%) at 12 weeks was a potential cut-off point of PSA progression and poor survival.

Arai et al. assessed the prognostic factors in 73 non-metastatic and metastatic prostate cancer patients treated with ADT and found that the patients who had a decrease in PSA levels of 80% or more within one month after the beginning of therapy experienced significantly longer free of disease progression [17]. The study was reported at 1990, when the treatment strategy markedly differed from those treated now, and it included the non-metastatic patients. In the current study, 25 patients (41.7%) received docetaxel chemotherapy during their treatment period. Our results suggest that the change in the PSA level at an early stage after the initiation of ADT may have been a risk factor for poor patient outcomes even in recent years when various treatment options including novel anti-androgens, chemotherapies and vaccines became available for advanced prostate cancer.

Regarding other serum biomarkers, Gravis et al. conducted a new prognostic model of mHSPC using a contemporary data set from the phase III study GETUG-15 study [18]. They found that the pre-treatment ALP level was the strongest factor for discriminating patients with a good prognosis; by contrast, in our study, a high level of ALP at 12 weeks was significantly associated with poor OS. Although the Gravis et al. study was a prospective study conducted with a larger number of patients, it could not eliminate the problems such as the impact of upfront docetaxel and/or ADT initiated up to two months before study entry. The combination of pre-treatment variables previously proposed as risk factors of poor OS and the early changes in serum biomarkers evaluated in the current study may be an intriguing option as a novel prognostic model for survival after initial ADT in mHSPC.

Visceral metastasis was one of the well-known prognostic factors for poor OS in metastatic prostate cancer [19]. Regarding the proportion of patients with visceral metastasis, only two (3.3%) patients initially had visceral metastasis in this study, whereas 15.6% of the patients had visceral metastasis at initial diagnosis in the CHAARTED trial [2]. Although the small number of patients with visceral metastasis is a limitation of the current study, OS of the two patients having visceral metastasis were very short (12 month and 21 months). Therefore, the impact of visceral metastases on OS needs to be re-assessed in future study. Severity and location of bone metastasis have also been known to be prognostic factors for poor survivals in a previous study [7]. In our study, the EOD score, which was significantly associated with PSA progression in univariable and multivariable analyses. A recent study showed the impact of more objective scoring of bone metastasis using bone scintigraphy called bone scan index (BSI) [20]. It is intriguing to know the impact of BSI as a novel biomarker in our model because the EOD score tended to be a subjective and semi-quantitative parameter, which may have affected the impact on survivals in the statistical analyses.

Other potential prognostic markers such as serum bone marker [21], circulating tumor cell [22], and single nucleotide polymorphism [23] were also interesting, but not investigated in this study due to lack of adequate data. Further studies should use more sophisticated models using these variables along with the factors established in the current study.

This study has several limitations. First, the major limitations were the retrospective study design. Bias from patients with extremely poor performance status, possibly not be referred to our hospital, which is a tertiary medical center, could have occurred. A larger multicenter prospective study is warranted to validate the results. Second, in spite of the study cohort spanning 15 years, the number of patients we assessed and the number of deaths were small with a short median follow-up. In addition, among our 80 consecutive patients, 20 (25%) patients were excluded from further analysis because of missing laboratory data at 12 weeks after the administration of ADT, thus, further prospective studies are warranted to validate the results using consecutive case series. Lastly, our study did not consider the impact of sequential treatments after initial ADT therapy. Although the continuous and categorical treatment years were not statistically associated with OS in the current study (data not shown), sequential treatments after ADT failure may have a role in patient's outcome.

Conclusion

Early changes in serum biomarkers may be associated with early PSA progression-free survival and poor OS in patients with mHSPC. In particular, an increased level of PSA at baseline was an independent predictor of PSA progression, whereas a high level of ALP at 12 weeks was a risk predictor of death for OS. A larger decline in PSA from the baseline until 12 weeks was associated with both PSA progression-free and OS time. The selection of the patients with mHSPC having poor OS by initial ADT using early changes in serum biomarkers, not only pretreatment risk factors, may be useful in adding upfront chemotherapy to these patients.

Abbreviations

ADT: Androgen deprivation therapy; ALP: Alkaline phosphatese; BSI: Bone scane index; ECOG-PS: Western cooperative oncology group performance status score; EOD score: Extent of bone disease score; Hb: Hemoglobin; MAB: Maximal androgen blockage; mHSPC: metastatic hormone-sensitive prostate cancer; OS: Overall survival; PSA: Prostate specific antigen

Declarations

This study was approved by the ethics committee of Akita University Hospital (Number: 1444). The study did not require additional informed consent due to the retrospective nature of the study.

Authors' contributions

HS, SN: Data collection, statistical analysis, manuscript writing. AK, TN, SK, KN (Kazuyuki Numakura), HT, AM: technical and material support. MS, TI, KN (Kyoko Nomura): Data analysis. NT, SS, TH: manuscript editing, supervision. All authors had read and approve of the final manuscript.

Competing interests

The authors declare that they have no competing interests.

Author details

[1]Department of Urology, Akita University School of Medicine, 1-1-1 Hondo, Akita 010-8543, Japan. [2]Department of Urology, Yamagata University School of Medicine, Yamagata, Japan. [3]Center for Kidney Disease and Transplantation, Akita University Hospital, Akita, Japan. [4]Department of Public Health, Akita University School of Medicine, Akita, Japan.

References

1. Siegel RL, Miller KD, Jemal A. Cancer statistics, 2015. CA Cancer J Clin. 2015; 65:5–29.
2. Sweeney CJ, Chen YH, Carducci M, Liu G, Jarrard DF, Eisenberger M, Wong YN, Hahn N, Kohli M, Cooney MM, et al. Chemohormonal therapy in metastatic hormone-sensitive prostate Cancer. N Engl J Med. 2015;373:737–46.
3. Vale CL, Burdett S, Rydzewska LH, Albiges L, Clarke NW, Fisher D, Fizazi K, Gravis G, James ND, Mason MD, et al. Addition of docetaxel or bisphosphonates to standard of care in men with localised or metastatic, hormone-sensitive prostate cancer: a systematic review and meta-analyses of aggregate data. The Lancet Oncology. 2016;17:243–56.
4. Kenmotsu H, Tanigawara Y. Pharmacokinetics, dynamics and toxicity of docetaxel: why the Japanese dose differs from the western dose. Cancer Sci. 2015;106:497–504.
5. Lee JL, Kim JE, Ahn JH, Lee DH, Lee J, Kim CS, Hong JH, Hong B, Song C, Ahn H. Efficacy and safety of docetaxel plus prednisolone chemotherapy for metastatic hormone-refractory prostate adenocarcinoma: single institutional study in Korea. Cancer Res Treat : official journal of Korean Cancer Association. 2010;42:12–7.
6. Grivas PD, Robins DM, Hussain M. Predicting response to hormonal therapy and survival in men with hormone sensitive metastatic prostate cancer. Crit Rev Oncol Hematol. 2013;85:82–93.
7. Glass TR, Tangen CM, Crawford ED, Thompson I. Metastatic carcinoma of the prostate: identifying prognostic groups using recursive partitioning. J Urol. 2003;169:164–9.
8. Park YH, Hwang IS, Jeong CW, Kim HH, Lee SE, Kwak C. Prostate specific antigen half-time and prostate specific antigen doubling time as predictors of response to androgen deprivation therapy for metastatic prostate cancer. J Urol. 2009;181:2520–4. discussion 2525
9. Mikah P, Krabbe LM, Eminaga O, Herrmann E, Papavassilis P, Hinkelammert R, Semjonow A, Schrader AJ, Boegemann M. Dynamic changes of alkaline phosphatase are strongly associated with PSA-decline and predict best clinical benefit earlier than PSA-changes under therapy with abiraterone acetate in bone metastatic castration resistant prostate cancer. BMC Cancer. 2016;16:214.
10. Scher HI, Halabi S, Tannock I, Morris M, Sternberg CN, Carducci MA, Eisenberger MA, Higano C, Bubley GJ, Dreicer R, et al. Design and end points of clinical trials for patients with progressive prostate cancer and castrate levels of testosterone: recommendations of the prostate Cancer clinical trials working group. J Clin Oncol. 2008;26:1148–59.
11. Soloway MS, Hardeman SW, Hickey D, Raymond J, Todd B, Soloway S, Moinuddin M. Stratification of patients with metastatic prostate cancer based on extent of disease on initial bone scan. Cancer. 1988;61:195–202.
12. Choueiri TK, Xie W, D'Amico AV, Ross RW, Hu JC, Pomerantz M, Regan MM, Taplin ME, Kantoff PW, Sartor O, Oh WK. Time to prostate-specific antigen nadir independently predicts overall survival in patients who have metastatic hormone-sensitive prostate cancer treated with androgen-deprivation therapy. Cancer. 2009;115:981–7.
13. Huang SP, Bao BY, Wu MT, Choueiri TK, Goggins WB, Huang CY, Pu YS, Yu CC, Huang CH. Impact of prostate-specific antigen (PSA) nadir and time to PSA nadir on disease progression in prostate cancer treated with androgen-deprivation therapy. Prostate. 2011;71:1189–97.
14. Ji G, Song G, Huang C, He S, Zhou L. Rapidly decreasing level of prostate-specific antigen during initial androgen deprivation therapy is a risk factor for early progression to castration-resistant prostate cancer: a retrospective study. Medicine. 2017;96:e7823.
15. Halabi S, Armstrong AJ, Sartor O, de Bono J, Kaplan E, Lin CY, Solomon NC, Small EJ. Prostate-specific antigen changes as surrogate for overall survival in men with metastatic castration-resistant prostate cancer treated with second-line chemotherapy. J Clin Oncol. 2013;31:3944–50.
16. Hussain M, Tangen CM, Higano C, Schelhammer PF, Faulkner J, Crawford ED, Wilding G, Akdas A, Small EJ, Donnelly B, et al. Absolute prostate-specific antigen value after androgen deprivation is a strong independent predictor of survival in new metastatic prostate cancer: data from southwest oncology group trial 9346 (INT-0162). J Clin Oncol. 2006;24:3984–90.
17. Arai Y, Yoshiki T, Yoshida O. Prognostic significance of prostate specific antigen in endocrine treatment for prostatic cancer. J Urol. 1990;144:1415–9.
18. Gravis G, Boher JM, Fizazi K, Joly F, Priou F, Marino P, Latorzeff I, Delva R, Krakowski I, Laguerre B, et al. Prognostic factors for survival in noncastrate metastatic prostate Cancer: validation of the glass model and development of a novel simplified prognostic model. Eur Urol. 2015;68:196–204.
19. Pond GR, Sonpavde G, de Wit R, Eisenberger MA, Tannock IF, Armstrong AJ. The prognostic importance of metastatic site in men with metastatic castration-resistant prostate cancer. Eur Urol. 2014;65:3–6.
20. Poulsen MH, Rasmussen J, Edenbrandt L, Hoilund-Carlsen PF, Gerke O, Johansen A, Lund L. Bone scan index predicts outcome in patients with metastatic hormone-sensitive prostate cancer. BJU Int. 2016;117:748–53.
21. Nozawa M, Hara I, Matsuyama H, Iki M, Nagao K, Nishioka T, Komura T, Esa A, Uejima S, Imanishi M, et al. Significance of baseline bone markers on disease progression and survival in hormone-sensitive prostate cancer with bone metastasis. World J Urol. 2015;33:1263–8.
22. Goodman OB Jr, Symanowski JT, Loudyi A, Fink LM, Ward DC, Vogelzang NJ. Circulating tumor cells as a predictive biomarker in patients with hormone-sensitive prostate cancer. Clin Genitourin Cancer. 2011;9:31–8.
23. Tsuchiya N, Wang L, Suzuki H, Segawa T, Fukuda H, Narita S, Shimbo M, Kamoto T, Mitsumori K, Ichikawa T, et al. Impact of IGF-I and CYP19 gene polymorphisms on the survival of patients with metastatic prostate cancer. J Clin Oncol. 2006;24:1982–9.

27

Progressive bladder remodeling due to bladder outlet obstruction: a systematic review of morphological and molecular evidences in humans

Ferdinando Fusco[1*], Massimiliano Creta[1], Cosimo De Nunzio[2], Valerio Iacovelli[3], Francesco Mangiapia[1], Vincenzo Li Marzi[4] and Enrico Finazzi Agrò[3]

Abstract

Background: Bladder outlet obstruction is a common urological condition. We aimed to summarize available evidences about bladder outlet obstruction-induced molecular and morphological alterations occurring in human bladder.

Methods: We performed a literature search up to December 2017 including clinical and preclinical basic research studies on humans. The following search terms were combined: angiogenesis, apoptosis, bladder outlet obstruction, collagen, electron microscopy, extracellular matrix, fibrosis, hypoxia, histology, inflammation, innervation, ischemia, pressure, proliferation, remodeling, suburothelium, smooth muscle cells, stretch, urothelium.

Results: We identified 36 relevant studies. A three-stages model of bladder wall remodeling can be hypothesized involving an initial hypertrophy phase, a subsequent compensation phase and a later decompensation. Histological and molecular alterations occur in the following compartments: urothelium, suburothelium, detrusor smooth muscle cells, detrusor extracellular matrix, nerves. Cyclic stretch, increased hydrostatic and cyclic hydrodynamic pressure and hypoxia are stimuli capable of modulating multiple signaling pathways involved in this remodeling process.

Conclusions: Bladder outlet obstruction leads to progressive bladder tissue remodeling in humans. Multiple signaling pathways are involved.

Keywords: Bladder outlet obstruction, Bladder remodeling, Systematic review

Background

Bladder outlet obstruction (BOO), clinically defined as high-pressure/low-flow micturition pattern at urodynamic investigations, is a common urological condition in humans with benign prostatic obstruction (BPO) being the most frequent causative factor. It represents a key pathophysiological link between benign prostate enlargement (BPE) and lower urinary tract symptoms (LUTS) [1–3]. Besides symptoms, BOO can also lead to progressive tissue remodeling of the bladder and of the upper urinary tract with subsequent serious functional impairments [1–4]. Based on the results from studies on animal models exposed to experimental partial outlet obstruction, the remodeling of the bladder involves the modulation of several signaling pathways as well as histological alterations occurring in almost all cellular compartments [5]. These changes are described to progress through three sequential stages: hypertrophy, compensation and decompensation [6]. In the hypertrophy stage, mechanical stress activates early signals that mediate bladder wall hypertrophy. At the same time, due to the occurrence of focal area of hypoxia, angiogenesis is stimulated thus enabling blood flow to increase relative to bladder mass [6]. In the compensated stage bladder growth and angiogenesis stop. At some point, if obstruction persists, the bladder shifts to a decompensated state as a result of cyclical

* Correspondence: ferdinando-fusco@libero.it
[1]Dipartimento di Neuroscienze e Scienze Riproduttive ed Odontostomatologiche, Università Degli Studi Di Napoli Federico II, Via Pansini, 5, 80131 Naples, Italy
Full list of author information is available at the end of the article

ischemia-reperfusion injury occurring during the micturition phase that leads to the activation of pathways involved in the progressive loss of smooth muscle, deposition of extracellular matrix and neuronal loss [6]. The duration of these stages varies considerably according to the experimental models and is unpredictably. Data about the reversibility of these alterations are also lacking. *H*uman detrusor differs significantly from animal models and most of the species used for research don't suffer from naturally occurring outflow obstruction [7]. *The aim of the present study was to summarize available evidences about BOO-induced morphological and molecular alterations occurring in the various compartments of human bladder.*

Methods

We performed a systematic review using the Preferred Reporting Items for Systematic Reviews and Meta-Analyses Statement as a guideline in the development of the study protocol and the report of the current study [8]. In December 2017 we used the National Library of Medicine PubMed search engine, the Scopus database, and the ISI Web of Knowledge official website to search for all published studies evaluating morphological and molecular alterations involved in BOO-induced bladder wall remodeling. The following search terms were combined: angiogenesis, apoptosis, bladder outlet obstruction, collagen, electron microscopy, extracellular matrix, fibrosis, hypoxia, histology, inflammation, innervation, ischemia, pressure, proliferation, remodeling, suburothelium, smooth muscle cells, stretch, urothelium. We included publications that met the following criteria: reporting original in vitro and in vivo research; English language; human studies. Reference lists in relevant articles and reviews were also screened for additional studies.

Results

The search strategy revealed a total of 159 results. Screening of the titles and abstracts revealed 44 papers eligible for inclusion. Further assessment of eligibility, based on full-text papers, led to the exclusion of 8 papers. This left 36 papers meeting our criteria for inclusion [9–44] (Fig. 1).

Alterations occurring in the urothelium and suburothelium

We identified one study describing BOO-induced alterations occurring in the context of urothelium and suburothelium [9]. Bladder biopsies were obtained from 33 men with urodynamic proven BOO and 10 control subjects. Authors demonstrated the occurrence of significant urothelial dysfunction and alterations of urothelial signaling and sensory transduction pathways in patients with BOO. In detail, the following alterations were found: significantly lower expression of the adhesion protein E-cadherin and of the muscarinic receptor M3, and significantly higher expression of the purinergic receptor P2X3 and of the muscarinic receptor M2. Interestingly, patients with detrusor underactivity had a significantly lower expression of E-cadherin and of inducible nitric oxide synthase as well as a significantly higher expression of β3 adrenoreceptors than patients with detrusor overactivity/hypersensitive bladder. Clinically, lower expression of E-cadherin was associated with lower voided volumes thus suggesting a more severe or decompensated status with more severe urothelial dysfunction. Alterations found in the suburothelium of BOO patients included: inflammation, with a significantly increased level of activated mast cells, and increased apoptosis.

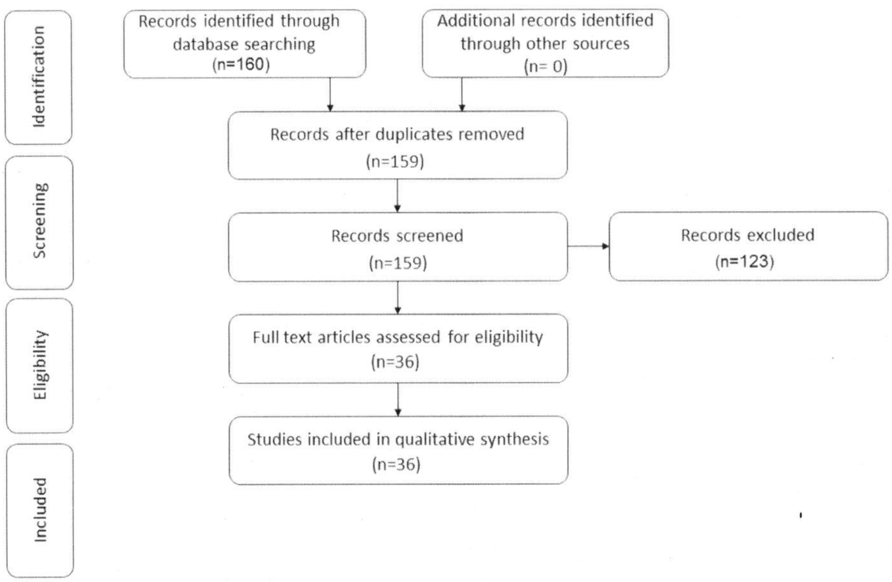

Fig. 1 Preferred Reporting Items for Systematic Reviews and Meta-analysis (PRISMA) flowchart

Alterations occurring in the detrusor muscle: morphological aspects

The detrusor muscle represents the bladder compartment more extensively investigated. Studies describing BOO-induced morphological alterations occurring in the detrusor are summarized in Table 1. Significant alterations involving both smooth muscle cells (SMCs) and extracellular matrix (ECM) have been demonstrated using light and electron microscopy studies.

SMCs alterations

Detrusor SMCs hypertrophy represents the most relevant morphological alteration occurring in BOO patients. Gilpin et al. compared the morphological and morphometric characteristics of detrusor specimens from patients with unequivocal urodynamic BOO accompanied by evidence of severe bladder trabeculation at cystoscopy and subjects with normal urodynamic assessment and absent trabeculation [10]. Although authors did not find morphological evidences of SMCs hyperplasia, the mean profile

Table 1 Summary of studies describing BOO-induced detrusor morphological alterations

Author, year	Study design	Subjects in the case group (n)	Main findings
Gosling, 1980 [15]	Case control	9	• ↑ intrafascicular and interfascicular collagen • ↓ SMCs diameter
Gilpin, 1985 [10]	Case control	14	• ↑connective tissue infiltration of some smooth muscle bundles in 12/14 patients • ↑ SMCs mean profile area
Elbadawi, 1993 [12]	Case control	7	• ↓ intermediate cell junctions • ↑intrafascicular collagen and elastic fibers • ↑ SMCs hypertrophy • ↑ SMCs and axons degeneration in patients with impaired detrusor contractility
Inui, 1999 [19]	Case control	26	• Significant positive linear relationship between C/M and estimated bladder weight in patients with bladder weight ≥ 60 g • ↑ C/M in patients with bladder weight ≥ 60 g
Tse, 2000 [13]	Case control	9	• Myohypertrophy pattern in all cases
Brierly, 2003 [14]	Case control	12	• Myohypertrophy pattern in 8/10 BOO patients. • Degenerative pattern in 4/10 BOO patients.
Holm, 2003 [22]	Case control	25	• Significant correlation between intra- and interfascicular elastin and BOO degree
Mirone, 2004 [15]	Case control	36	• ↑collagen content in BPO patients with respect to controls • ↑collagen content in patients with severe symptoms
Horn, 2004 [44]	Observational	54	• Correlation between abnormal morphology and impaired bladder compliance and decreased capacity
Collado, 2006 [11]	Case control	33	• ↑ intrafascicular and interfascicular collagen • ↑ intrafascicular fibrosis in BOO patients with history of AUR • ↑ SMCs diameter in BOO patients with respect to controls • Not significant differences in terms of SMCs diameter between BOO patients with and without AUR history • Positive correlation between SMCs diameter and symptoms duration
Rubinstein, 2007 [18]	Case control	10	• ↑ collagen and elastic fibers
Blatt, 2012 [16]	Case control	17	• Poor post-TURP voiding outcome in patients with detrusor ultrastructural pattern characterized by variable muscle cell size, muscle cell shape, abnormal fascicle arrangement and collagenosis.
Bellucci, 2017 [21]	Case control	19	• ↑ C/M • Significant negative correlation between C/M and bladder compliance • Significant correlation between the probability of urinary retention and C/M
Averbeck, 2017 [20]	Observational	38	• ↑ C/M in patients with PVR ≥ 200 mL and in those with reduced bladder compliance

AUR acute urinary retention, *BOO* bladder outlet obstruction, *C/M* connective tissue-to-smooth muscle ratio, *PVR* post void residual volume, *SMCs* smooth muscle cells, *TURP* trans urethral resection of the prostate area of SMCs was higher in BOO patients due to hypertrophy. Similarly, Collado et al. demonstrated that detrusor SMCs diameter was significantly higher in BOO patients with respect to controls [11]. Authors found a positive correlation between SMCs diameter and symptoms duration but no statistically significant differences between BOO patients with and without history of Acute Urinary Retention (AUR). Electron microscopy studies also confirmed the evidence of SMCs hypertrophy in many cases. Elbadawi et al. investigated the ultrastructural basis of obstructive detrusor dysfunction in a prospective case-control study enrolling 35 elderly subjects [12]. Authors described the "myohypertrophy" structural pattern in patients with urodynamic proven BOO. This pattern was characterized by 4 distinctive features, including SMCs hypertrophy, marked widening of intercellular spaces with reduced normal intermediate cell junctions, increased deposition of collagen and elastin between SMCs, and patchy distribution of the preceding features in various muscle fascicles. This ultrastructural pattern was confirmed by other authors in patients with urodynamic evidence of BOO [13, 14]. Of note, the evidence of SMCs hypertrophy has not been confirmed in all patients. In their light microscopy study, Gosling et al. failed to found evidences of SMCs hypertrophy or hyperplasia in a subset of patients with unequivocal BPO accompanied by trabeculated urinary bladder [15]. On the contrary, authors identified some muscle bundles containing SMCs characterized by a small diameter [15]. Elbadawi et al. showed degeneration of SMCs in the specimens of patients who had impaired detrusor contractility [12]. The degenerative pattern was confirmed by Brierly et al. in BOO patients with high post void residual volume [14].

ECM alterations

Detrusor ECM remodeling is characterized by increased accumulation of collagen and elastic fibers in both the interfascicular and intrafascicular compartments. This finding has been confirmed in several studies using both light and electron microscopy techniques [10, 11, 15–21]. Interestingly, Gilpin et al. found that patients with evidence of interfascicular connective tissue infiltration had the highest levels of SMCs mean profile area thus leading the authors to hypothesize that the deposition of connective tissue occurs at a later stage with respect to onset of SMCs hypertrophy [10]. This hypothesis has been confirmed by other studies. Inui et al. investigated the relationship between the amount of detrusor connective tissue in patients with BPH and the degree of bladder hypertrophy evaluated by ultrasound estimated bladder weight. In detail, authors compared the ratio of connective tissue-to-smooth muscle (C/M) between controls and BPE cases [19]. The study failed to found statistically significant differences between the two groups (27.3% in BPE patients and 24.7% in controls). However, a significant positive linear relationship between C/M and estimated bladder weight was evident in all BPE patients with estimated bladder weight ≥ 60 g [19]. Interestingly, 30% of BPE patients had C/M < 20% compared to only 7.7% of controls. Author hypothesized that the increase in ultrasound estimated bladder weight is caused at early stages by hyperplasia and/or hypertrophy of detrusor SMCs leading to a lower C/M and later to the additional increase of connective tissue with higher C/M. Other studies confirmed the occurrence of increased detrusor ECM accumulation with more advanced stages within the natural history of BOO. Collado et al. compared detrusor C/M of patients with urodynamic BOO and no history of AUR, patients with urodynamic BOO and history of AUR and non-obstructed controls [11]. Patients with BOO (obstruction and AUR groups) had a significantly higher intrafascicular and interfascicular collagen content than the control group. Patients with history of AUR had statistically significant higher levels of intrafascicular collagen than BOO patients without history of AUR. Moreover, authors found a statistically significant correlation between the amount of intrafascicular fibrosis and detrusor pressure at maximum urinary flow as well as with the Abrams-Griffiths number in BOO patients without history of AUR at pre-operative urodynamics. Additionally, a statistically significant negative correlation was found between intrafascicular fibrosis and postoperative bladder compliance in the same group of patients. Finally, a positive and significant correlation was found between intrafascicular fibrosis and both detrusor pressure at maximum urinary flow and the Abrams-Griffiths number in BOO patients with history of AUR at post-operative urodynamic evaluation [11]. Averbeck et al. evaluated the collagen content in the bladder wall of men undergoing open prostate surgery. Although BOO was not a predictor of increased collagen deposition, patients with reduced bladder compliance and those with a PVR ≥ 200 mL showed a significantly higher C/M [20]. Similarly, Bellucci et al. found a significant negative correlation between C/M and bladder compliance [21]. Moreover, the probability of urinary retention increased significantly with the C/M. Mirone et al. found higher detrusor collagen content in patients with BPO and severe symptoms with respect to patients with moderate symptoms [22]. Blatt et al. investigated the correlation between detrusor ultrastructural features of patients with urodynamic BOO or a hypocontractile detrusor and clinical outcomes after transurethral resection of the prostate [16]. Authors found that the morphological pattern characterized by variable SMCs size, SMCs shape, abnormal fascicle arrangement and collagenosis correlated with poor postoperative voiding outcome. Holm et al. investigated the correlation between ultrastructural findings and urodynamic parameters in patients with BOO [17]. SMCs hypertrophy, occurrence of abnormal cell junctions and configurations, variation in intercellular distances, and intracellular changes were investigated. The increase in intra- and interfascicular elastin was only parameter which was found to relate to the degree of obstruction in BOO patients.

Alterations occurring in the detrusor muscle: molecular aspects and signaling pathways

Data about molecular aspects and signaling pathways involved in BOO-induced detrusor remodeling mainly derive from in vitro cell culture models of human bladder SMCs (HBSMCs) exposed to stressful stimuli such as cyclic mechanical stretch, increased hydrostatic (HP) or cyclic hydrodynamic pressure (CHP), and hypoxia. Further evidences derive from genetic and molecular studies on tissue specimens from BOO patients. Table 2 summarizes evidences from these studies.

Effects of cyclic stretch

Yang et al. investigated the effects of cyclic stretch on HBSMCs gene expression [23]. Authors identified multiple mechano-responsive genes encoding *cytokine, growth-related factors, adhesive molecules, signal transduction molecules, cytoskeleton and extracellular matrix proteins, developmental, differentiation, and inflammatory factors.* Twelve of proteins encoded by these genes had interacting partners in the vascular system and were functionally involved in multiple aspects of angiogenesis and vascular development such as endothelial cell proliferation and migration, SMCs differentiation, and arterial-venous differentiation.

Effects of increased pressure

The effects of increased pressure on HBSMCs has been investigated by many authors. These studies demonstrated the existence of multiple pressure-dependent pathways involved into cellular processes such as adhesion, proliferation, inflammation, and ECM remodeling.

Effects of increased pressure on cell adhesion

Wang et al. demonstrated a significant decreased expression of the gap junction connexin 43 under hydrostatic pressures >60 cm H_2O for 24 h or pressures >40 cm H_2O for 72 h [24].

Effects of increased pressure on cell hypertrophy and hyperplasia

Lee et al. investigated the effects of HP on HBSMCs in terms of cell hypertrophy and hyperplasia and the potential role of muscarinic receptors [26]. HBSMCs proliferation and hypertrophy were measured by 3H-thymidine and leucine incorporation assays, respectively [25]. 3H-thymidine incorporation increased by 16.7, 25.9 and 39.4% after exposure to acetylcholine, 40 cmH_2O HP, and both, respectively. Similarly, leucine incorporation increased by 66.5, 66.5 and 81.8%, after exposure to acetylcholine, 40 cmH_2O HP, and both, respectively. These findings were consistent with increased proliferation and hypertrophy, respectively. Antimuscarinic agents determined a dramatic decrease in thymidine and leucine incorporation for cells exposed to increased HP, most pronounced when both M2 and M3 receptor antagonist were applied. In a subsequent study, authors found that M2 and M3 receptor expression increases in a time- and pressure-dependent manner in isolated HBSMCs [26]. Preis et al. investigated the role of platelet derived growth factor (PDGF) pathway in pressure-induced proliferation [27]. Exposure of HBSMCs to HP induced proliferation in a time dependent manner. Moreover, HBSMCs showed increased PDGF receptor (PDGFR) α and β expression. Interestingly, DNA synthesis in cells with intact PDGFR α was increased after short-term HP but cells lacking PDGFR α did not proliferate. All studies evaluating the effects of CHP on HBSMCs demonstrated increased proliferation under CHP > 100 cmH_2O. Involved signaling pathways include: phosphoinositide 3-kinase/serum-glucocorticoid regulated kinase 1, S-phase kinase-associated protein 2, p27, Ras-related C3 botulinum toxin substrate 1, miR-3180-5p and miR 4323 [28–32]. MiR-3180-5p promotes HBSMCs proliferation by the activation of the pro-proliferative cyclin-dependent kinase 2 pathway [29]. On the other hand, miR 4323 can promote HBSMCs proliferation by inhibiting LYN expression and activating the Erk1/2 pathway, also known as the mitogen activated protein kinase signaling pathway [30].

Effects of increased pressure on inflammatory pathways

Liang et al. investigated the effects of HP and acetylcholine on the release of inflammatory cytokines in HBSMCs to test the hypothesis that mechanical force and muscarinic receptors have pro-inflammatory effect in obstructed bladder [33]. HP produced a significant time-dependent and pressure-dependent increase in expressions of inflammatory genes. HP of 200 cm H_2O for 24 h was associated with a statistically significant increase of monocyte chemoattractant protein, IL-6, and RANTES. Both NFκB and ERK1/2 pathways were proved to be involved in pressure-induced inflammation.

Effects of increased pressure on ECM remodeling

Backhaus et al. applied HP to HBSMCs to determine the effect on matrix metalloproteinases (MMPs) and tissue inhibitors of metalloproteinases (TIMP) [34]. Exposure of HBSMCs to a sustained HP of 20 cm H_2O for 7 h

Table 2 Summary of studies evaluating BOO-induced molecular alterations and related cellular events in human detrusor

Author, year	Experimental conditions	Molecular alteration	Cellular events
Backhaus, 2002 [34]	HBSMCs exposed to HP (0.3, 20 and 40 cm H_2O) for 1, 3, 7 and 24 h	↓ MMP-1, 2, 9 after exposure to 20 cm H_2O for 7 h ↑TIMP-1 after exposure to 40 cm H_2O 3, 7 and 24 h	
Wang, 2013 [24]	HBSMCs exposed to HP (0, 20, 40, 60, 80 and 100 cm H_2O) for 6, 12, 24 and 72 h	↓expression of the gap junction connexin 43 under HP > 60 cm H_2O for 24 h or HP > 40 cm H_2O for 72 h.	
Chen, 2012 [28]	HBSMCs exposed to CHP (0, 100, 200, and 300 cm H_2O)	↑ SGK1 expression and activity	↑ proliferation in the 200 and 300 cm H_2O groups
Chen, 2014 [32]	HBSMCs exposed to CHP (0, 100, 200, and 300 cm H_2O)	↑ Skp2 expression and ↓ p27 expression under 200 and 300 cmH_2O CHP	
Wu, 2012 [31]	HBSMCs exposed to CHP (static, 100, 200, and 300 cm H_2O)	Ras-related C3 botulinum toxin substrate 1, mitogen-activated protein kinase kinase 1/2 and extracellular regulated protein kinases 1/2 activated by 200 and 300 cmH_2O CHP	↑proliferation under 200 and 300 cmH_2O CHP
Preis, 2015 [27]	HBSMCs exposed to HP of 136 cm H_2O for 1 h	↑ expression of PDGFR α and β	↑ proliferation
Sun, 2016 [29]	HBSMCs exposed to CHP up to 200 cm H_2O	↑ miR-3180-5p	↑ proliferation
Sun, 2017 [30]	HBSMCs exposed to CHP up to 200 cm H_2O	↑ miR 4323	↑ proliferation
Lee, 2006 [25]	HBSMCs exposed to HP (40 cm H_2O) and/or acetylcholine for 24 h	Activation of muscarinic receptors	↑ proliferation ↑ hypertrophy
Lee, 2008 [26]	HBSMCs exposed to acetylcholine in the presence or absence of HP (10, 20, and 40 cm H_2O)	↑ M2 and M3 receptors expression	↑ proliferation ↑ hypertrophy
Yang, 2008 [23]	HBSMCs exposed to cyclic stretch with maximum of 15% strain magnitude at a frequency of 0.3 Hz for either 1 h or 24 h.	30 genes upregulated and 59 downregulated after 1 h exposure 59 genes upregulated and 27 downregulated after 24 h exposure	
Backhaus, 2002 [34]	HBSMCs exposed to HP (0.3, 20 and 40 cm H_2O)	↓ MMP-1, 2, 9 ↑TIMP-1	
Liang, 2017 [33]	HBSMCs exposed to HP (100, 200, or 300 cm H_2O) and/or acetylcholine	↑ IL-6, monocyte chemoattractant protein, and RANTES	
Galvin, 2004 [7]	HBSMCs exposed to 1% O_2 tension for 24, 48, 72, and 96 h	↑ HIF-1α ↑ VEGF ↑ $p27^{kip1}$	↓ proliferation
Wiafe, 2017 [35]	HBSMCs exposed to 3% O_2 tension for 2, 24, 48, and 72 h	↑ HIF1α, HIF2α, and HIF3α ↑VEGF ↑TGFβ1 ↑CTGF ↑ collagens 1, 2, 3, 4 ↑ fibronectin ↑aggrecan ↑TIMP ↑ α-smooth muscle actin ↑vimentin, ↑desmin ↑TNFα, IL 1β, and IL 6 ↓ IL-10	
Boopathi , 2011 [38]		↑ expression of GATA-6 in cases	

Table 2 Summary of studies evaluating BOO-induced molecular alterations and related cellular events in human detrusor *(Continued)*

Author, year	Experimental conditions	Molecular alteration	Cellular events
	Bladder samples from subjects with BOO and controls	↓ Caveolin-1 expression	
Koritsiadis, 2008 [36]	Bladder samples from subjects scheduled for BPE-surgery and controls	↑ HIF-1α expression in stromal cells between muscle bundles and in connective tissue beneath the mucosal layer	
Barbosa, 2017 [37]	Bladder samples from subjects with obstructive BPE and controls	↑ collagens I and III ↓ MMP-9 and TIMP-1 ↑VEGF ↓ CD105	
Gheinani, 2017 [43]	Bladder samples from subjects with different states of urodynamic defined BOO-induced bladder dysfunction	Progressive increase in the number of altered mRNA and miRNAs from the detrusor overactive to the obstruction group to the underactive detrusor groups	

BOO bladder outlet obstruction, *BPE* benign prostatic enlargement, *CHP* cyclic hydrodynamic pressure, *CTGF* connective tissue transforming growth factor, *HBSMCs* human bladder smooth muscle cells, *HIF* hypoxia inducible factor, *HP* hydrostatic pressures, *IL* interleukin, *MMP* matrix metalloproteinases, *PDGFR* platelet derived growth factor receptor, *SGK1* serum-glucocorticoid regulated kinase 1, *Skp2* S-phase kinase-associated protein 2, *TGF* transforming growth factor, *TIMP* tissue inhibitor *of* metalloproteinases, *TNF* tumor necrosis factor, *VEGF* vascular endothelial growth factor

resulted in a significant time dependent decrease in MMP-1, 2 and 9 activities compared to controls maintained at atmospheric pressure. TIMP-1 levels increased an average of 10% after exposure to 20 cm H_2O. These changes became statistically significant when the cells were exposed to 40 cm H_2O.

Effects of hypoxia

Available evidences demonstrate that hypoxia can modulate signaling pathways involved in angiogenesis, proliferation and ECM remodeling.

Effects of hypoxia on hypoxia inducible factor and vascular endothelial growth factor

Galvin et al. demonstrated significant time-dependent upregulation of hypoxia inducible factor (HIF)-1α and vascular endothelial growth factor (VEGF) in HBSMCs exposed to hypoxia [7]. HIF-1α expression was maximal at 72 h while a twofold increase in VEGF production was evident after 24 h of hypoxia and this increase continued in a time-dependent manner. Wiafe et al. investigated the effects of hypoxia on HIF1α, HIF2α, HIF3α and VEGF expression [35]. Transcription of HIF1α and HIF2α demonstrated a time-dependent increased expression and were transiently upregulated in response to short-term hypoxia (2–24 h). HIF3α genes and protein were significantly expressed after 72 h of hypoxia when HIF1 and HIF2α proteins had resumed normoxic control levels. VEGF mRNA increased significantly after 24 and 72 h. The up-regulation of HIF and VEGF has been confirmed in bladder specimens from LUTS/BPE subjects. Koritsiadis et al. compared the expression of HIF-1alpha and carbonic anhydrase IX, a further cellular marker of hypoxia, in detrusor tissue retrieved from patients scheduled for surgery to treat BPE and controls [36]. The mean number of total cells immunoreactive to HIF-1α in the study group was significantly higher with respect to the control group. HIF-1α was expressed mainly in stromal cells between muscle bundles and in connective tissue beneath the mucosal layer, while urothelium and detrusor had no immunoreactivity [36]. Interestingly, the HIF-1α response was limited in a time-dependent manner. Indeed, the probability of HIF-1α immunoreactivity was four times greater in men with BOO for < 10 years, than in those with BOO for $>$ 10 years with an odds ratio of 4.25 thus suggesting that the bladder can compensate for the first few years after that the adaptive response declines [36]. Moreover, the risk of identifying a high expression of HIF-1α was four times higher in patients with urinary retention [36]. Barbosa et al. compared the gene expression of the angiogenic growth factor VEGF in bladder specimens from patients with obstructive BPH with grade IV or higher BOO as per Schäfer criteria and age-matched controls [37]. Patients with BOO presented a statistically significant overexpression of VEGF. Interestingly, upregulation of VEGF was particularly evident in subjects with risk factors for atherosclerosis.

Effects of hypoxia on HBSMCs proliferation

Galvin et al. demonstrated that HBSMCs exposed to hypoxia maintain their cell viability in culture and do not undergo cell death when placed under hypoxic conditions [7]. However, hypoxia significantly reduces the rate of proliferation in a time-dependent manner, associated with an increase in the cell cycle inhibitor $p27^{kip1}$ [7].

Effects of hypoxia on HBSMCs differentiation

Wiafe et al. found evidences in favor of HBSMCs dedifferentiation, as demonstrated by the increased expression of α-smooth muscle actin, vimentin, and desmin, and acquisition of a profibrotic phenotype [35]. Pro-fibrotic changes included the upregulation of SMAD 2, SMAD 3, and connective tissue growth factor (CTGF) genes as well as collagens 1, 2, 3, and 4, fibronectin, aggrecan, and TIMP-1 transcripts [35]. Collagen 1 transcripts exhibited a consistent increase over the entire time course, with a 3.4-fold increase after 2 h eventually reaching a maximum fold increase of 12 by 72 h. Collagen 2 transcript levels showed a 4-fold increase by 72 h; collagen 3 exhibited a similar increase, although a 5-fold increase was evident at 48 and 72 h. Collagen 4 transcripts rose by almost 8-fold following 72 h hypoxia. Total secreted collagen remained at control values until 24 h at which point levels rose by 100% and values remained consistently elevated during prolonged hypoxia. Fibronectin transcripts showed a consistent increase from 1.9 to 3.9-fold for values between 24 and 72 h.

Effects of hypoxia on inflammatory pathways

Wiafe et al. demonstrated that hypoxia can produce a robust inflammatory response in isolated HBSMCs [35]. Indeed, hypoxia induced increased expression of TNFα, IL 1β, and IL 6 which are all part of the acute phase proteins secreted in response to inflammation. Transcript levels of the anti-inflammatory cytokine, IL-10 exhibited a consistent decline [35].

Other SMCs molecular alterations

Boopathi et al. demonstrated the loss of caveolin-1, a protein that has a pivotal role in regulating SMCs contractile activity, in bladder wall smooth muscle from BPO subjects [38].

Alterations occurring in the neuronal compartment

We identified four studies describing BOO-induced morphological alterations involving bladder innervation and two studies investigating the potential role of tissue nerve growth factor (Table 3). Golsin et al. found a 56% reduction in the number of acetylcholine-positive nerves in the specimens from obstructed bladder with respect to controls [39]. Cumming et al. confirmed the significant reduction of detrusor innervation in bladder biopsies from patients with urodynamic confirmed BOO [40]. Interestingly, innervation level was normalized in 80% of patients after BOO relief. Chapple et al. demonstrated a reduction in the density of innervation by vasoactive intestinal polypeptide, calcitonin gene-related peptide, substance P and somatostatin-immunoreactive but not neuropeptide Y-immunoreactive nerve fibers in bladder specimens from BOO patients [41]. Elbadawi et al. showed axon degeneration at electron microscopy in specimens of patients who had impaired detrusor contractility [12]. The role of tissue nerve growth factor, a key signal in the regulation of nerve physiology, is controversial. Steers et al. found that the amount of nerve growth factor in grossly hypertrophied human bladders exceeded that in non-hypertrophied samples [42]. In the study by Barbosa et al. the levels of nerve growth factor and of nerve growth factor receptor in bladder tissue from the overall BPO population were not different with respect to controls [37]. However, the levels of nerve growth factor receptors were higher in the subgroup of smokers and dyslipidemic BPO patients [37].

Table 3 Summary of studies evaluating BOO-induced neuronal alterations

Author, year	Study design	Subjects in the cases group (n)	Findings
Gosling, 1986 [39]	Case-control	19	↓ autonomic nerve supply
Chapple, 1992 [41]	Case-control	19	↓ density of innervation by vasoactive intestinal polypeptide, calcitonin gene-related peptide, substance P and somatostatin immunoreactive nerve fibers in the obstructed bladder.
Cumming, 1992 [40]	Case-control	10	↓innervation
Elbadawi, 1993 [12]	Case control	7	↑axon degeneration in patients with impaired detrusor contractility
Steers, 1991 [42]	Case-control	–	↑ NGF in grossly hypertrophied human bladders
Barbosa, 2017 [37]	Case-control	43	↑ NGF receptor expression in smokers and dyslipidemic patients

NGF nerve growth factor

Discussion

To our knowledge, we performed the first systematic review of studies investigating BOO-induced morphological and molecular alterations in human bladder. Data summarized demonstrate the occurrence of a remodeling process involving multiple cellular compartments, namely urothelium, suburothelium, detrusor SMCs, detrusor ECM, and neurons. Based on evidences from in-vitro HBSMCs cultures, cyclical stretch, increased pressure and hypoxia can modulate several signaling pathways potentially involved in this process. Taken together, these data support the hypothesis that the natural history of BOO may be characterized, also in humans, by three morpho-functional stages: an initial hypertrophy phase, a subsequent compensation, and a late decompensation (Fig. 2). Increased intravescical pressure during bladder voiding, the pathognomonic urodynamic feature of BOO, can be considered the "primum movens". Indeed, it can stimulate compensatory SMCs hypertrophy and proliferation as demonstrated by in vitro studies. Tissue hypoxia subsequently intervenes as further critical stress factor. It is due to the imbalance between increased oxygen demand and lower oxygen delivery and may arise early in the natural history of BOO-induced bladder remodeling. Clinically, detrusor hypoxia has been confirmed in studies on human subjects with evidence of BOO [45–47]. Compensatory responses to hypoxia have been demonstrated in several human tissues, including the bladder. These include hypoxia-induced pathways such as HIF and VEGF. Available data suggest that, similar to animal models, these adaptive responses may counteract hypoxia only for a limited period of time. Persistent hypoxia also inhibits HBSMCs proliferation thus favoring the transition from the hypertrophy to the compensation phase, and activates signaling involved in ECM remodeling and collagen accumulation that characterize the transition from compensation to decompensation. Indeed, increased deposition of collagen and elastin in the interfascicular and intrafascicular detrusor compartments can alter the biomechanical properties of the bladder causing decreased compliance and impaired voiding function, which are feature considered by some authors as clinical marker of decompensation. Results from the present review have relevant clinical implications. In recent years evidences have emerged demonstrating that LUTS/BPO represent a progressive disorder in many patients [48–50]. Progression, however, has been defined based on clinical parameters such as deterioration of symptoms and health-related quality of life, decreased urinary peak flow rate, increased prostate size, and unfavorable outcomes such as AUR and BPE-related surgery [48–50]. Based on the results from the present study, clinicians should be aware of the fact that, beyond subjective symptoms, BPO also causes progressive morphological remodeling of the bladder with potential serious functional impairments. Consequently, this aspect should be carefully taken in account in the management of these patients and therapeutic outcomes should include not only the improvement of subjective symptoms but also the prevention of pathologic bladder remodeling. Evidences summarized in the present review suggest the existence of multiple signaling pathways that can represent potential targets for future therapies. Meantime, increased bladder pressure is the only pathophysiological mechanism that can be realistically improved in everyday clinical practice. Although multiple treatment options are available to treat LUTS/BPO, only surgery, alpha-1 adrenergic antagonists and 5-alpha reductase inhibitors have been reported to improve BOO by reducing bladder pressures. The progressive model of bladder remodeling

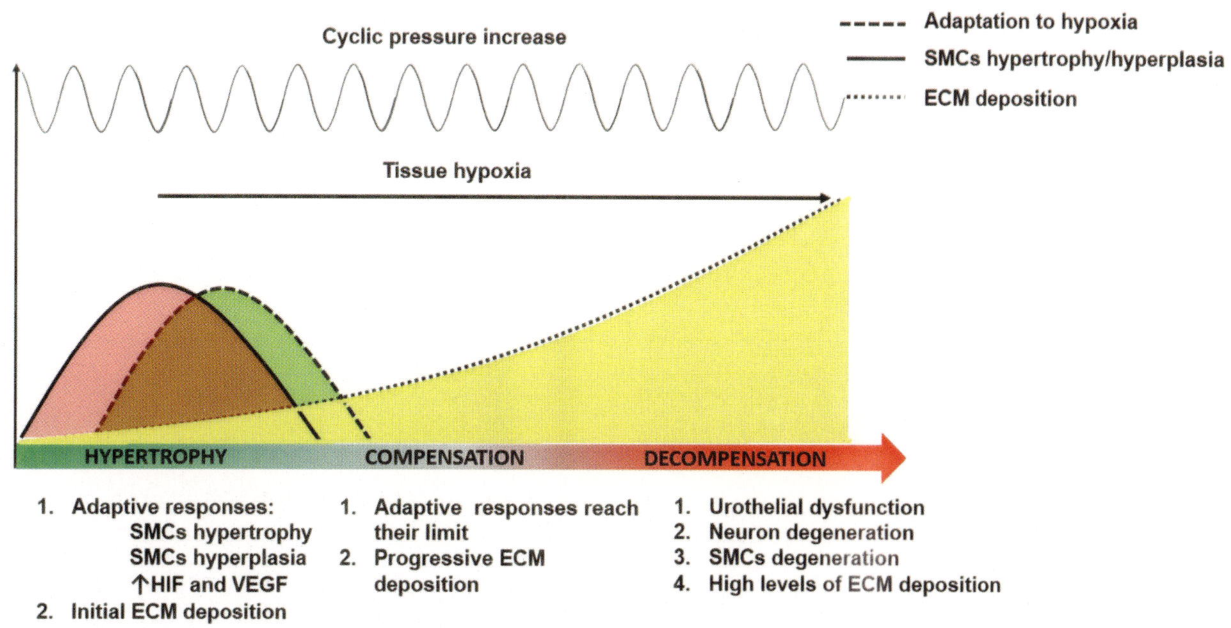

Fig. 2 Proposed three-stage model for BOO-induced bladder remodeling in humans

emerged from evidences summarized in the present study also contributes to explain the failures of surgical and medical therapies when prescribed later in the natural history of BOO and suggests to intervene early [48–50]. Although adherence to medical therapy for LUTS/BPO has been reported to prevent clinical disease progression the advantages in terms of morphological remodeling deserve further investigations [51]. At time, only few clinical markers of morphological bladder remodeling are available including increased estimated bladder weight and endoscopic evidence of bladder trabeculation. The role of bladder biopsies is controversial [44]. Results from the present study provide the basis for future investigations about urinary and/or serum markers of bladder remodeling. Some limits of the present study should be acknowledged: studies included are often outdated and enrolled a limited number of patients. Cultured cells may differ from fresh detrusor tissues as potential interactions among various compartments are not considered and cells are simply exposed to a single stress factor. Consequently, the molecular mechanism of bladder remodeling in BOO remains unclear and it remains difficult to establish an integrated signaling pathway. Further issues deserving investigations are the timing and the reversibility of BOO-induced bladder remodeling.

Conclusions

Evidences from available studies on human tissues demonstrate that BOO induces molecular and morphological alterations in multiple bladder compartments, namely urothelium, suburothelium, detrusor SMCs, detrusor ECM, and neurons. Cyclic stretch, increased pressure and hypoxia have been demonstrated to modulate multiple signaling pathways involved in these processes. A three-stages model can be hypothesized to characterize BOO-induced bladder remodeling also in humans: hypertrophy, compensation, decompensation.

Abbreviations

AUR: Acute urinary retention; BOO: Bladder outlet obstruction; BPE: Benign prostatic enlargement; BPO: Benign prostatic obstruction; C/M: Connective Tissue-to-Smooth Muscle Ratio; CHP: Chronic hydrostatic pressure; CTGF: Connective tissue growth factor; ECM: Extracellular matrix; HBSMCs: Human bladder smooth muscle cells; HIF: Hypoxia inducible factor; HP: Hydrostatic pressure; IL: Interleukin; LUTS: Lower urinary tract symptoms; MMPs: Matrix metalloproteinases; PDGF: Platelet derived growth factor; SMCs: Smooth Muscle Cells; TIMP: Tissue inhibitors of metalloproteases; TNF: Tumor necrosis factor; VEGF: Vascular endothelial growth factor

Acknowledgements

All authors belong to the Italian Society of Urodynamics (SIUD) Publication Group.

Funding

None to declare.

Authors' contributions

Conception and design: FF, MC, EFA. Drafting of the manuscript: MC, FF, VLM, VI. Analysis and interpretation of data: FM, CDN, VI. Supervision: EFA, FM, CDN. We confirm that all authors read and approved the final manuscript.

Competing interests

Ferdinando Fusco: Speaker and Consultant for Recordati, Bayer, Lilly, Pierre-Fabre.
Massimiliano Creta: Consultant and medical writer for Recordati.
Vincenzo Li Marzi: Invited speaker from Wellspect and Allergan.
Enrico Finazzi Agrò: Consultat for Laborie, Wellspect, Allergan; Speaker honorarium from: Astellas, Coloplast, Glaxo Smith Kline, Wellspect.
Cosimo De Nunzio (SE) and Enrico Finazzi Agrò (AE) are members of the editorial board of BMC Urology.

Author details

[1]Dipartimento di Neuroscienze e Scienze Riproduttive ed Odontostomatologiche, Università Degli Studi Di Napoli Federico II, Via Pansini, 5, 80131 Naples, Italy. [2]Dipartimento di Urologia, Ospedale Sant'Andrea, Università Degli Studi di Roma "La Sapienza", Rota, Italy. [3]Dipartimento di Medicina Sperimentale e Chirurgia, Università Degli Studi di Roma "Tor Vergata", Roma, Italy. [4]Dipartimento di Urologia, Ospedale Careggi, Università Degli Studi di Firenze, Firenze, Italy.

References

1. Fusco F, Creta M, Imperatore V, Longo N, Imbimbo C, Lepor H, et al. Benign prostatic obstruction relief in patients with lower urinary tract symptoms suggestive of benign prostatic enlargement undergoing endoscopic surgical procedures or therapy with alpha-blockers: a review of urodynamic studies. Adv Ther. 2017;34(4):773–83.
2. Fusco F, Palmieri A, Ficarra V, Giannarini G, Novara G, Longo N, et al. α1-blockers improve benign prostatic obstruction in men with lower urinary tract symptoms: a systematic review and meta-analysis of urodynamic studies. Eur Urol. 2016;69(6):1091–101.
3. Creta M, Bottone F, Sannino S, Maisto E, Franco M, Mangiapia F, et al. Effects of alpha1-blockers on urodynamic parameters of bladder outlet obstruction in patients with lower urinary tract symptoms suggestive of benign prostatic enlargement: a review. Minerva Urol Nefrol. 2016;68(2):209–21.
4. Mirone V, Imbimbo C, Longo N, Fusco F. The detrusor muscle: an innocent victim of bladder outlet obstruction. Eur Urol. 2007;51(1):57–66.
5. Komninos C, Mitsogiannis I. Obstruction-induced alterations within the urinary bladder and their role in the pathophysiologyof lower urinary tract symptomatology. Can Urol Assoc J. 2014;8(7–8):E524–30.
6. Levin R, Chichester P, Levin S, Buttyan R. Role of angiogenesis in bladder response to partial outlet obstruction. Scand J Urol Nephrol Suppl. 2004;215:37–47.
7. Galvin DJ, Watson RW, O'Neill A, Coffey RN, Taylor C, Gillespie JI, et al. Hypoxia inhibits human bladder smooth muscle cell proliferation: a potential mechanism of bladder dysfunction. Neurourol Urodyn. 2004; 23(4):342–8.
8. Moher D, Liberati A, Tetzlaff J, Altman DG. PRISMA Group Preferred reporting items for systematic reviews and meta-analyses: the PRISMA statement. BMJ. 2009;339:2535.
9. Jiang YH, Lee CL, Kuo HC. Urothelial dysfunction, suburothelial inflammation and altered sensory protein expression in men with bladder outlet obstruction and various bladder dysfunctions: correlation with Urodynamics. J Urol. 2016;196(3):831–7.
10. Gilpin SA, Gosling JA, Barnard RJ. Morphological and morphometric studies of the human obstructed, trabeculated urinary bladder. Br J Urol. 1985;57(5):525–9.
11. Collado A, Batista E, Gelabert-Más A, Corominas JM, Arañó P, Villavicencio H. Detrusor quantitative morphometry in obstructed males and controls. J Urol. 2006;176(6 Pt 1):2722–8.
12. Elbadawi A, Yalla SV, Resnick NM. Structural basis of geriatric voiding dysfunction. IV. Bladder outlet obstruction. J Urol. 1993;150(5 Pt 2): 1681–95.
13. Tse V, Wills E, Szonyi G, Khadra MH. The application of ultrastructural studies in the diagnosis of bladder dysfunction in a clinical setting. J Urol. 2000; 163(2):535–9.

14. Brierly RD, Hindley RG, McLarty E, Harding DM, Thomas PJ. A prospective evaluation of detrusor ultrastructural changes in bladder outlet obstruction. BJU Int. 2003;91(4):360–4.
15. Gosling JA, Dixon JS. Structure of trabeculated detrusor smooth muscle in cases of prostatic hypertrophy. Urol Int. 1980;35(5):351–5.
16. Blatt AH, Brammah S, Tse V, Chan L. Transurethral prostate resection in patients with hypocontractile detrusor–what is the predictive value of ultrastructural detrusor changes? J Urol. 2012;188(6):2294–9.
17. Holm NR, Horn T, Smedts F, Nordling J, de la Rossette J. The detrusor muscle cell in bladder outlet obstruction–ultrastructural and morphometric findings. Scand J Urol Nephrol. 2003;37(4):309–15.
18. Rubinstein M, Sampaio FJ, Costa WS. Stereological study of collagen and elastic system in the detrusor muscle of bladders from controls and patients with infravesical obstruction. Int Braz J Urol. 2007;33(1):33–9.
19. Inui E, Ochiai A, Naya Y, Ukimura O, Kojima M. Comparative morphometric study of bladder detrusor between patients with benign prostatic hyperplasia and controls. J Urol. 1999;161(3):827–30.
20. Averbeck MA, De Lima NG, Motta GA, Beltrao LF, Abboud Filho NJ, Rigotti CP, et al. Collagen content in the bladder of men with LUTS undergoing open prostatectomy: a pilot study. Neurourol Urodyn. 2017;25 https://doi.org/10.1002/nau.23418.
21. Bellucci CHS, Ribeiro WO, Hemerly TS, de Bessa J Jr, Antunes AA, Leite KRM, et al. Increased detrusor collagen is associated with detrusor overactivity and decreased bladder compliance in men with benign prostatic obstruction. Prostate Int. 2017;5(2):70–4.
22. Mirone V, Imbimbo C, Sessa G, Palmieri A, Longo N, Granata AM, et al. Correlation between detrusor collagen content and urinary symptoms in patients with prostatic obstruction. J Urol. 2004;172(4 Pt 1):1386–9.
23. Yang R, Amir J, Liu H, Chaqour B. Mechanical strain activates a program of genes functionally inolved in paracrine signaling of angiogenesis. Physiol Genomics. 2008;36(1):1–14.
24. Wang Y, Wang K, Li H, Chen L, Xu F, Wu T. Effects of different sustained hydrostatic pressures on connexin 43 in human bladder smooth muscle cells. Urol Int. 2013;90(1):75–82.
25. Lee SD, Akbal C, Jung C, Kaefer M. Intravesical pressure induces hyperplasia and hypertrophy of human bladder smooth musclecells mediated by muscarinic receptors. J Pediatr Urol. 2006;2(4):271–6.
26. Lee SD, Misseri R, Akbal C, Jung C, Rink RC, Kaefer M. Muscarinic receptor expression increases following exposure to intravesical pressures of < or =40 cm-H2O: a possible mechanism for pressure-induced cell proliferation. World J Urol. 2008;26(4):387–93.
27. Preis L, Herlemann A, Adam RM, Dietz HG, Kappler R, Stehr M. Platelet Derived Growth Factor Has a Role in Pressure Induced Bladder Smooth Muscle CellHyperplasia and Acts in a Paracrine Way. J Urol. 2015;194(6):1797–805.
28. Chen L, Wei TQ, Wang Y, Zhang J, Li H, Wang KJ. Simulated bladder pressure stimulates human bladder smooth muscle cell proliferation via the PI3K/SGK1 signaling pathway. J Urol. 2012;188(2):661–7.
29. Sun Y, Luo DY, Zhu YC, Zhou L, Yang TX, Tang C, et al. MiR 3180 5p promotes proliferation in human bladder smooth muscle cell by targeting PODN under hydrodynamic pressure. Sci Rep 2016; 9. 6:33042.
30. Sun Y, Luo D, Zhu Y, Wang K. MicroRNA 4323 induces human bladder smooth muscle cell proliferation under cyclic hydrodynamic pressure by activation of erk1/2 signaling pathway. Exp Biol Med (Maywood) 2017; 242(2):169–176.
31. Wu T, Chen L, Wei T, Wang Y, Xu F, Wang K. Effect of cyclic hydrodynamic pressure-induced proliferation of human bladder smooth muscle through Ras-related C3 botulinum toxin substrate 1, mitogen-activated protein kinase kinase 1/2 and extracellular regulated protein kinases 1/2. Int J Urol. 2012;19(9):867–74.
32. Chen L, Wu T, Wei TQ, Wei X, Li SF, Wang KJ, et al. Skp2-mediated degradation of p27 regulates cell cycle progression in compressed human bladder smooth muscle cells. Kaohsiung J Med Sci. 2014;30(4):181–6.
33. Liang Z, Xin W, Qiang L, Xiang C, Bang-Hua L, Jin Y, et al. Hydrostatic pressure and muscarinic receptors are involved in the release of inflammatory cytokines in human bladder smooth muscle cells. Neurourol Urodyn. 2017;36(5):1261–9.
34. Backhaus BO, Kaefer M, Haberstroh KM, Hile K, Nagatomi J, Rink RC, et al. Alterations in the molecular determinants of bladder compliance at hydrostatic pressures lessthan 40 cm. H2O. J Urol. 2002;168(6):2600–4.
35. Wiafe B, Adesida A, Churchill T, Adewuyi EE, Li Z, Metcalfe P. Hypoxia-increased expression of genes involved in inflammation, dedifferentiation, pro-fibrosis, and extracellular matrix remodeling of human bladder smooth muscle cells. In Vitro Cell Dev Biol Anim. 2017;53(1):58–66.
36. Koritsiadis G, Stravodimos K, Koutalellis G, Agrogiannis G, Koritsiadis S, Lazaris A, et al. Immunohistochemical estimation of hypoxia in human obstructed bladder and correlation with clinical variables. BJU Int. 2008; 102(3):328–32.
37. Barbosa JABA, Reis ST, Nunes M, Ferreira YA, Leite KR, Nahas WC, et al. The obstructed bladder: expression of collagen, matrix metalloproteinases, muscarinic receptors, and Angiogenic and neurotrophic factors in patients with benign prostatic hyperplasia. Urology. 2017;106:167–72.
38. Boopathi E, Gomes CM, Goldfarb R, John M, Srinivasan VG, Alanzi J, et al. Transcriptional repression of Caveolin-1 (CAV1) gene expression by GATA-6 in bladder smoothmuscle hypertrophy in mice and human beings. Am J Pathol. 2011;178(5):2236–51.
39. Gosling JA, Gilpin SA, Dixon JS, Gilpin CJ. Decrease in the autonomic innervation of human detrusor muscle in outflow obstruction. J Urol. 1986;136(2):501–4.
40. Cumming JA, Chisholm GD. Changes in detrusor innervation with relief of outflow tract obstruction. Br J Urol. 1992;69(1):7–11.
41. Chapple CR, Milner P, Moss HE, Burnstock G. Loss of sensory neuropeptides in the obstructed human bladder. Br J Urol. 1992;70(4):373–81.
42. Steers WD, Kolbeck S, Creedon D, Tuttle JB. Nerve growth factor in the urinary bladder of the adult regulates neuronal form and function. J Clin Invest. 1991;88(5):1709–15.
43 Gheinani AH, Kiss B, Moltzahn F, Keller I, Bruggmann R, Rehrauer H, et al. Characterization of miRNA-regulated networks, hubs of signaling, and biomarkers in obstruction-induced bladder dysfunction. JCI Insight. 2017;2(2):e89560.
44 Horn T, Kortmann BB, Holm NR, Smedts F, Nordling J, Kiemeney LA, et al. Routine bladder biopsies in men with bladder outlet obstruction? Urology. 2004;63(3):451–6.
45 Belenky A, Abarbanel Y, Cohen M, Yossepowitch O, Livne PM, Bachar GN. Detrusor resistive index evaluated by Doppler ultrasonography as a potential indicator of bladder outlet obstruction. Urology. 2003;62(4): 647–50.
46 Farag FF, Meletiadis J, Saleem MD, Feitz WF, Heesakkers JP. Near-infrared spectroscopy of the urinary bladder during voiding in men with lower urinary tractsymptoms: a preliminary study. Biomed Res Int. 2013;2013:452857.
47 Macnab AJ, Shadgan B, Stothers L, Afshar K. Ambulant monitoring of bladder oxygenation and hemodynamics using wireless near-infraredspectroscopy. Can Urol Assoc J. 2013;7(1–2):E98–E104.
48 Roehrborn CG. 5-alpha-reductase inhibitors prevent the progression of benign prostatic hyperplasia. Rev Urol. 2003;5(Suppl 5):S12–21.
49 Roehrborn CG. Alfuzosin 10 mg once daily prevents overall clinical progression of benign prostatic hyperplasia but not acute urinary retention: results of a 2-year placebo-controlled study. BJU Int. 2006;97(4):734–41.
50 Fusco F, Arcaniolo D, Creta M, Piccinocchi G, Arpino G, Laringe M, et al. Demographic and comorbidity profile of patients with lower urinary tract symptoms suggestive of benign prostatic hyperplasia in a real-life clinical setting: are 5-alpha-reductase inhibitor consumers different? World J Urol. 2015;33(5):685–9.
51 Cindolo L, Pirozzi L, Fanizza C, Romero M, Tubaro A, Autorino R, et al. Drug adherence and clinical outcomes for patients under pharmacological therapy for lower urinary tract symptoms related to benign prostatic hyperplasia: population-based cohort study. Eur Urol. 2015 Sep;68(3):418–25.

Non-ischemic laparoscopic partial nephrectomy using 1318-nm diode laser for small exophytic renal tumors

Martin Drerup[1], Ahmed Magdy[1], Martina Hager[2*], Daniela Colleselli[1], Thomas Kunit[1], Lukas Lusuardi[1], Günter Janetschek[1] and Michael Mitterberger[1]

Abstract

Purpose: Warm ischemia (WI) and bleeding constitute the main challenges for surgeons during laparoscopic partial nephrectomy (LPN). Current literature on the use of lasers for cutting and coagulation remains scarce and with small cohorts. We present the largest case series to date of non-ischemic LPN using a diode laser for small exophytic renal tumors.

Methods: We retrospectively evaluated 29 patients with clinically localized exophytic renal tumors who underwent non-ischemic laser–assisted LPN with a 1318-nm wavelength diode laser. We started applying the laser 5 mm beyond the visible tumor margin, 5 mm away from the tissue in a non-contact fashion for coagulation and in direct contact with the parenchymal tissue for cutting.

Results: The renal vessels were not clamped, resulting in a WIT (warm ischaemic time) of 0 min, except for one case that required warm ischemia for 12 min and parenchymal sutures. No transfusion was needed, with a mean Hemoglobin drop of 1,4 mg/dl and no postoperative complications. The eGFR did not significantly change by 6 months. Histologically, the majority of lesions ($n = 22/29$) were renal-cell carcinoma stage pT1a. The majority of malignant lesions ($n = 13/22$) had a negative margin. However, margin interpretation was difficult in 9 cases due to charring of the tumor base. A mean follow-up of 1.8 years revealed no tumor recurrence. The mean tumor diameter was 19.4 mm.

Conclusion: The 1318-nm diode laser has the advantages of excellent cutting and sealing properties when applied to small vessels in the renal parenchyma, reducing the need for parenchymal sutures. However, excessive smoke, charring of the surgical margin, and inability to seal large blood vessels are encountered with this technique.

Keywords: Renal cell carcinoma, Non ischaemic nephrectomy, Laparoscopy, Laser

Introduction

Renal cell carcinoma is one of the more frequent carcinomas, comprising 2–3% of all cancers. Within the last few years, the incidence has consistently increased in most Western countries. [1] A shift to more organ-confined tumors has been observed due to diagnostic changes, such as ultrasound and computer tomography. [2] The only feasible therapy to date is surgical extirpation. The surveillance for patients with SRM is under investigation. Currently, it is feasible strategy both for hereditary RCC patients and those with small renal masses with more indolent growth rates. Recent guidelines point out that NSS should be performed in all tumors < 7 cm whenever feasible. There are no differences in the overall survival and cancer-specific survival between radical nephrectomy and partial nephrectomy (PN), with the advantage of better renal function preservation in PN patients. [3] Therefore, it is a goal to perform nephron-sparing surgery whenever feasible by sparing the maximum amount of renal parenchyma and reducing warm ischemic time (WIT). In order

* Correspondence: m.hager@salk.at
[2]Department of Pathology, Paracelsus Medical University Salzburg, Salzburg, Austria
Full list of author information is available at the end of the article

to achieve a good surgical result with restricted blood loss, hilar clamping is the standard procedure. The interruption of renal blood flow leads to WIT, with a loss of renal function. [4] Patients who already suffer a chronic renal insufficiency have the highest risk to loose further renal function due to WIT. In these patients, hypoxic radicals formed in the hypoxic tissue after off clamping can lead to further damage within 5–8 min. [5] The most common complication in NSS remains bleeding, with a transfusion risk of 5%. [6] To optimize the surgical treatment of RCC, the technique is under continuous investigation. Improvements have been done over the years in reducing the risk of bleeding, as well as reducing WIT and complications of any cause. By changing the access from open to laparoscopic partial nephrectomy (LAPN), and more recently to robot-assisted partial nephrectomy (RAPN) the procedure was upgraded. [7] With laparoscopic access, the intraoperative blood loss is lower than with the open surgical approach, whereas the postoperative complications do not increase. [8] However, LAPN elevates the WIT, as the surgical steps in a crucial time frame are challenging, even for an experienced surgeon. [9] Therefore, different surgical techniques have emerged to reduce or eliminate the WIT, including targeted renal blood flow interruption, selective renal artery clamping, selective renal parenchymal clamping, laser supported MIPN, radio frequency assisted MIPN, hydro-jet assisted MIPN, and sequential preplaced suture renorrhaphy. [10] None of these techniques are widely accepted, and they are still under investigation. Thus, we chose to further investigate the laser for partial nephrectomy in this case-control study. Different wavelengths have different absorptions in different types of tissue, and finding the optimal wavelength is crucial. Experience in non-ischemic laparoscopic partial nephrectomy has been gained with a Ho:YAG-, Thulium-,and Diode-laser. Ho:YAG, Nd:YAG and KTP have good cutting and coagulation properties with the drawback of blood splashing and excessive smoke building due to the pulsating nature of the Ho:YAG laser. Thulium and Diode laser are the most recent investigated promising laser systems with excellent cutting and coagulation features. Smoke building and carbonization of the tissue is also observed [11].

As different types of lasers have already been tested, the aim of this study was to show the feasibility of laser laparoscopic partial nephrectomy (LLPN) using a 1318-nm diode laser. Tumor excision and the ability of pathological reporting after laser enucleation was also of interest when the oncological result coincided with the actual standard of care.

Materials and methods

Between May 2012 and June 2014, we retrospectively evaluated 29 patients with clinically localized exophytic renal tumors. All patients were operated on at the university clinic Salzburg using a 1318-nm laser. The ethics committee was consulted. The diagnosis of SRM and decision for surgery with laparoscopic laser enucleation was based on CT scans and/or magnetic resonance tomography. The patient who underwent surgery had mainly exophytic renal masses with a minimum distance of 5 mm to the renal calix. Renal masses were included in the study when radiologically suspected of malignancy. All patients were classified by PADUA score and R.E.N.A.L score [12] for an objective preoperative evaluation of the complexity of the intervention. Only single lesions were treated in this study, and only renal masses up to 4 cm in maximum dimension. Centrally located tumors were excluded, as well as patients with a single functional kidney.

Instruments and laser

The renal masses were enucleated by non-ischemic LLPN using the Eraser® laser (Rolle & Rolle, Salzburg, Austria), a semiconductor diode laser with a wavelength of 1318 nm. A continuous wave (CW) was used in all cases. For laparoscopic purposes, the flexible laser fiber with the bundled light was set into a laparoscopic instrument.

Surgical technique

The procedure was performed through a laparoscopic transperitoneal approach except for one case. All of the operations were performed by four different surgeons with different levels of surgical experience. By default, three trocars (Karl Storz, Tuttlingen, Germany) were set into the patient in the flank lateral position. They were inserted after achieving pneumoperitoneum with the Veress needle. The initial trocar was placed near the umbilicus with the camera port. The cranial trocar was set midway between the xiphoid and umbilicus, and the caudal trocar was placed at the edge of the rectus abdominus. In case of necessity, further trocars were put into place. After complete dissection of the kidney, we exposed the tumor outline with preservation of its overlying perinephric fat. If necessary a laparoscopic ultrasound was in standby. The surrounding fat was removed from the renal capsule. We than prepared the hilar vessels completely from the surrounding tissue, and a vessel-loop without pull was enlaced. Even while the enucleation occurred, the vessel loop was not closed. The laser fiber was introduced with a guidance instrument through a trocar. The laser power was adjusted to 45–65 W. We started applying the laser 5 mm beyond the visible tumor margin. For cutting, the laser fiber was applied in direct contact with the parenchymal tissue. For coagulation, the laser was applied 5 mm away from the tissue in a non-contact fashion and the velocity of the laser fiber was reduced (Fig. 1). Coagulation of the tumor feeding vessels before cutting was always

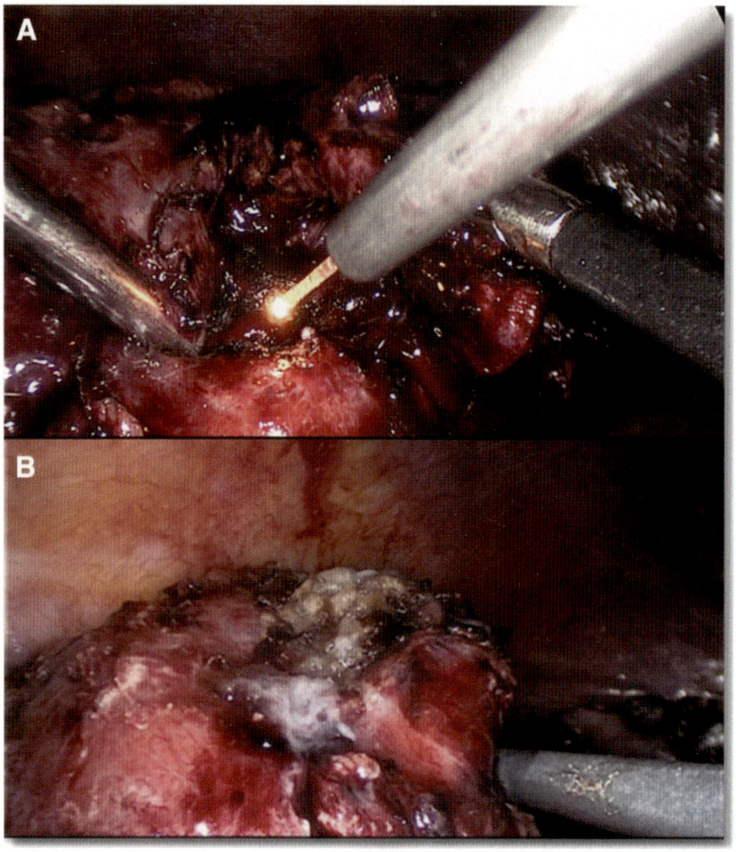

Fig. 1 Surgical steps. **a**, Laser enucleation of the tumor. **b**, The tumor bed after enucleation and coagulation with the 1318-nm diode laser

attempted using the laser. With a dissecting forceps the tumor was mobilized in order to cut and coagulate around the tumor similar to the enucleation of an exophytic renal mass with WIT in the normal manner. Attention was paid to an adequate resection margin. During enucleation, we opened one trocar in order to preserve a good view, as there was excessive smoke. Simultaneously, suction without opening a trocar was inadequate, as the view of the operative field was diminished because of dense smoke. After enucleation, the tumor was removed by a laparoscopic sac and the resection side of the kidney inspected for bleeding (Fig. 1) before the Gerota fascia was put back into place and the closure performed in the typical fashion. The coagulation property of the laser was adequate leaving renorrhaphy omitted except for one case. All specimens were fixed in formalin and histologically examined by our Department of Pathology. Drainage was not routinely inserted. The postoperative treatment was in line with our standard operating procedures.

Results

All patients in this study underwent tumor enucleation and coagulation with the laser only. The mean age of the patients was 67.6 (range 40–85) years, with a mean body mass index (BMI) of 27.7 (range 21.3–37.2). The mean tumor diameter was 19.4 (range 11–40) mm. Eleven of the tumors were located on the left side and 18 on the right side; 9 were in the upper pole, 6 in the midparenchymal area, and 14 in the lower pole. The Padua Score was low (6–7) in 27 patients and moderate (8–9) 2 patients. The renal nephrometry score was low (4–6) in 26 patients and moderate (7–9) in three patients. (Table 1).

The mean total operative time was 179.4 (range 90–300) minutes. The renal vessels were not clamped, except for one case in which hilar clamping had to be performed for 12 min and parenchymal sutures had to be placed because of insufficient coagulation. In all other cases, we had no WIT and parenchymal sutures were not necessary. No blood transfusions were needed perioperatively or postoperatively. The mean change in hemoglobin (Hb) from before surgery to discharge was 13.7 g/dl to 12.3 g/dl respectively, p-Value = 0.0001. No significant change in eGFR was measured at the 6-month follow-up; the mean decrease from before surgery to 6-month follow-up was 63,9 ml/min to 61,3 ml/min respectively p-Value = 0,27. We encountered excessive smoke when the laser was applied continuously for more than 1 min.

Table 1 Characteristics of the patients and tumor size

Characteristic Median (range)	
Age, years	67.6 (40–85)
BMI	27.7 (21–37)
R.E.N.A.L. Score	4.8 (4–9)
Low (4–6): $n = 26$	
Moderate (7–9): $n = 3$	
P.A.D.U.A. Score	6.3 (6–8)
Low (6–7): $n = 27$	
Moderate (8–9): n = 2	
Tumor diameter, mm	19.4 (11–40)

Intraoperatively, no immediate frozen sections were sent to pathology and the tumor bed was evaluated macroscopically. Histologically, the majority of lesions (22/29) were renal cell carcinoma stage pT1a. Four cases of angiomyolipoma and three of oncocytoma were found. The majority of malignant lesions (13/22) were margin negative (R0). However, the interpretation of the surgical margins included 7 cases with unknown surgical margin (RX) due to charring of the tumor base through the Laser. In two cases, were classified margin positive (R1) by the pathologist (Fig. 2). As the positive margins in these two cases were described as small, they were placed into strict follow-up and a second resection avoided (Table 2).

The mean hospital stay was 6.4 days, which is in line with the average duration of LPN in our department. No postoperative complications occurred. A mean follow-up of 1.8 years revealed no tumor recurrence.

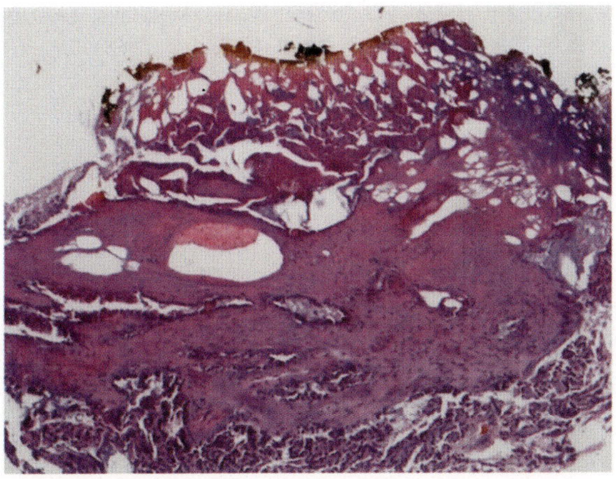

Fig. 2 Hematoxylin & eosin staining of papillary RCC, Type 1. Magnification 100x. Note the upper part of the coagulation zone without accessibility and an adjacent fibrous pseudo capsule with tumor proliferation

Table 2 Clinical results, histopathology, and pathological classification

Clinical results	
Mean operative time	179.3 min
Mean change Hb	1.4 g/dl
Without WIT	28 Pat.
WIT	1 Pat. (12 min)
Blood transfusion	0
eGFR after 6 months	2.6 ml/min
Mean follow-up	1.8 years
Histopathology	
Renal cell carcinoma	22
Angiomyolipoma	4
Oncocytoma	3
Residual tumor classification	
R0	13 (59%)
RX	7 (32%)
R1	2 (9%)

WIT warm ischemic time

Discussion

Laparoscopic surgery with off-clamping of the hilar vessels and enucleation with WIT is the standard procedure for enucleation of renal masses and SRM. As LPN is a demanding operation, the WIT is still longer than with the open approach. Especially in pre-damaged organs or in the case of a single kidney, the WIT is of issue [9]. Recently the robotic partial nephrectomy has emerged as an alternative to laparoscopic partial nephrectomy. The risk of renal damage is reduced as ischaemic time is significantly shorter when using robotic surgery compared to laparoscopic surgery [13]. As the reduction in warm ischemia seems to be the best modifiable risk factor for later renal insufficiency, we wanted to investigate the feasibility of a diode laser. Reduction or omission of WIT in laparoscopic surgery of the kidney is a future goal.

The laser is a widely used tool that has been well studied in various fields of medicine but still experimental in kidney surgery. As the effectiveness of the laser is dependent on the wavelength and portion of water in the tissue, its usefulness has to be investigated. The feasibility of using a laser in the kidney was previously shown. [11, 14–28] The property of the diode laser we used (1318-nm Eraser Rolle and Rolle) was a shallow penetration depth, which leads to strong carbonization on the surface without penetrating and damaging deeper structures as it is the risk with other laser systems, such as the Ho: YAG-laser. This could lead to accidental opening of the tumor capsule, damaging deeper renal tissue. Co2 lasers, which have been tested in the past, have even less penetration depth, which leads to insufficient coagulation of larger vessels and even stronger carbonization of the tissue. For this reason, the diode laser seemed to strike a balance between these laser systems, as Khoder et al. already published their promising results with the same laser system.

To the best of our knowledge, this is the largest series of laparoscopic laser-assisted partial nephrectomy published to date. The number of patients in the literature treated with laser without WIT is even smaller, and the variety of different wavelengths used is large (Table 1).

Still the Laser is experimental when it comes to renal surgery. One major drawback during the operation was the excessive smoke building due to the carbonization of the tissue. We tried to avoid this by rinsing, which did not avoid the smoke building and the visibility was reduced. The best visibility was achieved by opening one of the trocars as a fume hood. Still, this was not optimal because the intraabdominal pressure of the pneumoperitoneum is reduced, but suction alone did not achieve good visibility. Furthermore because of the strong carbonization the surgeon was hindered to discriminate between renal tissue and tissue of the RCC.

All tumors except one were enucleated without WIT, which is great progress in terms of reducing renal damage. The main drawback in our study was the number of unclassified resection margins and positive resection margins in the histopathological examination. To the best of our knowledge, this problem has not yet been published for renal tumor enucleation. Although our pathology department is familiar with resection margins from laser enucleation in the prostate and other organs, they could not make a definitive diagnosis in 32% of the renal samples and stated them as RX. The reason for the indistinct pathological report is the carbonization of the resection margin. In addition, we had 9% positive margins, whereas 0–4% positive margins after LPN is reported in the literature. [29] The small number of patients in our cohort does not allow the general assumption of a higher rate of Rx and R1 resections. One explanation of the positive margin is the excessive smoke building during laparoscopy, which leads to difficulties in identifying the capsule. Another reason is the small diameter of the renal tumor, which has been identified as a reason for a positive surgical margin in the past. [30]

All patients with an indistinct or positive surgical margin were followed up and have had no tumor recurrence to date.

Conclusion

Data on laser-assisted partial nephrectomy without WIT has been published for over a decade, [26] but so far this technical option is still regarded as experimental. In this retrospective study including the largest number of patients thus far, we show that the major problems are smoke building and indistinct surgical margins. In this context, we cannot promote the laser as a valid option for partial nephrectomy outside of clinical trials. As we have different results than previous clinical studies, further clinical trials are needed.

Abbreviations

BMI: Body mass index; CW: Continuous wave; eGFR: Estimated glomerular filtration rate; Hb: Hemoglobin; LAPN: Laparoscopic partial nephrectomy; LLPN: Laser laparoscopic partial nephrectomy; LPN: Laparoscopic partial nephrectomy; MIPN: Minimal invasive partial nephrectomy; NSS: Nephron sparing surgery; PN: Partial nephrectomy; RAPN: Robot-assisted partial nephrectomy; rn: Between radical nephrectomy; SRM: Small renal masses; WI: Warm ischemia; WIT: Warm ischemic time

Acknowledgments

Not applicable.

Funding

Not applicable.

Authors' contributions

MD: Data Collection, Manuscript writing, Project development. AM Collection. MH Data collection. DC, TK, LL, GJ Manuscript writing. MM Manuscript writing, Project development. All authors read and approved the final manuscript.

Competing interests

The authors declare that they have no competing interests.

Author details

[1]Department of Urology, Paracelsus Medical University Salzburg, Muellner-Hauptstrasse 48, 5020 Salzburg, Austria. [2]Department of Pathology, Paracelsus Medical University Salzburg, Salzburg, Austria.

References

1. Lindblad P. Epidemiology of renal cell carcinoma. Scand J Surg. 2004;93:88–96.
2. Palsdottir HB, Hardarson S, Petursdottir V, et al. Incidental detection of renal cell carcinoma is an independent prognostic marker: results of a long-term, whole population study. J Urol. 2012;187:48–53. https://doi.org/10.1016/j.juro.2011.09.025.
3. MacLennan S, Imamura M, Lapitan MC, et al. Systematic review of oncological outcomes following surgical management of localised renal cancer. Eur Urol. 2012;61:972–93. https://doi.org/10.1016/j.eururo.2012.02.039.
4. Volpe A, Blute ML, Ficarra V, et al. Renal Ischemia and Function After Partial Nephrectomy: A Collaborative Review of the Literature. Eur Urol. 2015. https://doi.org/10.1016/j.eururo.2015.01.025.
5. Adam S, Loertzer H, Fornara P, Brömme HJ. The carboxyproxyl-derived spin trap (CP-H) is an appropriate detector-compound for oxidative stress. Urol Res. 2010;38:179–86. https://doi.org/10.1007/s00240-010-0256-7.
6. Gratzke C, Seitz M, Bayrle F, et al. Quality of life and perioperative outcomes after retroperitoneoscopic radical nephrectomy (RN), open RN and nephron-sparing surgery in patients with renal cell carcinoma. BJU Int. 2009;104:470–5. https://doi.org/10.1111/j.1464-410X.2009.08439.x.
7. Laird A, Choy KCC, Delaney H, et al. Matched pair analysis of laparoscopic versus open radical nephrectomy for the treatment of T3 renal cell carcinoma. World J Urol. 2015;33:25–32. https://doi.org/10.1007/s00345-014-1280-y.
8. Gong EM, Orvieto MA, Zorn KC, et al. Comparison of laparoscopic and open partial nephrectomy in clinical T_{1a} renal tumors. J Endourol. 2008;22:953–8. https://doi.org/10.1089/end.2007.0300.
9. Muramaki M, Miyake H, Sakai I, Fujisawa M. Prognostic factors influencing postoperative development of chronic kidney disease in patients with small renal tumors who underwent partial nephrectomy. Curr Urol. 2012;6:129–35. https://doi.org/10.1159/000343526

10. Hou W, Ji Z. Achieving zero ischemia in minimally invasive partial nephrectomy surgery. Int J Surg. 2015;18:48–54. https://doi.org/10.1016/j.ijsu.2015.04.046.
11. Kyriazis I, Ozsoy M, Kallidonis P, et al. Current evidence on lasers in laparoscopy: partial nephrectomy. World J Urol. 2014:589–94. https://doi.org/10.1007/s00345-014-1343-0.
12. Kutikov A, Uzzo RG. The R.E.N.a.L. Nephrometry score: a comprehensive standardized system for quantitating renal tumor size, location and depth. J Urol. 2009;182:844–53. https://doi.org/10.1016/j.juro.2009.05.035.
13. Benway BM, Bhayani SB, Rogers CG, et al. Robot assisted partial nephrectomy versus laparoscopic partial nephrectomy for renal tumors: a multi-institutional analysis of perioperative outcomes. J Urol. 2009;182:866–73. https://doi.org/10.1016/J.JURO.2009.05.037.
14. Zhou X-F, Ding Z-S, Wang J-F, et al. Laparoscopic partial nephrectomy by diode laser with highly selective clamping of segmental renal arterial. Chin Med J. 2015;128:2262–4. https://doi.org/10.4103/0366-6999.162513.
15. Knezevic N, Kulis T, Maric M, et al. Laparoscopic partial nephrectomy with diode laser: a promising technique. Photomed Laser Surg. 2014;32:101–5. https://doi.org/10.1089/pho.2013.3646.
16. Khoder WY, Sroka R, Siegert S, et al. Outcome of laser-assisted laparoscopic partial nephrectomy without ischaemia for peripheral renal tumours. World J Urol. 2012;30:633–8. https://doi.org/10.1007/s00345-011-0807-8.
17. Khoder WY, Sroka R, Hennig G, et al. The 1,318-nm diode laser supported partial nephrectomy in laparoscopic and open surgery: preliminary results of a prospective feasibility study. Lasers Med Sci. 2011;26:689–97. https://doi.org/10.1007/s10103-011-0897-y.
18. Hsueh TY, Chiu AW, Huang AC, et al. Thulium laser laparoscopic partial nephrectomy without renal hilar control in a porcine model. Urol Sci. 2010; 21:126–31. https://doi.org/10.1016/S1879-5226(10)60027-9.
19. Gruschwitz T, Stein R, Schubert J, Wunderlich H. Laser-supported partial nephrectomy for renal cell carcinoma. Urology. 2008;71:334–6. https://doi.org/10.1016/j.urology.2007.09.060.
20. Barzilay B, Lijovetzky G, Shapiro A, Caine M. The clinical use of CO2 laser beam in the surgery of kidney parenchyma. Lasers Surg Med. 1982;2:81–7. https://doi.org/10.1002/lsm.1900020110.
21. Thomas AZ, Smyth L, Hennessey D, et al. Zero ischemia laparoscopic partial thulium laser nephrectomy. J Endourol. 2013;27:1366–70. https://doi.org/10.1089/end.2012.0527.
22. Sciarra A, Von Heland M, Minisola F, et al. Thulium laser supported nephron sparing surgery for renal cell carcinoma. J Urol. 2013;190:698–701. https://doi.org/10.1016/j.juro.2013.01.079.
23. Rosemberg SK. Clinical experience with carbon dioxide laser in renal surgery. Urology. 1985;25:115–8.
24. Merguerian PA, Seremetis G. Laser-assisted partial nephrectomy in children. J Pediatr Surg. 1994;29:934–6.
25. Mattioli S, Muñoz R, Recasens R, et al. What does Revolix laser contribute to partial nephrectomy? Arch Esp Urol. 2008;61:1126–9.
26. Malloy TR, Schultz RE, Wein AJ, Carpiniello VL. Renal preservation utilizing neodymium:YAG laser. Urology. 1986;27:99–103.
27. Loertzer H, Strauß A, Ringert RH, Schneider P. Laser-supported partial laparoscopic nephrectomy for renal cell carcinoma without ischaemia time. BMC Urol. 2013;13:31. https://doi.org/10.1186/1471-2490-13-31.
28. Korhonen AK, Talja M, Karlsson H, Tuhkanen K. Contact Nd:YAG laser and regional renal hypothermia in partial nephrectomy. Ann Chir Gynaecol Suppl. 1993;206:59–62.
29. Marszalek M, Carini M, Chlosta P, et al. Positive surgical margins after nephron-sparing surgery. Eur Urol. 2012;61:757–63. https://doi.org/10.1016/j.eururo.2011.11.028.
30. Yossepowitch O, Thompson RH, Leibovich BC, et al. Positive surgical margins at partial nephrectomy: predictors and oncological outcomes. J Urol. 2008;179:2158–63. https://doi.org/10.1016/j.juro.2008.01.100.

Adjustable single-incision mini-slings (Ajust®) versus other slings in surgical management of female stress urinary incontinence: a meta-analysis of effectiveness and complications

Fuding Bai, Jimin Chen, Zhewei Zhang, Yichun Zheng, Jiaming Wen, Xiawa Mao and Nan Zhang*

Abstract

Background: Adjustable single-incision mini-sling (SIMS) is a new category of SIMS for stress urinary incontinence (SUI). The aim of this study was to compare the efficacy and safety of adjustable single-incision mini-sling with other slings.

Methods: Literature search in databases such as Pubmed, and Conchrane Library was performed up to December, 2015. The outcomes including cure rate, operation time, postoperative pain score and complications were reanalyzed. The pooled relative risk (RR) and mean difference (MD) with their 95% confidence interval (95% CI) were calculated by RevMan v5.0.

Results: Eight studies with 1093 SUI female patients were included. There was no significant difference between adjustable SIMS and other slings (transobturator slings and MiniArc) in patients subjective cure rate and objective cure rate. In addition, adjustable SIMS was associated with a significantly shorter operative time and lower postoperative pain score when comparing adjustable SIMS with transobturator tape (MD = – 1.35; 95%CI: -2.24 to – 0.46, $P = 0.003$). For the complications, there was also no significant difference between adjustable SIMS and transobturator slings.

Conclusions: Adjustable SIMS had equally efficacy for SUI compared with transobturator slings and MiniArc. However, the significantly shorter operative time and lower postoperative pain score than transobturator tape supported the clinical application of adjustable SIMS.

Keywords: Ajust, Single-incision mini-slings, MiniArc, Transobturator slings, Meta-analysis

Background

Based on the definition of International Continence Society, stress urinary incontinence (SUI) is the complaint of involuntary leakage of urine on effort or exertion, or on sneezing or coughing [1]. SUI is a common problem in women, which accounts for nearly 50% of all incontinent women and affects the quality of life [2]. Surgical treatment is necessary for SUI after failure of conservative treatment [3]. The midurethral sling is the mainstay of SUI treatment over the last ten years [4]. Tension-free vaginal tape (TVT), which is the first generation of MUS and firstly reported by Ulmsten et al. in 1995, has been used as a standard minimally invasive procedure for SUI with a success rate of 84-95% [5]. However, it is associated with many serious complications because of the blind passage through the retropubic space, such as bladder perforation, vessel and bowel injuries, perioperative bleeding and hematoma formation [6, 7]. Subsequently, transobturator slings including tension-free vaginal tape-obturator (TVT-O) and

* Correspondence: nanzhang@zju.edu.cn
Department of Urology, School of Medicine Hangzhou, Second Affiliated Hospital, Zhejiang University, No.88 Jiefang Road, Hangzhou, Zhejiang Province, People's Republic of China

transobturator tape (TOT), were developed with comparable cure rates and relatively less complications compared with TVT [8, 9]. However, the transobturator approaches are associated with the risk of persistent groin and thigh pain [10]. Afterwards, a new tension-free midurethral vaginal sling, which is known as single-incision mini-slings (SIMS) and the third generation of midurethral sling, is developed with the advantage of avoiding both retropubic and groin muscle trajectories [11], such as TVT-Secur and MiniArc [12]. However, a previous meta-analysis, which compared the safety and efficacy of SIMS with standard midurethral sling (SMUS, including TVT, TOT and TVT-O), did not show the superior outcomes of SIMS to SMUS [13]. Thus, it is important to perform further investigations to find a more safety and efficacious approach for treatment of SUI.

Currently, the adjustable SIMS is a new category of SIMS [14], which provides a robust insertion into the obturator internus muscle/membrane and allows post-insertion adjustment of the tape [14, 15]. Recently, some studies have been performed for comparing the adjustable SIMS with other slings [16]. However, it still cannot determine whether the efficacy and safety of adjustable SIMS are superior to these slings due to the small sample size in single study and inconsistent results among these studies. Therefore, we performed this meta-analysis to comprehensively evaluate the efficacy and safety of adjustable SIMS comparing with other slings.

Methods

Literature search

This meta-analysis was conducted according to the Preferred Reporting Items for Systematic Reviews and PRISMA statement guidance [17]. The studies were searched in Medline, Embase, Pubmed, EBSCO, Conchrane Library, and Science, up to December, 2016, using the following key words: "Ajust" or "adjustable" and "urinary incontinence" or "stress urinary incontinence" and "female". No language restriction was applied.

Selection criteria

The studies included in this meta-analysis should meet the following criteria: (1) the study type was randomized controlled trial (RCT); (2) participants were females over 18 years old and diagnosed with SUI; (3) the studies investigated the primary SUI surgery and compared adjustable SIMS with other slings; (4) the outcomes such as operation time, postoperative pain score, postoperative complications, and/or patients subjective cure rate and objective cure rate were reported.

The studies were excluded according to the following criteria: (1) there was no available data for meta-analysis; (2) they were reviews, letters and comments. In addition, for the duplicated publications, only the one with the most complete data was included.

Data extraction and quality assessment

The literature search and data extraction were performed independently by two authors, and the disagreements were resolved by discussion or consulting a third reviewer. The following data were recorded from each study: first author's name; country, sample size, type of other slings, follow up, definition of patients subjective cure, definition of objective cure, as well as the clinical outcomes.

The Jadad score system was used to assess quality of the included studies [18]. There were three items in the score system and each item had one or two questions: randomization (two questions: was the study randomized? was the randomization method described and appropriate?), blinding (two questions: was the study described as double blind? was the method of blinding described and appropriate?) and description of withdrawals and dropouts (one question: was there a description of withdrawals and dropouts?). One score was assigned for each "yes" answer to each question. The studies with 3-5 scores were regarded as high-quality, while those with 0-2 scores were low-quality.

In addition, risk of bias of each study was assessed by the Cochrane Collaboration's tool [19].

Statistical analysis

Data were analyzed using RevMan v5.0. The relative risk (RR) and mean difference (MD) with their 95% confidence interval (95%CI) were used as the effect size to assess the effectiveness and complications of adjustable SIMS versus other slings. A Z-test was used to test the significance of RR and MD. $P < 0.05$ was considered statistically significant. The heterogeneity among studies was measured using the Cochran's Q-statistic and I^2 test. A significant Q-statistic ($P < 0.10$) or I^2-statistic ($I^2 > 50\%$) indicated significant heterogeneity across the studies, and then the random effects model was used to pool the data. Otherwise, the fixed effects model was applied.

Results

Characteristics of included studies

Initially, 284 articles were retrieved from the databases. After removing the duplicates, total 131 articles were remained. Subsequently, 79 obviously irrelevant studies were excluded by scanning the titles. Then, 44 articles were excluded by reviewing the full-texts and abstracts according to the inclusion and exclusion criteria. Finally, a total of 8 studies [16, 20–26] were included in the meta-analysis (Fig. 1).

As shown in Table 1, all the RCTs were published between 2012 and 2016. Based on the Jadad score system, five studies were identified as high quality and two were

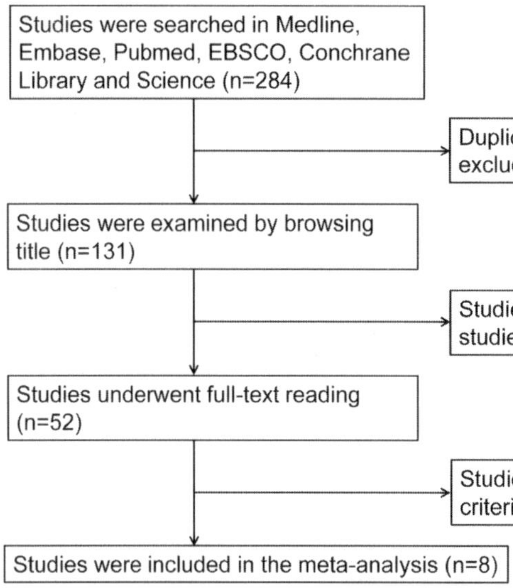

Fig. 1 Flow chart of study selection in the meta-analysis

low quality. In addition, a majority of the studies had a low risk of bias (Fig. 2), indicating a high quality of the included studies. Totally, 1093 females with SUI were included in this meta-analysis. There were differences in definitions of patients subjective cure rate and objective cure rate among the eight studies.

Comparison of subjective cure rate and objective cure rate for treating SUI patients

When comparing adjustable SIMS with transobturator slings or TVT-O alone, as no significant heterogeneity (I^2 = 0%, $P > 0.1$) was detected among the included studies for patients subjective cure rate and objective cure rate, thus the fixed effects model was used to combine the data. The pooled estimates showed that there was no evidence of significant differences in patients subjective cure rate (RR = 1.02, 95%CI: 0.97 to 1.07, $P = 0.95$, Fig. 3a) and objective cure rate (RR = 1.01, 95%CI: 0.97 to 1.06, $P = 0.94$, Fig. 3d) between patients received adjustable SIMS and transobturator slings. Likewise, no significant differences between adjustable SIMS and TVT-O alone were detected (patients subjective cure rate: RR = 1.01, 95%CI: 0.96 to 1.07, $P = 0.89$, Fig. 3b; objective cure rates: RR = 1.01, 95%CI: 0.96 to 1. 06, $P = 0.87$, Fig. 3e).

When comparing adjustable SIMS with MiniArc SIMS, significant heterogeneity between the two studies was found, so the random effects model was applied. Similarly, there was also no significant difference between adjustable SIMS and MiniArc SIMS in patients subjective cure rate (RR = 0.97, 95%CI: 0.86 to 1.08, Fig. 3c) and objective cure rate (RR = 0.97, 95%CI: 0.86 to 1.08, Fig. 3f).

Comparison of operation details

For operation time, there was significant heterogeneity (I^2 = 97%, $P < 0.00001$) among the three included studies. Thus, the random effects model was applied. The pooed estimate indicated that the adjustable SIMS had a shorter operation time than transobturator slings (MD = – 3.70; 95%CI: -8.57 to 1.17, $P = 0.14$, Fig. 4a) but without significance. However, after excluding the study of Xing et al. which reported the comparison between adjustable SIMS and TOT-V, the significant difference was detected (MD = – 1.35; 95%CI: -2.24 to – 0.46, $P = 0.003$, Fig. 4b) under a fixed effects model.

In addition, the postoperative pain score by visual analog scale was investigated in three of the included studies [24–26], which compared the adjustable SIMS and transobturator slings. However, the data in the study Schweitzer et al. (which reported the comparison between adjustable SIMS and TOT) were unavailable for meta-analysis [22], so this meta-analysis only assessed postoperative pain score of adjustable SIMS comparing with TVT-O. Significant heterogeneity (I^2 = 89%, $P = 0.0001$) was found among the three studies for the postoperative pain score, so the random effects model was used. The pooled results showed that patients received adjustable SIMS had significantly lower postoperative pain scores than those received TVT-O at the first (MD = 1.69, 95%CI: -2.84 to 0.53, $P = 0.0001$, Fig. 4c) and fourth (MD = – 0.73, 95%CI: 0.90 to – 0.55, $P < 0.0001$, Fig. 4d) day after operation.

Comparison of complications

The postoperative complications were also reanalyzed in this meta-analysis. No significant heterogeneity (I^2 <

Table 1 Characteristics of included studies

First author, year	Region	Sample size		Age	Follow up (months)	Definition of subjective cure	Definition of objective cure	Outcomes	Jadad score
Xing X, 2016	China	Adjustable SIMS	184	57.6 ± 6.8	12	Defined as "very much improved" or "much improved" on the PGI-I scale	Negative CST	(a) (b) (c)	3
		TVT-O	184	56.5 ± 5.7					
Mostafa, 2012 and 2013	UK	Adjustable SIMS	69	52.6 ± 11.2	4-6/12[a]	Responses of "very much/much improved" on PGI-I	Negative CST with comfortably full bladder	(a) (b) (c) (d)	3
		TVT-O	68	49.4 ± 8.8					
Grigoriadis, 2013	Greece	Adjustable SIMS	86	65.2 (47-81)	22.3 (12-36)	No loss of urine with exercise, coughing or weight lifting	Absence of stress urinary incontinence during CST	(a) (b) (c) (d)	3
		TVT-O	85	67.2 (49-82)					
Masata, 2016	Czech	Adjustable SIMS	50	55.8 ± 10.2	12	No stress leakage of urine after surgery based on the responses to the ICIQ-UI SF	Negative CST	(a)(a)(b)(c)	4
		TVT-O	50	58.9 ± 12.4					
Dati, 2012	Italy	Adjustable SIMS	57	NA	6	NA	Negative CST	(b) (c)	3
		TVT-O	57						
Schweitzer, 2015	Netherland	Adjustable SIMS	92	50.86 ± 9.6	12	A negative answer to the Urogenital Distress Inventory question	Negative CST at a bladder volume of at least 300 mL	(a) (b) (c)	4
		TOT	48	48.36 ± 10.2					
Martan, 2014	Czech	Adjustable SIMS	31	58.97 ± 8.40	28	A drop in the score of more than 50% compared to before the operation based on ICIQ-SF	Negative CST at a bladder volume of at least 300 mL	(a) (a) (b)	2
		MiniArc SIMS	32	60.19 ± 8.12	29				

SIMS Single-incision mini-slings, *TVT-O* Tension-free vaginal tape-obturator, *TOT* Transobturator tape, *PGI-I* Patient global impression of improvement, *ICIQ-SF* International Consultation on Incontinence Questionnaire – Short Form, *SUI* Stress urinary incontinence, *CST* Cough stress test, *NA* Not applicable. Outcomes:(a) subjective cure rate, (b) objective cure rate, (c) operative details (such as operation time postoperative pain score) and postoperative complications, (d) sexual function. [a]the subjective and objective cure rate at 12 months follow up in the study of Mostafa 2013 was used in this meta-analysis; the operative details and postoperative complications at 4-6 months follow up in the study of Mostafa 2012 was used for meta-analysis. [b]the study of Palomba et al. published in 2012 reported the operative details and postoperative complications and the study of Palomba et al. published in 2014 reported the data of patients subjective and objective cure rate

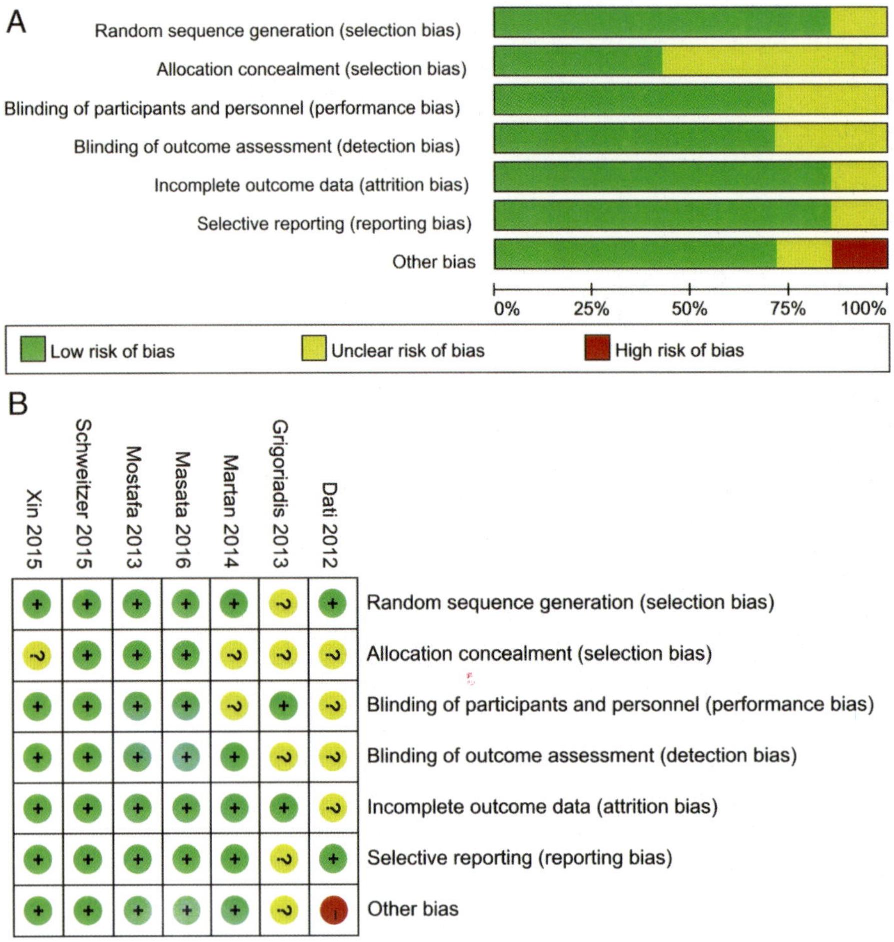

Fig. 2 Risk of bias assessed by the Cochrane Collaboration's tool. **a** Methodological quality item of all included studies; **b** Methodological quality item for each included study. +: low risk of bias; "?": unclear risk of bias; "-": high risk of bias

50%, $P > 0.1$) was found among the included studies for rates of repeated continence surgery, postoperative voiding difficulties, vaginal tape erosions and de novo urgency and/or worsening of preexisting urgency, so the fixed effects model was used to pool the data. However, random effects model was used to combine the data of groin pain due to significant heterogeneity ($I^2 = 62\%$, $P = 0.11$). The pooled estimates demonstrated that there was no significant difference between patients receiving adjustable SIMS and transobturator slings in the rates of repeated continence surgery (RR = 1.48, 95%CI: 0.45 to 4.89, $P = 0.52$, Fig. 5b), vaginal tape erosions (RR = 0.80, 95%CI: 0.26 to 2.45, $P = 0.69$, Fig. 3d) and de novo urgency and/or worsening of preexisting urgency (RR = 1.30, 95%CI: 0.81 to 2.09, $P = 0.28$, Fig. 5f). Moreover, results also showed that compared to the patients received TVT-O, the patients received adjustable SIMS had a similar incidence of groin pain (RR = 0.49, 95%CI: 0.02 to 15.59, $P = 0.69$, Fig. 5a), postoperative voiding difficulties (RR = 0.47, 95%CI: 0.22 to 1.02, $P = 0.06$, Fig. 5c), vaginal tape erosions (RR = 0.38, 95%CI: 0.09 to 1.63, $P = 0.619$, Fig. 5e) and de novo urgency and/or worsening of preexisting urgency (RR = 1.32, 95%CI: 0.78 to 2.25, $P = 0.30$, Fig. 5g).

Discussion

In this meta-analysis, we comprehensively compared the effectiveness and complications of adjustable SIMS and conventional slings for treating SUI patients. Reportedly, the efficacy of SUI correction is limited in those patients undergoing pelvic reconstructive surgery and corrective operation of pelvic organ prolapse is ineffective for 74.4% SUI [27], and previous continence surgery is independent risk factors for the lower success rate of TVT for SUI correction. Thus, in order to avoid the factor such as prior surgeries, concomitant prolapse associated, and surgical correction of prolapse to impact the assessment outcomes, we mainly focused on the primary SUI in females.

In our study, we found that the primary SUI patients received adjustable SIMS did not have superior outcomes to the primary SUI patients received other slings (including transobturator slings, TVT-O and MiniArc)

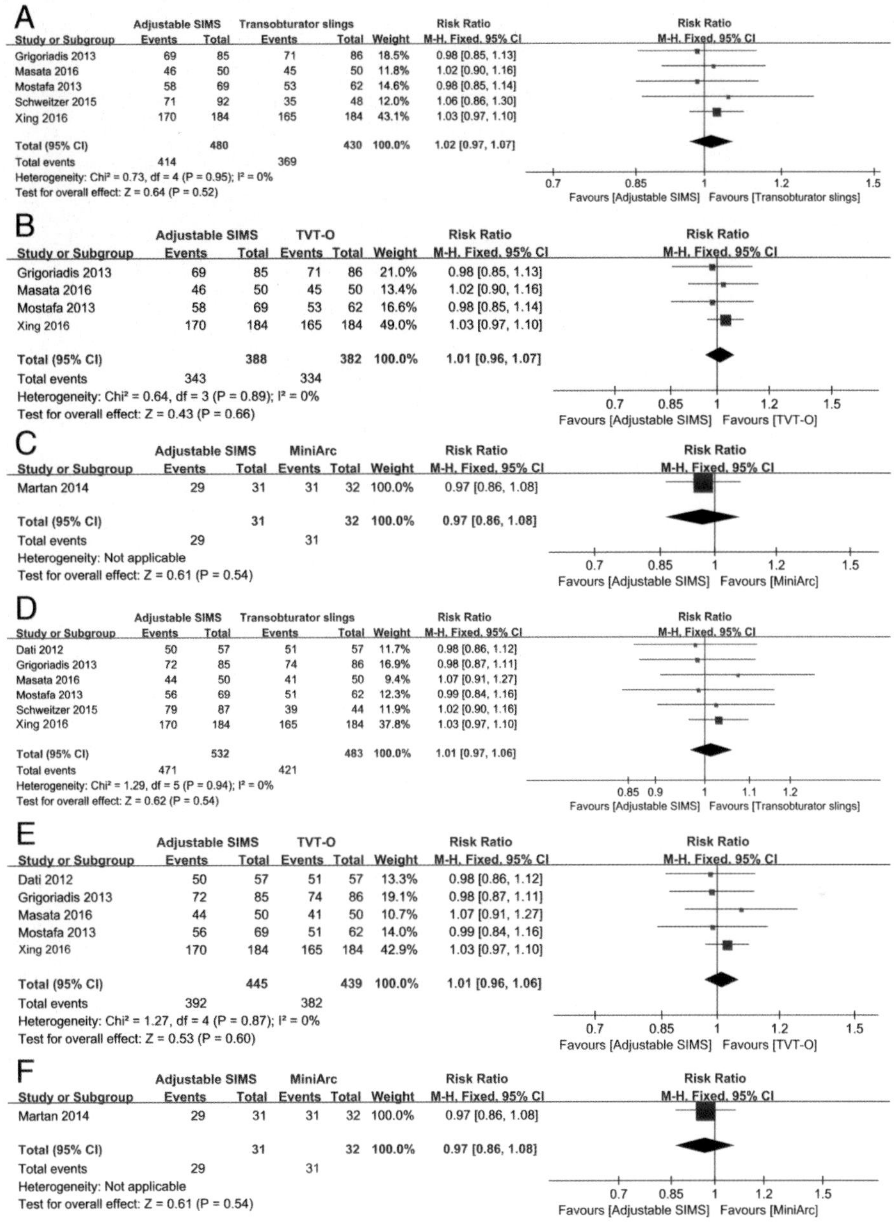

Fig. 3 The forest plots of meta-analysis for patients subjective cure rate and objective cure rate. **a** patients subjective cure rate of adjustable SIMS versus transobturator slings; **b** patients subjective cure rate of adjustable SIMS versus TVT-O; **c** patients subjective cure rate of adjustable SIMS versus MiniArc; **d** objective cure rate of adjustable SIMS versus transobturator slings; **e** objective cure rate of adjustable SIMS versus TVT-O; **f** objective cure rate of adjustable SIMS versus MiniArc

in patients subjective cure rate and objective cure rate. The possible explain for the no obvious difference outcomes of subjective and objective cure rates between adjustable SIMS and conventional slings groups were the same treatment principle for the surgical correction of SUI in female patients. These results were in line with the two previous meta-analyses [13]. Compared with the meta-analysis of Mostafa et al. [13], we especially concerned the adjustable SIMS including more relevant studies. Moreover, the differences in operation details and complications between adjustable SIMS and other slings were investigated in this study. By contrast, only the differences in patients subjective cure rate and objective cure rate between adjustable SIMS and SMUS was assessed in the meta-analysis of Mostafa et al. Compared with the meta-analysis reported by Zhang et al. [28], we specially analyzed the comparison between adjustable SIMS and TVT-O as well as between adjustable SIMS and MiniArc SIMS. In addition, the events of patients subjective cure rate and objective cure rate were

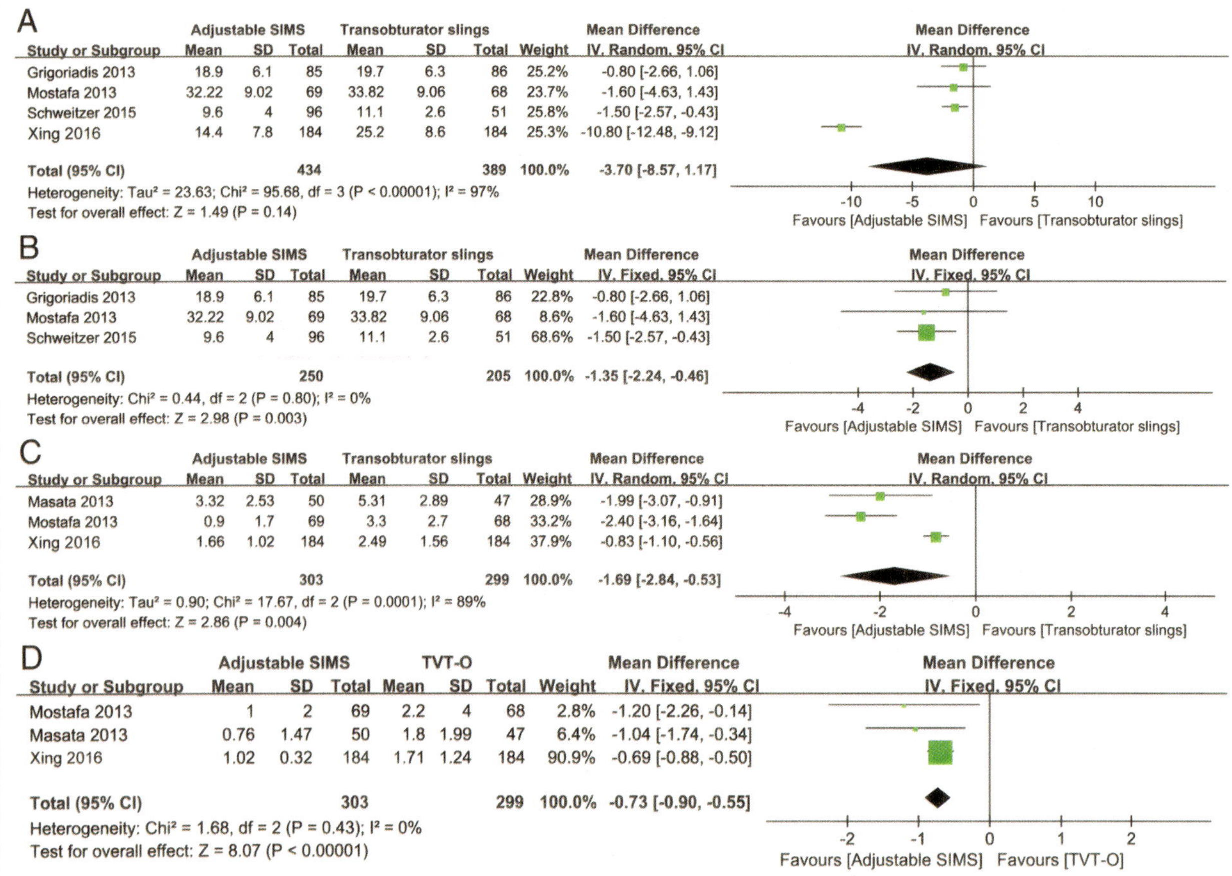

Fig. 4 The forest plots of meta-analysis for operation details. **a** operation time of adjustable SIMS versus transobturator slings; **b** operation time of adjustable SIMS versus TVT-O; **c** comparison of adjustable SIMS versus TVT-O in postoperative pain score at the first day after operation; **d** comparison of adjustable SIMS versus TVT-O in postoperative pain score at the fourth day after operation

recorded conversely in the two groups between one of the included studies of Zhang et al. and that meta-analysis [20, 28].

Based on the above mentioned, no obvious difference outcomes of subjective and objective cure rates between adjustable SIMS and conventional slings groups were found. Notably, it is reported that compared with conventional slings, the adjustable SIMS is a minimally invasive technique with less slings length and mesh material to reducing the foreign body in the patient's body [29].

Our results also showed that the patients underwent adjustable SIMS had a shorter operation time than the patients underwent transobturator slings but without significance. However, after excluding Xing's study that compared adjustable SIMS with TOT-V, the difference was significant. The change of results after excluding the study involving comparison of adjustable SIMS and TOT-V indicated that the operation time in adjustable SIMS may be significantly shorter than TOT but not TVT-O. The potential reason may be that the outside to inside technique in TOT takes more time than inside to outside in TVT-O. More studies were required to verify this speculation. In addition, the different measurement scheme of operation time among the included studies (such as the time from incision to its closure and the overall time spent in the operating theatre) may affect the results. Thus, more studies with larger sample size and unified measurement scheme should be performed to confirm the results of this study.

A previous study has confirmed that patients received SIMS significantly improved the postoperative pain profile than transobturator slings [21]. Consistent with this study, we found the postoperative pain score in patients received adjustable SIMS was significantly lower than that in patients received TVT-O. Although no available data of postoperative pain could be used for this meta-analysis in the study of Schweitzer et al., it also reported the lower early postoperative pain scores of adjustable SIMS than TOT [22]. These results indicated that, similar to SIMS, the adjustable SIMS also had the advantage of lower postoperative pain score than transobturator slings. Thus, the lower postoperative pain score of adjustable SIMS may be caused by the characteristics of SIMS. In SIMS, a single vaginal insertion approach was

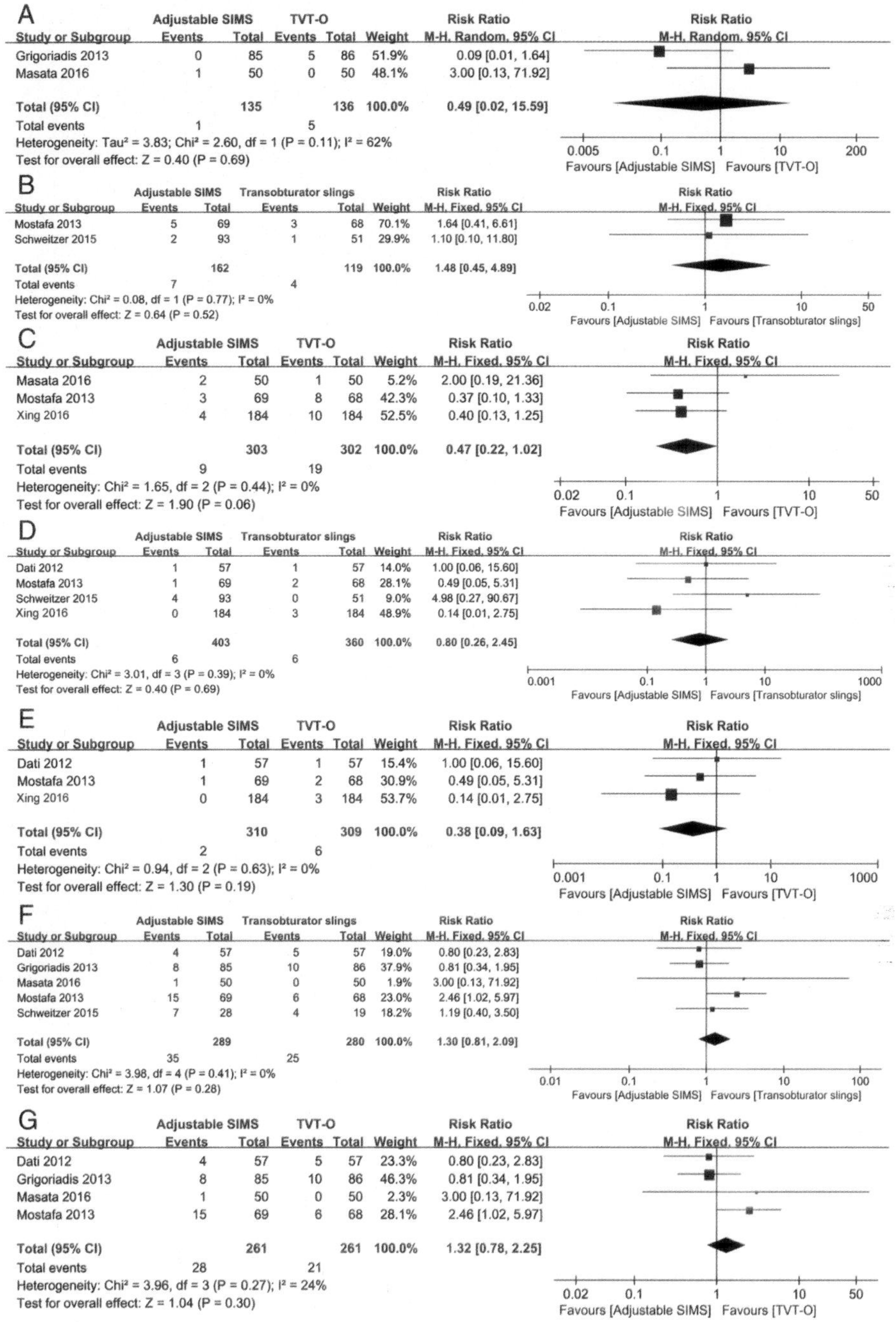

Fig. 5 The forest plots of meta-analysis for postoperative complications. **a** comparison of adjustable SIMS versus TVT-O in groin pain; **b** comparison of adjustable SIMS versus transobturator slings in repeated continence surgery; **c** comparison of adjustable SIMS versus TVT-O in postoperative voiding difficulties; **d** comparison of adjustable SIMS versus transobturator slings in vaginal tape erosion; **e** comparison of adjustable SIMS versus TVT-O in vaginal tape erosion; **f** comparison of adjustable SIMS versus transobturator slings in de novo urgency and/or worsening of preexisting surgery; **g** comparison of adjustable SIMS versus TVT-O in de novo urgency and/or worsening of preexisting surgery

utilized to avoid the blind passage of the trochars through the retropubic area and the groin/adductor muscles. The single vaginal insertion approach may be the main reason resulting in the lower postoperative pain score in SIMS and adjustable SIMS. However, the different anesthesia protocols among studies may affect the results of early postoperative pain score and further studies should consider this influence. Besides, Palomba et al. reported that there was no significant difference in postoperative pain score among the three SIMSs [30]. However, only this one study reported the comparison of adjustable SIMS and other SIMSs in postoperative pain [30], so the meta-analysis could not be performed. More studies were required to further investigate the postoperative pain in adjustable SIMS comparing with other SIMSs.

In addition, the analysis for complications indicated no significant difference between adjustable SIMS and transobturator slings or TVT-O alone. A previous meta-analysis reported that the SIMS was associated with the higher repeated continence surgery rates [13]. Moreover, the recent meta-analysis also found a nonsignificant trend of higher repeated continence surgery rates in patients received SIMS [28]. Considering the results in this meta-analysis (adjustable SIMS had similar repeated continence surgery rate to transobturator slings), we inferred that the adjustable SIMS might have less rates of repeated continence surgery than other SIMSs. More studies were required to prove this speculation.

Some limitations should be noted in this study. Firstly, the sample size and numbers of included studies were small. Secondly, the evaluation of publication bias was not assessed due to less than 10 included studies. Third, the heterogeneity was found in this study, the differences in race of participants, definitions of cure rate and types of transobturator slings may be the heterogeneity sources. However, subgroup analysis could not be performed to explore the heterogeneity sources due to inadequate data. Thus, these confounding factors may provide bias for the results of meta-analysis. Fourth, the follow up duration in these included studies were different and not long enough, thus more studies with long term follow up were required to further confirm the efficacy of adjustable SIMS. Fifth, we failed to compare all the indicators used in this meta-analysis between the adjustable SIMS and each slings method due to little involved studies was found. In addition, only two studies investigated the comparison between adjustable SIMS and other SIMSs. The comparison between adjustable SIMS and the TVT-Secur SIMS was not assessed due to only one study involving TVT-Secur SIMS. Thus, more RCTs with larger sample size and longer term follow up were required to further investigate the efficacy and safety of adjustable SIMS comparing with other slings, especially the other SIMSs.

Conclusions

This meta-analysis showed that the adjustable SIMS was as effective as transobturator slings and MiniArc in curing primary SUI patients in female. In addition, the adjustable SIMS was recommended due to shorter operative time and lower postoperative pain than TOT and TVT-O, respectively. However, the efficacy of adjustable SIMS approach needed to be further verified using multicenter, large sample, and long-term follow-up studies.

Abbreviations

95% CI: Confidence interval; MD: Mean difference; RCT: Randomized controlled trial; RR: Relative risk; SIMS: Single-incision mini-sling; SIMS: Single-incision mini-slings; SUI: Stress urinary incontinence; TOT: Transobturator tape; TVT: Tension-free vaginal tape; TVT-O: Tension-free vaginal tape-obturator

Funding

This work was supported by the National Natural Science Foundation of China (Grant No. 81400756 and No. 81202022), the Public Welfare Technology, project of Science Technology Department of Zhejiang Province (Grant No. 2014C33184), Zhejiang health Bureau (Grant No. 2016KYA093) and Zhejiang Provincial Natural Science Foundation of China (Grant No. LY16H160028).

Authors' contributions

JC participated in the design of this study. ZZ and JW performed the statistical analysis. YZ collected important background information. FB drafted the manuscript. NZ conceived of this study, and participated in the design and helped to draft the manuscript. All authors read and approved the final manuscript.

Competing interests

The authors declare that they have no competing interests.

References

1. Donkelaar CST, Rosier PFWM, Kort LMOD: 990 international continence society definition of detrusor underactivity; analysis of clinical parameters and comparison with contractility grading methods. Eur Urol Suppl 2016, 15(3):e975-e975.
2. Kavia R, Rashid T, Ockrim J. Stress urinary incontinence. J Clin Urol. 2013;6(6): 377–90.
3. Fritel X, Fauconnier A, Bader G, Cosson M, Debodinance P, Deffieux X, Denys P, Dompeyre P, Faltin D, Fatton B. Diagnosis and management of adult female stress urinary incontinence: guidelines for clinical practice from the French College of Gynaecologists and Obstetricians. Eur J Obstet Gynecol Reprod Biol. 2010;151(1):14–9.
4. Fong ED, Nitti VW. REVIEW ARTICLE: mid-urethral synthetic slings for female stress urinary incontinence. BJU Int. 2010;106(5):596–608.
5. Nilsson C, Palva K, Aarnio R, Morcos E, Falconer C. Seventeen years' follow-up of the tension-free vaginal tape procedure for female stress urinary incontinence. Int Urogynecol J. 2013;24(8):1265–9.
6. Kroon N, Smith K, Gill J: Bowel injury at TVT: an issue of consent. Journal of Obstetrics & Gynecology 2007, 27(7):741-741.
7. Agostini A, Bretelle F, Franchi F, Roger V, Cravello L, Blanc B. Immediate complications of tension-free vaginal tape (TVT): results of a French survey. Eur J Obstet Gynecol Reprod Biol. 2006;124(2):237–9.
8. Serati M, Braga A, Cattoni E, Siesto G, Cromi A, Ghezzi F, Salvatore S. Transobturator vaginal tape for the treatment of stress urinary incontinence in elderly women without concomitant pelvic organ prolapse: is it effective and safe? Eur J Obstet Gynecol Reprod Biol. 2013;166(1):107–10.
9. Potić M, Ignjatović I, Bašić D. Tension free vaginal tape (TVT) vs transobturator tape (TOT) complications and outcomes. Acta Chirurgica Iugoslavica. 2014;61(1):81–4.
10. Bozkurt M, Yumru A, Salman S. Assessment of perioperative, early, and late postoperative complications of the inside-out transobturator tape procedure in the treatment of stress urinary incontinence. Clin Exper Obstet Gynecol. 2014;42(1):82–9.
11. Neuman M, Sosnovski V, Kais M, Ophir E, Bornstein J. Transobturator vs single-incision suburethral mini-slings for treatment of female stress urinary incontinence: early postoperative pain and 3-year follow-up. J Minim Invasive Gynecol. 2011;18(6):769–73.
12. Oliveira R, Botelho F, Silva P, Resende A, Silva C, Dinis P, Cruz F. Exploratory study assessing efficacy and complications of TVT-O, TVT-Secur, and mini-arc: results at 12-month follow-up. Eur Urol. 2011;59(6):940–4.

13. Mostafa A, Lim CP, Hopper L, Madhuvrata P, Abdel-Fattah M. Single-incision mini-slings versus standard midurethral slings in surgical management of female stress urinary incontinence: an updated systematic review and meta-analysis of effectiveness and complications. Eur Urol. 2013;29:00860–9.
14. Meschia M, Barbacini P, Baccichet R, Buonaguidi A, Maffiolini M, Ricci L, Braghin C, Brusati V, Dell'Utri C, Spreafico L. Short-term outcomes with the Ajust™ system: a new single incision sling for the treatment of stress urinary incontinence. Int Urogynecol J. 2011;22(2):177–82.
15. Abdel-Fattah M, Agur W, Abdel-All M, Guerrero K, Allam M, Mackintosh A, Mostafa A, Yousef M. Prospective multi-Centre study of adjustable single-incision mini-sling (Ajust®) in the management of stress urinary incontinence in women: 1-year follow-up study. BJU Int. 2012;109(6):880–6.
16. Martan A, Krhut J, MAŠATA J, ŠVABÍK K, HALAŠKA M, HORČIČKA L, Zachoval R. Prospective randomized study of MiniArc and Ajust single incision sling procedures. LUTS. 2014;6(3):172–4.
17. Moher D, Liberati A, Tetzlaff J, Altman DG. Reprint—preferred reporting items for systematic reviews and meta-analyses: the PRISMA statement. Phys Ther. 2009;89(9):873–80.
18. Jadad AR, Moore RA, Carroll D, Jenkinson C, Reynolds DJM, Gavaghan DJ, McQuay HJ. Assessing the quality of reports of randomized clinical trials: is blinding necessary? Control Clin Trials. 1996;17(1):1–12.
19. Higgins JPT, Altman DG, Gøtzsche PC, Jüni P, Moher D, Oxman AD, Savović J, Schulz KF, Weeks L, Sterne JAC: The Cochrane Collaboration's tool for assessing risk of bias in randomised trials. BMJ 2011, 343(oct18 2):d5928-d5928.
20. Boyers D, Kilonzo M, Mostafa A, Abdel-Fattah M. Comparison of an adjustable anchored single-incision mini-sling, Ajust®, with a standard mid-urethral sling, TVT-OTM: a health economic evaluation. BJU Int. 2013;112(8): 1169–77.
21. Grigoriadis C, Bakas P, Derpapas A, Creatsa M, Liapis A. Tension-free vaginal tape obturator versus Ajust adjustable single incision sling procedure in women with urodynamic stress urinary incontinence. Eur J Obstet Gynecol Reprod Biol. 2013;170(2):563–6.
22. Schweitzer KJ, Milani AL, van Eijndhoven HW, Gietelink DA, Hallensleben E, Cromheecke G-J, van der Vaart CH. Postoperative pain after adjustable single-incision or Transobturator sling for incontinence: a randomized controlled trial. Obstet Gynecol. 2015;125(1):27–34.
23. Dati S, Rombolà P, Cappello S, Piccione E. M432 single-incision minisling (ajust) vs obturator tension-free vaginal shortened tape (tvt-abbrevo) in surgical management of female stress urinary incontinence. Int J Gynecol Obstet. 2012;119:S670.
24. Mostafa A, Agur W, Abdel-All M, Guerrero K, Lim C, Allam M, Yousef M, N'Dow J, Abdel-Fattah M. A multicentre prospective randomised study of single-incision mini-sling (Ajust®) versus tension-free vaginal tape-obturator (TVT-O™) in the management of female stress urinary incontinence: pain profile and short-term outcomes. Eur J Obstet Gynecol Reprod Biol. 2012; 165(1):115–21.
25. Masata J, Svabik K, Zvara K, Hubka P, Toman A, Martan A. Comparison of the efficacy of tension-free vaginal tape obturator (TVT-O) and single-incision tension-free vaginal tape (Ajust™) in the treatment of female stress urinary incontinence: a 1-year follow-up randomized trial. Int Urogynecol J. 2016; 27(10):1–9.
26. Xing X, Yue S, Xia Z. A comparison between adjustable single-incision sling and tension-free vaginal tape-obturator in treating stress urinary incontinence. Arch Gynecol Obstet. 2016;293(2):1–7.
27. Wang SM, Zhang ZY, Liu CD, Wang SZ. Study on concomitant surgical correction of pelvic organ prolapse and TVT-O for treatment of stress urinary incontinence. Zhonghua Fu Chan Ke Za Zhi. 2013;48(7):494–8.
28. Zhang P, Fan B, Han H, Xu Y, Wang B, Zhang X. Meta-analysis of female stress urinary incontinence treatments with adjustable single-incision mini-slings and transobturator tension-free vaginal tape surgeries. BMC Urol. 2015;15(1):64.
29. Zhang X. Initial study with the Ajust~(TM) system:a single incision adjustable sling for the treatment of female stress urinary incontinence. J Clin Urol. 2012;
30. Palomba S, Oppedisano R, Torella M, Falbo A, Maiorana A, Materazzo C, Tartaglia E, Tolino A, Mastrantonio P, Alio L. A randomized controlled trial comparing three vaginal kits of single-incision mini-slings for stress urinary incontinence: surgical data. Eur J Obstet Gynecol Reprod Biol. 2012;163(1):108–12.

30

What predicts emotional response in men awaiting prostate biopsy?

AnnMarie Groarke[1*], Ruth Curtis[1], Deirdre M. J. Walsh[1] and Francis J. Sullivan[2]

Abstract

Background: Incidence of prostate cancer is increasing as opportunistic screening becomes widespread and life expectancy rises. Despite screening availability, research reveals conflicting results on medical outcomes, for example, disease specific mortality. However the gold standard in early diagnosis of potentially curable organ confined prostate cancer is transrectal ultrasound-guided systematic prostate biopsy (TRUS-BX). While focus has been given to medical sequalae there is a paucity of research on the psychological impact of biopsy. Awaiting biopsy may be inherently stressful but no studies to date, have assessed men's perception of stress and its impact on emotional response. This study, therefore, examines the role of stress and also personal resources namely, self-efficacy and sense of coherence in emotional adjustment in men awaiting a prostate biopsy.

Methods: Men attending a Rapid Access Prostate Cancer Clinic for a transrectal prostate biopsy ($N = 114$) participated in the study. They completed self report questionnaires on perceived stress (PSS), generalised self-efficacy (GSES), and sense of coherence (SOC). Adjustment was measured by the Profile of Mood States (POMS-B) which assesses tension, depression, anger, fatigue, confusion and vigour.

Results: Hierarchical regression analyses demonstrated that the set of predictors accounted for 17%–34% of variance across six mood states and predicted 46% of total mood disturbance. Perceived stress explained variance on all domains (11%–26%) with high stress linked to poor functioning.

Conclusion: Perceived stress was the strongest and most consistent predictor of emotional adjustment. This is an important finding as stress appraisal has not been examined previously in this context and suggests that stress management is an important target to enhance emotional wellbeing of men attending for a prostate biopsy.

Keywords: Prostate biopsy, Stress, Self-efficacy, Sense of coherence, Emotional adjustment

Background

Prostate cancer is the most frequent malignant disease in older men and is the second most common cause of cancer-related death in this age group, after lung cancer [1, 2]. Prostate cancer rates in Ireland are the highest in Europe and Irish men have a 1 in 8 chance of developing prostate cancer [3].

Incidence of prostate cancer (PCa) worldwide is increasing as opportunistic screening becomes more widespread and average life expectancy rises [4]. Despite screening availability, research yields conflicting results on outcomes. A European trial examining disease specific mortality found benefits to population-based PCa screening [5, 6] but this was not replicated in a similar trial in the United States [7]. Furthermore, both over-diagnosis and resulting over-treatment are problematic sequelae of PCa screening due to low diagnostic specificity of prostate specific antigen (PSA levels) and prostatic biopsies [8, 9].

So the optimal management of screen-detected, localised prostate cancer remains controversial. However, the gold standard in early diagnosis of potentially curable and organ-confined prostate cancer is transrectal ultrasound-guided systematic prostate biopsy (TRUS-Bx), the most common form of investigation of raised PSA levels [10]. Biopsy can cause bleeding, pain, urinary and sexual symptoms [7, 11, 12] and it has been reported that up to 7% of men require hospital admission within 30 days of biopsy, most for febrile infections [13].

* Correspondence: annmarie.groarke@nuigalway.ie
[1]School of Psychology, National University of Ireland, Galway, Ireland
Full list of author information is available at the end of the article

While considerable focus has been given to medical sequelae, there is a relative paucity of empirical data examining the psychological impact of a prostate biopsy.

Existing qualitative research assessing the subjective experience of the procedure indicates that while some men find it merely uncomfortable, others report that it is stressful, exhausting, extremely painful [14] and view it as the worst aspect of their disease experience [15]. Further reports reveal that some men express fears post biopsy, for example, that cancer cells might pass from a man to his wife during ejaculation or that biopsy might spread cancer cells to other parts of the body [10]. The extant qualitative literature, therefore, indicates that men perceive biopsy as a stressful event.

Moreover, quantitative studies demonstrate that the negative impact of prostate biopsy on patient well-being can even begin while waiting for the scheduled procedure [16, 17] and that there is increased anxiety and worry reported immediately before undergoing biopsy [18, 19] with a minority (20%) suffering high levels of distress at this time [20]. In the main, studies used the Hospital Anxiety and Depression Scale (e.g. [17, 21]), which is designed to detect clinical cases of anxiety and depression. It has been recommended that more detailed, specific measures (e.g. Profile of Mood States) would better reflect changes in mood and distress of men undergoing biopsy [20]. The current study, therefore, uses the Profile of Mood States (POMS).

Awaiting biopsy may be inherently stressful given that it is an unexpected, uncontrollable event with potential for loss and harm, an important hallmark of a stressor [22, 23]. For example, uncertainty about diagnosis was associated with greater stress in women awaiting a breast biopsy than women awaiting more invasive and risky treatments [24]. The transactional model of stress and coping [23] provides a framework for understanding the impact of this stressor on adjustment. Stressful experiences in the model are construed as person-environment transactions in which the impact of an external stressor is mediated by a person's appraisal of the stressor and the psychological and social resources at his or her disposal. The model defines two types of appraisal, primary where the person asks himself, "is this stressful?" , and secondary where the person asks, "can I cope with this?" .

While it has been shown that emotional stress, as measured by elevated cortisol levels was higher in men called for a biopsy, than in a healthy matched control group [25], no studies to date have assessed men's perception of stress and its impact on mood awaiting biopsy. This warrants investigation given that perceived stress has been shown to be an important predictor of adjustment in men with a diagnosis of prostate cancer [26, 27]. Similarly personal resources, such as self-efficacy [28] and sense of coherence [29] have been shown to be important variables in coping with cancer [30–32], an aspect of secondary appraisal within the transactional model of stress.

Self-efficacy is a broad disposition rooted in the person's personality and life experience. It refers to both the perception of controllability of self-management tasks and sense of efficacy to use skills effectively under difficult circumstances [33]. Given a stressful situation, low self-efficacy can make people vulnerable to distress, whereas robust efficacy beliefs can serve to reduce anxiety [33–35]. Two studies to date have shown that self-efficacy beliefs have a positive impact on mood in men recently diagnosed with prostate cancer [26, 36] but less is known about its impact at biopsy stage. It would be of value, therefore, to examine if a sense of personal mastery enhances emotional response immediately prior to a biopsy. Sense of coherence, on the other hand, is conceptualised as a global orientation to life experience, including the degree to which life is viewed as comprehensible, manageable and meaningful. A strong sense of coherence is a health promoting factor that reflects a person's capacity to cope with health stressors [29] and is associated with less distress in cancer [37–39]. While a low sense of coherence predicted high levels of distress in women awaiting an examination for diagnosis of breast cancer [40] it has not yet been examined in the context of prostate biopsy.

So it is of interest to ascertain if this personality variable impacts men at the earlier stage, when facing an invasive procedure with an uncertain outcome.

This study, therefore, assesses for the first time the role of perceived stress and personal resources namely, generalised self-efficacy and sense of coherence in predicting emotional adjustment, in a group of Irish men immediately prior to a prostate biopsy.

Method

Participants

Consecutive men attending the Rapid Access Prostate Cancer Clinic in a University –affiliated hospital over a 6 month period were eligible to participate. The study protocol was approved by the Institutional Research Ethics Committee of the University Hospital. Written informed consent was obtained from all participants. Inclusion criteria were men awaiting biopsy for the first time who had completed at least second level education. Exclusion criteria were other comorbidities. Men were asked by the researchers to complete a questionnaire in the clinic while awaiting the procedure. Out of 215 men attending, 114 agreed to participate (53% response rate). The majority who declined, said they were unable to concentrate on the task or said they wouldn't have time before being called for the procedure.

Materials

The Perceived Stress Scale (PSS) [41] is a 14-item scale which measures the degree to which situations in one's life over a 1 month time frame are appraised as stressful. It taps the degree to which respondents find their life unpredictable, uncontrollable and overloaded. Respondents indicate how often they thought or felt a certain way on a five point Likert scale from 0 "never" to 4 "very often". Scores can range from 0 to 56 with higher scores indicating more perceived stress. In this study Cronbach's alpha coefficient was .67.

Generalised Self-Efficacy Scale (GSES) [35] includes 10 items (e.g. *'I can always manage to solve difficult problems if I try hard enough'*) and the responses for each item range from strongly disagree (1) to strongly agree (4). The scale provides one overall summmative score and has been shown to have high reliability ($\alpha = .96$). In this study Cronbach's alpha coefficient was .71.

The Sense of Coherence (SOC-13) scale [29] has three components: Comprehensibility (items 2, 6, 8, 9, 11), Manageability (items 3, 5, 10, 13) and Meaningfulness (items 1, 4, 7, 12). This scale is rated on a 7-point likert scale, a total score can also be used and the coding for items 1, 2, 3, 7 and 10 should be reversed. SOC scores range from 13 to 91. Antonovsky [42] concluded that content, construct and criterion validity were adequate. In the current study the total scale score reliability etimate was .52.

The Profile of Mood Scale-Brief (POMS-B) [43] is a 30 item indicator of psychological state, used to measure mood disturbance across 6 dimensions: tension/anxiety, depression/dejection, anger/hostility, fatigue/inertia, confusion/bewilderment and vigour/activity. It provides individual subscale scores and a total mood disturbance score. The POMS-B is made up of the 5 highest loading items per subscale based on six previous investigations of the POMS [44]. In this study Cronbach's alpha ranged from .60–.92. The total score reliability estimate was .92.

Statistical analyses

The statistical program G*Power was used to conduct power analysis. Adhering to Cohen's [45] guidelines for small ($r = 0.02$), medium ($r = 0.15$), and large ($r = 0.35$) effects, two-tailed alpha of .05 was assumed for all tests. With 4 predictors as well as a medium effect size and a power of 0.8, the recommended total sample size for linear multiple regression was 85.

Inspection of histograms and analysis of skewness showed that POMS subscales with the exception of tension and vigour were skewed. Outliers were windzorised which reduced the skewness to an acceptable level. Pearson correlation coefficients assessed relationships between predictors and outcomes. Missing data was less than or equal to 5% on all scale items (with the exception of two items where the proportion was 9.5% and 9.6%). Using Little's MCAR test, data was found to be missing competely at random ($p > .05$) and therfore, the Expectation Maximization algorithm was used to substitute missing values [46]. EM is considered an excellent procedure for handling missing data [47, 48], and is advised when data are MCAR or MAR [49] and the percentage of missing data is minimal (i.e., less than 5%) [48, 49]. Hierarchical regression was chosen as the study is based on the transactional model of stress [23]. Accordingly, age was entered in Step 1, the effect of primary appraisal, that is level of perceived stress, was entered in Step2. The effect of secondary appraisal was examined in subsequent steps with self-efficacy entered in Step 3 and sense of coherence entered in Step 4. Self-efficacy was entered before sense of coherence as previous literature has shown a link with distress at diagnosis of prostate cancer [26, 36].

Results

Descriptive data are presented in Table 1. The sample scored in the moderate range on perceived stress and sense of coherence and in the upper range in self-efficacy. The intercorrelations between predictors and the 6 outcomes are shown in Table 2 and reveal that relationships between stress and all mood variables are in the expected direction with stress linked to high tension, depression, anger, fatigue, confusion, and low vigour. Equally, low self-efficacy and low sense of coherence correlated with high tension, depression, anger, fatigue, confusion, and low vigour.

The results of the regression analysis are presented in Table 3. Age explained 3% of variance on vigour with older participants reporting lower vigour-activity. Age did not contribute to other mood states. Perceived

Table 1 Descriptive Statistics for predictor and outcome variable for 114 men attending for Biopsy

	Test Range	Sample Range	*M*	*SD*
Age		41–77	62.56	7.25
PSS	0–56	4–37	20.40	7.11
GSES	10–40	19–40	31.06	4.91
SOC	13–91	36–91	68.31	12.50
POMS				
Tension	0–20	0–14	5.31	4.07
Depression	0–20	0–9	2.77	3.04
Anger	0–20	0–10	2.72	3.22
Fatigue	0–20	0–15	4.53	4.14
Confusion	0–20	0–10	4.70	2.80
Vigor	0–20	0–20	9.33	4.52
POMS TMD		-15-42	10.63	15.48

GSES General Self-Efficacy Score. *PSS* Perceived Stress Scale. *SOC* Sense of Coherence Scale

Table 2 Intercorrelations between Age, Stress,Self-efficacy, Sense of coherence and Mood in 114 men attending for a bipsy

	1	2	3	4	5	6	7	8	9	10	11
1. Age	–										
2. PSS	.00	–									
3. GSES	–.03	–.49**	–								
4. SOC	.10	–.53*	.58**	–							
5. Anxiety	.00	.52**	–.36**	–.39**	–						
6. Depression	.01	.60**	–.41**	–.58**	.64**	–					
7. Anger	–.04	.513**	–.31**	–.50**	.56**	.78**	–				
8. Fatigue	.08	.48**	–.41**	–.47**	.64**	.64**	.59**	–			
9. Confusion	.01	.37**	–.30**	–.43**	.62**	.68**	.59**	.69**	–		
10. Vigor	–.20*	–.39**	.37**	.19*	–.16	–.13	–.08	–.23*	.13	–	
11. POMS TMD	.06	.64**	–.48**	–.56**	.82**	.83**	.78**	.84**	.73**	.40**	–

Note; * $p < .05$, ** $p < .01$, *** $p < .001$. $N = 115$. *GSES* General Self-Efficacy Score. *PSS* Perceived Stress Scale. *SOC* Sense of Coherence Scale

stress explained variance in all domains; tension (26%), depression (26%), anger (24%), fatigue (22%) confusion (11%) and vigour (15%), with the beta weights showing relationships in expected directions. Self-efficacy explained additional variance on the domain of vigour (4%) with high self-efficacy indicative of good status on this index. Sense of coherence significantly predicted four out of six mood outcomes; depression (8%), anger (6%), fatigue (3%) and confusion (6%). In all cases beta weights showed that sense of coherence was related to poorer function.

The total amount of variance explained by all predictors in the model for each mood index was as follows; Tension 26%, Depression 34%, Anger 29%, Fatigue 28%, Confusion 17%, and Vigour 22%. The model explained more than a quarter of the variance on four of the emotional states and 46% of variance on total mood disturbance.

Discussion

This current study examined the role of predictors of emotional adjustment in men attending for a prostate biopsy. An important finding is that perceived stress was the strongest and most consistent predictor of adjustment in men awaiting a biopsy. It explained variance ranging from 11 to 26% on all six emotional domains with higher levels of stress at biopsy linked to poor adjustment. Overall it explained 40% of variance on total mood distubance. This is in line with the finding by

Table 3 Hierarchical Multiple Regression of the Role of Age, Stress, Self-Efficacy and Sense of Coherence on Six Subscales and Total Score of the Profile of Mood States Questionnaire in 114 Men Attending for a Biopsy

Predictors	Tension – Anxiety			Depression – Dejection			Anger - Hostility			Fatigue - Inertion		
	β	Fchange	Adj R^2 ch	β	Fchange	Adj R^2 ch	β	Fchange	Adj R^2 ch	β	Fchange	Adj R^2 ch
(1) *Demographic Variables* (Age)	0.01	0.00	−0.01	0.05	0.01	−0.01	−0.01	0.18	−0.01	0.10	0.77	−0.00
(2) *Stress* (PSS)	0.42***	42.37***	0.26	0.40***	62.50***	0.26	0.36***	40.23***	0.24	0.28**	33.29***	0.22
(3) *Self-Efficacy* (GSES)	−0.08	2.02	0.01	0.01	3.20	0.01	0.06	0.75	0.00	−0.11	5.75*	0.03
(4) *Sense of Coherence* (SOC)	−0.12	1.21	0.00	−0.38***	16.22***	0.08	−0.34***	10.83***	0.06	−0.26*	6.24*	0.03
Total *Adj R^2*			0.26			0.34			0.29			0.28
Predictors	Confusion - Bewilderment			Vigour – Activity			Total Mood Disturbance					
(1) *Demographic Variables* (Age)	0.04	0.01	−0.01	−0.18*	4.68*	0.03	0.08	0.43	−0.01			
(2) *Stress* (PSS)	0.19	17.74***	0.11	−0.31**	20.81***	0.15	0.45***	79.97***	0.40			
(3) *Self-Efficacy* (GSES)	−0.01	2.35	0.01	0.30**	6.22*	0.04	−0.10	7.19**	0.03			
(4) *Sense of Coherence* (SOC)	−0.33**	8.54**	0.06	−0.13	1.47	0.00	−0.27**	8.91**	0.04			
Total *Adj R^2*			0.17			0.22			0.46			

Note; * $p < .05$, ** $p < .01$, *** $p < .001$. $N = 115$. GSES; General Self-Efficacy Score. PSS; Perceived Stress Scale. SOC; Sense of Coherence Scale. Standardised beta values are reported from the final model (Model 4). *F* change illustrates significance of each step over and above previous step

Curtis et al. [26] and Orom et al. [36] in men with newly diagnosed prostate cancer and so illustrates for the first time a similarly strong impact of stress in predicting mood states during the biopsy phase.

Of particular interest is that while stress best explained variability on tension and depression it also predicted a quarter of the variability in anger and fatigue, and over 10% of variance in vigour. This emphasises the need to extend assessment beyond anxiety and depression, which is the typical focus of adjustment in the biopsy literature, to include a more comprehensive analysis of mood in men awaiting biopsy. The PSS measured the extent to which patients found their lives uncontrollable and unpredictable within the previous month and so this suggests that the stress of waiting for a scheduled biopsy can impact on emotional responses. This concurs with previous findings [16, 17, 24] and pinpoints, moreover, the importance of adequate preparation for the upcoming procedure and its emotional aftermath [50]. Recent systematic reviews report that psychosocial interventions with men with prostate cancer have enhanced participants' cancer knowledge, quality of life and mood [51, 52]. In light of findings here, the effect of psychosocial interventions at the biopsy stage should be investigated. Further research, differentiating the particular sources of stress, whether related to fear of the procedure and or worry about a potential diagnosis, could usefully inform the design of such interventions.

In the present study sense of coherence explained some additional variance on four of the six emotional indices (depression, anger, fatigue and confusion) with low sense of coherence linked to poor functioning similar to women awaiting biopsy [40]. Such that those who viewed life as comprehensible, manageable and meaningful experienced better mood states in the face of this challenging medical procedure. While the amount of variance explained is small, these results for men awaiting biopsy are congruent with Antonovsky's model [29] and a recent meta-analysis [39], which purports consistency of the sense of coherence–distress association across medical subgroups of cancer patients. While further research is needed to confirm these relationships, findings suggest that the SOC scale could be a useful screening tool to detect those patients who are vulnerable and who would benefit from counselling to improve their coping capacities [38].

Self-efficacy had minimal effect on mood when awaiting biopsy but did explain a small amount of variance in domains which pertain to states concerning energy level (vigour). This is in contrast to the positive role of self-efficacy on mood (distress) in men diagnosed with prostate cancer [26, 36]. Perhaps the period prior to biopsy does not yet present symptom-related self management tasks and so self-efficacy beliefs are not as pertinent to emotional state.

Alternatively, the role of self-efficacy in adjustment may depend on the subjective appraisal of a potential diagnosis. A qualitative analysis, found that some men construed their prostate cancer as non-threatening, associated with few symptoms and a positive prognosis [15]. According to self-regulation theory [53] perceptions of an illness, for example, the extent to which it is seen as curable or incurable, can impact perceived ability to cope. Future research, could therefore, explore the interaction between threat appraisal, illness beliefs and self-efficacy to provide a more in depth understanding of emotional adjustment in men awaiting a prostate biopsy.

A limitation of the study is that it is cross-sectional and so does not allow for causal inferences among variables. Furthermore the modest sample size and response rate may influence generalisability of the findings, as may the low alpha reliability of the sense of coherence measure.

The study does, however, provide useful insight into predictors of adjustment in consecutive men attending for a biopsy at a prostate cancer clinic. It identifies that stress had an important explanatory role in mood disturbance with those higher in stress reporting poor adjustment across a range of mood states. This is an important finding as stress appraisal has not been examined previously in this context and it may be that stress management is a more important target than enhancement of personal resources to the emotional wellbeing of men attending for a biopsy. This fits with a growing consensus that intervening to reduce distress is an essential component of cancer care [54–56].

It is important that health professionals are fully cognizant of misconceptions held as well as the emotional impact of investigative procedures, such as transrectal prostate biopsy so that they can provide optimal information and psychological support at this time.

Acknowledgements

The authors wish to acknowledge the excellent collaboration of the medical and nursing staff at the Rapid Access Prostate Cancer Clinic at University Hospital Galway. The authors sincerely thank the men who gave their time to participate in the study.

Funding

This research was funded by Cancer Care West, Ireland a registered charity (CHY 11260).

Authors' contributions

AG and RC designed the study, analysed the data and wrote the manuscript. DW collected the data. FS assisted with patient recruitment. All authors approved the final manuscript.

Competing interests

The authors declare that they have no competing interests.

Author details
[1]School of Psychology, National University of Ireland, Galway, Ireland.
[2]Prostate Cancer Institute, National University of Ireland Galway, Galway, Ireland.

References

1. Greenlee RT, Hill-Harmon MB, Murray T, Thun M. Cancer statistics, 2001. CA Cancer J Clin. 2001;51:15–36.
2. Raja J, Ramachandran N, Munneke G, Patel U. Current status of transrectal ultrasound-guided prostate biopsy in the diagnosis of prostate cancer. Clin Radiol. 2006;61:142–53.
3. National Cancer Registry Ireland (2014). Cancer Projections for Ireland 2015–2040. Ireland.http://www.ncri.ie/sites/ncri/files/pubs/Cancer%20projections%20for%20Ireland%202015%20-%202040.pdf. Accessed 26 September 2016.
4. Ferlay J, Soerjomataram I, Dikshit R, Eser S, Mathers C, Rebelo M, Parkin DM, Forman D, Bray F. Cancer incidence and mortality worldwide: sources, methods and major patterns in GLOBOCAN 2012. Int J Cancer. 2015;136:E359–86.
5. Schröder FH, Hugosson J, Roobol MJ, Tammela TL, Ciatto S, Nelen V, Kwiatkowski M, Lujan M, Lilja H, Zappa M. Screening and prostate-cancer mortality in a randomized European study. N Engl J Med. 2009;360:1320–8.
6. Hugosson J, Carlsson S, Aus G, Bergdahl S, Khatami A, Lodding P, Pihl C-G, Stranne J, Holmberg E, Lilja H. Mortality results from the Göteborg randomised population-based prostate-cancer screening trial. The. Lancet Oncol. 2010;11:725–32.
7. Andriole GL, Crawford ED, Grubb IIIRL, Buys SS, Chia D, Church TR, Fouad MN, Gelmann EP, Kvale PA, Reding DJ. Mortality results from a randomized prostate-cancer screening trial. New Engl J Med. 2009;360:1310–9.
8. Bellardita L, Valdagni R, Van Den Bergh R, Randsdorp H, Repetto C, Venderbos LD, Lane JA, Korfage IJ. How does active surveillance for prostate cancer affect quality of life? A systematic review. Eur Urol. 2015;67:637–45.
9. Drummond FJ, O'Leary E, Gavin A, Kinnear H, Sharp L. Mode of prostate cancer detection is associated with the psychological wellbeing of survivors: results from the PiCTure study. Support Care Cancer. 2016;24:2297–307.
10. Chapple A, Ziebland S, Brewster S, McPherson A. Patients' perceptions of transrectal prostate biopsy: a qualitative study. Eur J Cancer Care. 2007;16:215–21.
11. Glaser AP, Novakovic K, Helfand BT. The impact of prostate biopsy on urinary symptoms, erectile function, and anxiety. Curr Urol Rep. 2012;13:447–54.
12. Ilic D, O'Connor D, Green S, Wilt TJ. Screening for prostate cancer: an updated Cochrane systematic review. BJU Int. 2011;107:882–91.
13. Loeb S, van den Heuvel S, Zhu X, Bangma CH, Schröder FH, Roobol MJ. Infectious complications and hospital admissions after prostate biopsy in a European randomized trial. Eur Urol. 2012;61(6):1110–4.
14. Medd JC, Stockler MR, Collins R, Lalak A. Measuring men's opinions of prostate needle biopsy. ANZ J Surg. 2005;75:662–4.
15. Appleton L, Wyatt D, Perkins E, Parker C, Crane J, Jones A, Moorhead L, Brown V, Wall C, Pagett M. The impact of prostate cancer on men's everyday life. Eur J Cancer Care. 2015;24:71–84.
16. Zisman A, Leibovici D, Kleinmann J, Siegel YI, Lindner A. The impact of prostate biopsy on patient well-being: a prospective study of pain, anxiety and erectile dysfunction. Journal Urol. 2001;165:445–54.
17. Awsare N, Green J, Aldwinckle B, Hanbury D, Boustead G, McNicholas T. The measurement of psychological distress in men being investigated for the presence of prostate cancer. Prostate Cancer and Prostatic Dis. 2008;11:384–9.
18. Saraçoglu T, Ünsal A, Taskin F, Sevinçok L, Karaman CZ. The impact of pre-procedural waiting period and anxiety level on pain perception in patients undergoing transrectal ultrasound-guided prostate biopsy. Diagn Interv Radiol. 2012;18:195.
19. Fowler FJ, Barry MJ, Walker-Corkery B, Caubet JF, Bates DW, Lee JM, Hauser A, McNaughton-Collins M. The impact of a suspicious prostate biopsy on Patients' psychological, socio-behavioral, and medical care outcomes. J Gen Intern Med. 2006;21:715–21.
20. Macefield R, Metcalfe C, Lane J, Donovan J, Avery K, Blazeby J. Down L, Neal D, Hamdy F, Vedhara K: impact of prostate cancer testing: an evaluation of the emotional consequences of a negative biopsy result. Br J Cancer. 2010;102:1335–40.
21. Wade J, Rosario DJ, Macefield RC, Avery KN, Salter CE, Goodwin ML, Blazeby JM, Lane JA, Metcalfe C, Neal DE. Psychological impact of prostate biopsy: physical symptoms, anxiety, and depression. J Clin Oncol. 2013;31(33):4235–4241.
22. Cohen S. Aftereffects of stress on human performance and social behavior: a review of research and theory. Psychol Bull. 1980;88:82.
23. Lazarus RS, Folkman S: Stress, appraisal, and coping. New York: Springer publishing company; 1984.
24. Flory N, Lang EV. Distress in the radiology waiting room. Radiology. 2011;260(1):166–73.
25. Gustafsson O, Theorell T, Norming U, Perski A, Öhström M, Nyman C. Psychological reactions in men screened for prostate cancer. Brit J Urol. 1995;75:631–6.
26. Curtis R, Groarke A, Sullivan F. Stress and self-efficacy predict psychological adjustment at diagnosis of prostate cancer. Sci Rep. 2014;4: 5569. https://doi.org/10.1038/srep05569
27. Steginga SK, Occhipinti S. Dispositional optimism as a predictor of men's decision-related distress after localized prostate cancer. Health Psychol. 2006;25(2):135.
28. Bandura A. Self-efficacy: the exercise of control. New York: Freeman; 1997.
29. Antonovsky A: Unraveling the mystery of health: How people manage stress and stay well. San Francisco: Jossey-Bass; 1987.
30. Taylor SE. Adjustment to threatening events: a theory of cognitive adaptation. Am Psychol. 1983;38:1161.
31. Haugland T, Wahl AK, Hofoss D, DeVon HA. Association between general self-efficacy, social support, cancer-related stress and physical health-related quality of life: a path model study in patients with neuroendocrine tumors. Health Quality Life Outcomes. 2016;14:1.
32. Sarenmalm EK, Browall M, Persson LO, Fall-Dickson J, Gaston-Johansson F. Relationship of sense of coherence to stressful events, coping strategies, health status, and quality of life in women with breast cancer. Psychooncology. 2013;22:20–7.
33. Lev EL, Eller LS, Gejerman G, Kolassa J, Colella J, Pezzino J, Lane P, Munver R, Esposito M, Sheuch J. Quality of life of men treated for localized prostate cancer: outcomes at 6 and 12 months. Support Care Cancer. 2009;17:509–17.
34. Bandura A. Exercise of personal agency through the self-efficacy mechanism. In: Schwarzer R, editor. Self-efficacy: thought control of action. Washington DC: Hemisphere Publishing Corp; 1992. p. 3–38.
35. Jerusalem M, Schwarzer R, Schwarzer R. Self-efficacy as a resource factor in stress appraisal processes. In: Self-efficacy: Thought control of action; 1992. p. 195–213.
36. Orom H, Nelson CJ, Underwood W, Homish DL, Kapoor DA. Factors associated with emotional distress in newly diagnosed prostate cancer patients. Psychooncology. 2015;24:1416–22.
37. Gustavsson-Lilius M, Julkunen J, Keskivaara P, Hietanen P. Sense of coherence and distress in cancer patients and their partners. Psychooncology. 2007;16:1100–10.
38. Hyphantis T, Papadimitriou I, Petrakis D, Fountzilas G, Repana D, Assimakopoulos K, Carvalho AF, Pavlidis N. Psychiatric manifestations, personality traits and health-related quality of life in cancer of unknown primary site. Psychooncology. 2013;22:2009–15.
39. Winger JG, Adams RN, Mosher CE. Relations of meaning in life and sense of coherence to distress in cancer patients: a meta-analysis. Psychooncology. 2016;25:2–10.
40. Gilbar O. Do attitude toward cancer, sense of coherence and family high risk predict more psychological distress in women referred for a breast cancer examination? Women & health. 2003;38(2):35–46.
41. Cohen S, Kamarck T, Mermelstein R. A global measure of perceived stress. J Health Soc Behav. 1983;24: 385–96.
42. Antonovsky A. The structure and properties of the sense of coherence scale. Soc Sci Med. 1993;36:725–33.
43. McNair D, Lorr M, Droppelman L. EDITS manual for the profile of mood states: manual. San Diego, Calif: Educational and Testing Service; 1992.
44. McNair DM, Heuchert P: Profile of mood states: POMS: technical update: multi-health systems; 2007.
45. Cohen J. Statistical power analysis for the behavioural sciences. Lawrence Earlbaum Associates: Hillside. NJ; 1988.
46. Tabachnick BG, Fidell LS. 6th ed. using multivariate statistics. Essex: Pearson Education limited; 2014.
47. Allison P. Missing data. Thousand Oaks, CA: Sage; 2001.

48. Graham JW. Missing data analysis: making it work in the real world. Ann. Rev Psychol. 2009;60:549–76.
49. Scheffer J. Dealing with missing data. Research Letters in the Information and Mathematical Sciences. 2002;31:53–160.
50. Tarhan H, Cakmak O, Unal E, Akarken I, Un S, Ekin RG, et al. The effect of video-based education on patient anxiety in men undergoing transrectal prostate biopsy. Can Urol Assoc J. 2014;8(11–12):894–900.
51. Parahoo K, McDonough S, McCaughan E, Noyes J, Semple C, Halstead EJ, Neuberger MM, Dahm P. Psychosocial interventions for men with prostate cancer: a Cochrane systematic review. BJU Intern. 2015;116:174–83.
52. Newby TA, Graff JN, Ganzini LK, McDonagh MS. Interventions that may reduce depressive symptoms among prostate cancer patients: a systematic review and meta-analysis. Psychooncology. 2015;24:1686–93.
53. Leventhal H, Nerenz DR, Purse J: Illness representations and coping with health threats; 1984.
54. Watson M, Jacobsen P. Editorial. Stress Health. 2012;28:353–4.
55. Cowens-Alvarado R, Sharpe K, Pratt-Chapman M, Willis A, Gansler T, Ganz PA, Edge SB, McCabe MS, Stein K. Advancing survivorship care through the National Cancer Survivorship Resource Center. CA: Canc J Clin. 2013;63:147–50.
56. Holland JC, Bultz BD. The NCCN guideline for distress management: a case for making distress the sixth vital sign. J National Compr Canc Netw. 2007;5:3–7.

Knowledge and attitude for overactive bladder care among women: development and measurement

Sumedha Chhatre[1*], Diane K. Newman[2], Alan J. Wein[2], Ashlie E. Jefferson[3], J. Sanford Schwartz[4] and Ravishankar Jayadevappa[5]

Abstract

Background: Overactive bladder (OAB) affects millions of women. It is important to assess knowledge and attitude in affected patients. The study objective was to develop surveys to assess OAB knowledge and OAB related attitude, and its association with OAB treatment status.

Methods: Systematic literature review and qualitative analysis of patient and provider focus groups helped identify OAB knowledge and attitude survey items. We determined psychometric properties of the two surveys in a cross-sectional sample of 104 women, 27% of whom had received OAB treatment.

Results: The OAB-knowledge survey consisted of 16 items and 3 condition-related concepts: perception of OAB; cause and information; and signs of OAB. The OAB-attitude survey consisted of 16 items and its concepts were treatment seeking; decision-making and effects. Both surveys demonstrated good construct validity and test-retest reliability (($\geq$ 0.60). In the cross-sectional validation sample, OAB-knowledge and attitude discriminated between those with different levels of ICIQ-UI scores. We observed some difference in the OAB knowledge, OAB attitude, and severity of symptoms between those treated for OAB vs. treatment naive.

Conclusions: OAB knowledge and attitude surveys provide a novel tool to assess OAB domains in women. Though we did not find statistical significance in OAB knowledge and attitude scores across treatment status, they may be potentially modifiable factors that affect OAB treatment uptake and treatment compliance. Refinement of these surveys in diverse sub-populations is necessary. Our study provides effect sizes for OAB knowledge and attitude. These effect sizes can help development of fully powered trials to study the association between OAB knowledge and attitude, type and length of treatment, treatment compliance, and quality of life, leading to interventions for enhancing OAB care.

Keywords: Overactive bladder, Women, Knowledge and attitude, Treatment uptake

Background

A common health concern for men and women of all ages, overactive bladder (OAB) is defined by the International Continence Society as urgency, with or without urge urinary incontinence (UI), frequently accompanied with frequency and nocturia in the absence of proven infection or other obvious pathology [1]. An embarrassing and debilitating condition with substantial health and economic consequences [1–3], OAB affects nearly 17% of women in the US. Prevalence of OAB increases with age and among women aged 65 and older, the prevalence of OAB is approximately 30% [2–5].

The symptoms of OAB can have negative effects on quality of life and necessitate lifestyle changes [6–9]. The National Overactive Bladder Evaluation (NOBLE) Program data showed that OAB with or without urgency urinary incontinence was associated with significantly lower quality of life and quality of sleep, and higher depression, compared to controls [2]. Total cost related to OAB in the US was more than $12 billion in 2000 using

* Correspondence: rasu@mail.med.upenn.edu
[1]Department of Psychiatry, Perelman School of Medicine, University of Pennsylvania, 3535 Market St., Suite 4051, Philadelphia, PA 19104, USA
Full list of author information is available at the end of the article

the NOBLE survey data. These costs are comparable to those of osteoporosis and gynecological cancers [5]. However, many women with OAB suffer in silence without seeking care [1–9], while attempting to manage their symptoms by developing coping mechanisms.

Conceptual framework

Our study conceptual model is based on the Theory of Planned Behavior (TPB) [10]. The TPB posits that human behavior results from intentions, which in turn are driven by attitude toward behavior; subjective norms; and perceived behavioral control. Knowledge plays an important role in each of these. In this study, the focus is on the assessment of knowledge of and attitude towards OAB. This information, when linked with the observed behavior, can inform interventions to influence OAB care seeking behavior (Fig. 1).

Knowledge regarding OAB and attitudes towards seeking care for OAB can affect the uptake of OAB care [11]. Therefore, the objective of this study was to develop psychometrically sound surveys to assess knowledge and attitudes among adult women from a large academic, urban healthcare system. We also studied if OAB knowledge and attitude was associated with OAB treatment and if those with higher level of OAB knowledge had more positive attitude towards OAB care.

Methods

In this study, we evaluated the knowledge and attitude among women with OAB. We used theory of TPB to postulate a conceptual framework of knowledge of and attitude toward OAB care. Two phases of our study were: (1) development of OAB knowledge and attitude items and surveys; and (2) psychometric testing of the surveys. The local Institutional Review Board approved the study.

Survey development

In Phase 1, we conducted in-depth literature review, and patient and provider focus groups to determine OAB-knowledge and OAB-attitude survey items [12]. As OAB symptoms in women often are associated with perceived social stigma, we included the term "stigma" in our literature review. We also searched for OAB related surveys to expand our framework for knowledge and attitude measurement. We conducted a comprehensive review of the literature published in English from 1990 to 2014 using Medline, PUBMED, CINAHL, and EMBASE. A key term search strategy was employed using "Overactive bladder (urgency, frequency and urge urinary incontinence)", "incontinence", "nocturia", "health related quality of life (HRQoL)", "symptoms", "attitude", and "knowledge".

Next, we conducted patient focus groups to explore their knowledge of OAB, experience of OAB symptoms and attitudes towards seeking OAB care. Prior to focus groups, we developed an interview guide with instructions, think-aloud exercises, and scripted probes. All focus group participants provided written consent. An experienced moderator led each focus group with assistance from co-facilitators (DK and RJ). Similarly, two provider focus groups yielded expert's perceptions of OAB care. Focus group discussions were audio taped and transcribed. Two reviewers (SC and RJ) analyzed the transcribed text using NVivo software, a qualitative

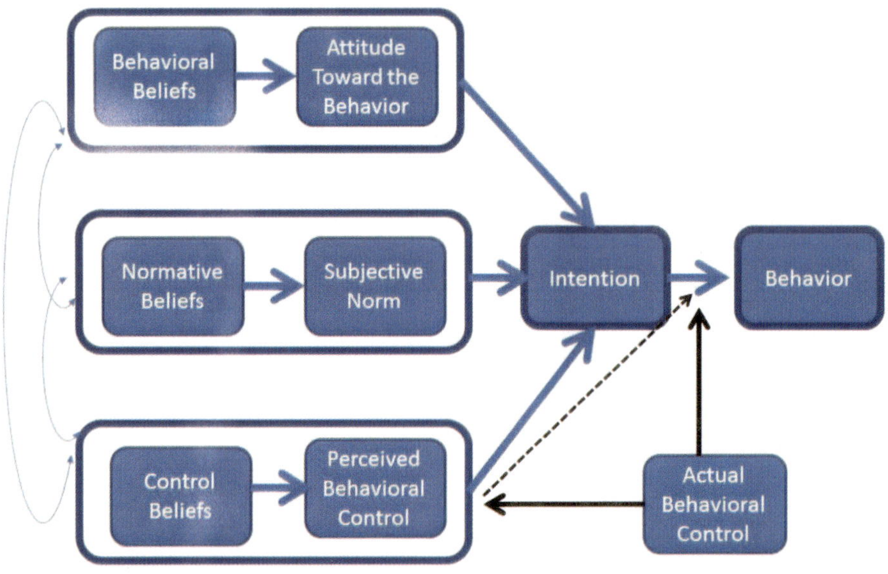

Fig. 1 Conceptual Model-Theory of Planned Behavior (Ajzen, 1991)

analysis program that allows coding and classification of text into major and minor concepts.

Informed by the literature review and focus groups, we assembled an initial pool of items for OAB-knowledge and OAB-attitude surveys. These items were reviewed by external and internal collaborators who gave feedback on the face validity (clarity and relevance) of the candidate items. The qualitative item review was initiated by developing draft OAB-knowledge and OAB-attitude surveys. We employed best practices [13–15] for creating new questions for the surveys, reviewing items to ensure that they: (1) did not exceed a sixth-grade reading level, as measured by the Flesch–Kincaid Grade Level standard; (2) minimized ambiguity or cognitive difficulty; (3) avoided multi-barreled questions; (4) were concisely and simply worded; and (5) were easy to translate into other languages.

Statistical analysis

The internal reliability of the OAB knowledge and attitude surveys was assessed by Cronbach's alpha (≥ 0.60) with items with low item-total correlations excluded. A random-effects, repeated measures analysis of variance was used to compute intra-class correlation coefficients (ICC) for the seven-day test–retest administration of the surveys. The minimum threshold for re-test was an ICC of 0.40 [12, 16]. We determined the number of participants required for test–retest reliability assessment based on a target of 0.80 (excellent) ICC for the pair of total scores on each measure against an ICC of 0.50 (fair). On this basis, we estimated that at least 21 participants would be needed [16]. Construct validity was evaluated by using confirmatory factor analysis; concurrent validity was evaluated by comparing the OAB knowledge and OAB attitude with ICIQ-UI scores. We also explored if OAB knowledge, OAB attitude and severity of symptoms (ICIQ-UI scores) varied by OAB treatment status.

Results

Literature review

From literature review we identified three preliminary OAB knowledge and attitude concepts: (1) OAB symptoms and treatment; (2) psychological symptoms (e.g., anxiety, depression, fear, frustration), and (3) social symptoms (e.g., disease stigma, intimacy and sexuality, embarrassment, diminished work productivity). We used these concepts and expert feedback to develop an initial conceptual model and focus group script.

Focus group

Five focus group meetings of patients (total $n = 62$) were conducted. Two focus groups consisted of participants recruited from a database of women who failed prescreening for enrollment in a urinary incontinence prevention study. The third and fourth focus group consisted of women who received care from a large urban academic healthcare system. The fifth focus group consisted of female members of the Living Independently for Elders program. Not all focus group participants reported having OAB. Average length of each focus group was 45 min. In addition, two provider focus groups were conducted. One consisted of primary care physicians, geriatricians, and geriatric nurse practitioners. The other one was among providers of the Living Independently for Elders program.

Data collection continued until saturation occurred [13–15]. Content analysis was performed through open coding by the same investigator [13–15]. Peer review and consistency of the analysis occurred whereby another investigator independently analyzed transcripts using open coding and then crosschecked for discrepancies.

Item Development

Informed by literature review and focus groups, we created an initial pool of 18 and 19 items for OAB-knowledge and OAB-attitude surveys, respectively. OAB-knowledge items were related to three general themes: perception of OAB; cause of and information about OAB; and signs of OAB. OAB-attitude items were related to three general themes of treatment seeking, decision making and effects of OAB.

Field versions of the measures were constructed as follows. The OAB-knowledge items used a 'yes'/'no' or 'don't know'; or 'true'/'false' or 'don't know' response format (each correct answer scored one and 'don't know' and incorrect responses scored zero). Responses to the OAB-attitude surveys were anchored by a five-point Likert type scale ('completely disagree', 'disagree', 'unsure', 'agree', and 'completely agree'). The order of the items was random. After eliminating the items that were duplicative, or unrelated to the constructs, we retained 16 items in each survey. Please see Additional file 1 for OAB knowledge and attitude surveys.

Cross sectional sample characteristics

To validate the OAB-knowledge and OAB-attitude surveys, we contacted 244 women in total. Of these 170 were from a database of women who failed prescreening for enrollment in a urinary incontinence prevention study; and the rest were identified from the administrative database of a large urban academic healthcare system. Of these 244 women, 115 provided written consent and 104 completed the assessments. A research coordinator administered the International Consultation of Incontinence Modular Questionnaire – Urinary Incontinence (ICIQ-UI) form, OAB-knowledge, and OAB-attitude surveys over telephone. Seven-day test–retest reliability was assessed among 21 randomly selected participants. More than 90%

of the participants were between the age of 56 and 75, about three-quarters were white, a large proportion were college educated, about half were retired and 60% were married.

In Tables 1 and 2, show the response distribution for the OAB-knowledge and OAB-attitude surveys. The average OAB knowledge score was 9.1 (±1.9). The possible range is 0 to 16 and higher score represents better OAB knowledge. The average attitude score was 42.8 (±6.6). The possible range for attitude score is 16–80, and lower score represents more positive attitude towards OAB care. Almost all participants had heard of OAB and were aware of treatment options for OAB (98%). Most agreed that treatment benefits outweigh its costs (76%), Slightly more than half said they were very likely to seek treatment for OAB (54%). The women in our sample were very likely to seek behavioral treatment (such as such as Kegel exercise) for OAB than pharmacological treatment (72% vs. 8%). A large proportion of women thought that OAB will very likely cause stigma (47%) and affect quality of life (40%).

The mean ICIQ score was 6.6 (SD 3.3). The total ICIQ score ranges from 0 to 21 and a higher score indicates greater severity of symptoms (Table 3). Factor analysis yielded a three-factor solution for the obliquely rotated factor pattern for the surveys. We identified three OAB knowledge factors - perception of OAB, cause and information, and signs of OAB; and three OAB-attitude factors - treatment seeking, decision-making, and effects of OAB. Inter-correlations of the sub-scales supported the validity of a single, higher order OAB-knowledge and OAB-attitude scales, which was not refuted by the confirmatory factor analysis, thus helping establish the construct validity of the surveys.

Table 1 Overactive Bladder (OAB) Knowledge ($n = 104$)

Have you heard of overactive bladder syndrome (OAB), which includes urinary urgency, frequency, and nocturia with or without urgency incontinence? (% yes)	98.1		
Knowledge items (%)	True	False	Don't know
OAB is a natural aging process	52.9	43.3	3.9
OAB happens mostly in women	59.6	34.6	5.8
There are no treatments for OAB	6.7	92.3	0.96
OAB is related to childbirth	44.2	53.9	1.9
My doctor can tell me if I have OAB	68.3	30.8	0.96
Any sickness can cause OAB	39.4	54.8	5.8
OAB has specific symptoms	91.4	7.7	0.96
Treatments for OAB have many side effects	27.9	70.2	1.9
OAB is a chronic disease	42.3	55.8	1.9
OAB can go away on its own	17.3	80.8	1.9
I can get all information about OAB from internet	34.6	63.5	1.9
Pharmacological (i., e drug) treatment is available for OAB	86.5	11.5	1.9
OAB is caused by an enlarged prostate	42.3	52.9	4.8
Insurance does not cover treatment for OAB	12.5	77.9	9.6
OAB medication is too expensive	23.1	63.5	13.5
The benefit of OAB medication is worth the cost	76.0	17.3	6.7
Total OAB knowledge score (mean, std)	9.1 (±1.9)		

The total scores of the OAB-knowledge and OAB-attitude surveys demonstrated statistically significant correlations with the ICIQ total scores, 0.3231 ($p = 0.0009$) and – 0.4454 ($p < 0.0001$), respectively. The OAB-knowledge and attitude scores varied significantly between patients with low ICIQ scores (0–7), moderate ICIQ scores (8–14) and high ICIQ scores (15–21). The mean knowledge scores were 8.6 (±1.6), 9.4 (±1.0) and 10.8 (±0.5) for the low, moderate and high ICIQ score groups, respectively. Similarly, the mean attitude scores were 44.8 (±5.2), 42.0 (±6.9) and 33.2 (±3.3) for the low, moderate and high ICIQ score groups, respectively. These associations between OAB knowledge scores, OAB attitude scores and ICIQ scores helped establish the concurrent validity of the surveys. Finally, all OAB-knowledge and OAB-attitude sub-scales demonstrated high test-retest reliability, with Cronbach's α for each exceeding our a priori threshold of ≥0.70, indicating good test-retest reliability of the surveys.

Seventy-six (73.1%) women were treatment naïve whereas 28 (26.9%) had either pharmacological or behavioral treatment for OAB. We did not obtain data on treatment length or treatment compliance. The mean OAB knowledge score was 9.0 (SD 8.7) for the treatment naïve group, and 9.3 (SD 8.4) for those with treatment ($p = 0.6446$; effect size 0.10). Mean attitude score was 42.6 (SD 6.6) for the treatment naïve group, and 43.3 (SD 6.4) for those with treatment ($p = 0.5956$; effect size 0.12). Finally, the severity of symptoms as measured by ICIQ-UI was 5.9 (Sd 3.3) for the treatment group, compared to 7.0 (SD 3.6) for the treatment naïve group ($p = 0.1812$; effect size 0.29).

Discussion

Our OAB-knowledge and attitude surveys are an important step in assessment of the association between OAB knowledge, attitude, and treatment uptake and treatment compliance. We observed some difference in the OAB knowledge, OAB attitude, and severity of symptoms across treatment status. Though we did not find statistical significance in these differences, they may be potentially modifiable factors that affect OAB treatment uptake and treatment compliance.

Approximately 33 million Americans (16.5% of the U.S. population) experience OAB [1–9]. The genesis of

Table 2 Overactive Bladder (OAB) Attitude ($n = 104$)

Attitude items (%)	Very likely	Somewhat likely	Neutral	Somewhat unlikely	Very Unlikely
How likely are you to ask your doctor about OAB?	45.2	24.0	4.8	14.4	11.5
If you have OAB, how likely are you to seek treatment?	53.9	28.9	3.9	6.3	6.3
How likely will you research about OAB?	52.9	29.8	5.8	3.9	7.7
How likely are you to seek pharmacological (drug) treatment for OAB?	7.7	33.7	10.6	25.9	22.2
How likely are you to seek behavioral (such as Kegel exercise) treatment for OAB?	72.1	23.1	1.9	0.96	1.9
How likely are you to seek surgery for OAB?	3.9	9.6	11.5	25.0	50.0
How likely will you seek other medical treatment for OAB? (e.g.acupuncture, yoga, meditation, herbal medicine, etc.)	32.7	34.6	14.4	13.5	4.8
How likely will side effects of a treatment affect your decision to seek treatment?	58.7	29.8	6.7	3.9	0.96
What is the likelihood OAB is causing you embarrassment?	47.1	31.7	4.8	7.7	8.9
How likely will OAB affect your quality of life?	40.4	30.8	7.7	13.5	7.7
How likely will cost affect your decision to seek treatment of OAB	10.6	27.9	9.6	29.0	27.9
What is the likelihood that wearing pads for protection will bother you?	17.3	25.9	12.5	20.2	24.0
How likely will you simply ignore the OAB problem?	5.8	11.5	2.9	26.9	52.9
How likely will you be to support a public health campaign about OAB awareness?	65.4	25.9	4.8	2.9	0.96
How likely would you be to discuss OAB with friends and family?	49.0	37.5	3.9	6.7	2.9
How likely would you be to continue with OAB treatment despite side effects?	11.5	27.9	22.1	25.0	13.5
Total OAB attitude score (mean, std)	42.8 (±6.6)				

symptoms of OAB commonly is multi-factorial, and thus multimodal therapy that includes pharmacologic and non-pharmacologic interventions may be necessary. However, OAB remains underdiagnosed and undertreated. A Finnish study analyzed the effects of frequency of urinary urgency and urge urinary incontinence on symptom-related bother, HRQoL, and the clinically meaningful prevalence of overactive bladder [17]. The study consisted of 6000 subjects (age 18–79 years) randomly identified from the Finnish population register in 2003–2004, with 62.4% responding. Urgency was reported by more than half, whereas urinary incontinence was reported by 25.7% of women. It was concluded that increased severity of urgency and urinary incontinence is associated with a statistically significant and clinically important decrease in HRQoL.

Older age, genetics, female sex, pregnancy, childbirth, stress and extreme physical activity are generally perceived as causes of OAB. Symptoms are under-reported in women, mainly due to limited understanding of or appreciation of the morbidity of the condition. Women tend to think of OAB as normal part of aging and develop coping mechanisms, rather than seeking care [3]. The cultural model constructed by women differs significantly from the professional model that emerged from media representations of female urinary incontinence [18]. Despite a wide variety of treatments for OAB, many women choose not to seek care [19–21]. Further exploration of the "disconnect" between the experiences of women who live with urinary incontinence and common public views of female urinary incontinence may lead to an increased appreciation and understanding of these issues [22]. A mixed-methods study conducted needs assessment of OAB patients. Significant time-gap was noted between the onset of OAB symptoms and diagnosis of OAB. This indicates need for better OAB screening and diagnosis [23].

Our results make important contribution to the existing research on OAB. Our cohort of women thought that OAB happens mostly in women. A large proportion had heard of OAB and was aware of treatments options for OAB. Also, most agreed that treatment benefits outweigh its costs, however, only half said they were very likely to seek treatment for OAB. The women in our sample were more likely to seek behavioral treatment or self-management for OAB than pharmacological treatment. A large proportion of women thought that OAB will likely cause stigma and affect quality of life.

Table 3 ICIQ UI Short Form ($n = 104$)

ICIQ items	
How often do you leak urine? (%)	
Never	26.9
About once a week or less	41.4
2–3 times a day	20.2
About once a day	7.7
Several times a day	3.9
All the time	0.0
How much urine do you think usually leaks (whether you wear protection or not)? (%)	
None	22.1
A small amount	69.2
A moderate amount	8.7
A large amount	0.0
Overall, on a scale from zero to 10, where zero is "not at all" and 10 is a "great deal", How much does leaking urine interfere with your everyday life?	Mean = 1.8 (±2.3)
Total ICIQ score	Mean = 6.6 (±3.3)
Does urine leak (% yes)	
Before you go to the toilet?	60.6
When you cough or sneeze?	51.9
When you are asleep?	7.7
When you are physically active or exercising?	27.9
When you have finished urinating and are dressed?	14.4
For no obvious reason	16.4
All the time?	0.96
Never – urine does not leak	22.2

We note following limitations to the study. First limitation is selection bias as participants were either self-selected to enroll in a urinary incontinence prevention study or were selected from a large urban academic healthcare system database. Hence, symptom severity of women in our cohort may not be representative of the general population of women with OAB. Participants were recruited via telephone during business hours and some of the focus groups also were held during those hours. As a result, the majority of those participated were retired, and older. Therefore, we may not have fully captured the experiences of younger adult women with OAB or of men with OAB. Additionally, the ICIQ-UI survey is not validated for telephone administration. Another limitation is that of discrepancies and biases in qualitative data analysis. To minimize this, two investigators analyzed the data separately. Finally, we did not collect information about length of OAB treatment, or treatment compliance that may affect overall association between treatment status, OAB knowledge and OAB attitude. While usually not life threatening, OAB has a significant negative impact on quality of life and can adversely affect self-esteem, resulting in embarrassment, diminished social relations, sexual satisfaction, professional and social life interactions, and overall wellbeing [22–28].

Our surveys must be refined for assessment among different subpopulations based on age, gender, and functional status. Knowledge plays an important role in shaping a person's attitude toward behavior, subjective norms, and perceived behavioral control. Our study provides effect sizes for OAB knowledge, OAB attitude and ICI UI scores. These effect sizes can form the basis for developing a fully powered trial to study the association between OAB knowledge and attitude, type and length of treatment, treatment compliance, and quality of life, leading to interventions for enhancing OAB care.

Funding
Asellas Pharma, Inc. (US).

Authors' contributions
SC - Conception and design, Acquisition of data, Data analysis, Manuscript writing/editing. DKN - Manuscript writing/editing. AJW - Manuscript writing/editing. AEJ - Data collection or management. JSS - Manuscript writing/editing. RJ - Obtaining funding, Conception and design, Acquisition of data, Data analysis, Manuscript writing/editing. All authors read and approved the final manuscript.

Competing interests
The authors declare that they have no competing interests.

Author details
[1]Department of Psychiatry, Perelman School of Medicine, University of Pennsylvania, 3535 Market St., Suite 4051, Philadelphia, PA 19104, USA. [2]Division of Urology, Department of Surgery, Perelman School of Medicine, University of Pennsylvania, Philadelphia, PA 19104, USA. [3]Department of Medicine, Perelman School of Medicine, University of Pennsylvania, Philadelphia, PA 19104, USA. [4]Departments of Medicine and Health Management, Leonard Davis Institute of Health Economics, University of Pennsylvania, Perelman School of Medicine and Wharton School of Business, Philadelphia, PA 19104, USA. [5]Departments of Medicine and Surgery, Divisions of Geriatrics and Urology, Perelman School of Medicine Leonard Davis Institute of Health Economics, University of Pennsylvania, Philadelphia, PA 19104, USA.

References

1. Abrams P, et al. The standardization of terminology of lower urinary tract function: report from the standardization sub-committee of the international continence society. Neurourol Urodyn. 2002;21:167–78.
2. Stewart WF, et al. Prevalence and burden of overactive bladder in the United States. World J Urol. 2003;20:327–36.
3. Diokno AC, et al. Perceptions and behaviours of women with bladder control problems. Fam Pract. 2006;23(5):568–77.
4. Irwin DE, et al. Population-based survey of urinary incontinence, overactive bladder, and other lower urinary tract symptoms in five countries: results of the EPIC study. Eur Urol. 2006;50:1306–15.
5. Milsom I, et al. Global prevalence and economic burden of urgency urinary incontinence: a systematic review. Eur Urol. 2014;65:79–95.

6. Anger JT, et al. Health literacy and disease understanding among aging women with pelvic floor disorders. Female Pelvic Med Reconstr Surg. 2012;18(6):340–3.
7. Anger JT, et al. Women's experience with severe overactive bladder symptoms and treatment: insight revealed from patient focus groups. Neurourol Urodyn. 2011;30:1295–9.
8. Burgio KL, et al. Impact of behavior and lifestyle on bladder health. Int J Clin Pract. 2013;67(6):495–504.
9. Coyne KS, et al. The prevalence of lower urinary tract symptoms (LUTS) and overactive bladder (OAB) by racial/ethnic group and age: results from OAB-POLL. Neurourol Urodyn. 2013;32(3):230–7.
10. Ajen I. The theory of planned behavior. Organ Behav Hum Decis Process. 1991;50:179–211.
11. Gagnon L, Simard A, Tu L. Knowledge about urology in the general population: alarming results. Can Urol Assoc J. 2009;3(5):388–91.
12. Borenstein M, Hedges L.V, Higgins J.P.T, Rothstein H.R. Introduction to meta analysis. Chichester, UK: Wiley; 2009.
13. DeWalt DA, et al. Evaluation of item candidates: the PROMIS qualitative item review. Med Care. 2007;45:S12–21.
14. Morgan DL. Focus groups as qualitative research. California: Sage University Press; 2009.
15. Reeve BB, et al. Psychometric evaluation and calibration of health-related quality of life item banks: plans for the patient-reported outcomes measurement information system (PROMIS). Med Care. 2007;45:S22–31.
16. Kraemer H, Thiemann S. How Many Subjects? Statistical Power Analysis in Research. California: Sage; 1987.
17. Tikkinen KAO, Tammela TLJ, Rissanen AM, Valpas A, Huhtala H, et al. Is the Prevalence of Overactive Bladder Overestimated? A Population-Based Study in Finland. PLoS ONE. 2007;2(2):e195. https://doi.org/10.1371/journal.pone.0000195.
18. Bradway CW, Barg F. Developing a cultural model for a long-term female urinary incontinence. Soc Sci Med. 2006;63:3150–61.
19. Hägglund D, et al. Reasons why women with long-term urinary incontinence do not seek professional help: a cross-sectional population-based cohort study. Int Urogynecol J. 2003;14:296–304.
20. Shaw C, et al. Barriers to help seeking in people with urinary symptoms. Fam Pract. 2001;18:48–52.
21. Wein AJ, Rovner ES. Definition and epidemiology of overactive bladder. Urology. 2002;60(suppl 5A):7–12.
22. Taylor DW, et al. The self-reported prevalence and knowledge of urinary incontinence and barriers to health care-seeking in a community sample of Canadian women. Am J Med Sci. 2013;3(5):97–102.
23. Filipetto FA, et al. The patient perspective on overactive bladder: a mixed-methods needs assessment. BMC Fam Pract. 2014;15:96.
24. Coyne KS, et al. An overactive bladder symptom and health-related quality of life short form: validation of the OAB-q SF. Neurourol Urodyn. 2015;34:255–63.
25. Hashim H, Brams P. How should patients with an overactive bladder manipulate their fluid intake? BJU International. 2008;102(1):62–6.
26. Kim TH, et al. Drug persistence and compliance affect patient-reported outcomes in overactive bladder syndrome. Qual Life Res. 2016;25:2021–9.
27. Wennberg AL, et al. A longitudinal population-based survey of urinary incontinence, overactive bladder, and other lower urinary tract symptoms in women. Eur Urol. 2009;55:783–91.
28. Willis-Gray MG, Dieter AA, Geller EJ. Evaluation and management of overactive bladder: strategies for optimizing care. Research and Reports in Urology. 2016;8:113–22.

With a new clip technique surgically inducing varicocele in Sprague-Dawley rats

Wen-bin Guo[1†], Cheng Yang[1†], Jun Bian[1†], Hui Xia[1], Jian-kun Yang[1], Qi-zhao Zhou[1], Ming-kun Chen[1], Kang-yi Xue[1], Wan-song Zhang[1], Peng Wang[1], Xin Li[2*] and Cun-dong Liu[1*]

Abstract

Background: We introduced and recreated a more consistent and effective experimental varicocele rat model by a new clip technique.

Methods: A total of 40 rats were numbered and randomly assigned to 5 groups of 8 each, including sham surgery (Group I), conventional (Group II) and clip groups with 0.7, 0.8, 0.9 mm gap widths, respectively (Group III, IV, V). All of the rats in each group were sacrificed at 8 weeks after initial surgery, and the rats forming out with less than 1 mm diameter of left spermatic vein or no presence of the pampiniform plexus dilation were excluded from the experimental groups. The left spermatic vein (LSV) diameter, testicular weight, left kidney weight to body weight coefficients, kidney and testicular histology were determined.

Results: The baseline mean diameter of the LSV in Group I, II and III was 0.22 ± 0.02, 0.23 ± 0.02 and 0.22 ± 0.03 mm, respectively ($P = 0.7504$). At 8 weeks after initial surgery, varicocele was successfully created in 6/8 (75%), 7/8 (87.5%), 3/8 (37.5%), 3/8 (37.5%) in GroupII-V, no varicocele was observed in Group I. In Group I, II and III, no pathological changes were observed and the left kidney weight to body weight coefficients showed no significant differences. The diameter of LSV was remarkably increased both in Group II and III compared to Group I (1.72 ± 0.13, 1.57 ± 0.19 and 0.25 ± 0.02, respectively), and Group II and III had a smaller testicular weight than the rats in Group I (1.67 ± 0.05, 1.62 ± 0.06, and 1.92 ± 0.12, respectively).

Conclusions: With a new clip technique, surgically inducing varicocele rat model becomes convenient and safe. This appears to improve the effectiveness of the model and this innovation may allow us to further understand the pathophysiology of varicocele.

Keywords: Clip, Varicocele, Spermatic vein, Rat model

Background

Varicocele (VC) is a condition characterized by the spermatic varicosity or abnormal dilation of testicular pampiniform venous plexus, and is present in 35% of men with primary infertility and in 70 to 81% with secondary infertility [1, 2]. Although it has been considered to be associated with male infertility, the exact pathophysiology of the varicocele is incompletely understood [3].

Specific questions regarding the pathophysiological of varicocele are even difficult to address in human. Several factors are often taken into account, such as limitedly acquisition of tissue, forbidden invasive experiment, or other indefinite characteristics [4]. Thus, this highlights the key role in the use of animal models. To date, the most widely used experimental varicocele rat model is to investigate the mechanisms underlying the varicocele-related male infertility. However, experimental rat model induced by the conventional technique has varied success [5–7]. In the present study, for the first time we used a clip technique mimicking the nutcracker phenomenon suffering a partial occlusion of the renal vein combined with ligation of the branches of the LSV to develop

* Correspondence: xinli268@gmail.com; cundongliu@163.com
†Wen-bin Guo, Cheng Yang and Jun Bian contributed equally to this work.
[2]Center for Clinical Research and Innovation, Shenzhen Hospital of Southern Medical University, Shenzhen, People's Republic of China
[1]Department of Urology, the Third Affiliated Hospital of Southern Medical University, No. 183 West Zhongshan Road, Tianhe District, 510630 Guangzhou, People's Republic of China

experimental rat varicocele model, which was more consistent and effective to help to create varicocele rat model.

Methods

Animal care

This study was approved by the animal care and ethics committee of the Southern Medical University. A total of 40 adult male specific-pathogen free (SPF) Sprague Dawley rats (*Rattus norvegicus*, age range from 7 weeks to 8 weeks, weighing 250–300 g) obtained from the animal center of Southern Medical University (certificate number: SYXK [Yue] 2011–0074), were housed in a climate controlled environment with free access to food and water under a 12-h day/night cycle. A 1-week acclimatization period was allowed prior to the experimental procedures.

Experimental design

The 40 rats were numbered and randomly assigned to 5 groups of 8 each, with the method of random digits table, including sham surgery (Group I), conventional group (Group II), clip groups (0.7 mm, 0.8 mm and 0.9 mm gap widths corresponding to Group III, IV, V, respectively) (obtained from ALCOTT BIOTECH, Shanghai, China). A sample size of 8 rats per group was sufficient according to our preliminary experiment and the previous study that the success rate of rat varicocele was ranged from 85 to 100% [8, 9]. At 8 weeks after initial surgery, all of the rats in each group were sacrificed. The postoperative outcomes were determined, including the left kidney histology, left kidney weight to body weight coefficients, the diameter of left spermatic vein (LSV), left testicular weight, histology and complications. The micrometer was used to measure the diameter of the LSV at the level of the crossing iliolumbar vein. All the operations were carried out by two skillful researchers, but they were not involved in the collection of data, analysis of results and evaluation of outcomes. All measurements were reviewed and based on agreement by 2 investigators independently. Other investigators and outcome assessors were blind to the groups.

Experimental procedures

In the present study, we created varicocele model in male Sprague-Dawley rats according to the procedures previously described by Turner TT [4], with partially occluding left renal vein and completely ligating the branches of the LSV. All experimental procedures were performed in a sterile environment. Briefly, after 12 h fasting, the rats were anesthetized using an intraperitoneal injection of 30 mg/kg sodium pentobarbital. The experimental rats were considered anaesthetized when holding and pressing the paw did not elicit a response from the rats. A midline laparotomy incision was made from xyphoid to pubis to visualize the left kidney, left adrenal vein, the left renal vein and the LSV and its collaterals. A tunnel was made around the left renal vein by careful blunt dissection, which was cleared of adhering tissue in a position medial to the insertion of the LSV and left adrenal vein. In Group II, a 4–0 silk suture was used for partially occluding of the left renal vein around a metal wire of 0.85 mm diameter at the point. The wire was then removed from the ligature, allowing the vein expand to an external diameter. In Group I, the rats with sham operation underwent a similar procedure that the left renal vein was dissected free but not ligated. In Group III, IV, and V, the clips with 0.7 mm, 0.8 mm and 0.9 mm gap widthsinstead of suture ligature was placed at the same point on the renal vein. Finally, the collaterals of the LSV were completely occluded and then the incision was closed in two layers with 3–0 silk sutures.

Histopathology assessment

After 8 weeks, the testes and kidneys were harvested and weighted. Half of each kidney and testis was fixed in 4% paraformaldehyde and modified Davidson's Fluid's solution [10], respectively. These were postfixed in 70% alcohol and embedded in paraffin blocks after tissue processing. Sections (5 μm) from testes were obtained, deparaffinized and stained with hematoxylin and eosin. Disintegration of the germinal epithelium and degenerative appearance in each group was observed by light microscopy. For kidney histology, sections were stained with periodic acid-Schiff (PAS) and Masson's trichrome (Baso, Zhuhai, China). Histopathology analysis was performed by two uropathologists independently.

Statistical analysis

Statistical analysis was performed using SPSS 20, and all data are presented as the mean ± SD. Comparisons of all 3 groups and 2 groups were made using the Kruskal-Wallis and the Games-Howell test for continuous variables, respectively. A value of $P < 0.05$ was considered statistically significance.

Results

The characteristics of experimental varicocele development in each group

Some complications occurred in study. For example, Group II had 1 rat tearing of vein or bleeding and 1 rat pyonephrosis, which lead to model failure. In Group IV and V, there were 3/8, and 5/8 clips showing slipping off the renal vein, respectively, while in Group III no severe complication happened and all rats had successful except for one rat failing to form varicocele. According to the criteria of VC model, the rats forming out with more than 1 mm diameter of left spermatic vein or presence of the pampiniform plexus dilation [4] in each group were included in the experimental groups [Fig. 1]. According to Table 1, we selected Group III for further analysis, excluding Groups IV and V because that the number of inducing varicocele is not enough to allow for extrapolations from the proposed statistics.

Baseline anatomy and outcomes

The mean baseline of total body weight of rats among Group I, II and III was 331.25 ± 8.27, 329.13 ± 13.66 and 326.75 ± 12.49 g, respectively ($P = 0.6992$). Baseline mean diameter of the left spermatic vein in these three groups was 0.22 ± 0.02, 0.23 ± 0.02 and 0.22 ± 0.03 mm, respectively ($P = 0.7504$). At 8 weeks after initial surgery, the size was remarkably increased when measuring the diameter of LSV both in Group II and III compared with Group I (1.72 ± 0.13, 1.57 ± 0.19 and 0.25 ± 0.02, respectively, $P < 0.0001$, Fig. 2a). No significant difference was observed between Group II and III ($P = 0.275$). Group II and III had smaller testicular weight compared with Group I (1.67 ± 0.05,1.62 ± 0.06, and 1.92 ± 0.12 respectively, $P < 0.0001$, Fig. 2b). There was also no difference between Group II and III ($P = 0.196$).

Evaluation of experimental varicocele model

After 8 weeks, macroscopic changes in the left kidney were carefully identified and compared with the right kidney. No pathological changes were observed in Group I, II and III [Fig. 3a]. The left kidney weight to body weight coefficients showed no significant differences among these three groups [Fig. 3b]. When calculating the numbers of degenerating tubules and compared the degenerating tubule percentages among these three groups, we found the percentage both in Group II and III were statistically significantly increased as compared with Group I [Fig. 4], which indicate impairment of spermatogenesis.

Table 1 The characteristics of experimental varicocele development in each group

Group	Number	Survival rate	Complications	Varicocele	Success rate
I[a]	8	100%	0	0	0
II[a]	8	100%	3[b]	6	75%
III[a]	8	100%	0	7	87.5%
IV[a]	8	100%	0	3	37.5%
V[a]	8	100%	0	3	37.5%

[a]I: Sham II: Conventional III: 0.7 mm clip IV: 0.8 mm clip V: 0.9 mm clip
[b]2 rats bleeding and 1 pyonephrosis

Discussions

Despite the fact that varicocele associated with male subfertility is widely accepted [11], the pathophysiology of varicocele has been poorly understood. With rare exception, varicocele does occur exclusively in humans, which are more difficult to address. Thus, the use of animal models has played an essential role in understanding this condition. In 1981, Saypol et al. [12] reported that surgically induced varicocele using partial left renal vein occlusion had influence on testicular blood flow, temperature, and histology in adult rats and dogs. Subsequently, many studies investigating on the pathophysiology underlying varicocele associated with infertility were conducted by this method [4, 13–15]. As similarities existed in venous anatomy between the rat and human when left varicocele occurs [16], since then experimental varicocele in rat has been the most widely used animal model. However, it has resulted in varied success except for interlaboratory and interoperator intrinsic variability [6, 7].

Previous studies on the variable vascular anatomy in rats may contribute to develop varicocele rat model [5, 17, 18]. In most rats, the left venous pampiniform plexus drains primarily into the left common iliac and a smaller internal spermatic vein to the left renal vein [5, 19]. In the present study, we created varicocele rat

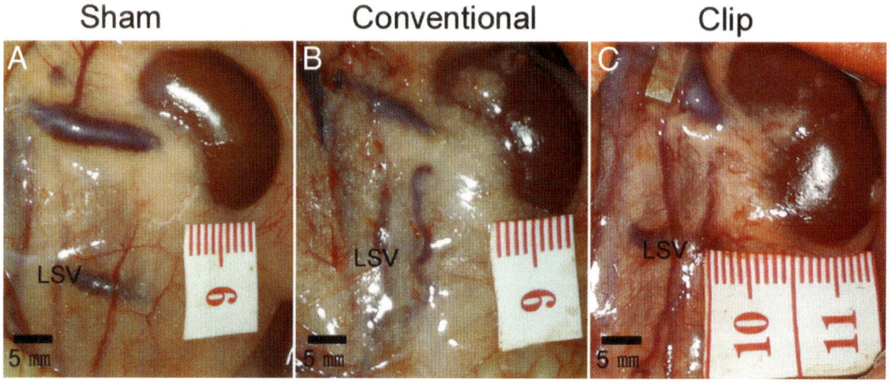

Fig. 1 The left spermatic vein (LSV) varicosity. At 8 weeks after initial surgery, (**a**, **b**, **c**) the LSV showed obvious dilatation in the conventional and clip groups compared to sham surgery. Scale bar = 5 mm

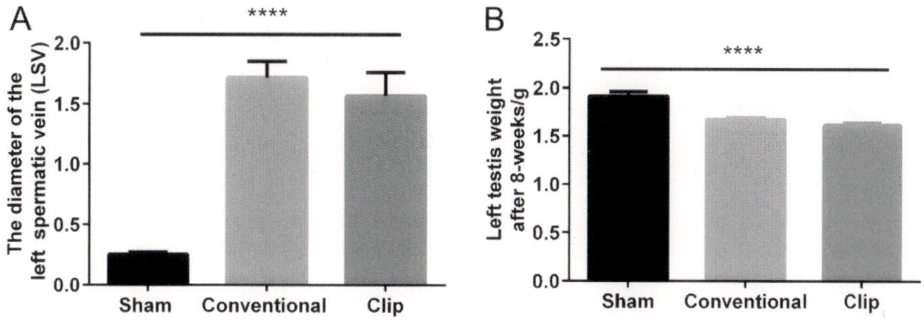

Fig. 2 The diameter of the left spermatic vein (LSV) **a** At 8 weeks after initial surgery, the diameter of LSV was remarkably larger and **b** the left testis weight was smaller in the conventional and clip groups when compared with sham surgery (****$P < 0.0001$)

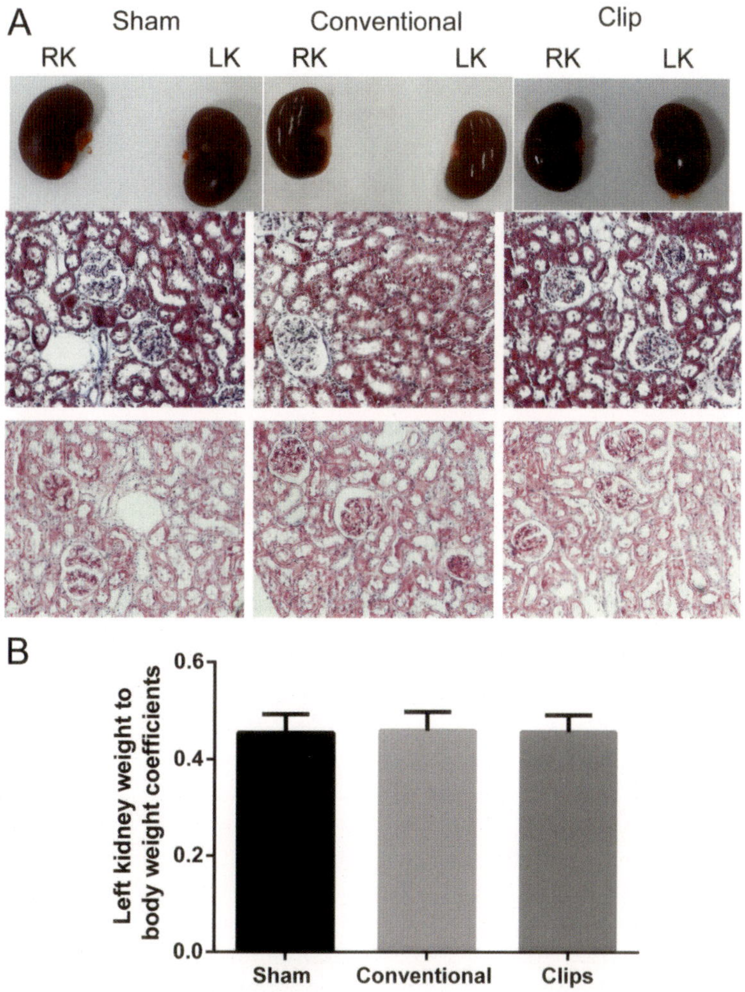

Fig. 3 Histopathology assessment of left kidney. (**a**) (a, b, c) Masson's Trichrome staining and (d, e, f) PAS staining of the left kidney showed no significantly pathological changes in the sham, conventional and clip groups after 8 weeks. Scale bar = 50 μm. Right kidney: RK, Left kidney: LK. (**b**) The left kidney weight to body weight coefficients showed no significant differences among these three groups

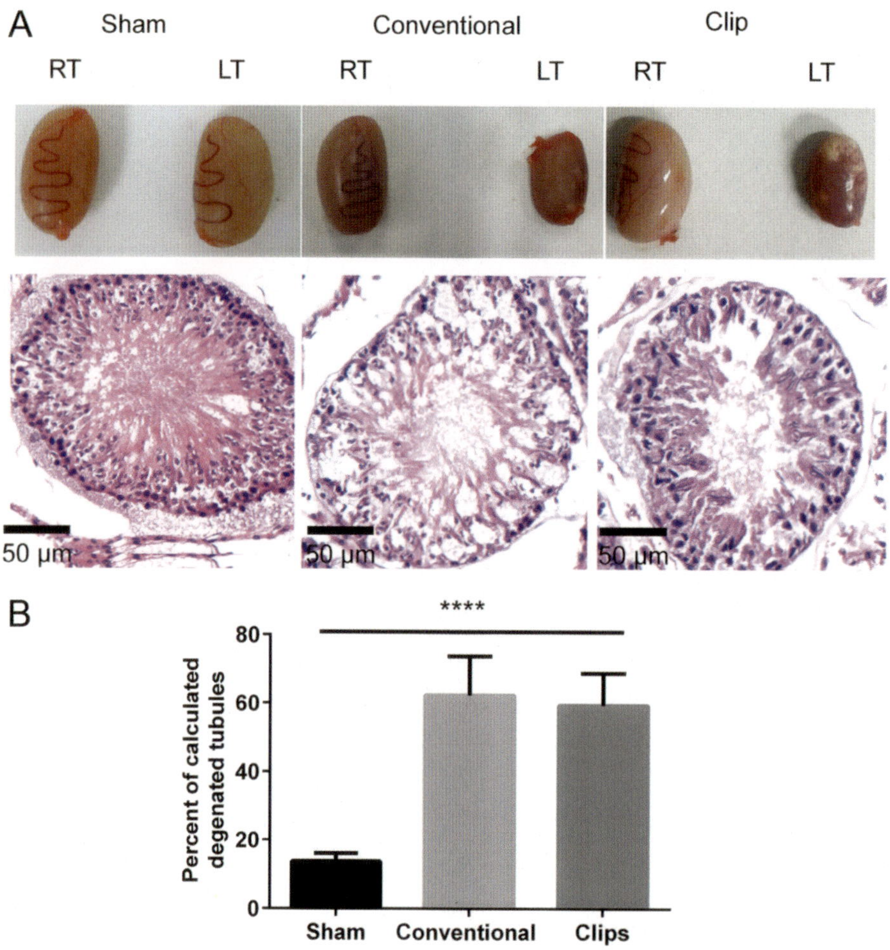

Fig. 4 Hematoxylin and eosin stained rat left testicular tissues after 8 weeks. **a** When compared with the sham group, rats showed an apparent degeneration of the tubules (magnification 40X) and **b** the percentage of degenerated tubules was significantly higher (****$P < 0.0001$) in the conventional and clip groups. Scale bar = 50 μm. Right testis: RT, Left testis: LT

model by partially occluded the renal vein combined with completely ligation of the collaterals of the left spermatic vein with minor modifications. Furthermore, to improve the efficacy and create a consistent rat varicocele model, we used a novel clip technique usually applied to produce hypertension in the 2K1C model (2-kidney, 1-clip) [20]. The clip has more advantages of accurate and consistent reduction of renal vein diameter than suture ligation. To date, a key factor in current varicocele model is the potential for a correct and consistent degree of obstruction as a result of too much reduction in renal vein resulting necrosis or too little construction failing to form varicocele. Thus, clips with 0.7, 0.8 and 0.9 mm gap widths were selected in our study according to the 0.85 mm diameter as criteria reported by Turner TT [4]. At 8 weeks after initial operation, clip with 0.7 mm gap widths was appropriate and selected for further analysis in the study. No macroscopic changes and histological findings in the kidneys were observed among Group I, II and III, indicating there was no renal lesion paralleling the clinical findings of varicocele in humans [21]. The Group III had larger mean diameter of left spermatic vein and worse testicular histology than the Group I, similar to Group II but showing no significant difference. These results were accordance with these studies previously reported [18, 22].

Moreover, success rate of experimental varicocele rat model, up to a certain extent, depends on the complications during the operation [9]. In this study, the success rate in group 2 is only 75% (6/8). Many factors may account for this, including vascular injury, pyonephrosis. Sometimes when blinded to dissect behind the renal vein, inadvertent puncture or tear of the vein often occurs, resulting in excessive bleeding. Vascular injury also happens just when ligating the left renal vein. In Group II, 1 rat with pyonephrosis is mainly due to mistakenly ligation of ureter adjacent to spermatic vein, leading to obstructive hydronephrosis and infection. Using clip technique, we found no complications in Group III, and the success rate is 87.5% (7/8) except for 1 rat failing to form a varicocele because of one clip dislodging from the renal vein. Although the effects of clip technique on varicocele in this study, the convenient and safe model constitutes a basis for investigating on male infertility underlying varicocele, which is still further evaluated in subsequent studies that also need to expand the sample size.

There were also some inadequacies in this model. In Group IV and V, these clips were slipped off or dislodged from the renal vein, resulting in failing to form varicocele. The clip needs to be designed to eliminate the possibility of dislodgement after implantation with some modifications. In addition, although clip with 0.7 mm gap widths was appropriate in this model, the different diameters of clips should be further investigated in different characteristics of species, age, and weight in rat.

Conclusion

With a new clip technique, surgically inducing varicocele rat model becomes convenient and safe. This appears to improve the effectiveness of the model and this innovation may allow us to further understand the pathophysiology of varicocele.

Abbreviations

2K1C: 2-kidney, 1-clip; LSV: Left spermatic vein; PAS: Periodic acid-Schiff; SD: Standard deviation; SPF: Specific-pathogen free; VC: Varicocele

Acknowledgements

The authors thank Dayu Han and Bing Yao for their contributions to the technique support of the model.

Funding

This study was supported in part by the Guangdong Provincial Science and Technology Program (No.2014A020212204; No.2013B021800317), Guangdong Provincial Natural Science Foundation of China (No.2015A030310027), Science and Technology Innovation Project of Southern Medical University (QD2014N005), Medical Scientific Research Foundation of Guangdong Province (A2014430) and National Natural Science Foundation of China (81772257).

Authors' contributions

CDL and XL designed the study. QZZ, MKC and KYX carried out the experiments of animal surgery. WSZ and PW conducted the PAS and Masson's trichrome assays, HX and JKY participated in acquisition of data. CY and WBG analyzed the experimental data and drafted the manuscript. WBG also participated in revising the manuscript critically for important intellectual content and made substantial contributions to conception and design of the study. XL and JB participated in the revising of the manuscript. All authors read and approved the final manuscript.

Competing interests

The authors declare that they have no competing interests.

References

1. Dubin L, Amelar RD. Etiologic factors in 1294 consecutive cases of male infertility. Fertil Steril. 1971;22(8):469–74.
2. Gorelick JI, Goldstein M. Loss of fertility in men with varicocele. Fertil Steril. 1993;59(3):613–6.
3. Naughton CK, Nangia AK, Agarwal A. Pathophysiology of varicoceles in male infertility. Hum Reprod Update. 2001;7(5):473–81.
4. Turner TT. The study of varicocele through the use of animal models. Hum Reprod Update. 2001;7(1):78–84.
5. Pascual JA, Lemmi C, Rajfer J. Variability of venous anatomy of rat testis: application to experimental testicular surgery. Microsurgery. 1992;13(6):335–7.
6. Hsu HS, Chang LS, Chen MT, Wei YH. Decreased blood flow and defective energy metabolism in the varicocele-bearing testicles of rats. Eur Urol. 1994;25(1):71–5.
7. Li H, Dubocq F, Jiang Y, Tiguert R, Gheiler EL, Dhabuwala CB. Effect of surgically induced varicocele on testicular blood flow and Sertoli cell function. Urology. 1999;53(6):1258–62.
8. Yao B, Zhou WL, Han DY, Ouyang B, Chen X, Chen SF, Deng CH, Sun XZ. The effect of the degree of left renal vein constriction on the development of adolescent varicocele in Sprague-Dawley rats. Asian J Androl. 2016;18(3): 471.
9. Zhou T, Cao H, Chen G, Yang B, Sun Y. Outcomes of experimental rat varicocele with and without microsurgery. BMC Urol. 2015;15(1):19.
10. Tu L, Yu L, Zhang H. Morphology of rat testis preserved in three different fixatives. J Huazhong Univ Sci Technolog Med Sci. 2011;31(2):178–80.
11. RUSSELL JK. Varicocele in groups of fertile and subfertile males. Br Med J. 1954;1(4873):1231–3.
12. Saypol DC, Howards SS, Turner TT, Miller EJ. Influence of surgically induced varicocele on testicular blood flow, temperature, and histology in adult rats and dogs. J Clin Invest. 1981;68(1):39–45.
13. Rajfer J, Turner TT, Rivera F, Howards SS, Sikka SC. Inhibition of testicular testosterone biosynthesis following experimental varicocele in rats. Biol Reprod. 1987;36(4):933–7.
14. Barqawi A, Caruso A, Meacham RB. Experimental varicocele induces testicular germ cell apoptosis in the rat. J Urol. 2004;171(1):501–3.
15. Sahin Z, Celik-Ozenci C, Akkoyunlu G, Korgun ET, Acar N, Erdogru T, Demir R, Ustunel I. Increased expression of interleukin-1alpha and interleukin-1beta is associated with experimental varicocele. Fertil Steril. 2006;85(Suppl 1): 1265–75.
16. Turner TT, Howards SS. The venous anatomy of experimental left varicocele: comparison with naturally occurring left varicocele in the human. Fertil Steril. 1994;62(4):869–75.
17. Turner TT, Caplis LA, Brown KJ. Vascular anatomy of experimentally induced left varicocele in the rat. Lab Anim Sci. 1996;46(2):206–10.
18. Zhang LT, Kim HK, Choi BR, Zhao C, Lee SW, Jang KY, Park JK. Analysis of testicular-internal spermatic vein variation and the recreation of varicocoele in a Sprague-Dawley rat model. Andrology. 2014;2(3):466–73.
19. Lewis MH, Moffat DB. The venous drainage of the accessory reproductive organs of the rat with special reference to prostatic metabolism. J Reprod Fertil. 1975;42(3):497–502.
20. Dussaule JC, Michel JB, Auzan C, Schwartz K, Corvol P, Menard J. Effect of antihypertensive treatment on the left ventricular isomyosin profile in one-clip, two kidney hypertensive rats. J Pharmacol Exp Ther. 1986;236(2):512–8.
21. Takemura T, Iwasa H, Yamamoto S, Hino S, Fukushima K, Isokawa S, Okada M, Yoshioka K. Clinical and radiological features in four adolescents with nutcracker syndrome. Pediatr Nephrol. 2000;14(10–11):1002–5.
22. Yao B, Zhou W, Han D, Ouyang B, Chen X, Chen S, Deng C, Sun X. The effect of the degree of left renal vein constriction on the development of adolescent varicocele in Sprague-Dawley rats. Asian J Androl. 2016;18(3):471.

Changes in renal papillary density after hydration therapy in calcium stone formers

Pietro Manuel Ferraro[1,5*†], Matteo Vittori[2,5†], Giuseppe Macis[3,5], Alessandro D'Addessi[2,5], Gianmarco Lombardi[1,5], Claudia Palmisano[3,5], Jacopo Gervasoni[4,5], Aniello Primiano[4,5], Pier Francesco Bassi[2,5] and Giovanni Gambaro[1,5]

Abstract

Background: Previous studies have shown that, compared with non-stone formers, stone formers have a higher papillary density measured with computer tomography (CT) scan. The effect of increased hydration on such papillary density in idiopathic calcium stone formers is not known.

Methods: Patients with recurrent calcium oxalate stones undergoing endourological procedures for renal stones at our Institution from June 2013 to June 2014 were considered eligible for enrolment. Enrolled patients underwent a baseline unenhanced CT scan before the urological procedure; after endoscopic removal of their stones, the patients were instructed to drink at least 2 L/day of a hypotonic, oligomineral water low in sodium and minerals (fixed residue at 180 °C < 200 mg/L) for at least 12 months. Finally, the patients underwent a follow-up unenhanced CT scan during hydration regimen.

Results: Twenty-five patients were prospectively enrolled and underwent baseline and follow-up CT scans. At baseline, mean papillary density was 43.2 ± 6.6 Hounsfield Units (HU) (43.2 ± 6.7 for the left kidney and 42.8 ± 7.1 HU for the right kidney). At follow-up and after at least 12 months of hydration regimen, mean papillary density was significantly reduced at 35.4 ± 4.2 HU (35.8 ± 5.0 for the left kidney and 35.1 ± 4.2 HU for the right kidney); the mean difference between baseline and follow-up was − 7.8 HU (95% confidence interval − 10.6 to − 5.1 HU, $p < 0.001$).

Conclusions: Increased fluid intake in patients with recurrent calcium oxalate stones was associated with a significant reduction in renal papillary density.

Keywords: Kidney stones, CT scan, Randall's plaque, Hydration therapy

Background

Kidney stones are an increasingly common condition, with an estimated prevalence in the United States of about 10%; [1] similar figures have been reported in European populations. [2] This condition is characterized by a relatively high frequency of recurrence [3] and elevated direct and indirect costs. [4] Kidney stones are most commonly composed of calcium; [5] a frequently seen lesion in calcium stone formers is the presence of suburothelial deposits of calcium phosphate known as Randall's plaques, which are thought to be the precursor lesion of idiopathic calcium oxalate stones. [6] Previous studies have shown that, compared with non-stone formers, stone formers have a higher papillary density measured with computer tomography (CT) scan, [7–11] likely reflecting the amount of calcium deposition within the renal parenchyma; it has also been suggested that papillary density values might correlate with first incident stones [12] and recurrent stones [13]. To date however, the effect of increased hydration on such papillary density in idiopathic calcium stone formers is not known. In our study, we analyzed changes in papillary density in recurrent idiopathic calcium stone formers before and after recommendations to increase fluid intake following urological stone removal.

* Correspondence: pietromanuel.ferraro@unicatt.it
†Pietro Manuel Ferraro and Matteo Vittori contributed equally to this work.
[1]U.O.C. Nefrologia, Fondazione Policlinico Universitario A. Gemelli IRCCS, Roma, Italia
[5]Università Cattolica del Sacro Cuore, Roma, Italia
Full list of author information is available at the end of the article

Methods

Patients undergoing endourological procedures for renal stones at our institution from June 2013 to June 2014 were considered eligible for enrolment. Inclusion criteria were recurrent stone disease and calcium oxalate stones (> 50% of the stone made of calcium oxalate). Stone composition was determined by Fourier transform infrared spectroscopy. Exclusion criteria were systemic conditions causing stones (hyperparathyroidism, intestinal malabsorption, renal tubular acidosis) and non-calcium oxalate stones. After signing written informed consent, patients underwent a baseline unenhanced CT scan before the urological procedure; the CT scans were performed using General Electric, Siemens, Philips and Toshiba equipment with a tube voltage variable from 120 to 140 kV, 80–643 mA and slices collimation from 1 to 5 mm. After endoscopic removal of their stones, the patients were instructed to drink at least 2 L/day of a hypotonic, oligomineral water low in sodium and minerals and rich in bicarbonate (fixed residue at 180 °C < 200 mg/L) for at least 12 months (Table 1). During follow-up, patients were contacted by phone every 3–4 months in order to maintain their adherence to increased hydration; at the first follow-up phone contact, patients were also asked to quantify the amount of fluid increase in terms of glasses per day (a glass would correspond to about 200 mL of water). Finally, the patients underwent a follow-up unenhanced CT scan during hydration regimen; this second CT was performed using similar technical specifications to the baseline CT scan. At that time point, blood and 24-h urine samples were also collected. Renal papillary density values were evaluated on baseline and follow-up CT scans and recorded as Hounsfield Unit (HU) values.

Six papillae were measured in each renal unit by randomly choosing two papillae from each of the major renal calyces (upper, middle and lower), as such that the densities of 12 renal papillae per patient were measured, and their means calculated. The images were magnified to 5× to prevent contamination of the region of interest with the fat in the renal sinus. The measurements of the renal papillae were made taking an area of 10 mm^2.

Table 1 Composition of the study water

Sodium	4.7
Calcium	57
Magnesium	3.5
Potassium	0.5
Bicarbonate	178
Fixed residue at 180 °C	178
pH	7.47

All values expressed as mg/L except for pH

All urine and serum analytes were measured in the central laboratory of Fondazione Policlinico Universitario Gemelli IRCCS on a Siemens ADVIA chemistry XPT with the following exceptions: urine citrate and oxalate were measured with LTA kit for enzymatic colorimetric determination.

Statistical analysis

Continuous variables were reported as means and standard deviations; categorical variables as frequencies and percentages. Arithmetic means of right and left renal papillary density measurements for each patient were calculated and used for statistical analysis. Differences between baseline and follow-up papillary density values were analyzed with paired t-tests; correlations between continuous variables were analyzed with Spearman tests. A p-value < 0.05 was considered statistically significant. Statistical analyses were performed with Stata 13.1 (StataCorp, TX, USA).

Results

Twenty-five patients were prospectively enrolled and underwent baseline and follow-up CT scans. Mean age at enrollment was 57 ± 17 years (range 18 to 78 years), 20 (80%) were males; average follow-up time was 22 ± 5 months (range 13 to 32 months); 22 patients received ureteroscopy and 3 percutaneous nephrolithotomy. All patients underwent measurements of papillary density on both kidneys except for one patient who had measurements taken only on the right kidney. At baseline, mean papillary density was 43.2 ± 6.6 HU (43.2 ± 6.7 for the left kidney and 42.8 ± 7.1 HU for the right kidney). At follow-up and after at least 12 months of hydration regimen, mean papillary density was significantly reduced at 35.4 ± 4.2 HU (35.8 ± 5.0 for the left kidney and 35.1 ± 4.2 HU for the right kidney); the mean difference between baseline and follow-up was − 7.8 HU (95% confidence interval − 10.6 to − 5.1 HU, $p < 0.001$). Individual changes in papillary density are represented in Fig. 1. The median self-reported increase in fluid intake during follow-up was 3 glasses (range 0 to 5 glasses). Blood and 24-h urine measurements performed at the time of follow-up CT scan are reported in Table 2. There was no correlation between the absolute change in papillary density and any of the laboratory measurements.

Discussion

In our study, we found that a course of hydration with oligomineral water after urological procedures of stone removal was associated with a significant reduction in renal papillary density as assessed with CT scan in a group of patients with recurrent calcium oxalate stones.

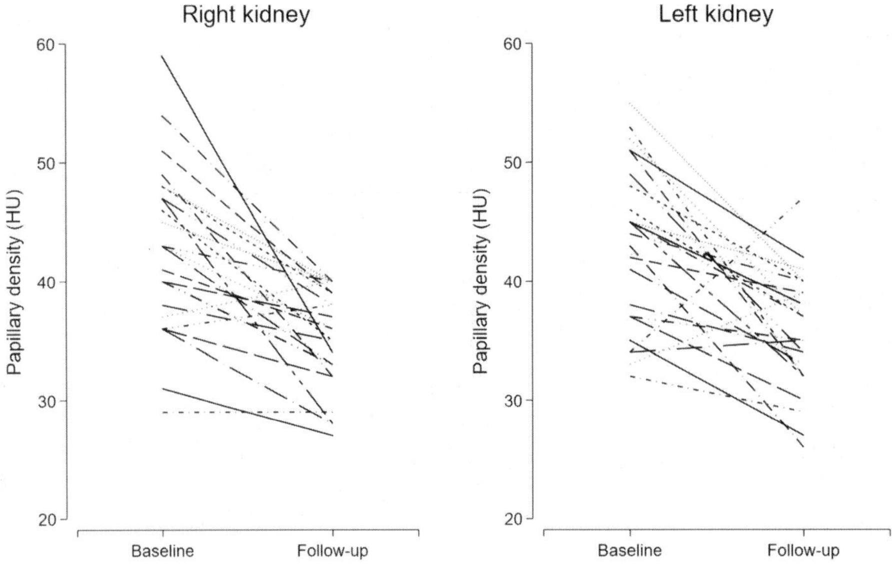

Fig. 1 Individual changes in renal papillary density before and after hydration

Several studies have investigated the association between kidney stones and increased renal papillary density. [7–11] Most studies found that the higher papillary density in stone formers is similar in affected and unaffected kidneys; it also seems to be independent of stone composition. [14] A few, retrospective, studies have also linked higher papillary density to higher likelihood of developing a first stone [12], as well as recurrent stones [13]. Only one study looked at the relationship between papillary density and the urinary metabolic profile, particularly urinary calcium excretion, and found no association, [11] which is consistent with our findings of a lack of association between changes in papillary density and blood and urine chemistries. Average HU values in previous studies ranged from 37 to 54 for stone formers and from 21 to 37 for controls, with some degree of heterogeneity likely explained by different study populations. Baseline HU values in our study (43.2 HU) were similar to those reported for stone formers in previous studies (average 42.1 HU, range 35.6 to 54.4 HU); [7–11] interestingly, follow-up HU values in our study (35.4 HU) were closer to the range of HU values previously reported for non-stone formers in those studies (average 29.5 HU, range 21.0 to 36.6 HU).

Table 2 Blood and 24 h urine chemistries

Blood	
Creatinine (mg/dL)	0.98 (0.23)
Calcium (mg/dL)	9.9 (0.3)
Phosphate (mg/dL)	3.4 (0.8)
Magnesium (mg/dL)	2.1 (0.1)
Sodium (mEq/L)	141 (2)
Potassium (mEq/L)	4.6 (0.7)
24 h urine	
Volume (mL/24 h)	2005 (765)
Creatinine (mg/24 h)	786 (340)
Calcium (mg/24 h)	98 (58)
Citrate (mg/24 h)	459 (208)
Oxalate (mg/24 h)	19 (13)
Uric acid (mg/24 h)	425 (192)
Phosphate (mg/24 h)	439 (164)
Magnesium (mg/24 h)	56 (27)
Sodium (mEq/24 h)	83 (30)
Potassium (mEq/24 h)	31 (12)

Data are expressed as means (standard deviation)

An adequate intake of fluids is regarded as one of the mainstays of treatment for stone disease; [15, 16] a randomized controlled trial on patients at their first episode of idiopathic calcium stone showed that increasing water intake to obtain 2 L of urine per day or more reduced the risk of recurrence at 5 years by about 55%. [17] Despite the proven efficacy of hydration in stone disease, changes in renal papillary density associated with increased water intake have not been investigated before. The results of our study suggest that increased fluid intake is likely to modify the concentration of lithogenic salts in the renal tissue; whether these changes would reflect in an actual reduction in risk of recurrence remains to be elucidated. Our study also highlights the need to include the HU of the renal papillae in future studies investigating interventions for stone prevention.

Our study has several strengths: a cohort composed of phenotypically homogeneous patients (recurrent calcium oxalate stone formers), whose stone composition was assessed by means of the gold-standard infrared spectroscopy; [18] all patients underwent the same urological procedure and the radiological images were obtained and analyzed prospectively; they all received the same indication in terms of hydration (e.g., at least 2 L per day of hypotonic oligomineral water) and the follow-up was relatively long (at least 12 months); furthermore, patients were asked and reminded about their increased fluid intake through phone contacts. We also had available data on blood and 24 h urine chemistries.

Our study also has limitations. First, we did not have a control group; however, it would not have been ethical nor feasible to not recommend increased hydration after urological removal of stones. Second, follow-up time was not identical for all participants, as it was performed on routine clinical follow-up visits based on the clinicians' judgement; however, all participants had at least 12 months of follow-up before the follow-up CT scan was performed. Third, adherence to the recommended fluid regimen was not assessed through changes in urine volume; however, the urine volume at follow-up was on average greater than 2 L, a figure higher than expected without intervention in a group of recurrent stone formers and thus likely increased compared with baseline. Fourth, we did not have a mean to assess long-term hydration habits of the patients. Fifth, the radiologist who assessed the HU value was not blinded to the patient status; this was done in order to allow the radiologist to sample the same ROI in baseline and follow-up CT scans. Finally, the documented changes in renal papillary density could not necessarily translate into reduced risk of recurrence, despite initial evidence for a predictive role of renal papillary density in stone development; future studies are warranted to investigate whether renal papillary density and changes thereof are independent predictors of incident stone formation.

Conclusions

Increased fluid intake in patients with recurrent calcium oxalate stones is associated with a significant reduction in renal papillary density.

Abbreviations

CT: Computer tomography; HU: Hounsfield Units

Acknowledgements

Authors would like to thank the patients for their important contribution to this study.

Funding

This research did not receive any specific grant from funding agencies in the public, commercial, or not-for-profit sectors.

Authors' contributions

GG, PMF and AD designed the study; MV and AD performed the urological procedures; GM and CP performed the radiological studies and HU measurements; MV and GL performed the follow-up by phone contacts; JG and AP performed the stone composition and biochemical analyses; PMF conducted the statistical analysis; PMF, MV, GM, GL, CP and GG drafted the manuscript; PB, JG and AP reviewed the manuscript for important intellectual content. All authors read and approved the final manuscript.

Competing interests

The authors declare that they have no competing interests.

Author details

[1]U.O.C. Nefrologia, Fondazione Policlinico Universitario A. Gemelli IRCCS, Roma, Italia. [2]U.O.C. Clinica Urologica, Fondazione Policlinico Universitario A. Gemelli IRCCS, Roma, Italia. [3]U.O.C. Radiologia, Fondazione Policlinico Universitario A. Gemelli IRCCS, Roma, Italia. [4]U.O.C. Biochimica Clinica, Fondazione Policlinico Universitario A. Gemelli IRCCS, Roma, Italia. [5]Università Cattolica del Sacro Cuore, Roma, Italia.

References

1. Scales CD, Smith AC, Hanley JM, Saigal CS. Prevalence of kidney stones in the United States. Eur Urol. 2012;62:160–5.
2. Croppi E, Ferraro PM, Taddei L, Gambaro G. Prevalence of renal stones in an Italian urban population: a general practice-based study. Urol Res. 2012;40:517–22.
3. Ferraro PM, Curhan GC, D'Addessi A, Gambaro G. Risk of recurrence of idiopathic calcium kidney stones: analysis of data from the literature. J Nephrol. 2017;30:227-33.
4. Saigal CS, Joyce G, Timilsina AR. Direct and indirect costs of nephrolithiasis in an employed population: opportunity for disease management? Kidney Int. 2005;68:1808–14.
5. Coe FL, Evan A, Worcester E. Kidney stone disease. J Clin Invest. 2005;115: 2598–608.
6. Matlaga BR, Coe FL, Evan AP, Lingeman JE. The role of Randall's plaques in the pathogenesis of calcium stones. J Urol. 2007;177:31–8.
7. Eisner BH, Iqbal A, Namasivayam S, Catalano O, Kambadakone A, Dretler SP, et al. Differences in computed tomography density of the renal papillae of stone formers and non-stone-formers: a pilot study. J Endourol. 2008;22:2207–10.
8. Bhuskute NM, Yap WW, Wah TM. A retrospective evaluation of Randall's plaque theory of nephrolithiasis with CT attenuation values. Eur J Radiol. 2009;72:470–2.
9. Baran I, Voyvoda N, Tokgöz Ö, Tokgöz H. Can Hounsfield unit values of the cortex and papillae determined by computed tomography demonstrate the possibility of kidney stone formation? Eur J Radiol. 2012;81:1446–9.
10. Ciudin A, Luque Galvez MP, Salvador Izquierdo R, Diaconu MG, de Castro AF, Constantin V, et al. Validation of Randall's plaque theory using unenhanced abdominal computed tomography. Urology. 2013;81:246–9.
11. Shavit L, Girfoglio D, Kirkham A, Allen D, Ferraro PM, Moochhala S, et al. Increased renal papillary density in kidney stone formers detectable by CT scan is a potential marker of stone risk, but is unrelated to underlying hypercalciuria. Urolithiasis. 2016;44:471–5.
12. Ciudin A, Luque MP, Salvador R, Diaconu MG, Franco A, Collado-Belvis A, et al. The evolution of CT diagnosed papillae tip microcalcifications: can we predict the development of stones? J Endourol. 2014;28:1016–21.
13. Ciudin A, Luque MP, Salvador R, Diaconu MG, Franco A, Constantin V, et al. Abdominal computed tomography--a new tool for predicting recurrent stone disease. J Endourol. 2013;27:965–9.
14. Deshmukh S, Kambadakone A, Sahani DV, Eisner BH. Hounsfield density of renal papillae in stone formers: analysis based on stone composition. J Urol. 2015;193:1560–3.
15. Cheungpasitporn W, Rossetti S, Friend K, Erickson SB, Lieske JC. Treatment effect, adherence, and safety of high fluid intake for the prevention of incident and recurrent kidney stones: a systematic review and meta-analysis. J Nephrol. 2016;29:211–9.
16. Gambaro G, Croppi E, Coe F, Lingeman J, Moe O, Worcester E, et al. Metabolic diagnosis and medical prevention of calcium nephrolithiasis and its systemic manifestations: a consensus statement. J Nephrol. 2016;29:715-34.
17. Borghi L, Meschi T, Amato F, Briganti A, Novarini A, Giannini A. Urinary volume, water and recurrences in idiopathic calcium nephrolithiasis: a 5-year randomized prospective study. J Urol. 1996;155:839–43.
18. Primiano A, Persichilli S, Gambaro G, Ferraro PM, D'Addessi A, Cocci A, et al. FT-IR analysis of urinary stones: a helpful tool for clinician comparison with the chemical spot test. Dis Markers. 2014;2014:176165.

Risk factors for urinary tract infection in patients with urolithiasis—primary report of a single center cohort

Li Yongzhi[1], Yan Shi[2], Liu Jia[1], Liu Yili[1*], Zhu Xingwang[1] and Gong Xue[1]

Abstract

Background: Urinary tract infection (UTI) is very common in patients with urolithiasis, which makes the treatment of urolithiasis complicated, even dangerous. The objective of this study was to determine the risk factors for UTI in patients with urolithiasis.

Methods: Eight hundred six patients with urolithiasis were retrospectively evaluated in the fourth affiliated hospital of China Medical University. All patients admitted to the study were divided into either a UTI infection group or a non-infection group. Sex, age, smoking, stone shape, alcohol consumption, position of stones, and presence of obstruction were used as exposure factors for the cross-sectional study.

Results: One hundred seventy-eight patients (22.0%) had UTI. Through a urine culture test, gram-negative bacilli were the most common pathogen, followed by gram-positive bacilli and fungi.

Conclusions: Sex, age, obstruction, stone shape, and multiple sites of stones could be considered the independent factors for UTI in patients with urolithiasis; smoking and drinking had no statistically significant correlation with the condition. Gram-negative bacilli are the most common pathogen in UTI in patients with urolithiasis.

Keywords: Urinary tract infection, Risk factors, Urolithiasis, Urine culture test

Background

Urolithiasis is one of the most common urological diseases, the prevalence of which ranges from 2.0 to 20% throughout the world based on the geographic and socioeconomic characteristics of different populations, and > $2 billion is spent on treatment each year [1, 2]. The prevalence of urolithiasis appears to have increased in recent years for both men and women [3, 4].

Urinary tract infection (UTI) is very common in patients with urolithiasis. Persistent infections caused by urease-producing bacteria will form infection stones consisting of monoammonium urate, struvite (magnesium ammonium phosphate), and/or carbonate apatite [5], which makes the treatment of urolithiasis complicated. Complications from urolithiasis, such as asymptomatic bacteriuria, UTI, and sepsis, have been recognized after treatment with extracorporeal shockwave lithotripsy [6]. Patients with severe or multiple stones might develop postoperative systemic inflammatory response syndrome after a percutaneous nephrolithotomy (PCNL), with a small percent progressing to urosepsis, which could lead to a catastrophic even, such as septic shock [7]. Of all infections of the urogenital tract, pyelonephritis is the most severe and leads to dangerous complications [5].

Few studies have been published on the risk factors for infection in patients with urolithiasis. In their studies, Schwartz [8] and Wong [9] found catheter, pouches, urinary tract obstructions, neurogenic bladder voiding disruptions, medullary sponge kidney, and distal renal tubular acidosis to be the risk factors for UTI and the development of infection stones. Li [10] and Liu [11] found that of the study patients with urolithiasis, females and those with diabetes mellitus were more prone to septic shock after PCNL treatment. In addition to these factors, there might be some others related to stone

* Correspondence: 44577492@qq.com
[1]Department of Urology, Urologic Minimally Invasive Treatment Center in Liaoning Province, The Fourth Affiliated Hospital of China Medical University, No4, Chongshan East Road, Shenyang 110032, China
Full list of author information is available at the end of the article

formation. For example, smoking, alcohol consumption [12], and other patient characteristics might influence UTI in patients with urolithiasis. The primary aim of our retrospective cross-sectional study was to analyze the risk factors for UTI in patients with urolithiasis; therefore, we chose sex, age, smoking, alcohol consumption, position of stones, presence of obstruction, and stone shape (whether staghorn stones) as risk factors.

Methods

Patients

In our study, data on all patients with urolithiasis were collected from September 2006 to February 2009 in the Fourth Affiliated Hospital of China Medical University. All the experiments were performed in accordance with the guiding principle of Fourth Affiliated Hospital of China Medical University Human Ethics Committee and were approved by the Human Care Committee of the Fourth Affiliated Hospital of China Medical University. Exclusion criteria were antibiotic usage within the previous 3 d; urinary tract instrumentation; and cardiac, renal, or hepatic failure.

Methods

Ultrasound, X-ray, CT, and intravenous pyelography were used to diagnose and classify the position of the stones, presence of an obstruction, and stone shape (whether staghorn stones) in the radiology department, and a routine urinalysis and urine culture test were performed to diagnose a UTI. UTI was defined as presenting one of the following signs or symptoms: fever of > 37.8 °C with dysuria, frequent urination, urgent urination, and/or suprapubic pain with growth of $> 10^5$ colony-forming units (CFUs)/mL from a properly collected midstream "clean-catch" urine sample [13].

Subjects were defined as alcohol drinkers and/or cigarette smokers if they had regularly consumed any alcoholic beverage one or more times per week or had smoked 10 or more cigarettes per week for at least 6. 0 months [14].

All patients included in our study were divided into either a UTI infection group or a non-infection group. Sex, age, smoking, alcohol consumption, position of stones, presence of obstruction, and stone shape (whether staghorn stones) were used as risk factors in our study.

Statistical analyses

All analyses were performed using SPSS version 15.0 (SPSS Inc., Chicago, IL, USA). All data are reported as the mean ± SD. Univariate analyses were performed using Student's t-test for parametric variables and the Kruskal–Wallis test for nonparametric variables to detect influencing factors for UTI. The chi-squared test and Fisher's exact test were used for comparing ratios. A post-hoc statistical analysis was used for comparing 3 subgroups in age group. $P < 0.05$ was considered statistically significant.

Results

Eight hundred six patients were included in our study of whom 178 (22.0%) had UTI. The general results are provided in Table 1. Ureteral calculi were the most common type of condition, followed by renal calculi, bladder stones, and urethral stones.

Table 2 shows the results of the urine cultures. Gram-negative bacilli isolates were the most common pathogen, followed by gram-positive bacilli isolates and strains of fungi (93.3 vs 4.5 vs 2.3%, respectively). Among the gram-negative bacilli, *Escherichia coli* was the most common, followed by *Pseudomonas aeruginosa*, *Klebsiella pneumoniae*, *Proteus mirabilis*, and "other" (52.80, 15.16, and 12.35% respectively).

Female patients had a higher rate of infection than male patients (32.0 vs 15.8%, $P < 0.001$) and patients > 60 years old were more prone to be infected, followed by those < 40 years old and 40–60 years old (31.0 vs 23.0 vs 18.3%, respectively; $P = 0.009$). Patients with obstructions were more prone to be infected than those without obstructions (26.1 vs 18.2%; $P = 0.006$). Patients with multiple stones had a higher rate of infection than those with a single stone (41.3 vs 16.0%, $P = 0.001$). Patients who smoked had a higher rate of infection than those who did not smoke (25.8 vs 20.1%, $P = 0.063$), but patients who drank alcohol had a lower rate of infection than those who did not drink alcohol (21.8 vs 22.2%, $P = 0.906$). Patients with staghorn stones had a higher rate of infection than those without staghorn stones (48.4 vs 19.8%, $P < 0.001$). (see Table 3).

Besides, we did separate analysis of patients with staghorn stone in comparison with non-staghorn stone, and we found the results were almost the same. However, there are two differences.

The first difference is that age does not have a statistically significant relationship to UTI in staghorn stone group ($P = 0.2150$), however, age does have a statistically significant relationship to UTI in non-staghorn stone group ($P = 0.0215$). (see Tables 4 and 5). We guess the

Table 1 Different locations of urolithiasis

Stone position	Number of cases	%
Renal stone	274	34.00
Ureteral stone	280	34.74
Bladder stone	50	6.20
Urethral stone	11	1.36
Multiple sites	191	23.70
Total	806	100.00

Table 2 Bacterial species and ratio in total

Bacterial species	Isolates count	%
Gram-negative bacteria	166	93.25
Escherichia coli	94	52.80
Pseudomonas aeruginosa	27	15.16
Klebsiella pneumoniae	22	12.35
Proteus mirabilis	7	3.93
Miscellaneous	16	8.98
Gram-positive bacteria	8	4.49
Fungus	4	2.24

reason may be that the number of patients with staghorn stone is a little small.

The second difference is that the first three gram-negative bacteria in staghorn stone are *Escherichia coli, Pseudomonas aeruginosa and Klebsiella pneumoniae.* However, the first three gram-negative bacteria in non-staghorn stone are *Escherichia coli, Klebsiella pneumoniae and Pseudomonas aeruginosa.* (see Tables 6 and 7).

Through the results of the chi-squared tests, sex, age, obstruction, multiple stones, and stone shape each had a statistically significant relationship to UTI (all $P < 0.05$); however, this was not true of smoking and alcohol consumption (all $P > 0.05$).

Discussion

In our retrospective study, the independent effects of risk factors on the development of UTI were investigated. Sex, age, obstructions, stone shape, and multiple sites of stones were found to be the independent risk factors for UTI in patients with urolithiasis, which might be helpful in their treatment.

Previous reports showed that females had a higher rate of infection stones than males [15, 16]. In Li and Liu's study [10, 11], females with urolithiasis were found to be more prone to septic shock after PCNL treatment. These results were comparable to ours. The reason might be that women have a shorter urethra, which predisposes them to ascending infections. Nearly 10% of women experience infections of the urinary tract within 1.0 year

Table 3 Different risk factors for urinary tract infection

Risk Factors	Number	Without Infection		With Infection		χ^2	P
		N	%	N	%		
Sex						28.49	<.0001
Male	492	414	84.15	78	15.85		
Female	314	214	68.15	100	31.85		
Age group[a]						9.35	0.0093
<40	252	194	76.98	58	23.02		
40-60	409	334	81.66	75	18.34		
>60	145	100	69.66	45	31.03		
Stone site						54.06	<.0001
Single stone	615	516	83.90	99	16.10		
Multiple sites	191	112	58.64	79	41.36		
Obstruction						7.38	0.0066
Yes	394	291	73.86	103	26.14		
No	412	337	81.80	75	18.20		
Staghorn calculi						28.06	<.0001
Staghorn stones	64	33	51.56	31	48.44		
Non-Staghorn stones	742	595	80.19	147	19.81		
Smoking						3.44	0.0638
Yes	279	207	74.19	72	25.81		
No	527	421	79.89	106	20.11		
Alcohol Drinking						0.016	0.9006
Yes	293	229	78.16	64	21.84		
No	513	399	77.78	114	22.22		

[a]Age group,
<40 versus 40-60, $\chi^2 = 3.08$, $P = 0.0793$;
<40 versus >60, $\chi^2 = 2.12$, $P = 0.1451$;
40-60 versus >60, $\chi^2 = 10.17$, $P = 0.0014$;

Table 4 Different risk factors for urinary tract infection in Staghorn stones

Risk Factors	Number	Without Infection		With Infection		X^2	P
		N	%	N	%		
Sex						37.16	<.0001
Male	39	32	82.05	7	17.95		
Female	25	1	4.00	24	96.00		
Age group						3.07	0.2150
<40	20	9	45.00	11	55.00		
40-60	32	20	62.50	12	37.50		
>60	12	4	33.33	8	66.67		
Smoking						0.03	0.8563
Yes	22	11	50.00	11	50.00		
No	42	22	52.38	20	47.62		
Alcohol Drinking						0.35	0.5521
Yes	23	13	56.52	10	43.48		
No	41	20	48.78	21	51.22		

of PCNL treatment, including cystitis and pyelonephritis [17], and as many as 26% of UTIs recur within 6.0 months [18].

In our study, the patients < 40 years old and > 60 years old were more prone to infections than those from 40 to 60 years old. Thomas [16] found that infection stones were most common in each sex at ages from 60 to 69 years compared with that in other age groups, which was nearly the same as indicated from our results. Daudon et al. [15] reported that struvite was especially low in ages 40 to 49 years, but the frequency peak of ammonium urate stones was observed in ages 0 to 9.0 years. Thereafter, the proportion declined rapidly. In our study, patients between the ages of 40 and 60 years showed a low rate of infection compared with that of the other two groups.

It has been proved that urinary tract obstruction is a risk factor for UTI and the development of infection stones urine cannot pass smoothly. In addition, the inflamed narrowing of the ureter or injuries made by stones when moving down the ureter could easily cause infection. In our study, obstructions were confirmed by CT scan and intravenous pyelography, and 26.14% of patients with obstructions were prone infection compared with 18.20% of patients without obstructions, the results of which were the same as those in the previous study [5]. In addition, those with multiple stones are more likely to be infected than those with a single stone,

Table 5 Different risk factors for urinary tract infection in Non-Staghorn stones

Risk Factors	Number	Without Infection		With Infection		X^2	P
		N	%	N	%		
Sex						12.53	0.0004
Male	453	382	84.33	71	15.67		
Female	289	213	73.70	76	26.30		
Age group						7.68	0.0215
<40	232	185	79.74	47	20.26		
40-60	377	314	83.29	63	16.71		
>60	133	96	72.18	37	27.82		
Smoking						3.81	0.0509
Yes	257	196	76.26	61	23.74		
No	485	399	82.27	86	17.73		
Alcohol Drinking						0.01	0.9223
Yes	270	216	80.00	54	20.00		
No	472	379	80.30	93	19.70		

Table 6 Bacterial species and ratio in Staghorn stones

Bacterial species	Isolates count	%
Gram-negative bacteria	31	100.00
Escherichia coli	12	38.70
Pseudomonas aeruginosa	11	35.48
Klebsiella pneumoniae	5	16.12
Miscellaneous	3	9.67

which could be because multiple stones have more of a chance to cause an obstruction, which could easily cause urinary retention after which the chance of UTI increases significantly.

Staghorn calculi are branched stones that occupy a large portion of the collecting system. Typically, they fill the renal pelvis and branch into several or all of the calices. However, there is no consensus regarding the precise definition of staghorn calculus, such as the number of involved calices required to qualify for a staghorn designation. In our study, the term staghorn stone refer to any branched stone occupying more than one portion of the collecting system, ie renal pelvis with one or more caliceal extensions [19]. A staghorn calculus has traditionally been synonymous with infection stones. Typically, UTI with urease-producing bacteria promote the crystallization and formation of branching stones that encompass the renal pelvis and calyces [20]. It was reported that in 59–68% of cases, the majority of infectious constituents were staghorn calculi [21], which suggests that patients with staghorn calculi are more easily infected. In our study, patients with staghorn calculi were also more likely to be infected, which confirmed the results of previous reports.

There was no statistical significant correlation between smoking and/or alcohol consumption and infection, which indicates that smoking and alcohol consumption could not be considered as independent risk factors for UTI in patients with urolithiasis; however, recently, cigarette smoking has been identified as an important risk factor for the development and progression of urolithiasis [12]. Decreasing urinary flow [22] and increasing serum cadmium [23] might be two reasons for urolithiasis that are associated with smoking and alcohol consumption. In healthy subjects, smoking has been found to significantly increase the antidiuretic plasma arginine vasopressin, resulting in a decrease in urinary flow and possibly promoting the development of calcium urolithiasis [12]. Hamano et al. [24] reported that cigarette smokers have a 4.29-fold risk of developing calcium urolithiasis; however, they did not report any correlation between smoking and UTI.

Table 7 Bacterial species and ratio in Non-Staghorn stones

Bacterial species	Isolates count	%
Gram-negative bacteria	135	91.83
Escherichia coli	82	55.78
Klebsiella pneumoniae	17	11.56
Pseudomonas aeruginosa	16	10.88
Proteus mirabilis	7	4.76
Miscellaneous	13	8.84
Gram-positive bacteria	8	5.44
Fungus	4	2.72

Typically, gram-negative bacteria are the most common pathogen of UTI, among which, *E. coli* has a high frequency rate [25]. In epidemiology and antimicrobial susceptibility profiles of gram-negative bacteria causing UTIs in the Asia-Pacific region, Lu et al. [26] reported that *E. coli*, *K. pneumoniae*, and *P. aeruginosa* were the three most common species of pathogens found in UTIs. In our study, gram-negative-bacteria were the most common, followed by gram-positive bacteria and fungus. Among the gram-negative-bacteria, *E. coli* was the most common pathogen following by *P. aeruginosa*, *K .pneumoniae* and *P. mirabilis*.

Our study had a number of limitations. First, we lacked the data on stone composition, which could be useful for analysis of infection stones. Second, we lacked the details of antimicrobial susceptibility testing. Thus, the relationship between stone composition and bacterial colonization received our attention and might be the subject of our next study.

Conclusions

Sex, age, obstruction, multiple sites of stones, and stone shape (whether staghorn stones) could be considered as independent factors for UTI in patients with urolithiasis. Gram-negative bacilli are the most common bacteria found in UTIs in patients with urolithiasis.

Abbreviations

CFUs: Colony-Forming Units; PCNL: Percutaneous Nephrolithotomy; SD: Standard Deviation; UTI: Urinary Tract Infection

Acknowledgements

We here acknowledge Dr. Li Zizheng for the help of statistical analysis.

Funding

The study was funded by the Fourth Affiliated Hospital of China Medical University, which had no influence over the design of the study, the collection, analysis, interpretation of data and the writing of the manuscript.

Authors' contributions

SY, XG and XWZ collected the patients' information. YZL wrote the manuscript and participated in the design of the study, JL performed the statistical analysis. YLL conceived of the study and participated in its design and coordination. All authors read and approved the final manuscript.

Competing interests
The authors declare that they have no competing interests.

Author details
[1]Department of Urology, Urologic Minimally Invasive Treatment Center in Liaoning Province, The Fourth Affiliated Hospital of China Medical University, No4, Chongshan East Road, Shenyang 110032, China. [2]Department of Urology, Sheyang Red Cross Hospital, No4, Chongshan East Road, Huanggu District, Shenyang 110032, China.

References
1. Pak CY. Kidney stone. Lancet. 1998;351:1797–801.
2. Pearle M, Calhoun E, Curhan GC. Urological diseases in America project. J Urol. 2005;173:848–57.
3. Stamatelou KK, Francis ME, Jones CA, Nyberg LM, Curhan GC. Time trends in reported prevalence of kidney stones in the United States: 1976-1994. Kidney Int. 2003;63:1817–23.
4. Hesse A, Brändle E, Wilbert D, Köhrmann KU, Alken P. Study on the prevalence and incidence of urolithiasis in Germany comparing the years 1979 vs. 2000. Eur Urol. 2003;44:709–13.
5. Bichler KH, Eipper E, Naber K, Braun V, Zimmermann R, Lahme S. Urinary infection stones. Int J Antimicrob Agents. 2002;19:488–98.
6. Bierkens AF, Hendrikx AJ, Ezz el Din KE, de la Rosette JJ, Horrevorts A, Doesburg W, Debruyne FM. The value of antibiotic prophylaxis during extracorporeal shock wave lithotripsy in the prevention of urinary tract infections in patients with urine proven sterile prior to treatment. Eur Urol. 1997;31:30–5.
7. Korets R, Graversen JA, Kates M, Mues AC, Gupta M. Post-percutaneous nephrolithotomy systemic inflammatory response: a prospective analysis of preoperative urine, renal pel-Vic urine and stone cultures. J Urol. 2011;186: 1899–903.
8. Schwartz BF, Stoller ML. Nonsurgical management of infection-related renal calculi. Urol Clin N Am. 1999;26:765–78.
9. Wong HY, Riedl CR, Griffith DP. The effect of iontophoresis on bacterial growth in urine. J Urol. 1995;154:1944–7.
10. Li K, Liu C, Zhang X, Liu Y, Wang P. Risk factors for septic shock after mini-percutaneous nephrolithotripsy with holmium laser. Urology. 2013;81:1173–6.
11. Liu C, Zhang X, Liu Y, Wang P. Prevention and treatment of septic shock following mini-percutaneous nephrolithotomy: a single-center retrospective study of 834 cases. World J Urol. 2013;31:1593–7.
12. Liu CC, Huang SP, Wu WJ, Chou YH, Juo SH, Tsai LY, Huang CH, Wu MT. The impact of cigarette smoking, alcohol drinking and betel quid chewing on the risk of calcium urolithiasis. Ann Epidemiol. 2009;19:539–45.
13. Cope M, Cevallos ME, Cadle RM, Darouiche RO, Musher DM, Trautner BW. Inappropriate treatment of catheter-associated asymptomatic bacteriuria in a tertiary care hospital. Clin Infect Dis. 2009;48:1182–8.
14. Lee CH, Wu DC, Lee JM, Wu IC, Goan YG, Kao EL. Anatomical subsite discrepancy in relation to the impact of the consumption of alcohol, tobacco and betel quid on esophageal cancer. Int J Cancer. 2007;120:1755–62.
15. Daudon M, Dore J-C, Jungers P. Changes in stone composition according to age and gender of patients: a multivariate epidemiological approach. Urol Res. 2004;32:241–7.
16. Knoll T, Schubert AB, Fahlenkamp D, Leusmann DB, Wendt-Nordahl G, Schubert G. Urolithiasis through the ages: data on more than 200,000 urinary stone analyses. J Urol. 2011;185:1304–11.
17. Nicolle LE. Uncomplicated urinary tract infection in adults including uncomplicated pyelonephritis. Urol Clin North Am. 2008;35:1–12.
18. Foxman B. Recurring urinary tract infection: incidence and risk factors. Am J Public Health. 1990;80:331–3.
19. Preminger GM, Assimos DG, Lingeman JE, Nakada SY, Pearle MS, Wolf JS Jr. AUA guideline on Management of Staghorn Calculi: diagnosis and treatment recommendations. J Urol. 2005;173:1991–2000.
20. Vargas AD, Bragin SD, Mendez R. Staghorn calculus: its clinical presentation, complications and management. J Urol. 1982;127:860–2.
21. Preminger GM, Assimos DG, Lingeman JE. Chapter 1: AUA guideline on management of staghorn calculi: diagnosis and treatment recommendations. J Urol. 2005;173:1991–2000.
22. Mooser V, Burnier M, Nussberger J, Juillerat L, Waeber B, Brunner HR. Effects of smoking and physical exercise on platelet free cytosolic calcium in healthy normotensive volunteers. J Hypertens. 1989;7:211–6.
23. Scott R, Cunningham C, McLelland A, Fell GS, Fitzgerald-Finch OP, McKellar N. The importance of cadmium as a factor in calcified upper urinary tract stone diseaseda prospective 7-year study. Br J Urol. 1982;54:584–9.
24. Hamano S, Nakatsu H, Suzuki N, Tomioka S, Tanaka M, Murakami S. Kidney stone disease and risk factors for coronary heart disease. Int J Urol. 2005;12: 859–63.
25. Zhanel GG, DeCorby M, Adam H, Mulvey MR, McCracken M, Lagacé-Wiens P, Nichol KA, Wierzbowski A, Baudry PJ, Tailor F, Karlowsky JA, Walkty A, Schweizer F, Johnson J, Canadian Antimicrobial Resistance Alliance, Hoban DJ. Prevalence of antimicrobial resistance pathogens in Canadian hospitals: results of the Canadian ward surveillance study (CANWARD 2008). Antimicrob Agents Chemother. 2010;54:4684–93.
26. Lu PL, Liu YC, Toh HS, Lee YL, Liu YM, Ho CM, Huang CC, Liu CE, Ko WC, Wang JH, Tang HJ, Yu KW, Chen YS, Chuang YC, Xu Y, Ni Y, Chen YH, Hsueh PR. Epidemiology and antimicrobial susceptibility profiles of gram-negative bacteria causing urinary tract infections in the Asia-Pacific region: 2009-2010 results from the study for monitoring antimicrobial resistance trends (SMART). Int J Antimicrob Agents. 2012;40(S1):S37–43.

35

Expression and clinical significance of Caveolin-1 in prostate Cancer after transurethral surgery

Xiaoming Wang[1,2*], Zhigui Liu[1] and Zhanbin Yang[1]

Abstract

Background: Prostate cancer is a common malignancy of the male genitourinary system that occurs worldwide. The current research aims to investigate caveolin-1 expression in prostate cancer tissue and its relationship with pathological grade, clinical pathologic staging, and preoperative prostate-specific antigen (PSA) levels.

Methods: From January 2012 to December 2014, samples from 47 patients with prostate cancer who had received transurethral prostatic resection (TURP) and 20 patients with benign prostatic hyperplasia were collected at the First Affiliated Hospital of Guangxi Medical University. Caveolin-1 was detected by streptavidin-perosidase (SP) immunohistochemical staining in pathological tissue slices. The results were statistically analyzed for pathological grade, clinical stage, and preoperative PSA level.

Results: The expression of caveolin-1 was significantly higher in prostate cancer samples than in benign prostatic hyperplasia samples ($P < 0.05$), and caveolin-1 expression was significantly different among the pathological grades of poorly, moderately and well-differentiated prostate cancer ($P < 0.05$). The difference in caveolin-1 expression was significant for different clinical stages (T1-T2 and T3-T4) of prostate cancer ($P < 0.05$). The difference in caveolin-1 expression was not significant among samples with different preoperative PSA levels (0–10, 10–100 and > 100 μg/L) ($P > 0.05$).

Conclusions: Caveolin-1 is closely related to the pathological grade and clinical stage of prostate cancer after transurethral surgery, and it may be a novel tumor marker for prostate cancer. The expression of caveolin-1 is not associated with preoperative serum PSA levels.

Keywords: Prostate cancer, Benign prostatic hyperplasia, Caveolin-1, Immunohistochemistry

Background

Prostate cancer is a common malignancy of the male genitourinary system. In recent years, there has been a continuous rise in the incidence of prostate cancer cases, and it is becoming the first cancer to threaten male health [1, 2]. Screening for prostate cancer relies mainly on PSA testing. However, because of low PSA specificity and the very low serum PSA levels in some patients with prostate cancer, there is a possibility of missed diagnosis [3, 4]. Therefore, finding new screening markers is essential for providing powerful evidence for the early detection, early diagnosis, and early treatment of prostate cancer [5].

At present, the pathogenesis and relevant molecular biological basis of prostate cancer are not yet fully understood [6]. Recent studies have proved that caveolin-1 is associated with the incidence and progression of prostate cancer [7], but the specific mechanism is not clear.

Caveolin (Cav) is a special vesicle-like structure on the surface of the cell membrane and is an important structural-functional protein. It has been found that mammals have three caveolin genes (caveolin-1, caveolin-2 and caveolin-3). Caveolin-1 and caveolin-2 are widely present in a variety of normal human cells, and caveolin-3 is expressed specifically in muscle. Caveolin interacts with

* Correspondence: wangxiaomingcn@126.com
[1]Department of Urology, The First Affiliated Hospital of Guangxi Medical University, Nanning 530021, China
[2]Department of Urology, The Second Affiliated Hospital of Guangxi Medical University, No 166 DaXueDong Road, Nanning 530007, Guangxi, China

specific lipids, such as glycosphingolipids or cholesterols, thereby leading to the formation of caveolae. In the sub-cell, caveolin-1 is positioned at the cytoplasm, mitochondria, caveolae, and other related secretion channels [8]. Caveolin-1 is involved mainly in the interaction of signaling molecules and the regulation of signaling channels, as well as the regulation of cell proliferation, differentiation, migration, apoptosis, and angiogenesis signaling pathways. Caveolin-1 is also closely related to the occurrence, progression, invasion, and metastasis of tumors [9].

A large number of studies have shown that caveolin-1 is expressed at a low level in most tumors and is present as a tumor suppressor gene [10]. However, it has been found that caveolin-1 protein expression is not consistent in different tumor tissues and cell lines; in a small number of malignant tumors, specifically urinary tract tumors (prostate cancer, kidney cancer, and bladder cancer), it is highly expressed and is thus a gene related to cancer and cancer metastasis [11].

In this study, caveolin-1 was detected in pathological tissue slices of prostate cancer by streptavidin-peroxidase (SP) immunohistochemical staining. Statistical analysis was performed on the immunohistochemistry results for the tissue slices to investigate the correlation of caveolin-1 with the prostate cancer pathological grade, clinical stage, and preoperative serum PSA level to provide new information for the clinical diagnosis and treatment of prostate cancer.

Materials and methods

General information

Inpatients who received transurethral resection of prostate in the Urology Department of the First Affiliated Hospital of Guangxi Medical University between January 2012 and December 2014 were included in this study. The inclusion criteria were patients who had undergone surgical resection for prostate cancer and had benign prostatic hyperplasia that had been diagnosed pathologically. The exclusion criteria included 1) patients with non-prostate cancer and benign prostatic hyperplasia; 2) patients without pathological reports; 3) patients with incomplete clinical data; and 4) patients who had received preoperative radiotherapy, chemotherapy or endocrine treatment. Forty-seven samples from patients with transurethral electrocision of the prostate and a pathological diagnosis of prostate cancer were included in the experimental group. In the experimental group, the patients' ages ranged from 55 to 91, and the average age was 71.15 ± 9.60 years old. In addition, 20 patients with benign prostatic hyperplasia were selected as the control group. In the control group, the patients' ages ranged from 48 to 79, and the average age was 69.63 ± 8.24 years old. All specimens were from patients who were admitted to the Urology Department of the First Hospital Affiliated of Guangxi Medical University after transurethral electrocision of the prostate. The clinical data collected from all patients included general information (including name, age, inpatient number, admission diagnosis, and contact information) and the results of auxiliary examination, including the preoperative serum PSA level, tumor node metastasis (TNM) staging, pathological findings (including Gleason score), and treatment.

Immunohistochemical detection

Cav-1 protein was detected by the standard streptavidin-peroxidase (SP) immunohistochemical staining method. The tissue slices were processed and incubated with a rabbit anti-human caveolin-1 polyclonal antibody (1:200 dilution; cat. no. SC-894; Santa Cruz Biotechnology Inc., CA, USA) overnight at 4 °C; then, the slices were incubated with biotin-labeled goat anti-rabbit IgG (1:200; Histostain-SP Kit; cat. no. SPN-9001; Zsbio, Beijing, China) at room temperature for 20 min; next, the slices were incubated with peroxidase-labeled streptavidin at room temperature for 20 min and stained with a Tris-HCl solution containing 0.02% 3,9-diaminobenzidine for 5 to 7 min; finally, the slices were stained with hematoxylin, washed with water, dehydrated, removed, sealed, detected and photographed under a microscope.

Result analysis

Positive results were analyzed using an Olympus optical microscope, and double-blind randomized observations were made by two chief physicians. Positive caveolin-1 expression was located in the cell membrane and cytoplasm and was indicated by yellowish-brown or brown granules. The scores were calculated according to the staining intensity of positive-staining cells and the number of positive-staining cells (percentage of positive cells) in the tissue slice. (1) The staining intensity was calculated as follows: negative - 0 points; weak positive - 1 point; positive - 2 points; and strong positive - 3 points. For the tissue slices, the staining intensity was calculated as follows: colorless - 0 points; light yellow - 1 point; yellowish-brown - 2 points; and brown - 3 points. (2) The percentage of positive cells were calculated as follows: $< 5\%$ - 0 points; ≥ 5 to 25% - 1 point; > 25 to 50% - 2 points; > 50 to 75% - 3 points; and $> 75\%$ - 4 points. The final score was calculated by multiplying the staining intensity score by the positive cell percentage. When the final score was ≥ 4 points, it was considered

Table 1 Clinical and pathological data in 47 cases of patients with prostate cancer

	Item	Cases (percentage)
Age	< 70	19 (40.4%)
	≥70	28 (59.6%)
Preoperative PSA	0–10	6 (12.8%)
level (ng/ml)	10–100	22 (46.8%)
	> 100	19 (40.4%)
Clinical stage	T1-T2	26 (55.3%)
	T3-T4	21 (44.7%)
Gleason score	2–6	11 (20%)
	7	16(37.4%)
	8–10	20(42.6%)

positive; when the final score was < 4 points, it was considered negative.

Statistical analysis

All statistical analyses were performed using the SPSS 16.0 software (SPSS Inc., Chicago, IL). Group comparisons were performed using the Chi-square test. Differences were considered statistically significant when $p < 0.05$.

Results

Experimental group: Clinical and pathological data

As shown in Table 1, in the experimental group, 19 patients (40.4%) were younger than 70 years old, and 28 patients (59.6%) were older than or equal to 70 years old. The preoperative PSA level was 0–10 ng/ml in 6 cases (12.8%), 10–100 ng/ml in 22 cases (46.8%), and > 100 ng/ml in 19 cases (40.4%). The clinical stage was T1-T2 in 26 cases (55.3%) and T3-T4 in 21 cases (44.7%). According to the 2016 World Health Organization (WHO) classification of tumors of the urinary system and male genital organs and the risk classification, which is based on the D'amico classification system, the Gleason score was categorized as follows: low risk 2–6, intermediate risk 7, and high risk 8–10. This study found 2–6 points in 11 cases (23.4%), 7 points in 16 cases (34.0%), and 8–10 points in 20 cases (42.6%).

Tissue expression of caveolin-1 in prostate cancer and benign prostatic hyperplasia

Caveolin-1 positive staining was found in the cell membrane and cytoplasm of prostate cancer (PCa) cells, presenting as yellowish-brown or brown particles. In 47 cases of prostate cancer, positive expression was found in 29 cases, and negative expression was found in 18 cases; the positive expression rate was 61.70%. In 20 cases of benign prostatic hyperplasia, positive expression was found in 2 cases, and negative expression was found in 18 cases; the positive expression rate was 10.0% (Fig 1). The difference between the two groups was statistically significant (Table 2).

Correlation of the expression of caveolin-1 and pathological grading

As shown in Fig. 2, the positive expression rate of caveolin-1 in PCa tissue was 61.70%. The positive expression rate of caveolin-1 was 80.0% in poorly differentiated PCa tissue, 68.8% in moderately differentiated PCa tissue, and 18.2% in well-differentiated PCa tissue. The higher the differentiation of the prostate cancer tissue was, the stronger the staining intensity of caveolin-1, the higher the percentage of positive cells, and the higher the positive rate were. The inter-group difference was statistically significant (Table 3). Therefore, prostate cancer is closely related to caveolin-1 since prostate cancer of a high pathological grade was often accompanied by the high expression of caveolin-1.

Correlation of the expression of caveolin-1 and the clinical stage of prostate cancer

The positive rates of caveolin-1 expression in T1-T2 and T3-T4 PCa tissues were 46.15 and 80.95%, respectively.

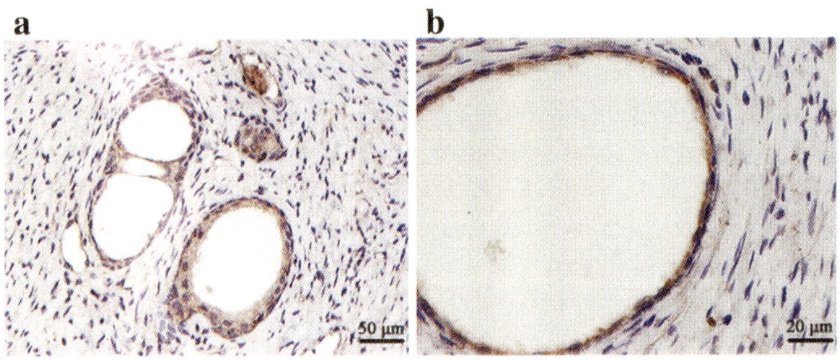

Fig. 1 Caveolin-1 expression in benign prostatic hyperplasia. a: SP × 200; b: SP × 400

Table 2 Tissue caveolin-1 expression in prostate cancer and benign prostatic hyperplasia

	Cases	Positive	Negative	Positive rate	X^2	*P* value
Prostate cancer	47	29	18	61.70%	15.085	0.000
Benign prostatic hyperplasia	20	2	18	10%		

The expression rate of caveolin-1 increased with the clinical stage. The difference between the two groups was statistically significant (Table 4), suggesting that caveolin-1 was related to prostate cancer invasion ($P < 0.05$).

Correlation of the expression of caveolin-1 and the preoperative PSA level in patients with prostate cancer

The positive expression rates of caveolin-1 in preoperative PSA groups (0–10 μg/L, 10–100 μg/L, and > 100 μg/L) were 16.67, 68.18 and 68.42%, respectively. The difference was not statistically significant ($P > 0.05$) (Table 5), suggesting that caveolin-1 and preoperative PSA levels in patients may be two independent markers.

Discussion

The occurrence and progression of prostate cancer as well as its surrounding infiltration plus distant metastasis are closely related to abnormal gene and protein expression. In cases where the tumor suppressor gene is an inactivator and the oncogene is an activator, protein expression will be abnormal, resulting in the deregulation of cell differentiation and growth disorders and eventually leading to the occurrence of prostate cancer [12].

The expression of caveolin-1 is low in most tumors, indicating its role as a tumor suppressor, but the specific mechanism is still unclear. It is generally believed that caveolin-1 can inhibit the malignancy of cells by inhibiting the activity of the cyclin D1 gene promoter, thereby inhibiting the MAPK pathway and the phosphorylation of the Src tyrosine kinase [13]. The reduced expression of caveolin-1 can promote the activation of gastric cancer-related fibroblasts, resulting in gastric cancer [14]. The expression of caveolin-1 in leukemia HL-60 cells can inhibit tumor cell proliferation, induce apoptosis, block PI3K/AKT signaling pathway activation and enhance chemotherapeutic agent sensitivity [15]. The expression of caveolin-1 is also reduced in many primary tumors, such as colorectal cancer, ovarian cancer, and breast cancer [10, 16, 17]. The above evidence suggests that the reduced expression of caveolin-1 is closely related to tumorigenesis. In contrast to the above studies, the expression of caveolin-1 was significantly higher in some tumor tissues than in normal tissues. Tse et al. [18] found that caveolin-1 was not expressed in normal livers and normal liver cell lines, but it is positively expressed in hepatocellular carcinoma and related cell lines. In addition, the high expression level of caveolin-1 was associated with venous infiltration and tumor metastasis, indicating that high caveolin-1 expression promoted the occurrence, progression, infiltration, and metastasis of tumors. Caveolin-1 can interact with transcription factor Fox M1 to promote epithelial-to-mesenchymal cell transformation and the metastasis of pancreatic cancer cells [19]. The downregulation of caveolin-1 expression can also inhibit STAT3 signaling pathways to block lung cancer cell metastasis [20]. High levels of caveolin-1 expression can also be seen in

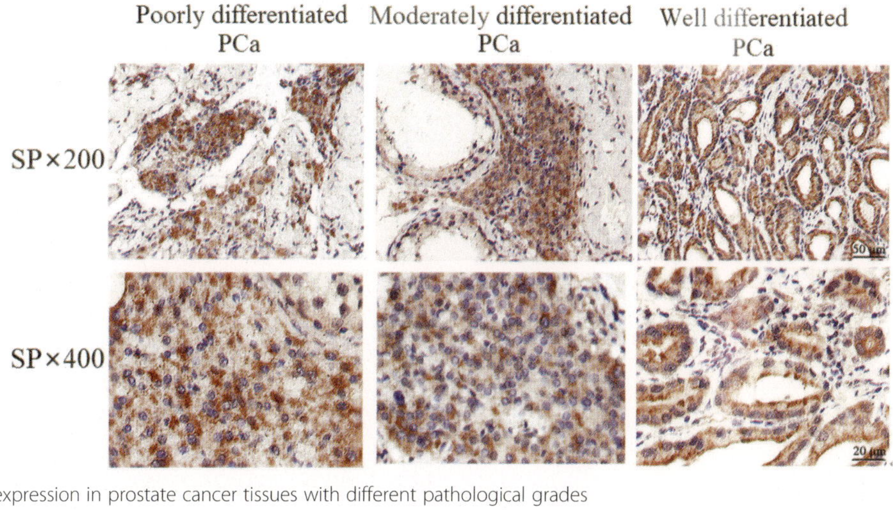

Fig. 2 Caveolin-1 expression in prostate cancer tissues with different pathological grades

Table 3 Correlation of caveolin-1 expression with pathological grade of prostate cancer

Pathological grade	Cases	Positive	Negative	Positive rate	X^2	*P* value
poorly differentiation	20	16	4	80.0%	8.773	0.012
Moderately differentiation	16	11	7	68.8%		
Well differentiation	11	2	7	18.2%		

hand and neck squamous cell carcinoma and kidney cancer cells that have metastasized [21, 22]. Thus, caveolin-1 exhibits a high degree of upregulation in early tumor cells that metastasize to lymph nodes and is closely related to poor prognosis [23], indicating that in different stages of tumor development, the effects of caveolin-1 as an important molecule in the regulation of growth are also very different; that is, caveolin-1 is not only a tumor suppressor protein but also a transfer-related molecule.

In this study, the expression of caveolin-1 was significantly higher in prostate cancer than in benign prostatic hyperplasia. The positive rates of caveolin-1 expression in poorly, moderately, and well-differentiated prostate cancer were 80.0, 68.8 and 18.2%, respectively. The positive rates of caveolin-1 expression in T1-T2 and T3-T4 prostate cancer were 46.15 and 80.95%, respectively; there were no significant differences between the different clinical stages. In groups with different preoperative PSA levels (0–10 μg/L, 10–100 μg/L, and 100 μg/L), the positive rates of expression were 16.67, 68.18 and 68.42%, respectively; there were no significant differences among the three groups. It is assumed that the high expression of caveolin-1 in prostate cancer may be related to the interaction between the phosphorylation and dephosphorylation of scaffolding and multiple signaling pathways and to gene mutation and promoter methylation, but it is not related to serum PSA levels; these results suggest that caveolin-1 may play an important role in the progression of prostate cancer. The results from Mohammed, D.A. [24] also suggest that the expression of caveolin-1 in prostate cancer is significantly higher than in BPH and high-grade PIN, indicating that caveolin-1 plays an important role in the occurrence and metastasis of prostate cancer and is not related to the invasion of prostate cancer. Caveolin-1 expression is upregulated in the terminal development stages of various tumors

Table 4 Correlation of caveolin-1 expression with clinical stage of prostate cancer

Clinical grade	Cases	Positive	Negative	Positive rate	X^2	P value
T1-T2	26	12	14	46.15%	5.953	0.015
T3-T4	21	17	4	80.95%		

and in various stages of urinary tumors, and it increases with tumor malignancy. The high expression of caveolin-1 is closely related to prostate cancer, promoting the occurrence, progression, and infiltration of the tumors. Possible mechanisms include gene site mutations, heterozygous deletions, and promoter hypermethylation. Paracrine caveolin-1 can promote the release of various growth factors by regulating their transcription, upregulating their mRNA and protein expression levels, stimulating tumor angiogenesis, and promoting tumor formation and proliferation. It can be used as a new biomarker for prostate cancer that can be used in the clinical diagnosis, treatment and prognosis of prostate cancer [25, 26].

How does caveolin-1 lose its inhibitory function as a tumor suppressor and instead promote tumor growth? It is generally believed that the mechanism of action may have three points: 1) point mutations [27]; 2) tyrosine phosphorylation [28]; and 3) serine phosphorylation. Under normal circumstances, caveolin-1 is an integrated membrane protein. However, if Ser is phosphorylated, caveolin-1 will be transformed into secreted proteins, which can improve its autocrine or paracrine function. Tahir et al. [29] demonstrated that androgen-insensitive prostate cancer cells could secrete caveolin-1 in autocrine or paracrine form and directly stimulate the growth and survival of prostate cancer cells. It is also believed that caveolin-1 activates the PI3-K-Akt signaling pathway in prostate cancer cells and promotes cancer cell metastasis by interacting with transfer molecules such as VEGF, TGF-β1 and FGF2 [30]. The absence of interstitial caveolin-1 expression is related to the activation of AKT, which leads to the upregulation of TGF-β1 and SNCG expression and results in the transfer of prostate cancer cells [31]. Caveolin-1 is upregulated in prostate cancer, and its high expression in most prostate cancer tissues can promote the proliferation of cancer cells and metastasis to lymph nodes. Caveolin-1 can be used as a biologically active molecule to promote tumorigenesis and tumor angiogenesis in the prostate cancer microenvironment. Caveolin-1 overexpression exists in primary and metastatic prostate cancer [32]. At present, caveolin-1 can be detected in the peripheral blood, and its expression level can be used to improve the diagnosis of prostate cancer and is related to prognosis.

Table 5 Correlation of caveolin-1 expression with preoperative PSA levels in patients with prostate cancer

Preoperative PSA level	Cases	Positive	Negative	Positive rate	X^2	*P* value
0–10	6	1	5	16.67%	5.904	0.052
10–100	22	15	7	68.18%		
>100	19	13	6	68.42%		

Conclusion

In this study, it was found that high caveolin-1 expression is closely related to prostate cancer after transurethral surgery and has a role in promoting tumorigenesis, development, and infiltration.

In conclusion, caveolin-1 is highly expressed in prostate cancer and is closely related to the pathological grade and clinical stage of prostate cancer. It may be a novel tumor marker for prostate cancer and has potential clinical value. The expression of caveolin-1 is not related to preoperative serum PSA levels.

Abbreviations

BPH: Benign prostatic hyperplasia; Cav: Caveolin; FGF2: Factor fibroblast growth factor 2; MAPK: Mitogen-activated protein kinase; PCa: Prostate cancer.; PIN: Prostatic intraepithelial neoplasia.; PSA: Prostate specific antigen.; TNM: Tumor node metastasis.; VEGF: Vascular endothelial growth factor

Acknowledgments

We thank Prof. Dianzhong Luo from the Department of Pathology, the First Affiliated Hospital of Guangxi Medical University, for his kind help with the tissue sections and related assistance.

Funding

None.

Authors' contributions

XMW planned the study and wrote the manuscript. ZGL and ZBY acquired and analyzed the data. All authors read and approved the final manuscript, and author contributions are in accordance with ICMJE guidelines.

Authors' information

Not applicable.

Competing interests

The authors declare that they have no competing interests.

References

1. Wong ECL, Kapoor A. Epidemiology of prostate and kidney cancer in the aboriginal population of Canada: a systematic review. Can Urol Assoc J. 2017;11:E222–E32.
2. Trama A, Botta L, Nicolai N, Rossi PG, Contiero P, Fusco M, et al. Prostate cancer changes in clinical presentation and treatments in two decades: an Italian population-based study. Eur J Cancer. 2016;67:91–8.
3. Rainato G, Fabricio AS, Zancan M, Peloso L, Dittadi R, Barichello M, et al. Evaluating serum insulin-like growth factor 1 and insulin-like growth factor binding protein 3 as markers in prostate cancer diagnosis. Int J Biol Markers. 2016;31:e317–e23.
4. Stephan C, Jung K, Miller K, Ralla B. New biomarkers in serum and urine for detection of prostate cancer. Aktuelle Urol. 2015;46:129–43.
5. Dickinson J, Shane A, Tonelli M, Connor GS, Joffres M, Singh H, et al. Trends in prostate cancer incidence and mortality in Canada during the era of prostate-specific antigen screening. Cmaj Open. 2016;4:E73–E9.
6. Terada N, Akamatsu S, Kobayashi T, Inoue T, Ogawa O, Antonarakis ES. Prognostic and predictive biomarkers in prostate cancer: latest evidence and clinical implications. Ther Adv Med Oncol. 2017;9:565–73.
7. Sugie S, Mukai S, Yamasaki K, Kamibeppu T, Tsukino H, Kamoto T. Significant Association of Caveolin-1 and Caveolin-2 with prostate Cancer progression. Cancer Genomics Proteomics. 2015;12:391–6.
8. Yang HJ, Feng P, Wang L, Li ZC, Ma SP, Wang M, et al. Caveolin-1 mediates gene transfer and cytotoxicity of polyethyleneimine in mammalian cell lines. Mol Cell Biochem. 2015;402:203–11.
9. Anwar SL, Wahyono A, Aryandono T, Haryono SJ. Caveolin-1 in breast Cancer: single molecule regulation of multiple key signaling pathways. Asian Pac J Cancer Prev. 2015;16:6803–12.
10. Simpkins SA, Hanby AM, Holliday DL, Speirs V. Clinical and functional significance of loss of caveolin-1 expression in breast cancer-associated fibroblasts. J Pathol. 2012;227:490–8.
11. Garnett DJ. Caveolae as a target to quench autoinduction of the metastatic phenotype in lung cancer. J Cancer Res Clin Oncol. 2016;142:611–8.
12. Reis ST, Viana NI, Leite KR, Diogenes E, Antunes AA, Iscaife A, et al. Role of genetic polymorphisms in the development and prognosis of sporadic and familial prostate Cancer. PLoS One. 2016;11:e0166380.
13. Bocci G, Fioravanti A, Orlandi P, Di DT, Natale G, Fanelli G, et al. Metronomic ceramide analogs inhibit angiogenesis in pancreatic Cancer through up-regulation of Caveolin-1 and Thrombospondin-1 and Down-regulation of cyclin D1. Neoplasia. 2012;14:833–45.
14. Shen X-J, Zhang H, Tang G-S, Wang X-D, Zheng R, Wang Y, et al. Caveolin-1 is a modulator of fibroblast activation and a potential biomarker for gastric Cancer. Int J Biol Sci. 2015;11:370–9.
15. Ma W, Wang DD, Li L, Feng YK, Gu HM, Zhu GM, et al. Caveolin-1 plays a key role in the oleanolic acid-induced apoptosis of HL-60 cells. Oncol Rep. 2014;32:293–301.
16. Friedrich T, Richter B, Gaiser T, Weiss C, Janssen KP, Einwächter H, et al. Deficiency of caveolin-1 in Apc(min/+) mice promotes colorectal tumorigenesis. Carcinogenesis. 2013;34:2109–18.
17. Xu J, Agyemang S, Qin Y, Aysola K, Giles M, Oprea G, et al. A novel pathway that links Caveolin-1 Down-regulation to BRCA1 dysfunction in serous epithelial ovarian Cancer cells. Enliven Challenges in cancer detection and therapy. 2014;1:004.
18. Tse EY, Ko FC, Tung EK, Chan LK, Lee TK, Ngan ES, et al. Caveolin-1 overexpression is associated with hepatocellular carcinoma tumourigenesis and metastasis. J Pathol. 2012;226:645–53.
19. Huang C, Qiu Z, Wang L, Peng Z, Jia Z, Logsdon CD, et al. A novel FoxM1-caveolin signaling pathway promotes pancreatic cancer invasion and metastasis. Cancer Res. 2012;72:655–65.
20. Pancotti F, Roncuzzi L, Maggiolini M, Gaspericampani A. Caveolin-1 silencing arrests the proliferation of metastatic lung cancer cells through the inhibition of STAT3 signaling. Cell Signal. 2012;24:1390–7.
21. Masuelli L, Budillon A, Marzocchella L, Mrozek MA, Vitolo D, Di Gennaro E, et al. Caveolin-1 overexpression is associated with simultaneous abnormal expression of the E-cadherin/α-β catenins complex and multiple ErbB receptors and with lymph nodes metastasis in head and neck squamous cell carcinomas. J Cell Physiol. 2012;227:3344–53.
22. Steffens S, Schrader AJ, Blasig H, Vetter G, Eggers H, Tränkenschuh W, et al. Caveolin 1 protein expression in renal cell carcinoma predicts survival. BMC Urol. 2011;11:25.
23. Steiner I, Jung K, Miller K, Stephan C, Erbersdobler A. Expression of endothelial factors in prostate cancer: a possible role of caveolin-1 for tumour progression. Oncol Rep. 2012;27:389–95.
24. Mohammed DA, Helal DS. Prognostic significance of epithelial/stromal caveolin-1 expression in prostatic hyperplasia, high grade prostatic intraepithelial hyperplasia and prostatic carcinoma and its correlation with microvessel density. J Egypt Natl Canc Inst. 2017;29:25–31.
25. Bennett NC, Hooper JD, Johnson DW, Gobe GC. Expression profiles and functional associations of endogenous androgen receptor and caveolin-1 in prostate cancer cell lines. Prostate. 2014;74:478–87.

26. Nassar ZD, Moon H, Duong T, Neo L, Hill MM, Francois M, et al. PTRF/Cavin-1 decreases prostate cancer angiogenesis and lymphangiogenesis. Oncotarget. 2013;4:1844–55.
27. Lee H, Park DS, Razani B, Russell RG, Pestell RG, Lisanti MP. Caveolin-1 mutations (P132L and null) and the pathogenesis of breast cancer: caveolin-1 (P132L) behaves in a dominant-negative manner and caveolin-1 (–/–) null mice show mammary epithelial cell hyperplasia. Am J Pathol. 2002;161: 1357–69.
28. Lee H, Volonte' D, Galbiati F, Iyengar P, Lublin DM, Bregman DB, et al. Constitutive and growth factor-regulated phosphorylation of caveolin-1 occurs at the same site (Tyr-14) in vivo: identification of a c-Src/Cav-1/Grb7 signaling cassette. Mol Endocrinol. 2000;14:1750–5.
29. Tahir SA, Yang G, Ebara S, Timme TL, Satoh T, Li L, et al. Secreted caveolin-1 stimulates cell survival/clonal growth and contributes to metastasis in androgen-insensitive prostate cancer. Cancer Res. 2001;61:3882–5.
30. Li L, Ren C, Yang G, Goltsov AA, Tabata K, Thompson TC. Caveolin-1 promotes autoregulatory, Akt-mediated induction of cancer-promoting growth factors in prostate cancer cells. Mol Cancer Res. 2009;7:1781–91.
31. Wang S, Zhang C, Liu Y, Xu C, Chen Z. Functional polymorphisms of caveolin-1 variants as potential biomarkers of esophageal squamous cell carcinoma. Biomarkers. 2014;19:652–9.
32. Karam JA, Lotan Y, Roehrborn CG, Ashfaq R, Karakiewicz PI. Caveolin-1 overexpression is associated with aggressive prostate cancer recurrence. Prostate. 2007;67:614–22.

Permissions

All chapters in this book were first published in UROLOGY, by BioMed Central; hereby published with permission under the Creative Commons Attribution License or equivalent. Every chapter published in this book has been scrutinized by our experts. Their significance has been extensively debated. The topics covered herein carry significant findings which will fuel the growth of the discipline. They may even be implemented as practical applications or may be referred to as a beginning point for another development.

The contributors of this book come from diverse backgrounds, making this book a truly international effort. This book will bring forth new frontiers with its revolutionizing research information and detailed analysis of the nascent developments around the world.

We would like to thank all the contributing authors for lending their expertise to make the book truly unique. They have played a crucial role in the development of this book. Without their invaluable contributions this book wouldn't have been possible. They have made vital efforts to compile up to date information on the varied aspects of this subject to make this book a valuable addition to the collection of many professionals and students.

This book was conceptualized with the vision of imparting up-to-date information and advanced data in this field. To ensure the same, a matchless editorial board was set up. Every individual on the board went through rigorous rounds of assessment to prove their worth. After which they invested a large part of their time researching and compiling the most relevant data for our readers.

The editorial board has been involved in producing this book since its inception. They have spent rigorous hours researching and exploring the diverse topics which have resulted in the successful publishing of this book. They have passed on their knowledge of decades through this book. To expedite this challenging task, the publisher supported the team at every step. A small team of assistant editors was also appointed to further simplify the editing procedure and attain best results for the readers.

Apart from the editorial board, the designing team has also invested a significant amount of their time in understanding the subject and creating the most relevant covers. They scrutinized every image to scout for the most suitable representation of the subject and create an appropriate cover for the book.

The publishing team has been an ardent support to the editorial, designing and production team. Their endless efforts to recruit the best for this project, has resulted in the accomplishment of this book. They are a veteran in the field of academics and their pool of knowledge is as vast as their experience in printing. Their expertise and guidance has proved useful at every step. Their uncompromising quality standards have made this book an exceptional effort. Their encouragement from time to time has been an inspiration for everyone.

The publisher and the editorial board hope that this book will prove to be a valuable piece of knowledge for researchers, students, practitioners and scholars across the globe.

Contributors

Jibril Oyekunle Bello
Department of Surgery, University of Ilorin Teaching Hospital, Ilorin, Nigeria

Karol Axcrona
Department of Urology, Akershus University Hospital, Lørenskog, Norway

Rasmus Nilsson
Department of Urology, Telemark Hospital, Skien, Norway

Bjørn Brennhovd
Department of Urology, Oslo University Hospital, The Norwegian Radium Hospital, Oslo, Norway

Øystein Sørebø
School of Business and Social Sciences, University College of Southeast Norway, Hønefoss, Norway

Sophie D. Fosså and Alv A. Dahl
National Resource Center for Late Effects after Cancer Treatment, Oslo University Hospital, The Norwegian Radium Hospital, P.O. Box 4453, Nydalen, 0424 Oslo, Norway
Faculty of Medicine, University of Oslo, Oslo, Norway

Ji Yun Lee, Su Jin Lee, Ho Yeong Lim and Se Hoon Park
Division of Hematology-Oncology, Department of Medicine, Samsung Medical Center, Sungkyunkwan University School of Medicine, 81 Irwon-Ro Gangnam-gu, Seoul 135-710, South Korea

Hae Su Kim
Division of Hematology-Oncology, Department of Medicine, Samsung Medical Center, Sungkyunkwan University School of Medicine, 81 Irwon-Ro Gangnam-gu, Seoul 135-710, South Korea
Department of Hematology-Oncology, Department of Medicine, Veterans Health Service Medical Center, Seoul, South Korea

Hyun Hwan Sung, Hwang Gyun Jeon, Byong Chang Jeong, Seong Il Seo, Seong Soo Jeon, Hyun Moo Lee and Han-Yong Choi
Department of Urology, Samsung Medical Center, Sungkyunkwan University School of Medicine, Seoul, South Korea

Qing Zhang, Shiwei Zhang, Shun Zhang, Wei Wang, Xiaozhi Zhao, Yongming Deng, Huibo Lian and Hongqian Guo
Department of Urology, Drum Tower Hospital, Medical School of Nanjing University, Institute of Urology, Nanjing University, 321 Zhongshan Road, Nanjing 210008, Jiangsu, People's Republic of China

Guoqing Chen, Limin Liao, Zhaoxia Wang, Xing Li and Wenjuan Du
Department of Urology, China Rehabilitation Research Center, Beijing 100068, China
Department of Urology, Capital Medical University, Beijing, China

U-Syn Ha, Kyu Won Lee, Sun Wook Kim and Sung-Hoo Hong
Department of Urology, Seoul St. Mary's Hospital, College of Medicine, The Catholic University of Korea, 222, Banpo-daero, Seocho-gu, Seoul 06591, Republic of Korea

Seung Hyun Jeon
Department of Urology, School of Medicine, Kyung Hee University, Seoul, Republic of Korea

Tae Gyun Kwon
Department of Urology, College of Medicine, Kyungpook National University, Daegu, Republic of Korea

Hyung Keun Park
Department of Urology, Asan Medical Center, University of Ulsan College of Medicine, Seoul, Republic of Korea

Faruk Kucukdurmaz, Erkan Efe and Sefa Resim
Department of Urology, Sutcu Imam University, Avsar Kampusu, 46100 Kahramanmaras, Turkey

Ahmet Çelik, Hasan Dagli and Metin Kılınc
Department of Biochemistry, Sutcu Imam University, Kahramanmaras, Turkey

F. Grases
Laboratory of Renal Lithiasis Research, University Institute of Health Sciences Research-(IUNICS), University of Balearic Islands, Palma of Mallorca, Spain

O. Söhnel
University of J.E. Purkyně, Faculty of Environmental Studies, Ústí n.L, Czech Republic

Rita de Cássia Oliveira, Renato Fidelis Ivanovic, Katia Ramos Moreira Leite, Nayara Izabel Viana, Ruan César Aparecido Pimenta, Vanessa Ribeiro Guimarães, Denis Reis Morais, Daniel Kanda Abe, Miguel Srougi and Sabrina Thalita Reis
Laboratory of Medical Investigation (LIM55), Urology Department, University of Sao Paulo Medical School, Av. Dr. Arnaldo 455, 2° floor, room 2145, Sao Paulo 01246-903, Brazil

José Pontes Junior
Laboratory of Medical Investigation (LIM55), Urology Department, University of Sao Paulo Medical School, Av. Dr. Arnaldo 455, 2° floor, room 2145, Sao Paulo 01246-903, Brazil
Uro-Oncology Group, Urology Department, University of Sao Paulo Medical School and Institute of Cancer Estate of Sao Paulo (ICESP), Sao Paulo, Brazil

Adriano João Nesrallah and William Nahas
Uro-Oncology Group, Urology Department, University of Sao Paulo Medical School and Institute of Cancer Estate of Sao Paulo (ICESP), Sao Paulo, Brazil

Rajan Veeratterapillay, Antonia Voysey, Katherine Kelly, Mark I. Johnson and Jonathan Aning
Department of Urology, Freeman Hospital, Newcastle-upon-Tyne Hospitals NHS Foundation Trust, Newcastle-upon-Tyne, UK

Ashwin Sachdeva and Naeem A. Soomro
Department of Urology, Freeman Hospital, Newcastle-upon-Tyne Hospitals NHS Foundation Trust, Newcastle-upon-Tyne, UK
Northern Institute for Cancer Research, Newcastle University, Newcastle-upon-Tyne, UK

Yiwei Lin, Qiqi Mao, Bin Chen, Liujiang Wang, Ben Liu, Xiangyi Zheng and Liping Xie
Department of Urology, The First Affiliated Hospital, School of Medicine, Zhejiang University, Qingchun Road 79, Hangzhou 310003, Zhejiang Province, China

Seung Woo Yang and Ki Hak Song
Department of Urology, School of Medicine, Chungnam National University Hospital, Chungnam National University, 282 Monwha-ro, Jung-gu, Daejeon, Republic of Korea35015

Seong Woo Jeong
Department of Physiology, Yonsei University Wonju College of Medicine, Wonju, Republic of Korea

Martin Pilskog and Oddbjørn Straume
Centre for Cancer Biomarkers CCBIO, University of Bergen, Bergen, Norway
Department of Oncology, Haukeland University Hospital, 5021 Bergen, Norway

Lars A. Akslen
Centre for Cancer Biomarkers CCBIO, University of Bergen, Bergen, Norway
Department of Pathology, Haukeland University Hospital, 5021 Bergen, Norway

Åse Haug
Department of Oncology, Haukeland University Hospital, 5021 Bergen, Norway

Christian Beisland and Karin M. Hjelle
Department of Urology, Haukeland University Hospital, 5021 Bergen, Norway
Department of Clinical Medicine, University of Bergen, Bergen, Norway

Leif Bostad
Department of Pathology, Haukeland University Hospital, 5021 Bergen, Norway

Daniel Heinrich
Department of Oncology, Akershus University Hospital, 1478 Lørenskog, Norway

Xiaofei Zhu
Department of Urology, Beijing Jishuitan Hospital, Beijing, China

Kui Zhai and Guangju Ji
National Laboratory of Biomacromolecules, Institute of Biophysics, Chinese Academy of Sciences, 15 Datun Road, Beijing 100101, China

Yue Mi
Department of Urology, Peking University First Hospital, Beijing, China

Vera Y. Chung and Benjamin W. Turney
Oxford Stone Group, Department of Urology, Nuffield Department of Surgical Sciences, University of Oxford, Oxford, UK

Muhammad Ali Chaudhary, Jeffrey J. Leow, Ritam Chowdhury, Wei Jiang and Joel S. Weissman
Center for Surgery and Public Health, Department of Surgery, Brigham and Women's Hospital, Harvard Medical School, Harvard T H Chan School of Public Health, Boston, MA, USA

Matthew Mossanen and Steven L. Chang
Division of Urology, Brigham and Women's Hospital, Harvard Medical School, Boston, MA, USA

Peter A. Learn
Department of Surgery, Uniformed Services University of Health Sciences, Bethesda, MD, USA

Christopher Naugler
Department of Pathology and Laboratory Medicine, University of Calgary, Calgary, AB, Canada
Department of Family Medicine, University of Calgary, Calgary, AB, Canada

Thomas P. Griener and Wilson W. Chan
Department of Pathology and Laboratory Medicine, University of Calgary, Calgary, AB, Canada
Division of Microbiology, Department of Pathology and Laboratory Medicine, University of Calgary, Calgary, AB, Canada

Deirdre L. Church
Department of Pathology and Laboratory Medicine, University of Calgary, Calgary, AB, Canada
Division of Microbiology, Department of Pathology and Laboratory Medicine, University of Calgary, Calgary, AB, Canada
Department of Medicine, University of Calgary, Calgary, AB, Canada
1W-410, Diagnostic and Scientific Centre, 9-3535 Research Road NW, Calgary, AB T2L 2K8, Canada

Johannes Bründl, Sabine Wallinger, Johannes Breyer, Bernd Rosenhammer, Maximilian Burger and Wolfgang Otto
Department of Urology, Caritas St Josef Medical Center, University of Regensburg, Landshuter Straße 65, 93053 Regensburg, Germany

Peter Rubenwolf
Department of Urology, Caritas St Josef Medical Center, University of Regensburg, Landshuter Straße 65, 93053 Regensburg, Germany
Department of Urology, Frankfurt University Medical Center, Frankfurt, Germany

Florian Weber and Matthias Evert
Institute of Pathology, University of Regensburg, Regensburg, Germany

Nikolaos Theodoros Georgopoulos
Department of Biological Sciences, School of Applied Sciences, University of Huddersfield, Huddersfield, UK

Alexander Andreev-Andrievskiy and Anfisa Popova
Lomonosov Moscow State University, Biology faculty, 1-12 Leninskie gory, Moscow 119234, Russia
Institute for biomedical problems RAS, 76A Khoroshevskoe shosse, Moscow 123007, Russia
MSU Institute for mitoengeneering, LLC, 1-73A Leninskie gory, Moscow 119234, Russia

Evgeniia Lagereva
Institute for biomedical problems RAS, 76A Khoroshevskoe shosse, Moscow 123007, Russia
MSU Institute for mitoengeneering, LLC, 1-73A Leninskie gory, Moscow 119234, Russia

László Pajor and Zoltán Bajory
Department of Urology, University of Szeged, Hungary, Semmelweis u. 1, Szeged H-6725, Hungary

Zoltán Fekete
Department of Urology, University of Szeged, Hungary, Semmelweis u. 1, Szeged H-6725, Hungary
Department of Obstetrics and Gynaecology, University of Szeged, Hungary, Semmelweis u. 1, Szeged H-6725, Hungary

Szilvia Kőrösi and Gábor Németh
Department of Obstetrics and Gynaecology, University of Szeged, Hungary, Semmelweis u. 1, Szeged H-6725, Hungary

Zoltan Kozinszky
Department of Obstetrics and Gynaecology, Blekinge Hospital, Karlskrona, Sweden

Shijun Zhang, Jing Du, Shaowei Xie and Fenghua Li
Department of ultrasound, Renji Hospital, School of Medicine, Shanghai Jiaotong University, 160 Pujian RD, Shanghai 200127, China

Ruhui Tian and Zheng Li
Department of Andrology, Shanghai General Hospital, Shanghai Jiaotong University, 100 Haining RD, Shanghai 200080, China

Runqi Guo, Yuze Zhu, Gengyan Xiong, Xuesong Li, Kai Zhang and Liqun Zhou
Department of Urology, Peking University First Hospital and Institute of Urology, National Research Center for Genitourinary Oncology, Beijing 100034, China

Sheng Xue, Qing-wen Li, Sheng Wang, Jian Li and Shuai Yang
Department of Urology, The First Affliated Hospital of Bengbu Medical College Bengbu, Bengbu, Anhui, China

Sheng-Qun Jiang
Department of Ophthalmology, The First Affliated Hospital of Bengbu Medical College Bengbu, Bengbu, Anhui, China

Hai-Min Zhang, Yun-Fei Xu and Long-Sheng Wang
Department of Urology, Shanghai Tenth People's Hospital, Tongji University, Shanghai, China

Jun-Hua Zheng
Department of Urology, Shanghai General Hospital, Shanghai Jiao Tong University School of Medicine, Shanghai 200072, China

Paul Nkemtendong Tolefac
Specialized Internship Program, Faculty of Medicine and Biomedical Sciences, University of Yaoundé 1, Yaoundé, Cameroon

Marcelin Ngowe Ngowe and Neville Alemnju Telelen
Department of Surgery, Faculty of Health Sciences, University of Buea, Buea, Cameroon

Jacqueline Ze Minkande
Department of Anaesthesia and Intensive Care, Faculty of Medicine and Biomedical Sciences, University of Yaoundé 1, Yaoundé, Cameroon
Department of Anaesthesia and Intensive Care, Yaoundé Gynaeco-Obstetric and Paediatric Hospital, Yaoundé, Cameroon

Georgette Guemkam
Paediatric Nephrology Unit, Mother and Child Centre, Chantal Biya Foundation, Yaoundé, Cameroon

Aurelien Maurice Sosso
Departmennt of Surgery and Subspecialties, Faculty of Medicine and Biomedical Sciences, University of Yaoundé 1, Yaoundé, Cameroon

Faustin Felicien Mouafo Tambo and Fru Fobuzshi Angwafo III
Departmennt of Surgery and Subspecialties, Faculty of Medicine and Biomedical Sciences, University of Yaoundé 1, Yaoundé, Cameroon
Paediatric Surgery Unit, Yaoundé Gynaeco-Obstetric and Paediatric Hospital, Yaoundé, Cameroon

Landry Mbouche
Paediatric Surgery Unit, Yaoundé Gynaeco-Obstetric and Paediatric Hospital, Yaoundé, Cameroon

Lu Zhang, Jin Hu, Robert P.A. Wallin and Ola Winqvist
Department of Medicine, Immunology and Allergy Unit, Karolinska University Hospital, SE-171 76 Stockholm, Sweden

A. Ali Zirakzadeh
Department of Medicine, Immunology and Allergy Unit, Karolinska University Hospital, SE-171 76 Stockholm, Sweden
Department of Surgical and Perioperative Sciences, Urology and Andrology, Umeå University, Umeå, Sweden

Jesper Rosvall and Mats Hedlund
Department of Urology, South General Hospital, Karolinska Institutet, Stockholm, Stockholm, Sweden

Ping Sheng Hu
Cancer Biotherapy Center, Affiliated Hospital of Guizhou Medical University, Guiyang, China

Amir Sherif
Department of Surgical and Perioperative Sciences, Urology and Andrology, Umeå University, Umeå, Sweden

Hiromi Sato, Shintaro Narita, Atsushi Koizumi, Taketoshi Nara, Sohei Kanda, Kazuyuki Numakura, Hiroshi Tsuruta, Atsushi Maeno, Mitsuru Saito, Takamitsu Inoue and Tomonori Habuchi
Department of Urology, Akita University School of Medicine, 1-1-1 Hondo, Akita 010-8543, Japan

Norihiko Tsuchiya
Department of Urology, Yamagata University School of Medicine, Yamagata, Japan

Shigeru Satoh
Center for Kidney Disease and Transplantation, Akita University Hospital, Akita, Japan

Kyoko Nomura
Department of Public Health, Akita University School of Medicine, Akita, Japan

Ferdinando Fusco, Massimiliano Creta and Francesco Mangiapia
Dipartimento di Neuroscienze e Scienze Riproduttive ed Odontostomatologiche, Università Degli Studi Di Napoli Federico II, Via Pansini, 5, 80131 Naples, Italy

Cosimo De Nunzio
Dipartimento di Urologia, Ospedale Sant'Andrea, Università Degli Studi di Roma "La Sapienza", Rota, Italy

Valerio Iacovelli and Enrico Finazzi Agrò
Dipartimento di Medicina Sperimentale e Chirurgia, Università Degli Studi di Roma "Tor Vergata", Roma, Italy

Vincenzo Li Marzi
Dipartimento di Urologia, Ospedale Careggi, Università Degli Studi di Firenze, Firenze, Italy

Martin Drerup, Ahmed Magdy, Daniela Colleselli, Thomas Kunit, Lukas Lusuardi, Günter Janetschek and Michael Mitterberger
Department of Urology, Paracelsus Medical University Salzburg, Muellner-Hauptstrasse 48, 5020 Salzburg, Austria

Martina Hager
Department of Pathology, Paracelsus Medical University Salzburg, Salzburg, Austria

Fuding Bai, Jimin Chen, Zhewei Zhang, Yichun Zheng, Jiaming Wen, Xiawa Mao and Nan Zhang
Department of Urology, School of Medicine Hangzhou, Second Affiliated Hospital, Zhejiang University, No.88 Jiefang Road, Hangzhou, Zhejiang Province, People's Republic of China

AnnMarie Groarke, Ruth Curtis and Deirdre M. J. Walsh
School of Psychology, National University of Ireland, Galway, Ireland

Francis J. Sullivan
Prostate Cancer Institute, National University of Ireland Galway, Galway, Ireland

Sumedha Chhatre
Department of Psychiatry, Perelman School of Medicine, University of Pennsylvania, 3535 Market St., Suite 4051, Philadelphia, PA 19104, USA

Diane K. Newman and Alan J. Wein
Division of Urology, Department of Surgery, Perelman School of Medicine, University of Pennsylvania, Philadelphia, PA 19104, USA

Ashlie E. Jefferson
Department of Medicine, Perelman School of Medicine, University of Pennsylvania, Philadelphia, PA 19104, USA

J. Sanford Schwartz
Departments of Medicine and Health Management, Leonard Davis Institute of Health Economics, University of Pennsylvania, Perelman School of Medicine and Wharton School of Business, Philadelphia, PA 19104, USA

Ravishankar Jayadevappa
Departments of Medicine and Surgery, Divisions of Geriatrics and Urology, Perelman School of Medicine Leonard Davis Institute of Health Economics, University of Pennsylvania, Philadelphia, PA 19104, USA

Wen-bin Guo, Cheng Yang, Jun Bian, Hui Xia, Jian-kun Yang, Qi-zhao Zhou, Ming-kun Chen, Kang-yi Xue, Wan-song Zhang, Peng Wang and Cun-dong Liu
Department of Urology, the Third Affiliated Hospital of Southern Medical University, No. 183 West Zhongshan Road, Tianhe District, 510630 Guangzhou, People's Republic of China

Xin Li
Center for Clinical Research and Innovation, Shenzhen Hospital of Southern Medical University, Shenzhen, People's Republic of China

Pietro Manuel Ferraro, Gianmarco Lombardi and Giovanni Gambaro
U.O.C. Nefrologia, Fondazione Policlinico Universitario A. Gemelli IRCCS, Roma, Italia
Università Cattolica del Sacro Cuore, Roma, Italia

Matteo Vittori, Alessandro D'Addessi and Pier Francesco Bassi
U.O.C. Clinica Urologica, Fondazione Policlinico Universitario A. Gemelli IRCCS, Roma, Italia
Università Cattolica del Sacro Cuore, Roma, Italia

Giuseppe Macis and Claudia Palmisano
U.O.C. Radiologia, Fondazione Policlinico Universitario A. Gemelli IRCCS, Roma, Italia
Università Cattolica del Sacro Cuore, Roma, Italia

Jacopo Gervasoni and Aniello Primiano
U.O.C. Biochimica Clinica, Fondazione Policlinico Universitario A. Gemelli IRCCS, Roma, Italia
Università Cattolica del Sacro Cuore, Roma, Italia

Li Yongzhi, Liu Jia, Liu Yili, Zhu Xingwang and Gong Xue
Department of Urology, Urologic Minimally Invasive Treatment Center in Liaoning Province, The Fourth Affiliated Hospital of China Medical University, No4, Chongshan East Road, Shenyang 110032, China

Yan Shi
Department of Urology, Sheyang Red Cross Hospital, No4, Chongshan East Road, Huanggu District, Shenyang 110032, China

Zhigui Liu and Zhanbin Yang
Department of Urology, The First Affiliated Hospital of Guangxi Medical University, Nanning 530021, China

Xiaoming Wang
Department of Urology, The First Affiliated Hospital of Guangxi Medical University, Nanning 530021, China
Department of Urology, The Second Affiliated Hospital of Guangxi Medical University, No 166 DaXueDong Road, Nanning 530007, Guangxi, China

Index

P

R

S

T

U